An Illustrated Dictionary of
Hairdressing
& Wigmaking

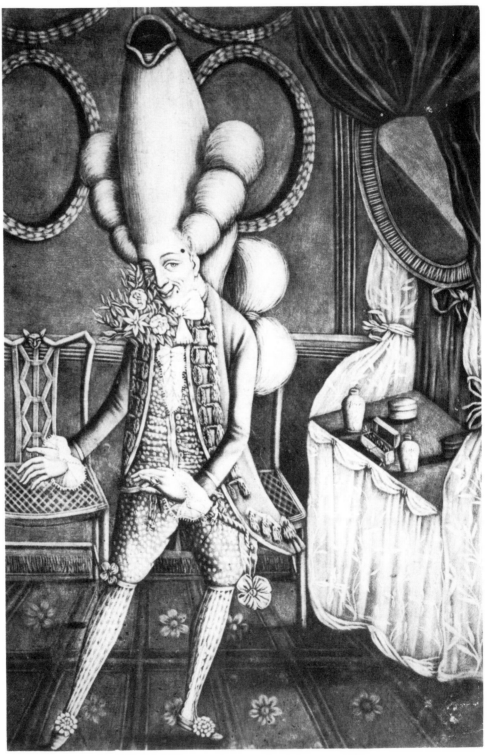

The Macaroni, 3 July 1773. Published by J. Bowles. Note the Cadogan or Club Wig and the queue doubled back and tied in the middle, as worn by fashionable rakes from 1760 to 1800

An Illustrated Dictionary of
Hairdressing & Wigmaking

Containing words, terms and phrases (current and obsolete),
dialectal, foreign, and technical, used in Britain and America
pertaining to the crafts of hairdressing and wigmaking; also
words derived from these crafts having a wider use.

WITH 1136 ILLUSTRATIONS, and A FULL BIBLIOGRAPHY

J Stevens Cox, FSA

*Extra-Mural Tutor, Bristol University and W.E.A.; Contributor to the
Encyclopaedia Britannica; Chairman of the Hairdressers' Registration
Council 1960–63; Late Examiner in Hairdressing (theory and practice) for
The Hairdressers' Technical Council and The City and Guilds of London
Institute; Late Member of The Advisory Committee for Hairdressing, City
and Guilds of London Institute; Lecturer in Hairdressing for the Guernsey
Education Council; 1966–1979 Visiting lecturer to universities and
technical colleges*

Batsford Academic and Educational, London

In loving memory of my father,
William George Cox, born at Ilchester,
and my mother,
Annie Eugenia Cox, née Stevens,
born at Bristol

© James Stevens Cox 1984
First published 1966
New revised edition 1984

Typeset by Deltatype, Ellesmere Port
and printed in Great Britain by
R. J. Acford
Chichester, Sussex
for the publishers
Batsford Academic and Educational
an imprint of B T Batsford Ltd
4 Fitzhardinge Street
London W1H 0AH

British Library Cataloguing in Publication Data

Stevens Cox, James
    An illustrated dictionary of hairdressing and
    wigmaking.
    1. Hairdressing-Dictionaries
    I. Title
    646.7′242′0321   TT957
ISBN 0 7134 4208 5

Other titles on hairdressing by James Stevens Cox

Curriculum and Synopsis of Training for Hairdressing Apprentices used by Stevens Hair Artists, Bristol, 1927

The Wave-Cut, 1938

Surrealism and The Coiffure, 1938

Hair Styles for Men, 1949

The Art of the Wigmaker, 1961

Examination Notes for Hairdressing Students, 1963

The Physical Reason for Hair Curl and Wave, 1964

The Wigmaker's Art in the 18th Century, 1965

The Hair Pedlar in Devon, 1968

Shampoos and Shampooing: notes for apprentices, 1969

Marcel Waving and Curling: an elementary treatise, 1970

Hair and Beauty Secrets of the 17th Century, 1971

The Story of Wigs Through the Ages, 1974

The Construction of an Ancient Egyptian Wig (c 1400 bc) *in the British Museum*, 1975

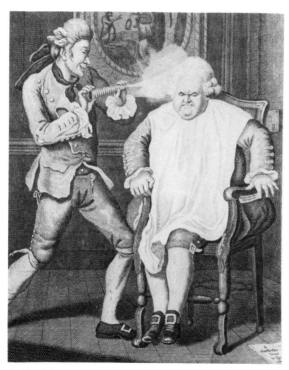

An Englishman in Paris has his wig powdered, 1770

PREFACE

Speaking generally, knowledge is of two kinds: the knowledge we already have of a subject and the knowledge of where to look for more. And Mr J Stevens Cox's new work 'containing words, terms and phrases, current and obsolete; dialectal, foreign and technical, used in Britain pertaining to the crafts of hairdressing and wigmaking' admirably fulfills the second of these functions, being an almost untapped source of information.

At first glance, the appeal of such a book might seem to be mainly for specialists, but the up-to-date hairdresser should be armed at every point, and thus an insight into hairdressing and wigmaking, as practised not only today but in days gone by, will give him a wider grasp of its potentialities and may prove invaluable. The basis of all business is the capacity to earn a livelihood, but the man who, together with technical skill and unfailing tact (an essential adjunct), can find it a fascinating study, is the man who, with his enlarged horizon, is likely to impress his clients and add to their number. It has been said that knowledge is power, and one never can tell when the most unexpected word may come in useful. Many people are prepared to jog along as their fathers did, but over-cautious conservatism can be as dangerous as wild gambling, and though the modern era offers great rewards to the wisely adventurous, it holds out little promise to the man without imagination.

It must be borne in mind that hairdressing and wigmaking are among the most ancient of the minor arts, as may be judged from this book's 1136 illustrations, which range over the centuries. And, as with women's fashions in hats, these fashions, too, are constantly changing and, as again with women's fashions in hats, often hark back to the past. Therefore the informed and alert hairdresser, with an eye on the future as well as on the present, must not alone keep in touch with current trends, but should endeavour to foresee and take advantage of any signs and hints of change. By adopting this attitude, he may himself become an innovator, thus increasing his prestige and his income.

As with all Mr Cox's writings on hairdressing and wigmaking, this is both an erudite work and a practical one. His primary aim is to render service, and so, according to their significance from that angle, some of the entries are brief and some detailed. Indeed, in certain aspects his book might be called a dictionary and in others a cyclopaedia.

Nobody was better fitted to compile it than Mr Cox, for not only was he a practising hairdresser for thirty years, with an hereditary background of several generations of hairdressers, but with energetic enthusiasm undimmed, he still keeps abreast of its ramifications and acts in various high capacities to forward the interests of the craft which was once his profession and is now his hobby.

Moreover, as an ardent bibliophile, he has collected a fine library of books on hairdressing and wigmaking, some of which are very rare, and without them it would have been virtually impossible to include such countless terms and such ample illustrations. In fact, quite apart from their practical application, hairdressing and wigmaking are absorbing subjects in themselves and contribute a vivid chapter to the social history of mankind.

Richard Curle

ABBREVIATIONS

AD	*Anno Domini*, in the year of our Lord
adj.	adjective
adv.	a single sheet advertisement
BC	Before Christ
cf	*conferatur*, compare
c	about
ed	edition
Fr	French, Heraldic usage
inf	information
ME	Middle English AD 1100–1500
ND	no date
NY	New York
OE	Old English AD 700–1100
OT	Old Testament
pl	plural
qv	*Quod vide* which see
Scot.	Scottish usage.
sic	Latin so, thus. To call attention to the supposition of misquotation
STC	A Short-Title Catalogue of Books Printed in England, 1475–1640, by A W Pollard and G R Redgrave, 1926
Subs	Substantive
WING	Short-Title Catalogue of Books Printed in England, 1641–1700, by Donald Wing, New York, 1945–1951

Hyphenated words have been regarded as a single word for alphabetical convenience.

The numbers at the end of each entry refer to the figure numbers on the pages of illustrations.

INTRODUCTION

If any there be that are desirous to be strangers in their owne soile and forrainers in their owne citie, they may continue and therein flatter themselves. For such like I have not written these lines, nor taken these pains.

William Camden, *16th century*

Dictionaries are like watches, the worst is better than none, and the best cannot be expected to go quite true.

Samuel Johnson, *18th century*

The compiler of this dictionary was a practising wigmaker and ladies' hairdresser for 30 years in the family business at Bristol, founded in 1850 by his maternal grandfather, John Stevens. Some of the implements and tools used by the writer until he retired from active hairdressing were of the 18th century and had been used by several generations of wigmakers. The manuscript work-books of John Stevens and his wife Frances have provided important evidence of terms, usages and processes of the Victorian period.

This collection and annotation of craft words was started in 1927 and from that beginning the present dictionary slowly grew over the intervening years as time and opportunity permitted.

All crafts have their specialized vocabularies. Their words are rarely recorded in literary use, and even the great dictionaries fail to notice them. Such hairdressing words as clumping, creoling, and jigger, either do not appear, or the sense in which they are used in the hairdressing craft is not given.

Until the 20th century France was the richest source for our foreign word importations. They often started as affectations, but became, after habitual use over many years, Anglicized to the extent that they were used freely with an English accent and accepted by their users as English words, their origin being popularly forgotten. Examples are postiche, salon, blond and croquignole.

Words are the tools of our thoughts, and custom, the sole arbiter of verbal propriety, is for ever accepting new words into the craft's vocabulary, abandoning others for which there is no longer need and re-adapting old words to new meanings. The mould of language never sets, but is ever changing by use. Since the first World War, hair fashion magazines have crossed the Atlantic in a week, and since the advent of air travel, in a few hours; consequently American fashions and expressions are quickly adopted in Britain and vice versa. The one-time dominance of French words has long since been replaced by the intrusive influence of Americanisms, and during the past forty years for every French craft word that has been adapted to English needs, four American have been accepted into current English usage.

Scope

The aim of the present work is to list and describe not only the literary, vernacular and technical craft words of the 20th century, but also archaic, dialectal and obsolete words, their uses and meanings. Words of foreign origin that are and were habitually used in the hairdressing craft in Britain to describe processes or coiffures are also noticed. The compilation is based on English and Foreign printed and manuscript sources

and the writer's own observations as a practising hairdresser and wigmaker. Reference to all sources used will be found in the bibliography. Included also are words such as allergy, that are not exclusively relevant to this craft, but which nevertheless are in frequent and necessary use by hairdressers. In addition words derived from hairdressing terms, but adapted to other, non-hairdressing subjects, are given.

Although this is not a biographical dictionary, a few names of outstanding interest or importance have been included such as Marcel Grateau, the inventor of Marcel waving, and J M W Turner, the famous artist and son of a barber. With a few necessary exceptions, modern proprietary names have been excluded. No attempt has been made to include the immense number of named hair styles that are born to die within days or at the best weeks. Each year sees thousands of such christenings. The task of collecting would be well nigh impossible and useless when done. Corson records a work entitled *L'Eloge des coiffures adresse aux Dames*, Paris 1772, in 39 volumes, which contained illustrations of no less than 3,744 hair styles.

As the same name is often given by different hairdressers to entirely dissimilar styles at the same period, the reader will perceive the impossibility of the total inclusion of named coiffures. The following new styles were noted by the writer in less than a week during an American tour in 1965: Butterfly, Champagne, China Doll, Chloe, Curly Kap, Do-do, Ecstasy, Fanfare, Glamour Girl, High Jinks, Irish Maid, Jingle Bells, Lazy Baby, Kewpie, Lulu, Miami, Night Life, Oriental Doll, Princess, Rose Petal, Suzette, Syrenette, Teena, Vera, Willow Flower, and Winsome. And these could be mutliplied by hundreds yearly. Nor are any of the invented colour names included here, attractive as some are, such as Bashful Blond, True Steel, Chocolate Kiss, Silvery Slate, Shy Violet, and dozens more. Colours are ill-defined in words and need direct comparisons with a colour chart of named shades.

The selection of entries has sometimes been difficult and at times arbitrary. Some words have been included that may seem of doubtful value, and certain it is that others of importance which should have been included have been inadvertently omitted, and for such omissions the writer asks for the reader's understanding forgiveness, this being a pioneer work. Additions and corrections would be welcome so that in the event of a further edition being printed, it could be made more complete.

Method of compilation

Before the editorial work was attempted a survey was made of every printed work that could be identified as being devoted in whole or part to some aspect of hairdressing, or wigmaking and directly associated subjects. In the course of its preparation more than 25,000 printed books (including periodicals) and manuscripts from the 14th century to 1965 were searched for material and most of those that have provided references are listed in the bibliography after this introduction. A few however, are given under the word to which they refer.

For most entries in the dictionary the authority is indicated in brackets, but where no authority is given it should be understood that the writer is the authority as a result of his hairdressing experience.

Many of the objects and chemicals used by hairdressers rejoice in several names. An example is: Potassium Carbonate (K_2CO_3), a constituent of some permanent waving reagents and liquid 'dry' shampoos (*qv*). This has been known by the following names: Subcarbonate of Potash, Salt of Tartar, Salt of Wormwood, Pearlash, Fixed Nitre, Kali Praeparatum and Alkali Tartari. In such cases only those variant names that have been used in hairdressing circles are included here.

The part of speech is indicated only when there could be some doubt in the reader's mind. Two or more meanings of an entry are separated and numbered. Many of the entries are illustrated by means of quotations from published sources, or from expressions heard and recorded by the writer, and they are given within inverted commas.

Cross references are frequently given and should always be consulted, as a word may be more fully discussed under another indicated entry.

Some groups of craft words
Some groups of words that have been used in the craft are given here to assist literary composition and to facilitate the expression of ideas. The lists are by no means exhaustive, but are suggestions to enrich the word power of the hairdresser.

1 Words which, when used in conjunction with the word *hair*, are descriptive of either the length, quality, condition, arrangement, form, quantity, or combinations thereof, of a *collection of Hairs*: Ball, Braid, Bun, Bunch, Coil, Curl, Gathering, Group, Hand, Hank, Head, Knot, Lock, Mane, Mat, Mop, Parcel, Pinch, Plait, Portion, Puff, Queue, Ribbon, Ringlet, Shock, Strand, Switch, Tail, Tête, Tress, Tuft, Weft, Wisp eg a strand of hair.

2 Words which, when used in conjunction with the word *curls*, are indicative of either the quantity, length, quality, condition or arrangement of a *group of curls*: Arch, Bounce, Bouquet, Bunch, Burst, Bush, Chaplet, Cluster, Cupola, Flop, Floss, Flounce, Fluff, Frill, Froth, Fuzz, Gathering, Grape, Group, Halo, Hang, Mane, Mop, Mound, Pompon, Posy, River, Rondeau, Rondel, Roundel, Ruff, Ruffle, Snuggle, Soufflé, Spray, Swish, Tail, Tumble, Verge, Welter eg a cluster of curls.

3 Words denoting a *person engaged in some aspect of the Hairdressing or Wigmaking crafts*: Barber, Barberess, Beautician, Bleacher, Boardsman, Boardworker, Children's hairdresser, Coiffeur, Coiffeuse, Colourist, Cosmetologist, Dyer, General hand, Gentlemen's hairdresser, Hair artist, Hair colourist, Hair cutter, Hairdresser, Hair dyer, Hair preparer, Hair setter, Hair specialist, Hair stylist, Hair weaver, Ladies' hairdresser, Marceller, Marcel waver, Permanent waver, Posticheur, Shampoo girl, Shampooer, Tinter, Tonsor, Tonsorial artist, Waver, Wig cleaner, Wig comber, Wig dresser, Wigmaker, Plococosmist, Friseur.

4 *The components of a hair style*. These may include: a Band, Bend, Braid, Coil, Crisp, Curl, Fall, Fillet, Fold, Fringe, Halo, Loop, Ringlet, Roll, Plait, Turn, Twist, Wave.

5 Words denoting a *dressed head of hair*: Coif, Coiffure, Hairdo, Hairdress, Head, Headdress, Tête, Hairdressing.

6 Some *slang terms for head hair*: Down, Moss, Straw, Thatch, Top, Top knot, Wig, Wool.

7 Words denoting different *methods of putting on colour or bleach*: Application, pack, rinse, shampoo, spray.

8 *Shampoo containers* named according to shape, size or substance: Beaker, Bottle, Carafe, Decanter, Ewer, Flask, Gourd, Jar, Jug, Mug, Tankard.

Other collections could be made by any interested student of hairdressing, and the exercise would beneficially extend the vocabulary.

The development of word power and the facility of fluent speech are necessary accomplishments of every qualified hairdresser, and it is hoped that this dictionary will be a useful aid to those ends.

A Note on the 2nd Edition

There still remain many words among us undefined, which are very necessary to be rightly understood and which produce very mischievous mistakes when they are erroneously interpreted.

Johnson, No. 100 *The Idler*

The first edition of this Dictionary of Hairdressing and Wigmaking has been out-of-print for many years. This second, revised and enlarged edition, with over a thousand additional entries, has been undertaken to meet the steady and continuing demand for the book.

As a pioneer work it was well received by the craft,

the hairdressing colleges, universities and public libraries and the world of the theatre, cinema and television. It is hoped that this second edition will enjoy an even wider circulation.

JSC 1984

Acknowledgment

To record my indebtedness to all those who, over the years, by their help and advice assisted me would be an impossible task.

Nevertheless I should be singularly remiss if I did not put on record how much I owe to the following: my mother and father, and indirectly through them, to my grandparents, who were the primary source for a large number of words and sayings; the late A E R Dyer, for many years the Editor of *Hair and Beauty*, who encouraged me to complete this dictionary for publication; the late Ivor Westlake, who finished reading through the final manuscript only a week before his death in January, 1966, and fruitfully exchanged ideas with me; Dr C H Clough for the entry under Lucrezia Borgia's hair; Dr Lois Morrison of San Antonio, Texas, for giving me unrestricted access to her fine library of 18th century books, which provided three important and hitherto unnoticed hair references; Mrs M Finn, of the Halifax County Vocational School, Nova Scotia, for much helpful information in January, 1965; Warren Boas, Deputy Librarian, Syracuse University, New York, for several American hair words; Michael Birkett, fca for calling my attention to the modern Italian use of the merkin; and J W Merrington of Washington, dc, for a practical demonstration of Flat-Topping and other kindnesses.

Others who have earned my thanks include Nigel Symonds; Sam Flitman, Frank Austin, J H Boudou, Mrs J Savage, Theo Brown, H F V Johnstone, Ernest Partridge, mbe, Miss E J Barker, E G French, P K Sartory, John Edwards, W Y Carman, fsa, The Hon. Rachel B Kay-Shuttleworth, mbe, jp, the late Gaston Boudou, Taylor Briggs, W F Scowcroft, Leslie Foan, Richard Curle, R W Chalmers, H S Beardow, R J Kennett, mbe, Professor Saburo Minakawa, Major R E Austin and D S E Tilley.

Libraries and their Librarians in Great Britain and Ireland, who have unstintingly given me worthy service, include Weymouth Town Library, Dorset Natural History and Archaeological Society, Dorset County Library, Devon and Exeter Institution, National Library of Ireland, Bristol University and Southampton University. In the Americas I remember with gratitude the Universities of Mexico, New York, Toronto, Yale, Harvard, and Chicago; the public libraries of Miami, Toronto, Norwalk, NY, Victoria, bc, Los Angeles, Salt Lake City, and San Antonio, Texas; also the Folger Library, and Smithsonian Institute, Washington dc.

Finally it is a pleasure to acknowledge a particular debt of gratitude to my wife, Adele, for typing the manuscript, and to Mrs Joyce Mansfield, Mrs Theo Downing and Miss Beryl Powell for their drawings. All other illustrations, unless otherwise indicated on the plate, are from original prints and paintings in the writer's collection, photographed by Reg Vincent of Portland, Dorset.

J Stevens Cox

A

A L'ADORABLE Man's wig style *c* 1757. (*Marchand*)   *1*

A L'ALLEMANDE Man's hair style of early 19th century. (*GMF*)

A L'ANGLAISE
(1) Man's hair style of early 19th century. (*GMF*)
(2) Woman's hair style of *c* 1813. (*R de N*)
(3) After the English custom. (*Creer*)

A L'ANVIEU Man's wig style *c* 1757. (*Marchand*)   *2*

A L'AVENTURE Man's wig style *c* 1757. (*Marchand*)   *3*

A L'AYLE DE PIGEON Man's wig style *c* 1757. (*Marchand*)   *4*

AU BANDEU D'AMOUR Woman's 18th century coiffure. (*Uzanne*)

A LA BEAUMONT Man's wig style *c* 1757. (*Marchand*)   *5*

A LA BELLE POULE An 18th century hair style for women dressed with a three-masted ship fixed to the top of the wig. Named after a famous 18th century French Man o' War.   *6*

A LA BORDAGE (the corded buckle) A man's wig style of the 18th century. (*London Magazine, 1764*)

A LA BROSSE The hair brushed from the forehead, sides and back in an upward direction towards the crown of the head.

A LA BRUSH A short cut hair style for men, 18th century. (*Stewart*)

A LA CABRIOLET Man's wig style *c* 1757. (*Marchand*)   *7*

A LA CANDEUR An 18th century hair style for women.   *8*

A LA CAPRICIEUSE An 18th century woman's wig style. The hair of the wig dressed high, with a cascade of curls and two ringlet curls hanging down the neck.   *9*

A LA CAVALIERE Man's wig style *c* 1757. (*Marchand*) 10

A LA CERES A woman's hair style of the 18th century. (*Villermont*)   *11*

AUX CHARMES DE LA LIBERTE A high dressed wig style for women, decorated with ribbons, feathers and grasses. Late 18th century.   *12*

AU CHASSEUR Man's wig style *c* 1757. (*Marchand*)   *13*

A LA CHINOISE See Chinese style.

A LA CHOISY Man's wig style *c* 1757. (*Marchand*)   *14*

A LA CIRCASSIENNE Woman's 18th century coiffure. (*Uzanne*)   *15*

A LA CLOTILDE Two or more plaits worn looped over the cheeks, *c* 1835.   *16*

A LA COLOMBE 18th century coiffure for women. (*Uzanne*)   *17*

AU COMBATANT Man's wig style *c* 1757. (*Marchand*) 18

A LA COMMETTE Man's wig style *c* 1757. (*Marchand*)19

A LA CONCIERGE A woman's long-hair style in which the hair is drawn up to the top of the head and pinned in a knot. Named after a style favoured by the concierges of Paris. 19th/20th century.

A LA CONQUERANT Man's wig style *c* 1757. (*Marchand*)   *20*

A LA CONSEILLEUR A woman's hair style, 1786, dressed with long loose tresses hanging down the back 'Behind it flows loosely à la conseilleur'. (*Ipswich Journal, 1788*)   *21*

A LA CYBELLE An 18th century hair style for women in which the hair was dressed about a foot high, towerwise, as the goddess Cybele is represented with her hair dressed in rising turrets. Both the natural hair and wigs were worn in this fashion. (*Elegant Arts*)

A LA DAUPHINE 1788. A high dressed French hair style for women, having a chignon with the form of a *croix de chevalier* with a curl à la Sultane falling onto the neck, two side curls and two shoulder curls; the whole coiffure being adorned with a ribbon and rose of diamonds crossed by a row of pearls.   *22*

AU DESIRE DE PLAIRE 18th century coiffure for women. (*Uzanne*)   *23*

A LA DISTINCTION An 18th century French hair style for women.   *24*

A LA DRAGONNE Man's wig style *c* 1757. (*Marchand*) 25

A LA DRIADE A French hair style for women, *c* 1778.   *26*

A L'ECONNOMME (*sic*) Man's wig style *c* 1757. (*Marchand*)   *27*

A L'ELEPHANT Man's wig style *c* 1757. (*Marchand*)   *28*

A L'ENFANT A man's wig style, 1770. Flat top, curls at front on each side, long straight hair at back with curls at end hanging *au naturel*.

A L'ENTIQUITEE Man's wig style *c* 1757. (*Marchand*) 29

A L'ESPAGNOLE A chignon style of the 18th century. (*Uzanne*)   *30*

A L'EURIDICE An 18th century hair style for women. (*Uzanne*)   *31*

AU FAVORIE Man's wig style *c* 1757. (*Marchand*)   *32*

A LA FELICITE Man's wig style *c* 1757. (*Marchand*)   *33*

A LA FLORE Woman's 18th century coiffure. (*Uzanne*) 34

A LA FRANCAISE After the French mode. (*Creer*)

A LA FRANCOISE Man's wig style *c* 1757. (*Marchand*) 35

A LA GENDARME Man's wig style *c* 1757. (*Marchand*) 36

A LA GENTILLY Man's wig style *c* 1757. (*Marchand*) 37

A LA GIRAFE A woman's high dressed hair style of 1832. (*Bysterveld, p 36*)

A LA GRECQUE (1) Man's hair fashion, 18th century. 'The hair is dressed in two long curls on each side and a grecque behind, like a horseshoe. It is tied behind in a long tail à la Panurge'. (*Ipswich Journal*, Oct 1787)
(2) a woman's hair style of the 18th century.   *263, 266*

A LA HERISSON Woman's hair style of extreme frizziness, introduced from France in 1777. 'Hair carried one storey higher and projects with a high peak over the forehead. It is called *à la hérisson* – hedgehog fashion – and is quite new from Versailles'. (*Gentleman's and London Magazine, 1777*)   *38*

A L'IMPASSIANT Man's wig style *c* 1757. (*Marchand*) 39

A L'IMPERATRICE BANDEAU Consisted of rolled hair divided in the centre and worn around the front of the head. Fashionable in mid-Victorian period and popularised by the Empress of the French. (*Moniteur de la Coiffure*)

A L'INCONSTANCE Man's wig style *c* 1757. (*Marchand*)   *40*

A L'INDEPENDANCE (*sic*) Man's hair style of early 19th century. (*GMF*)

A L'INDIFERENCE (*sic*) Man's wig style *c* 1757. (*Marchand*)   *41*

A L'ITALIENNE Man's wig style *c* 1757. (*Marchand*)   *42*

A LA JACOBINE A short and simple hair style worn by women *c* 1791. Named after the French political club founded 1789 at Versailles, which determined the radical trend of the French Revolution. (*Wraxall*)   *43*

A LA JALOUSIE Man's wig style *c* 1757. (*Marchand*)   *44*

A LA JANOT Late 18th century hair style for women.   *45*

A LA JUNON A French hair style for women, 1774. (*Moniteur de la Coiffure*)   *46*

A LA LEGERE Man's wig style *c* 1757. (*Marchand*)   *47*

AU LEVER DE LA REINE Woman's 18th century coiffure. (*Uzanne*)   *48*

A LA LUNATIQUE Man's wig style *c* 1757. (*Marchand*)   *49*

A LA MADONNA See Madonna hairdress.

A LA MAITRE D'HOTEL Man's wig style *c* 1757. (*Marchand*)   50

A LA MALIBRAN A hair style consisting of two partings, both starting separately from near the centre of the forehead and continuing to behind the ears, giving the hair between a heart shape. (*Cooley* p 259)

A LA MAPPEMONDE An 18th century woman's coiffure that depicted the five continents of the world.

A LA MAURESQUE Woman's 18th century coiffure (*Uzanne*)   51

A LA MINERVE 18th century high dressed wig style for women, adorned with 10 ostrich feathers. Worn by Marie Antoinette.

A LA MODE According to the fashion. (*Creer*)

A LA MOUSQUETAIRE Man's wig style *c* 1757. (*Marchand*)   52

A LA NATION A woman's hair style of 1790. (*Villermont*)   53

A NAUD ESPAGNOL Wig style worn by Marshal Vileron at battle of Ramillies and claimed by the Duke of Marlborough as final mark of his crowning triumph.

A LA NOUVELLE MODE Man's wig style *c* 1757. (*Marchand*)   54

A L'ORDINAIRE Man's wig style *c* 1757. (*Marchand*)   55

A L'OYSEAU ROYAL Man's wig style *c* 1757. (*Marchand*)   56

A LA PARESSEUSE Man's wig style *c* 1757. (*Marchand*)   57

A LA PARISIENE Man's wig style *c* 1757. (*Marchand*)   58

AU PARTERRE GALANT An 18th century hair style for women. (*Uzanne*)   59

A LA PERSANE An 18th century French hair style for women.   60

AU PETIT MAITRE Man's wig style *c* 1757 (*Marchand*)   61

A LA PLUS TOT FAIR Man's wig style *c* 1757. (*Marchand*)   62

A LA PORT MAHON Man's wig style *c* 1757. (*Marchand*)   63

A LA PRUDENCE Man's wig style *c* 1757. (*Marchand*) 64

A QUATRE BOUCLES AVEC UNE BARRIERE DE PERLES Woman's 18th century coiffure. (*Uzanne*)   65

A QUATRE BOUCLES DROITES SEPAREES Woman's 18th century coiffure. (*Uzanne*)   66

A LA QUINOT Woman's 18th century coiffure. (*Uzanne*)   67

A LA RANCOUR Woman's 18th century coiffure. (*Uzanne*)   68

A RAVIR Man's wig style *c* 1757. (*Marchand*)   69

A LA REINE A late 18th century French hair style for women.   70

A LA RINOXERROS (*sic*) Man's wig style *c* 1757 (*Marchand*)   71

A LA ROYALE Man's wig style *c* 1757. (*Marchand*)   72

A LA SACRIFICE A woman's short hair style popularised by Madame Tallier towards the end of the French Reign of Terror. Upon her rescue from prison she adopted a hair style short all round the head like that of a man. Similar to *à la Jacobine*. (*Ladies' Companion*, 1851)

AUX SENTIMENTS REPLIES Woman's 18th century coiffure. (*Uzanne*)   73

A LA SINGULIERRE (*sic*) Man's wig style *c* 1757. (*Marchand*)   74

A LA SOUVAROFF A beard-cut in which the moustache meets the side-whiskers, the chin being clean shaven.
                                                                                                                                                   75, 76

A LA SYLPHIDE An 18th century French hair style for women.   77

A LA SYRIENNE A woman's hair style of 1775 similar to a *hérisson* or hedgehog style, *qv*.

A TROIS BOUCLES EN ARRIERE 18th century coiffure for women. (*Uzanne*)   78

A TROIS GRANDES BOUCLES LACHES 18th century hair style for women. (*Uzanne*)   79

A LA TRONCHIN Man's wig style *c* 1757. (*Marchand*) 80

AU VAL D'AMOUR Woman's 18th century coiffure. (*Uzanne*)   81

A LA VENUS An 18th century hair style for women in which the hair was dressed with a few curls hanging loosely in imitation of the hair of Venus as depicted in the painting 'Venus rising from the sea' by Botticelli. (*Elegant Arts*)   82

A LA VICTIME A woman's hair style resulting from the influence of the French Revolution, in which the hair was combed up at the back in loose disarray baring the neck as if for decapitation by the guillotine. A blood red ribbon was worn about the neck. French *c* 1795. (*Wraxall*)

AU VIEILLARD Man's wig style *c* 1757. (*Marchand*)   458

A LA ZODIAQUE Woman's hair style dressed high and decorated with stars, moon and sun, and the head-dress encircled by the signs of the Zodiac. 18th century. (*Ladies' Magazine*, 1777)   459

AARON'S BEARD A large flowered St John's Wort.

ABBES WIG 18th century wig style with three rows of rolled curls covering the neck, and tonsure at crown. (*Garsault*)
                                                                                                                                            91 (12, 13)

ABBOTT, Charles. First Baron Tenterden (1762–1832), Lord Chief Justice, son of a barber.

ABNORMAL COLOUR A hair colour that is not found naturally in human hair.

ABRAHAM 16th century name for the colour auburn. 'Our heads are some brown, some black, some abram, some bald'. (*Coriolanus*, 1623)

ABRAHAM COLOURED BEARD Auburn beard. (See Abraham)

ABSALOM'S HAIR Is said to have weighed 200 shekels (*Samuel XIV 25, 26*). Absalom had an uncommonly fine head of hair, of unusual weight, which is all we know with certainty about it. Absalom in Dryden's poem 'Absalom and Achitophel' is the Duke of Monmouth (1649–1685).

ABUNDANCE OF HAIR in women is supposed to indicate wantonness. Abundance of hair in man or woman denotes sexual energy (*Porta*). An abundance of body hair on a man signifies an amourous disposition. (*Venette*, *Génération de l'homme*)

ACACIA GUM See Gum arabic. The gum of the acacia tree. (*Verrill*)

ACADEMY A place where art or learning is practised or displayed. By the 19th century academies of hairdressing had been founded in London, Bristol and several other English towns. Originally the name given to the garden where Plato taught. Later extended to a place of study, and by the 14th century there were academies of art at Venice. See also Hairdressing Academy.

ACARUS A mite that causes scabies.

ACCELERATOR An apparatus or chemical that speeds up a process or an action.

ACCENT COMB A hair comb usually tortoise-shell with a decorated top of gold, silver or precious stones, used to embellish a hair-dress, drawing attention to, or accentuating, the coiffure. Of Spanish origin, it became fashionable decoration in Latin America. American usage, 20th century.

ACCROCHE-COEUR Flat curl on temples, often gummed. (*Elegant Arts*)

ACETATE OF LEAD See Lead acetate.

ACETIC ACID (GLACIAL) ch₃cooh At a concentration of 2% to 3% by weight in distilled water is used as a hair rinse. (*Merck*)

ACETONE ch₃co.ch₃ A colourless, highly inflammable liquid solvent for fat, oils, resins, rubber, lacquers, varnishes, etc. It should be kept away from fire, plastic eyeglass frames, rayon stockings, etc. Used in manufacture of nail varnishes and as nail varnish remover. (*Merck*)

ACHILLES Bravest of all Greeks in Trojan war. Was described by Homer as having a fine head of hair. Martial refers to the most beautiful hair as Achilles' hair.

ACHILLES' HAIR A term descriptive of very beautiful hair. (See Achilles)

ACID BATH A solution of glacial acetic acid (ch₃cooh) and distilled water, used for treating heavily bleached hair to reconstitute it and facilitate combing. The usual mix is by volume 3% glacial acetic acid and 97% distilled water. The pure acid will produce burns on the skin.

ACID HAIR RINSE Weak solution in water of either acetic, tartaric, citric or amino-sulphamic acids, etc. In the hair-dressing salon vinegar and lemon juice are commonly used in an aqueous solution.

ACID RINSE See Acid hair rinse.

ACNE Inflammation of the sebaceous glands of the skin, giving rise to papules or pustules.

ACOMOUS Hairless. (*Roget Thesaurus*, 1929 ed)

ACRIFLAVINE An acridene dye with powerful germicidal and antiseptic properties.

ACRYLIC STRETCH WIG A wig made with acrylic hair on an extensile foundation that will conform to most normal sized skulls.

ACRYLIC WIG A wig made of a man-made acrylic fibre as a substitute for hair.

ADAPTOR (Hair) A tail of hair made on 2″–3″ weft, macramé running through. Popular late 1920s when many women wanted to revert to long hair. *93, 94*

ADDED-ON HAIR Postiche.

ADHESIVE Several types of adhesive are used to attach hair pieces to the scalp and face, such as spirit gum for beards and moustaches; and diachylon for toupets.

ADHESIVE HAIR-SET TAPE See Tape.

ADHESIVE PATCH A small patch of waterproofed material secured to the head-side of a toupet by stitching or sticking, and having adhesive on its exposed surface to secure the toupet to the scalp.

ADJECTIVE DYE A hair dye that requires the use of a mordant to fix and develop the colour.

ADJUSTABLE BLOCK HOLDER A metal or wooden adjustable tapered peg to hold a moveable block. The peg swivels on a clamp that can be secured to the work bench. *95*

ADJUSTABLE WIG A stock wig that can be adjusted to the head size of the wearer. Many theatrical wigs hired out to amateur groups come within this category.

ADOLPH MENJOU MOUSTACHE A style of moustache named after the film star Adolph Menjou. A popular style in the 1920s. *101M*

ADONIS WIG An effeminate white powdered wig in a flowing bushy dressing worn by fashionable young men *c* 1734–1775, 'powdered and appearing like the twigs of a gooseberry bush in a deep snow'. (*London Mag*, 1734). 'A fine flowing Adonis or white Periwig'. (*Graves, R, The Spiritual Quixote*, 1773)
Adonis was a youth of rare beauty and a favourite of Venus.

ADSCITITIOUS-HAIR False hair; a wig. (*Good*)

AESCULAP SCISSORS A proprietary brand of thinning scissors *qv*. *106*

AESCULAPIAN SNAKE A harmless snake associated with the god of health and medicine in Greek mythology. Today's symbol of medicine, the Caduceus, depicts two Aesculapian snakes entwined around a staff.

AESCULAPIUS Son of Apollo, God of Medicine, was represented with a large beard and abounding hair. Hygiea was one of his daughters.

AESTHETICS The study and appreciation of the beautiful.

AETAS CRITICA ALOPECIA The middle-age baldness of women. (*Wheeler*)

AETOLIAN TONSURE A curious hair style affected by the men of Aetolia in the 17th century. (*Bulwer*) *102C*

AFRICAN HAIR (1) Woolly hair from the head of an African. (2) Fibre from the leaves of the palm *Chamaerops humilis*.

AFRO HAIR-DO A hair style suitable for very frizzy hair, usually of a bouffant character, or straight hair that has been frizzed or crimped to imitate such styles.

AFRO-WIG A black-haired frizzy wig.

AFTER-SHAVE APPLICATION Any face treatment that takes place immediately after a shave, such as powdering, face massage, spirit spray, etc.

AFTER-SHAVE LOTION A refreshing, stimulating, deodorizing lotion for application to the face after shaving. These lotions are often perfumed with a 'manly' scent such as tweed or new mown hay.

AGATIZED SOAP A soap on which cameos, bas-reliefs and other designs appear. American usage. (*Morfit*)

AGG To cut clumsily, to hack. Wilts. usage. (*Akerman*)

AGGLUTINANT Any substance that causes adhesion such as hair lacquers that when dry hold dressed hair in position, or coloured powders that are sprayed upon the undried, lacquered hair.

AGGRAVATORS Half curls combed into the proximity of the outer corner of each eye. 'His hair carefully twisted into the outer corner of each eye, till it formed a variety of that description of semi-curls, usually known as *haggerawators*.' (*Dickens, C, Sketches by Boz*, 1839 ed, p 245)

AGNES TEUMEL'S DEPILATORY A 19/20th century 'secret' preparation that consisted chiefly of melted pine resin. (*Koller*)

AGRIPPINA A woman's hair style *c* 1803 inspired by the coiffure of Agrippina, the wife of the Roman Emperor Tiberius; she died AD 26. (*Lafoy*)

AIGRETTE (1) A bouquet of precious stones in a very light setting, used as a hair ornament, 17/18th century. (*Smith, H C*)
(2) A tuft or plume of feathers (originally from the Egret, a bird) worn as a head-dress, 19/20th century. (*Creer*) *124*

AILE DE PIGEON See Pigeon-wing periwig.

AILES DE PAPILLON See Butterfly wings.

AINU (pronounced eye-ne) The hairy indigenous inhabitants of Japan. (See N G Munro, *Ainu Creed and Cult*, 1962)

AIR BRUSH A pressurized spray used for blowing atomized colour on fantasy hair styles. (*N and N*)

AIR-CUSHION BRUSH A hair brush in which the bristles are set in rubber with a cushion of air behind to give resilience to the bristles.

AIREDALE Slang term for a film extra with a natural beard. American usage. (*BB*)

AIR-JET STYLING The shaping of hair by means of a warm jet of air as from a hand hair dryer with a constricted nozzle.

AIRY LEVANT An early 18th century wig style for men.

ALBERMARLE Wig style for men 18th century. A popular colonial style.

ALBINISM Congenital absence of colour in the hair and skin, which is white or creamy, and the eyes, which are pink.

ALBINISMUS See Albino. (*Wheeler*)

ALBINO A person with hair that has no pigment; the hair being white, creamy or flaxen, and the eyes pink. See also Albinism. (*Wheeler*)

ALBUMEN BASE SHAMPOO An egg shampoo, *qv* or a shampoo incorporating either powdered or fresh egg.

ALCIBIADES A man's hair style of *c* 1803 inspired by the hairdress of Alcibiades, the Athenian General, 5th century BC. (*Lafoy*)

ALCOHOL ANHYDROUS c_2h_5oh A colourless, clear, very mobile and highly flammable liquid with a pleasant odour and burning taste. Miscible with water. Used as an antiseptic and germicide at 70% to 95% alcohol.

ALCOHOL STOVE A small spirit stove convenient for travellers for heating curling or waving irons. (*A H 1915*)

ALDERMANIC WIG An 18th century full-bottom periwig of an inordinately impressive appearance, mainly worn by city aldermen to add to their dignity.   *125*

ALEXANDER'S BEARD Alexander the Great lacked a beard worthy of the name and the phrase Alexander's beard turned into a proverb. 'Disguised yet with Alexander's bearde.' (*Gascoigne*)

ALEXANDRA CURL A long spiral drop curl usually worn behind the ear; named after Her Royal Highness Alexandra, Princess of Wales, later Queen of Edward VII, who wore these curls and greatly influenced fashion. *122, 315*

ALEXANDRA HAIR WAVER A double pronged wire with a detachable metal stop that fitted over the two ends to secure the interlaced hair. (*Creer*)

ALFALFA The beard. Slang. American usage. (*B and B*)

ALGERNON Man's christian name meaning 'the whiskered'. From the Norman als gernons. (*Partridge Name this Child*)

ALICANT SOAP Manufactured by a similar method to that of Castile soap, *qv*, but made at Alicante and considered superior to Marseilles and Castile and in the 19th century was regarded the best soap for the perfumer's use. (*Lillie*)

ALICE BAND A flat swathe of hair or a ribbon worn over the front of the head. Name derived from the band depicted by Tenniel as worn by Alice in his drawings for Dodgson's *Alice in Wonderland*, 1866.

ALICE-IN-WONDERLAND PONY TAIL The front hair from ear to ear and forehead to crown tied into a pony tail that falls over the loose back hair. 20th century.

ALIGNING HAIR The disentangling of a ball of matted hair by means of the fingers and ranging the constituent hair in line, preparatory to carding. Picking combings. 'By picking combings the hair is aligned.'

ALKALI BLEACH A hydrogen peroxide bleach preparation incorporating ammonia.

ALKALI TARTARI See Potassium carbonate.

ALKALINE HAIR RINSE A hair rinse that contains a weak alkaline solution.

ALKANET The dried root of a plant alkanna tinctoria. Alkannin, its colouring matter is used for tinting pomades red. (*Verrill*)

ALL-AROUND HAIRBRUSH A brush having bristles set all round its head. 20th century.

ALL-OVER DESIGN A repeat hair design, *qv*, that covers the whole head.

ALL-PURPOSE COMB A comb that is suitable for use in hair cutting, setting, dressing, disentangling or back combing, etc.

ALL-ROUND FRISETTE or PAD A sausage shaped pad of crêped hair 20″–23″ long and 1½″–2″ in diameter; used as a foundation for a hair style. (See also Frisette)   *126*

ALL-ROUND POMPADOUR FRAME A circular frame of wire and crêpe hair 20″–23″ in circumference used as a foundation for postiche that is to be dressed pompadour. (See Pompadour frame)

ALL-ROUND TRANSFORMATION See Transformation.

ALLEGRECK An 18th century wig style for men. (*Fenton* p. XIV)

ALLEN'S HAIR RESTORER See Plumbiferous Hair Water.

ALLEN'S WORLD'S HAIR RESTORER See Plumbiferous Hair Water.

ALLERGIC Relating to an allergy, *qv*, sensitive to something.

ALLERGY Sensitivity to the effect or action of dye, food, pollen, insect bite, etc. For example, some persons are allergic to certain hair dyes which induce dermatitis, a troublesome disease, characterised by eruption, redness, swelling, blisters, oozing, etc, of the head, face and neck.

ALLIARIA (*Sisymbrium alliara*) Also called Jack of the Hedge in the vernacular. The hedge-garlic used as a hair restorer in the 18th century. (*Lady's Magazine*, Dec 1759 and *Kersey, English Dictionary*, 1715)

ALLONGE A man's Baroque style wig with long full curls and dressed high over the forehead. First worn at the court of Louis XIV. (*De Zemler*)   *190*

ALMAN COMB The fingers and thumb of the hand used as a comb to disentangle the hair. 17th century.

ALOE Pith of the stem of the aloe used by barbers in South America to sharpen razors. (*Orton, J, 'The Andes and the Amazon,'* NY 1870)

ALOPECIA Baldness. See Alopecia areata, etc. (*McCarthy*)

ALOPECIA ADNATA Baldness at or soon after birth. (*McCarthy*)

ALOPECIA AREATA A disease in which certain areas of the scalp or of other hairy regions of the body suddenly or gradually lose their hair. Sometimes referred to as 'patchy' baldness. (*McCarthy*)

ALOPECIA ATROPHICANS See Alopecia Cicatrisata. (*McCarthy*)

ALOPECIA CALVA Baldness (*Wheeler*)

ALOPECIA CICATRISATA A rare disease of the scalp producing in its early stages pinhead to split-pea sized areas of baldness. (*McCarthy*)

ALOPECIA COMPRESSIO Baldness resulting from unduly straining the hair roots by too tightly tying the hair. (*Wheeler*)

ALOPECIA CONGENITALIS See Alopecia Adnata. (*McCarthy*)

ALOPECIA DIFFUSA Diffuse loss of hair resulting from fever, use of drugs, childbirth, etc. Usually curable. (*Flitman*)

ALOPECIA DYNAMICA Baldness due to the destruction of the hair follicle by disease. (*Thorpe*)

ALOPECIA FOLLICULARIS Baldness due to inflammation of the hair follicles. (*Thorpe*)

ALOPECIA LOCALIS See Alopecia Neurotica. (*McCarthy*)

ALOPECIA MALIGNA A severe type of baldness extending to eyebrows, eyelids and bearded regions. (*McCarthy*)

ALOPECIA NEUROTICA A type of baldness brought on by shock, injury or emotional disturbance. (*McCarthy*)

ALOPECIA ORBICULARIS See Alopecia Cicatrisata. (*McCarthy*)

ALOPECIA PARVIMACULATA A type of alopecia in which hair is lost in very small irregularly shaped patches. (*McCarthy*)

ALOPECIA PITYROIDES Baldness or loss of hair by *pityriasis capitis* (dandruff). (*McCarthy*)

ALOPECIA PREMATURA Baldness of youth. (*McCarthy*)

ALOPECIA PREMATURA IDIOPATHICA A slow thinning of the head hair before middle age. (*McCarthy*)

ALOPECIA PREMATUREA SYMPTOMATICA Baldness, often temporary, caused by illness. (*McCarthy*)

ALOPECIA PUBERTATIS Loss of hair by teenage girls. (*Wheeler*)

ALOPECIA PUERPERA A woman's hair fall after confinement. (*Wheeler*)

ALOPECIA SEBORRHEICA Loss of hair caused by a seborrheic condition of the scalp. (*McCarthy*)

ALOPECIA SENILIS Baldness of old age. (*McCarthy*)

ALOPECIA SYPHILITICA Partial alopecia of the scalp, beard or eyebrows caused by syphilis. (*McCarthy*)

ALOPECIA TOTALIS Total baldness of the scalp. (*McCarthy*)

ALOPECIA UNIVERSALIS Complete baldness of the scalp and entire body. (*Savill*)

ALOPECIAN An early 19th century proprietary ointment for the cure of alopecia. Also called Fox ointment.

ALPACA Hair of the alpaca goat.

ALPHA KERATIN The substance of human hair; a protein of outstanding stability and high sulphur content. (*Savill*)

ALUM A double sulphate of aluminium and potassium. An astringent used as a styptic by the barber.

ALUM POWDER Used to treat face cuts in the barber's saloon.

ALUM STICK Prepared alum in the form of a stick for convenience in applying to razor cuts, etc. See Alum.

AMBERGRIS HAIR POWDER A starch hair powder scented with ambergris perfume. 18/19th century. (*Lille*)

AMBERGRIS WASH-BALLS Wash-balls perfumed with civet, musk and ambergris, 19th century. (*Lillie*)

AMERICAN CLOTH A glazed cloth used for covering work benches in the boardwork room. The smooth surface prevents the hair catching in the table splinters. Now largely superseded by formica and other plastic substances. (See also Oil cloth)

AMERICAN HAIR-DYE A 19th century preparation. Nitrate of silver 1 oz; nitrate of bismuth 1 oz; distilled water 6 oz. The hair was moistened with this solution and one hour later touched with sulphydric acid. (*Dussauce*)

AMERICAN INDIAN See Mongolian.

AMERICAN PATTERN SCISSORS Haircutting scissors with a finger rest for the little finger.

AMERICAN SHAMPOO LIQUID A 19/20th century 'secret' preparation that consisted of rum 1000 parts, spirit of wine 120 parts, cantharides tincture 3 parts, ammonium carbonate 5 parts, and potash 10 parts. (*Koller*)

AMERICAN SHAVING CHAIR A comfortably upholstered and adjustable chair on a cast iron frame designed to swing the client for shaving into that position most convenient for the barber to perform his task.

AMERICAN TAPER WAVE CUT See Wave cut.

AMINE DYE See Aniline dye.

AMISH HAIR STYLES See Mennonite hair styles.

AMMONIA WATER A solution of 10% NH_3 in water; a colourless liquid with very pungent odour used in hair bleaching processes. About 18 drops are added to ¼ pint preparation of hydrogen peroxide to:
(1) Act as a catalyst.
(2) Neutralize traces of acid in the H_2O_2 which is used as a stabilizer, and
(3) Destroy any trace of grease on the surface of the hair which could prevent effective action by the hydrogen peroxide.
Human toxicity: Ingestion could lead to inflammation and sloughing, followed by constrictive scarring. Death could result from shock and irritation to mucous membranes.

AMMONIUM HYDROXIDE A solution of 28–29% NH_3 in water. Colourless liquid with pungent, suffocating odour, showing alkaline reaction. Keep cool in strong glass, rubber-stoppered bottles about two thirds full. Used in hair bleaching processes (see Ammonia water), but half a dozen drops only to ¼ pint of prepared bleach.
Human toxicity: as ammonia water, qv.

AMMONIUM THIOGLYCOLATE Used for cold permanent waving lotions. See Thioglycolic acid.

AMOROUS HAIR Long hair, flowing style. 17th century. (*Prynne*, 1628)   129

AMYL ACETATE (Isoamyl acetate) A colourless neutral liquid with a pear-like odour. Soluble in 400 parts water, miscible with alcohol, either, ethyl acetate, amyl alcohol. Used as a solvent nail varnishes, lacquers, etc.
Human toxicity: Can cause headache, fatigue and irritation to the mucous membranes.

ANACARDIUM HAIR DYE See Cashew dye.

ANADEME A floral or leaved garland for adorning the head c 1600.

ANAPHALACROSIS Baldness extending to the crown. (*Wheeler*)

ANCHOR, V To secure postiche to a block with pins.

ANCHOR BEARD A short pointed beard on the edge of the chin, with a fringe running up to the middle of the lower lip.   98C

ANCHOR STICK See weaving stick and back stick.

ANDROPOGONIS CITRATE Verbena oil.

ANGEL HAIR (1) Crêpe hair; (2) Glass fibre as used to decorate Christmas trees.

ANGEL'S HAIR (*Calliandra eriophylla*) A Mexican desert plant. The name is descriptive of its ethereal hair-like stamens. See also Hair flower.

ANGNAIL Skin torn at the root of a fingernail. Not hangnail.

ANGORA See Mohair.

ANGORA GOAT Source of mohair, qv. Originally bred in neighbourhood of Angora, Asia Minor. The long silky hair or wool is a valuable economic commodity.

ANGORA WOOL See Mohair.

ANILINE A chemical base, the source of many hair dyes. Usually a product of coal tar. Discovered in 1826. First prepared from indigo by means of caustic potash. Found in coal in 1834.

ANIMAL NET See Horsehair and hair net.

ANIMAL OIL POMADE A mid-19th century proprietary preparation manufactured by W T Cooper, Oxford Street, London. 'Does not dry on the hair, which is the case with all pomatums made with vegetable oils'. (*Turnley, J, The Language of the Eye*, 1856)

ANIMATING BUCKLE A man's wig style introduced by a French wigmaker, Mons de la Papillote, in 1764. It gave the wearer 'a most warlike fierceness'. (*London Magazine*, 1764)

ANNATTO A red colouring substance obtained from the coating of the buds of a tropical American tree. Used to colour soap, pomades and other cosmetics. (*Verrill*)

ANNEAU Small flat curl, usually arranged upon the cheek. Sometimes called a kissing curl.

ANNULAR SLIDE Ring-shaped hair slide.

ANOGENITAL HAIR The pubic and anal hair, qv.

17

ANTEBELLUM LOOK A hair style reminiscent of the fashionable coiffures before the American Civil War, 1861–1865. American usage exclusively.

ANTECEDENT BLEACH A hair bleach before the application of a dye, a pre-dye bleach.

ANTHEMIS NOBILIS See Chamomile.

ANTHOS See Rosemary.

ANTHRAX A malignant boil or pustule induced in man by infection from animals so infected. Frequently carried by untreated animal hair.

ANTI-CLOCKWISE Opposite to a clock-wise direction.

ANTI-DANDRUFF SHAMPOO A shampoo that contains a chemical such as a selenium-sulphide-bentonite that is claimed to relieve itching and dandruff. (*Sagarin*)

ANTI-KINK A substance or process for removing the kink or frizz from the hair of the negro. American usage.

ANTIMACASSAR A covering, usually oblong in shape, to cover and protect from macassar oil and other hair oils, the backs of chairs and sofas. 'Anti-Macassar materials . . . crochet cotton . . . drab crochet twine'. (*Lady's Newspaper*, 1852)

ANTI-PERSPIRANT Opposed to perspiration. Preparations of an astringent nature that deflect the sweat from the area treated, such as the armpits, to some other part of the body. (*Wall*)

ANTIQUITTEE See *A l'Entiquitée*.

ANTISEPTIC A substance which will prevent the growth of micro-organisms. (*PPB*)

ANTISEPTIC BOWL The bowl in which is kept the antiseptic solution for immersing hairdressing tools, such as combs, etc.

ANTISEPTIC PENCIL See Styptic pencil.

ANTISEPTIC SHAMPOO A hair shampoo containing an antiseptic substance.

ANTOINE Internationally famous hair artist, born Antek Cierplikowski, in Poland. (*Johnson*)

ANTOINE BOB A short hair style that is dressed back from the face with curls or rolls at the back giving the appearance of long hair. Named after and introduced by Antoine, the famous international hairdresser. American usage   *128*

ANVIEU See *A l'anvieu*.

APEX (of a wave) See Crest (of a wave).

APHRODITE The Grecian name of Venus, Goddess of beauty, Mother of love, the Queen of laughter, the Mistress of the Graces and of pleasure and the Patroness of courtesans.

APHRODITE HAIR DYE A 19/20th century 'secret' preparation that contained free hydrochloric acid, cupric chloride, ferric chloride and pyrogallic acid. It could have been injurious to health. (*Koller*)

APLASIA PILORUM INTERMITTENS See Monilethrix.

APOLLO (1) Son of Jupiter and Latona, god of youth and manly beauty, was depicted with long hair. The Romans were fond of imitating his figure and in their youth were remarkable for their fine heads of hair, which they cut at the age of 17 or 18. Apollo was always depicted as a tall, beardless young man. The only other beardless Roman deity was Mercury *qv*. (*Lemprière*)

(2) Name given in the late 18th century to University students who wore their own hair. At this time it was usual for the University student to wear a wig.

(3) A woman's hair style of 1866 inspired by hairdressings of Greek antiquity. (*Bysterveld*, p. 74)

APOLLO AND THE RAZOR The barber shop sign of Nello in George Eliot's *Romola*, 1862.

APOLLO BOW A bow of hair 19th century.   *131, 132*

APOLLO KNOT False hair looped, plaited or coiled and looped, and wired to cause the loop to stand erect in the hairdress. Fashionable from 1826.   *127, 140*

APOTHECARY'S BUSH Facetious name for the full curled wig of the apothecary. 18th century. (*L C March*, 1762)

APOTHECARY'S GRIZZLED WIG Grey wig worn by apothecaries. See Apothecary's bush. (*Graves*)

APPLICATOR (1) The glass, rubber or ebony removable extremity of an apparatus used in contact with the hair or scalp in treatments such as vibratory massage, high frequency application, etc.

(2) A small brush or cotton-wool covered rod, etc, used to apply hair bleach or dye, or permanent waving lotion, etc.

APPLICATOR BRUSH A small brush used for applying dyes and bleaches to the hair.

APPOINTMENT BOOK Usually a 4to sized book in which the hairdresser records his business engagements with his clients for hair service. This is still a rarity in the men's salon but always used in the ladies' salon.

APPOINTMENT CARD A small card given to the hairdresser's client on which is noted the time and date of the hair appointment.

APPRENTICE An indentured learner. One who is bound by indenture, or otherwise to another person for a term of years, to learn his or her art or mystery. (*Phillips*) As early as 1388 an Act of Parliament refers to apprentices.

APRON (of hair) A short length of hair weft.

AQUA COLONIENSIS See Eau de Cologne.

AQUA DESTILLATA Distilled water.

ARABESQUE COIFFURE A hair style that incorporates intricate surface decoration such as geometrical patterns of curls, curves, swirls, etc.

ARC Arrangement of hair in the shape of an arc.

ARC CURL A part of the complete circumference of a curl.

ARCH Arrangement of hair in the shape of an arch.

ARCHAIC A style of antiquity.

ARCHING Plucking the eyebrows to an arched shape.

ARCHITECTURAL STYLE A mid–19th century mode of dressing a woman's hair to a centre parting, with both sides matching and hanging heavily upon the cheeks. Regarded at the time as one of the monstrosities of the fashions for females. (*HTATH*)   *130*

AREA CELSI A type of baldness that leaves a growth of hair only on the crown of the head.

ARGENT (1) English hair style for men. 20th century. (*Foan*)

(2) Silver (Heraldic).

ARGENTIC POMADE A 19th century preparation for dyeing the hair. It consisted of: nitrate of silver 2 drachms, cream of tartar 2 drachms, ammonia 4 drachms, lard 4 drachms. (*Dussauce*)

ARGENTINE HAIR DYE See Columbian hair dye.

ARGYRIA A greyish-blue discolouration of the skin due to the use of silver hair dyes. (*Phillips*)

ARISTOMENES A young Messenian of the royal line who when captured and cut up by the Spartans was found to have hair growing upon his heart. Plutarch, King of Sparta and Hermogenes, the rhetorician, also had hair growing on their hearts. (*Pliny and Valerius Maximus* are the authorities)

ARKWRIGHT, SIR RICHARD (1732–1792) A barber at Bolton until *c* 1767, when he turned his attention to mechanical inventions. Invented a spinning-mill; knighted 1786. High Sheriff of Derbyshire 1787. (*DNB*)

ARMORACIA RADIX Horse-radish root. As an infusion with a few grains of capsicum, used in the 19th century as a stimulating hair-wash. (*Gurney*)

ARMY CROP Short cut all over the head except at the front part, which was left 1½" long and brushed to the left hand side of the head and back to accommodate the forage cap, the front or point of which was centred in line with the right eyebrow. From Boer War to 1916.

ARMY WIG See Military wig.

ARRECTOR MUSCLE See *Arrectores pilorum*.

ARRECTORES PILORUM The small involuntary muscle associated with the hair follicle that causes the hair to stand erect as a result of cold or fright. Not usually present at the follicles of the lip hairs or in the axillae, which have no muscle as part of the follicular structure.

ARSLOCK Bottom end (furthest from head) of a tress of hair. The entangled or knotted ends of the head hair. *Arse* = bottom; *lock* = knotted. 17th century usage. (*Holme*)

ARTICHOKE (1) 18th century man's wig style.
(2) Teenage hair style, 1962.

ARTICHOKE-BOTTOM See *En-cue-d'artichaeux*

ARTICHOKE LEAF Beard style of 16/17th century. (*Mitchell*)

ARTIFICIAL BALDNESS In the province of Baske in the 17th century those women were accounted fairer who shaved their heads. The hair was regarded as an abject excrement, an unprofitable burden and an uncomely covering. There are other examples of this curious taste. (*Bulwer*) 102A

ARTIFICIAL BORDER False hair piece that encircled the head, 17/18th century, ('*Miscellaneous Works of George, Duke of Buckingham*' 1707, p. 27).

ARTIFICIAL EYELASHES (1) False eyelashes manufactured from human hair and woven on fine silk or white hair, and stuck in position to replace a natural deficiency.
(2) Single hairs stuck on existing eyelashes that are too short to suit the lady's taste. They are then cut to the required length. See also Eyelashes.

ARTIFICIAL HAIR Any manufactured hair, derived from nylon or certain grass fibres, etc. Not natural hair.

ARTIFICIAL HAIR-LINE The visible hair-line after the neck hair has been cut to a contour other than the natural hair-line.

ARTILLERY WHISKERS (Dundreary whiskers) Probably because affected by artillery officers 1865. (*Leech, J, Pictures of Life and Character*, 1865)

ARTIST A man's hair style of the 1920s, popularized by Paul Glaus of the London Gentlemen's Hairdressing Academy.

ARTISTIC COVERING A well-made and skilfully dressed postiche that defies detection. A euphemism for an attractive wig.

ARYBALLOS An oil jar used by Greek athletes. (*Torr, C, Rhodes in Ancient Times, Cambridge*, 1885)

ASEPSIS Absence of bacteria.

ASEPTIC Free from harmful bacteria.

ASH A shade that has no red or yellow tones.

ASHENING The removal of red or yellow tones in hair. (*Anderson*)

ASIATIC HAIR Dark, straight hair from the head of Asiatics especially Chinese. Used in the manufacture of theatrical wigs.

ASPASIA A woman's hair style *c* 1803 inspired by the coiffure of Aspasia, the daughter of Hermotimus of Phocaea, famous for her charm and elegance. She was priestess of the sun, mistress to Cyrus and later to his brother Artaxerxes. (*Lafoy*)

ASPIDOSPERMA (also called Guebracho) The dried bark of Aspidosperma Guerbracho-blanco, infusions of which have been used as a hair dye. (*Wall, Merck*)

ASSASSIN, L' A name suggested by Horace Walpole (1757) for a hair style. He wrote: 'Did you hear that, after their conquest (the French, of Port Mahon), the French ladies wore little towers for pompons, and called them *des Mahonnoises*! I suppose, since the attempt on the King, all their fashions will be *à l'assassin*'. (*Stone*, p 427)

ASSASSIN PERRUQUIER A Parisian barber who murdered clients and delivered the bodies to a neighbouring pastrycook, whose shop in the Rue de la Harpe became famous for its savoury patties. (*Procter*)

ASSYRIAN BEARD A long beard dressed in spiral curls or plaits. 103G

ASSYRIAN LOOK A hair style for women imitative of an Assyrian style in which the hair was worn flat on the top of the head and bunched out at the back, 1967.

ASTEATOSIS A condition brought on by the improper functioning of the sebaceous glands.

ASTLEY, MRS An 18th century actress and wife of 'Old Astley', who had 'such luxuriant hair that she could stand upright and it covered her to her feet like a veil'.

ASTRINGENT LOTION A lotion that causes contraction. Used in toilet waters for application to the skin.

ASYMMETRIC STYLE A hair style with a want of symmetry. (*Ingerid*)

ASYMMETRICAL STYLE A hair style wanting symmetry.

ASYMMETRY Irregularity, imbalance in the physical arrangement of materials. The opposite of symmetry, *qv*.

AT THE BOARD See On the board.

AT THE CHAIR A reference to work at barbering, the barber stands in the salon, as opposed to the boardworker, who sits in the workroom. 133, 156

ATOMIC HAIRDO A woman's hair style, 1954, dressed high with loose curls cascading over a band of ribbon around the drawn up hair on top of the head. Symbolizing the mushroom effect of the atomic cloud. Featured on model Terry Tune at Las Vegas, USA.

ATOMIZER A spray operated by compressed air from which the liquid to be sprayed emerges in an atomized condition.

ATRICHIA CONGENITA The congenital absence of hair. (*Savill*)

ATROPOS Daughter of Nox and Erebus and one of the goddesses who presided over the birth and life of mankind. She was represented by the ancients in a black veil, with a pair of scissors in her hand. (*Lemprière*)

ATTAR The concentrated essential oil of a flower, especially roses. (*Verrill*)

ATTIRE A jewelled head-dress, 15th century and later.

AU REPENTIR A woman's hair style resulting from the effect of the French Revolution, in which the hair was worn combed away from the neck. French *c* 1795. See *A la victime*. (*Wraxall*)

AUBREY TRESS A long-haired style for men 17th century 'the dancing of his aubrey tresses about'. (*Ladies' Dictionary*, p 373) Possibly the name was derived from John Aubrey, the Antiquary, 1626–1697.

AUDITORY HAIR Epithelial hair of the inner ear.

AUBURN (1) Adj (from Latin *alburnus*: whitish). From 16–17th century the word appears as abron, abroun, abrune, etc, which suggests a derivation from brown. Until *c* 1700 this name denoted a yellowish or whitish brown colour possibly what we would call a light grey coloured hair, but later the meaning changed to golden or ruddy brown colour without reference to white in it.
'Faire aburne or chesten colour' 1576.
'His hair was abourn in colour between white and red' 1649.
Probably the best colour effectively to display a fine coiffure. (2) Subs A red-haired woman. 20th century slang.

19

AUREOL A 19/20th century 'secret' hair dye. It consisted of 1% methol, 0.3% amidophenol hydrochlorate and 0.6% of monoamidophenylamine, the whole dissolved in 50% spirit containing 0.5% of sodium hyposulphite. The hair was first cleansed of all grease, then Aureol was mixed with an equal quantity of hydrogen peroxide (20 vols) and applied to the hair. After 2 or 3 hours a dark brown colour developed. (*Koller*)

AUREOLE BEARD A rounded beard. (*Wells*)

AUREOLE RAMBAUD A pompadour style set for a standard Marcel waving test. Named after René Rambaud, an esteemed French hairdresser, writer, and craft historian.

AURICOMOUS (*Auricomus*) Pertaining to golden hair. (*Mixing in Society*, 1874)

AURICOMUS GOLDEN HAIR WASH A 19/20th century 'secret' hair preparation for bleaching the hair. It was an aqueous solution of hydrogen peroxide. (*Koller*)

AURORA Greek goddess. Depicted, by the ancients, with hair dishevelled and hanging loose about the shoulders, being of the colour of purest gold. (*Salmon*)

AURELIA A celtic woman's name meaning 'gold-tressed'. (*Long*)

AUSTRALIAN ABORIGINE HAIR Wavy and black.

AUTOKUREUS A self-shaver. (*Southey, The Doctor*)

AWNIE (Scot) Bearded, 18th century (*Burns*)

AXILLARY HAIR Hair that grows in the armpit. (*Montagna*)

AYLE DE PIGEON See A *l'Ayle de pigeon.*

AYRO'S HAIR INVIGORATOR See Plumbiferous hair water.

B

BABY The small curl on the tail of a judge's wig.

BABY BRUSH A small hairbrush with soft bristles 1½" to 1¾" long, for use on the hair of babies.

BABY COMB A comb with blunt, rounded teeth for use on young children.

BABY CURL (1) The curl in a baby's hair. This sometimes disappears or lessens with age.
(2) A small curl.
(3) One of the two small curls near the end of the tail of a barrister's wig.

BABY SHAMPOO A shampoo so prepared that it can cause no irritation or ill effect to either the scalp, eyes or hair of a baby.

BACCHUS God of Wine, son of Jupiter and Semele, depicted with long unshorn locks. The Bearded Deity.

BACILLUS Microscopic rod-shaped vegetable organism.

BACK-AND-CURL See Backward curl.

BACKBRUSH, TO Brushing some of the hair in a lock back towards the roots. Similar to backcombing, *qv.*, but using a brush instead of a comb.

BACK-COMB A hair comb for decoration or for securing hair at the back of the hairdress.

BACKCOMB, TO See Backcombing.

BACKCOMBING The combining of the shorter hairs in a tress or lock back towards the roots. This gives the lock fullness. See also Backbrush.

BACKCOMBING COMB A comb composed of alternating long and short teeth, used for backcombing hair.

BACK-DRESSING A chignon or other form of hairdress for the back part of the head.

BACK FLUFF See Backcomb

BACK HAIR The hair that grows at the back of the head.

BACK NET A net for the back of the head.

BACK PIECE Similar to a chignon, *qv.*

BACK-ROOM HAIRDRESSER A term of opprobrium used by hairdressers when referring to other members of their craft who conduct their business in an ill-adapted or unsuitable room on domestic premises. The Back-room Hairdresser is disliked by the Craft because of the suspicion that he has a financial advantage by paying insufficient rates and avoiding income tax. This is not necessarily true.

BACK SHAMPOO A shampoo for which the subject leans backward over a basin, shampoo board or shute; the advantage being that the make-up of the subject is less likely to be disturbed. The term Backward Shampoo is to be preferred, *qv.*

BACK-SHAMPOO BOARD The board or shute on which the subject rests the back of her neck during the process of a backward shampoo. 19/early 20th century.

BACK-SHAMPOO STAND The stand that supports and holds in position the back-shampoo board, *qv.*

BACK STICK Left hand weaving stick, also called anchor stick or anchor peg.

BACK-STITCHING The stitching of the wig net to the galloon in wig-making. On the completed wig these stitches will be visible on the inside and covered with hair on its outside. (*B and S*)

BACK-STREET BARBER Term of professional contempt used by snob main street hairdressers when referring to other members of the craft whom they consider inferior socially and in hairdressing skill to themselves. Needless to write, most hairdressers who conduct their business in side streets are in all ways the equals of their 'main-street' fellow craftsmen. 20th century.

BACK-TOOTH COMB Teeth on one side only of the spine of the comb. 17th century. (*Holme*)

BACK WIND (1) Subs. The kind of hair wind in which the hair-ends are wound back towards the roots in a spiral wind.
(2) Verb The action of winding the hair-ends back towards the roots in a spiral wind. (*Smith*)

BACKWARD CURL A curl wound towards the back of the head. On the right-hand side of the model it is a clockwise curl and on the left-hand side an anti-clockwise curl. Also called Back-and-up-Curl. 20th century.

BACKWARD SHAMPOO See Back shampoo. Backward shampoo is to be preferred to avoid any confusion with the shampooing of a back.

BACTERICIDE A disinfectant substance which will destroy bacteria. (*PPB*)

BACTERIOLOGY The study of, and knowledge of, bacteria.

BACTERIOSTATIC An antiseptic substance used to prevent the growth of bacteria. (*PPB*)

BACTERIUM (plur Bacteria) A microscopic unicellular vegetable organism, some types of which are the cause of disease.

BADGER HAIR Hair from the badger, a grey-coated, nocturnal, plantigrade quadruped. This is the most favoured kind of hair for shaving brushes as it is soft, hard-wearing and long lasting. (*HWJ* 2nd June 1928, p 1792)

BAD-GIRL COIFFURE See Veronica Lake coiffure.

BAG (1) 18th century term for a wig of any kind, also for a bag wig (*qv*). Presumably as a shortened form of bag wig it was applied vernacularly to all other types of wig.
(2) The silk bag in which the queue of an 18th century wig was enclosed when being worn. See Bagwig.

135

BAG COMB A small dressing comb for carrying in a handbag.

BAGNOLETTE A head-dress for ladies. (*Creer*)

BAGOT, RICHARD Bishop of Bath and Wells, 1845–1854. The first Bishop to discontinue the use of the episcopal wig. (*Notes and Queries*, 27th Feb 1858)

BAG WIG Man's wig in which the tail or queue was enclosed in a bag of black satin or silk called a 'bourse', bag, purse or crapaud. The open end of the bag was enclosed around the top of the queue by a drawstring that was concealed beneath a stiff black decorative bow. From *c* 1737. (*Dodsley*). Also called a purse wig. See also Rose bag. 91 (3, 4, 9), 258

BAIRD beard. Scottish usage.

BAKER A curling iron heater. American usage. (*Rohrer*)

BAKING Drying wet dressed postiche at low temperatures in a metal wig oven, (*qv*). In permanent waving, heating wound hair enclosed in a sachet.

BALBO BEARD A short chin beard after that worn by Balbo, the Italian General. American usage. 97–i

BALD With the scalp wholly or partly hairless.

BALD CHIEF Benjamin Louis Eulalie de Bonneville (1796–1878). United States Army Officer who, during a two year leave led an expedition to the Rocky Mountains. Bonneville was completely bald and received the name Bald Chief from the Indians. (*Washington Irving, Adventures of Captain Bonneville*, 1837)

BALD DOME A bald head. Slang 18th/20th century.

BALD MEN (FAMOUS) Francis Bacon, Cicero, Homer, Socrates, Confucius, Aristotle, Plato, Pliny, Maecenas, Julius Caesar, Horace, Shakespeare, Napolean Bonaparte, Dante, Pope, Cowper, Goldsmith, Wordsworth, John Quincy Adams, Patrick Henry.

BALD PATE A bald head.

BALD TOP A wig with a bald crown. Theatrical usage.

BALD WIG A theatrical wig incorporating a bald crown. 'Making a bald wig for the Lisbon gentleman, 42/-, 1891, (*Stevens, MS*)

BALDCOOT A bald-headed man. Slang. (*B and B*) Presumably from the saying 'as bald as a coot'. The coot being an aquatic bird with a frontal head patch of white skin.

BALD FACE A man without whiskers. Somerset usage. (*Elworthy*)

BALD-FACED STAG A bald-headed man. American slang. (*B and B*)

BALDHEAD (1) A term of reproach made to an empty headed person.
(2) A bald-headed man. Slang. (*B and B*)

BALD-HEADED ROW The front seats of the orchestra stalls; so named on the assumption that they are taken by old or middle-aged men anxious to get as close as possible to their female favourites of the foot-lights. (*Walsh*)

BALDNESS The condition of being bald.

BALDNESS Old-age type. See Alopecia senilis.

BALDNESS Patchy type. See Alopecia areata.

BALDNESS Traction type. See Traction alopecia.

BALDWIN IV See Handsome beard.

BALDY Street urchins' cry after a bald-headed man, common in the 19th century and heard often by the writer in Bristol before *c* 1922. See Baldhead.

BALE OF STRAW (1) Blonde hair, especially bleached hair. American slang. (*B and B*)
(2) A blonde haired woman. Slang.

BALL-POINTED HAIR PIN Hair pin with small balls on the points to prevent scratching the head.

BALL-TIP BRUSH ROLLER A nylon or metal hair curler with implanted spikes like a cylindrical brush, each spike having a small ball tip. The hair is wound wet and after drying is ready for dressing out.

BALL-TOOTHED COMB A comb for the use on the hair of babies with very small balls on the tips of the teeth.

BALM OF COLUMBIA A proprietary preparation for strengthening the hair, manufactured by C and A Oldridge since 1822. 19th century. (*Wooton*)

BALM OF EGYPT Synonym for Balm of Mecca, *qv*.

BALM OF GRAND CAIRO Synonym for Balm of Mecca, *qv*.

BALM OF JUDEA Synonym for Balm of Mecca, *qv*.

BALM OF MECCA A liquid resin of whitish colour with a pungent lemon-like aromatic taste used in the east to render the skin white, soft and smooth. Described in the 18th century by Lady Mary Wortley Montague as having agreed very ill with her. Apparently it gave her dermatitis, although she added that all the women of Turkey 'make use of it, and have the loveliest bloom in the world'. (*Toilette*, 1832)

BALSA WIG BLOCK A light wig block of balsa wood, used to store wigs on. Storage blocks are also made of foam rubber, wood, plastic and wire mesh.

BAND OF HAIR A 1″ to 2″ wide strip of postiche. See Bandeau.

BAND, SLIP-ON Subs. A band with dressed hair attached; worn on the head for a quick change of style, also called quick switch.

BAND WIG A partial wig which is worn sewn on a ribbon, covering the natural hair line; the hair of the 'wig' covering and mingling with the natural hair. (*N and N*)

BANDEAU (plural bandeaux) (1) A fillet for the hair, 18th century.
(2) A postiche, narrow or wide but not extending beyond the crown, worn on the front of the head and secured by a ribbon of galloon tied at the nape. It embraced a variety of designs to suit different requirements. Some were made plain with a patent parting of silk or skin; others had net, gauze or human hair foundations, on which were sewn the wefts of waved or curled hair and fringe; while still others had long hair attached for combing in with the natural hair at the back. (*Creer*) See also semi-transformation, head-band, fillet or frontlet. 139, 206, 403, 407

BANDEAU A LA VIERGE A mid-Victorian bandeau, *qv* worn straight, parted in the centre and named after traditional paintings of the Virgin Mary.

BANDEAU D'AMOUR, LE A French high dressed hair style for women with frizzed toupee, high standing crochet curls and hanging curls, *c* 1780. 141

BANDEAU GRECQUE Long hair formed in waves and brought down flat upon the forehead, the ends of the short hair being allowed to go loose, imparting a lightness to the coiffure. The hair upon the temples is combed upwards and fixed to the tie of the back hair. (*Creer*) 142

BANDEAU RUSSE The hair is divided upon each side and rolled as shewn in figure, the flattened ends of the rolls resting upon the forehead. The temple hair should be puffed and combed away from the face. (*Creer*) 143

BANDEAU SLIP-ON A small postiche attached to an elastic band.

BANDELETTE (1) Little band, fillet. (*Creer*) 144–3
(2) Bandeau or front hair. (Coiffeur Européen)

BANDHOUSE CLIP A prison hairdo in which the whole head is shaven. American usage. (*Goldin*)

BANDOLINE A thick sticky hair dressing usually prepared from gum tragacanth, Iceland moss, linseed or quince seeds. A typical formula was: quince seeds 1 part, steeped in hot water 4 parts. Popular in the late Victorian period. (*Wooton*)

BANDROWSKY'S BASE A product resulting from the action of hydrogen peroxide on paraphenylenediamine.

BANG (1) Subs. 'hair cut bang off'. A horse tail cut horizontally across. American use 1880. Hence a bang was always a club-cut, never a taper cut, but today, by an extension of its original meaning it is used in American usage to denote all types of fringes. See Fringe.
(2) Verb To cut the front hair straight across the forehead. American usage. 1882 (*OED*)

BANG POMPADOUR A pompadour hair style with a fringe. American usage. (*AH*, 1915)

BANGING CHIGNON A wide flat loop of hair in a woman's hairdress, tied in the middle and hanging from the top of the head down to the nape of the neck. Late 18th century.

BARB, TO (verb) The verb to barb meaning to shave is rare. It was used in the 17th century and occurs in *Pepy's Diary* when on 27 November 1665, he wrote: 'To Sir G Smith's, it being now night, and there up to his chamber and sat talking and I barbing against to-morrow'. From the Latin *barba*: a beard.

BARBA Face hair.

BARBAROSSA Red Beard. Frederick I (1123–1190), King of Germany and of Holy Roman Empire (1152–1190).

BARBE (Fr) Beard.

BARBE DE CAPUCIN Chicory.

BARBED HAIR Bobbed hair. Slang, American usage. (*B and B*)

BARBED WIRE A tough beard. Slang. (*B and B*)

BARBEL A fresh water fish with filaments or feelers hanging from its mouth suggestive of a beard, hence its name, derived from latin *barba*, a beard.

BARBER (1) A person who shaves and trims hair and beards. For some thirty or so years the usual term for barber has been Gentlemen's Hairdresser. Derived from the Latin word *barba*: a beard. Barbers have practised their craft from the earliest recorded period. Ezekiel, verse 1, chapter 5, 'and thou, son of man, take thee a barber's razor and cause it to pass upon thy head and upon thy beard'. Randle Holme in 1688 gave a description of a barber at that time; 'A barber is always known by his checque parti-coloured apron; neither can he be termed a barber, or poler, or shaver till his apron is about him. His instrument case contains his looking-glass, a set of horn combs with teeth on one side and wide for the combing and readying of long, thick and strong heads of hair, a rasp to file the end of a tooth, etc,' In the 16th and 17th centuries, the barber in England was popularly regarded as somewhat of a foul knave. 'If thou art not an arrant stinking fellow then, but what do such people signifie but to maintain fools, whores, mercers, barbers and fiddlers.' (*Shadwell*, 1691). 'And cry up checkered-apron men: There is no trade but shaves, for, Barbers are trimme knaves.' 1592 (*Lyly*)
(2) A long faggot of wood. Origin from the barber's pole? Winchester College slang. 19th/20th century.
(3) Figuratively. A person who clips or cuts short anything.
(4) A storm accompanied by snow and spray which freezes on the face. Canadian usage.
(5) The water vapour that rises from water on a frosty day. Canadian usage.
(6) The name of the prevailing wind at Greymouth, New Zealand. (*Barr*)

BARBER CHIRURGEON A barber surgeon.

BARBER, DEMON See Sweeney Todd.

BARBERESS A woman barber. (*Cotgrave*)   176

BARBERING The work and art of a barber; shaving, haircutting, shampooing, and hairdressing. 'An important part of the barbering business.' (*Smiles, Self-Help*)

BARBERISH Of or appertaining to a barber. 'Barberish behaviour.'

BARBERLY In the manner of a barber.

BARBER MONGER (1) An Elizabethan term of reproachful contempt, conjectured by Dr Farmer to have been derived from the practice of stewards taking fees from barbers and other tradesmen for recommending them to the family the steward served. 'Draw you whoreson cullionly barber-monger, draw.' (*Shakespeare, King Lear*, ii, 2, 1605)
(2) A fop, 17/18th century. (*Partridge*)

BARBER MUSIC In the 16th century the barber shop not only offered barber service, dental treatment and minor surgery, but music as well. The Elizabethan dramatists allude to barber music. Dekker wrote, 'a barbers cittern for every serving man to play upon'; Ben Jonson refers to the virginal: 'I can compare him to nothing more happily than a barber's virginal; for every man may play upon him'. There are many other such references making it clear that the waiting clients had access to the musical instruments kept at the barbers for song and music. The most popular tune with the barbers at that time was a dance tune of that staid kind called 'pavan' and its nick-name was Gregory Walker for, as Morley in his *Introduction to Practical Musicke*, 1597, wrote 'it walketh among barbers more than any other'. As late as 1700 barber music was still very popular and intensively practised. In Browne's Amusements, Serious and Comical, 1700, we read 'the barber all the while keeping time on his cittern; for you know a cittern to a barber is as natural as milk to a calf, or bears to be attended by bagpipes'. By the 19th century the cittern had nearly died out but it lingered until later in America. Barber choirs and Barber quintets, etc, were a regular feature of some American barber shops in the 19th century.

BARBER OF LONDON Mr Tuffnell Trigge, a character in W H Ainsworth's, Revelations of London. (*Ainsworth's Magazine, 1844–5*)

BARBER OF SEVILLE, THE A comedy by Beaumarchais (1775); also two operas, one by Rossini (1816) and the other by Giovanni Paisiello (1776), both based on Beaumarchais's comedy.

BARBER POET Jacques Jasmin (1798–1864), last of the troubadours, a barber of Gascony, France.

BARBER'S APRON In the 19/20th century it was made from a plain or striped, dark coloured, shiny surfaced material to deflect hairs and had a commodious pocket in the middle front for the accommodation of the barber's tools. This most unhygienic garment is no longer seen in England, it having been superseded by white and grey tailored 'surgeon's' coats. The writer's grandfather's apron had a pocket 15" wide and 12" deep.   159

BARBER'S BASIN A shallow pewter, latten or pottery basin with a semi-circular cut-out in part of the flat rim, used in bleeding to catch the blood and for the soapsuds and whiskers in shaving. In the 16/17th century commonly of latten or pewter. 'With eyes as big as sawcers, nostrils wider then (*sic*) barbers basons.' (Randolph, *Muses Looking Glasse*, 1643)
'Barbers . . . throwing all their suddes out of their learned Latin★ Basons.' (*Dekker*)
★Latin – *Latten* a kind of brass, 'arrived at Vlacque before Remmakes (Holland) for account of the chamber of Zealand, which departed from Canton in China the 17 of December 1731 and brought cargo that included 50 ps Barber's basons, blue and white; 279 ps spilling pots, blue and white.' (*The Whitehall Evening Post* No. 2209, June 23–June 27, 1732)
In the 17th and 18th centuries the barbers' pottery basins

were extensively manufactured at Delft (Holland), Bristol and Lambeth (England). Other potteries also produced them. *86 (1–2), 177*

BARBER'S BIRDS In England and on the continent from at least as early as the 15th century until the early 20th century it was a common practice for barbers to keep cages of singing birds in their barber shops. Those most commonly kept included the linnet, goldfinch, chaffinch, blackbird, thrush, canary, magpie and, in London from the 18th century the Pekin Robin. The budgerigar did not become a fashionable pet until the 20th century. Until 1914, in Bristol, there were still more than thirty barbers, who regularly exhibited their song birds at local bird shows. *133*

BARBER'S BLEEDING BOWL See barber's basin.

BARBER'S BLOCK (1) A dummy head for displaying, dressing, or making wigs. See Malleable block, Wood block, Display block, etc.

113–118, 121, 182, 183, 185, 186, 187

(2) The head. 19th century slang. (*Partridge*)

(3) An overdressed man. 20th century slang. (*Partridge*)

BARBER'S BROTH Soap suds.

BARBER'S CAT A sickly-looking person. Slang. (*Partridge*)

BARBER'S CHAIR Usually a chair with arms and often an adjustable headrest for comfort during shaving. Since the late 19th century chairs of cast iron, comfortably upholstered and so constructed that they could be adjusted to a variety of positions for ease of operation became increasingly popular. These have been superseded since the 1930s by tubular chromium plated steel. *170*

BARBER'S CHAFER A deep, round, leaden or pewter or brass vessel, with a handle at the top. It held about a quart of boiling water and was carried by the flying barber, *qv*, on visits to his clients. The last mould in which they, chafers, were cast was sold at the sale of Richard Joseph's moulds for pewter utensils in January, 1815. It was of brass and was broken up for metal. (*Hone, EDB Vol 1*)

BARBER'S CHECK Brass tokens stamped with monetary denominations from 1^d to 2/6^d and on the reverse the chair number. They were used in Barber's shops as a check on the amount of money each assistant earned during the day. They are now replaced by paper slips. Both Osborne Garrett and Co, Frith Street, London, and R Hovenden and Sons, Berners Street, London, catalogued them before the First World War. (*Seaby, Coin Bulletin*, May 1968, p 176)

BARBER'S CHRISTMAS-BOX RHYME In the early 19th century and probably earlier, it was common practice at Christmas time for the apprentice to nail a box decorated with mistletoe and holly beneath the mirror in the barber shop. On this box was appended a doggerel verse such as: 'My Christmas-Box, kind gentlemen,
I hope you will remember,
And I will shave and lather well
Until the next December.'

(*Procter*)

BARBER'S CISTERN A pendant brass cistern with a tap to release water as it is needed during the hair washing process. 16th/late 18th century.

BARBER'S CITTERN The cittern hung in the barber's shop of the 15/16th century for the diversion of the customers. The cittern was a musical instrument rather like a guitar. It usually had a head grotesquely carved at the extremity of the neck and fingerboard.

'I have married his cittern that's common to all men.' (*Ben Jonson, Epicoene or the Silent Woman,* 1616)

Matheo, in *Dekker* and *Middleton's The Honest Whore* (1604) calls his wife 'a barber's citterne' for every serving man to play upon. See also Barber music.

BARBER'S CLERK An overdressed man. (*Partridge*)

BARBER'S COMPANY, THE See Barber surgeons.

BARBER'S DANCE A traditional European pantomimic dance performed in Austria, Bulgaria, Germany, Switzerland and Scandinavia, in which shaving, blood-letting, an operation and finally the revival of the customer were mimed. (*Henningsen*, p 136)

BARBER'S FLYING JACKASS The Opinicus, *qv*.

BARBER'S ITCH *Folliculitis barbae*, also *Tinea sycosis*. 'A chronic staphyloccocic inflammation of the upper third of the follicles of that part of the skin surface which produces long stiff hairs.' (*McCarthy*)

A disease affecting the face caused by a fungoid organism often resulting from the use of insanitary shaving materials.

BARBER'S KNIFE A razor.

BARBER'S KNOCK A double knock, the first hard and the second soft, as if by accident. (*F and H*)

BARBER'S KNOT A knot used for cawls of wigs. (*Hutton, Math. Dict*, 1795)

BARBER'S MASK A square of protective material worn over the nose and mouth by barbers to protect themselves against germs or bad breath from their clients. It also acts in reverse and protects the client from similar dangers which might emanate from the barber. 20th century.

BARBER'S POLE (1) When bleeding was a customary practice for most illnesses it was the barber who performed this minor operation during which the patient was required to grip a pole or staff which the barber kept for this purpose. After bleeding, the patient's arm was tied with a bandage. When the pole was not in use the bandages were secured to, and tied around it, and the pole was stood outside the barber's shop as a sign of the service offered within. Later, instead of displaying the actual pole used in the operation, a pole painted to imitate the original and the bandages thereon, was used and thus originated this characteristic sign. Lord Thurlow, in a speech in the House of Lords, 17 July, 1707, said that 'by statute still in force barbers and surgeons were each to use a pole (as a sign). The barbers were to have theirs blue and white, striped, with no other appendage; but the Surgeons' which was the same in other respects, was likewise to have a galley-pot, and a red rag, to denote the particular nature of their vocation'. (*Edwards*)

'. . . and Barbers hang out poles of a great huge length, almost as long as a missen-mast.' (*Sorbière*, 1698)

(2) A venomous snake of Honduras, Central America.

BARBER'S RASH See Barber's itch.

BARBER SHOP Common American usage for a hairdressing establishment which includes, at times, service for man and woman. In England the term is and was applied only to a man's hairdressing saloon and since *c* 1945 it has become increasingly prevalent and the earlier 'Gentlemen's Hairdressing Saloon' is not now in such general use. *472*

BARBER'S SHOP FORFEIT Formerly barber's shops were places of resort for idle persons, in addition to those who needed their service. In order to keep good order rules of conduct were displayed with penalties for non-compliance, these consisted of forfeitures such as paying for drinks. 'Laws for all faults, but laws as countenanc'd that the strong statutes stand like the forfeits in a barber's shop, as much in mock as mark.' (*Measure for Measure*, ii, 2)

BARBER SHOW A public and trade exhibition by manufacturers and wholesalers of hairdressing equipment and barber appliances and cosmetics, many of which are offered for sale; as well as competition in hairdressing as an added attraction. American usage.

BARBER'S SIGN (1) In England a standing pole decorated with two spiral lines of red and white. In France it is three basins, with a kind of circular notch for convenience of holding it under the chin for soaping. (*Holloway*) See Barber's pole.

(2) A barber's sign in the 18th century was a standing pole and two washballs. (*Grose*)

(3) The virile member. Slang derived from (2) above, 18th century.

BARBER'S STONE Pumice stone anciently used as a depilatory. (*Forbes*)

BARBER'S TWEESE A barber's case of instruments, 17th century. (*Robertson*)

BARBER SURGEON In medieval times the barber also acted as a minor surgeon and tooth-drawer. The Barber-Surgeon's Company was founded in 1461 and was re-incorporated in 1540. In 1745 it was decided that the trades of barber and surgeon should be independent of each other and the two branches were separated, but the ancient company or guild, was allowed to retain its charter and its hall still stands in Monkwell Street, Cripplegate. The last operative barber-surgeon in London was one Middleditch of Great Suffolk Street who died in 1821. (*Lambert*)

BARBER-SURGEONS ARMS The arms of the Barber-Surgeons of London are blazoned as follows: Quarterly first and fourth sable, a chevron between three fleames argent, second and third, per pale argent and vert, a spatula in pale azure surmounted of a rose gules charged with another of the first; the first rose regally crowned proper between the four quarters of a cross of St George gules charged with a lion passant guardant or. *Crest:* An opinicus with wings indorsed or and the supporters two lynxes.   *145*

BARBET (1) A small beard.

(2) A family of birds with tufts of beard-like bristles at the base of the bill.

(3) A poodle.

BARBETTE A small beard.

BARBICHE A small tuft of hair on the under-lip. 19th century. (*The Globe* newspaper, 23 May, 1892). Similar to Barbula, *qv*.

BARBIGEROUS Bearded. Usually used botanically to describe petals covered with hairs.

BARBING Trimming. 17th century. (*Robertson*)

BARBING CLOTH A gown to cover and protect the client whilst receiving attention to the hair. 17th century. (*Miege*)

BARBON A grey beard.

BARBOURE A barber. (*Levens*, 1570)

BARBULA A small beard, 17th century. (From Latin *barba*: beard) 'Barbula or pick-a-divant, or the little tuft of hair just under the middle of the lower lip.' (*Holme*) Similar to Barbiche, *qv*   *100(20)*

BAREFOOTED HEAD A bald head. Slang. American usage. (*B and B*)

BARKIT Dirt hardened on hair and hence forming a kind of bark. 18th century slang. (*Grose*, Prov. Glos)

BARLEY-SUGAR CURL Long drop curls worn by children in the 19th century.   *325*

BARNET HAIR Also Barnet Fair, *qv*. Rhyming slang. (*Partridge*)

BARNET FAIR 19th century thieves' rhyming slang for 'hair'. (*Vulg Tong*)

BAROQUE STYLE A 16/18th century art style of the Counter Reformation, which was a reaction from Renaissance classicism, characterised by a grotesque use of ornament and a theatrical expression in painting, sculpture and architecture, etc (including hairstyles). Michelangelo (1475–1564) is regarded as the father of the Baroque style.

BAROQUE COIFFURE A hairdress in the Baroque style, *qv*.   *190*

BARREL See Iron-barrel.

BARRELLING Overlapping hair on a curler in such a way that the wound curler is shaped like a barrel, ie tapering at both ends, with a bulge in the middle.

BARREL CURL Barrel-spring curl, *qv* and buffer curl.

BARREL CURLER A curler of large diameter ¾" to 2". Also caller roller.

BARREL-SPRING CURL A point wound, open-centre curl with all circinations of approximately equal diameter, *cf* clock-spring curl.   *198*

BARRETTE (1) A small bar-shaped hair slide.

(2) A metal pin approximately 3" long with a beaded head and guard cap, used to secure the hair. Mid-19th century. Specimen in Citadel Museum, Halifax, Nova Scotia.

(3) A decorated metal hair grip, similar to a kirbigrip, *qv*.

(4) A small flat cap (12th-14th century) worn by both sexes.   *103i*

BARRIER CREAM A cream used to protect the face, neck, forehead, etc, by acting as a barrier against hair dyes and permanent waving lotion.

BARRISTER'S WIG Wig customarily worn by barristers in the Law Courts. Mainly constructed of horsehair. First worn in the 17th century at the time of the Restoration as a French novelty. This wig is composed of a frizzy crown with 3 rows of 7 curls, then 1 row of 4 curls, 1 perpendicular curl, row of 2 curls and 2 tails with a baby curl near the end of each. It is worn in hair from the horse's mane only, tail hair being too coarse. This wig is worn by all barristers who plead. (*Pall Mall*)   *207*

BAR-SLIDE A hair slide in the form of a bar.

BASE (1) The foundation of a haircut or hair style. (*Trusty*, 136)

(2) The foundation of a wig or similar type of postiche. See Wig foundation. American usage. (*N and N*)

(3) The bulk ingredient of a cosmetic.

(4) A term including but wider than alkali.

BASIC CUT The removal of the unwanted head hair leaving only hair that in length and thickness is necessary for the projected style. The art of cutting does not lie in the removal of hair, but in the choice of hair that is to be left on the head and its disposition after cutting.

BASIN A large pottery, porcelain, earthenware, marble or stainless steel bowl with an outlet for water at the bottom, over which heads of hair are shampooed.

BASIN CUT Name applied to a haircut performed by placing a round bowl on the head and cutting off the hair to the edge of the bowl. Used in all ages by the unskilled public on their families when short hair styles were worn. Commonly employed as late as 1928 when the method was used on children's and women's hair at Ilchester, Somerset and seen in use in 1965 ·at Whitechurch Canonicorum, Dorset.

BASKET BRAID Composed of four small strands of hair, of which three are plaited and woven over and under the fourth, which is kept straight and serves to draw the chain up. (*Godey*)

BASKET HILT A 16th century rough beard style.

BASKET PLAIT See Basket braid.

BASKET-PLAIT CHIGNON A ready-made chignon of plaited hair, coiled and secured in the shape of a shallow, round basket. Fashionable in the 1880s.

BASKET-PLAIT HEADDRESS A coiffure prominently incorporating a basket plait.

BASKET WEAVE PLAIT See Basket braid.

BASTING STITCH A large loose stitch used in alterations to wigs.

BATCH Group of persons who go to their meal at the same time. Bristol usage, late 19th/early 20th century. A word commonly used in hairdressing salons when the shop did not close for lunch and the assistants had their meals in two groups, one after the other. 'I am going to dinner with the second batch today.'

BATHROOM HAIRDRESSER See Back-room hairdresser.

BATON FIXATEUR A bandoline of hard pomatum containing wax used to stick down smoothly little unwanted feathers of hair. 18th/19th century. (*Piesse*)

BAUME CIRCASSIENNE See Plumbiferous hair water.

BAWN White, fair. Generally applied to hair. Gaelic origin. (*Macneill*)

BAYONET HAIR A hair with part of its shaft near the hair's point bayonet shaped; said to occur in the initial stages of baldness. (*Savill, p 22*)

BAY RUM A hair wash and hair dressing believed to stimulate hair growth. Typical formula: Tincture of bay leaves 5 oz, otto of bay 1 drachm, bicarbonate of ammonia 1 oz, biborate of soda (borax) 1 oz, rosewater 1 quart; mix and filter. First introduced in New York early in the 19th century. The plant then used was the Indian bayberry, *Pimenta Acris*. Its fame and supposed efficiency rapidly spread through Europe. (*Piesse*)
Genuine Bay Rum was imported from the West Indies where a crude kind of alcohol, obtained in connection with the manufacture of rum from molasses was distilled with the fresh leaves of the bay tree – *Laycria acris*. (*Askinson*)

BAY TREE LEAF Once used by barbers in their washbasins, probably as a phrophylactic, 16th/18th century. 'The bay tree leafe which they (barbers) put in their basons.' (*Clerk, 1602*)
An infusion of bay leaves in hot water was used for hair treatments in the 19th century and probably earlier also.

BEADED HAIR See Monilethrix.

BEARD (1) The hair growing on the chin and adjacent parts of the face of a man; exceptionally and distressingly on a woman's face. Ancient writers have written honourably of the fine beards of antiquity. Homer praised the white beards of Nestor and King Priam. Until modern times the Chinese considered a long beard an inestimable adornment. The Turks thought it more infamous to have the beard removed than to be publicly whipped. A beard is a symbol of wisdom. (*Willick*, also *Creer*)
Beards were worn by the ancient Assyrians but not by the ancient Egyptians; worn by the Jews from at least 1490 BC. 'Ye shall not round the corners of your heads, neither shalt thou mar the corners of thy beard.'
The ancient Persians wore beards and the Tartars waged a long war upon them, declaring them infidels because they would not cut their beards after the custom of Tartary. The Greeks wore the beard until 330 BC when Alexander the Great (356–323 BC) ordered the Macedonians to shave in order to deprive their enemies of a convenient handle to facilitate their decapitation in battle. Scipio Africanus was the first Roman to shave daily. Under Hadrian the beard was allowed to grow and the practice remained fashionable until the time of Constantine the Great. Beards were worn by the Romans from about 390 BC. In AD 361 the Emperor Julian (*c* AD 331–363) wrote a diatribe called *Misopogon* against the wearing of beards. Beards were worn by the Saxons in England but from the Norman Conquest (1066) the Normans introduced short hair styles and beardless faces, which styles remained fashionable until the 13th

century when beards again became fashionable, and were worn until Charles II's reign when they again went out. At Lincoln's Inn in the reign of Elizabeth I the growth of beards was regulated by statute. In the first year of her reign (1558) it was ordered that no fellow of that house should wear a beard above a fortnight's growth, upon penalty of fine, loss of commons and finally expulsion; but by November of the following year all previous orders touching beards were repealed. In France the custom of shaving arose in the time of Louis XIII, who was young and beardless when he came to the throne. Beard dyeing was a common practice in the 16th/17th century for fashion and to disguise age – 'Now for a wager. What colour'd beard comes next by the window?'
Adr. A black man's, I think.
Taff. I think not so,
I think a red for that is most in fashion.' (*Barry*, 1611) '. . . and dyes his beard that did his age bewray.' (*sic*). (*Hall*)
In the 17th century so much care was taken with the beard that some were covered at night with pasteboard cases lest they should rumple during the wearer's sleep. (*Hudibras, Gray's ed, Notes*). From 1851 the custom of wearing beards became widespread but the advent of the safety razor and the influence of the World War were powerful factors, combined with the advertising of safety razor blades, manufacturers produced an almost complete return to a clean shaven look. After the Second World War a significant increase in beard wearing has taken place. There are early references to beards where it is clear that only the growth on the upper lip (or moustache, as we should say) is indicated.
(Significance in dreams) That one has a great beard, in a young man, signifies wisdom; in an old man, length of years; but in a woman, that she shall be a furious vixen and a scold, and wear the breeches. (*Little Gipsy Girl, 1799*)
The longest beard of a man recorded was 11' 11.7" on the face of Jules Dumont (b1856), a Frenchman.
The beard of a bearded woman, Janice Deveree (b 1842) of Kentucky, USA, was 14" in 1884. (*McWhirter*)
75, 97 (A–L), 98 (A–L), 99(1–19), 100(20–38), 102 (Gi), 103 (G.H.), 188, 189, 193, 196, 213, 469
(2) An adult man. 'Boyes and Beardes with dishes and platters'. (*Dekker, The Meeting of Gallants, 1604*)
(3) An egghead or intellectual person. Slang *c* 1958.
(4) Beard has also been a common English surname from at least as early as 13th century.
(5) An indistinct talker. American radio slang. (*B and B*)
(6) A verbal blunder on the radio. American radio slang. (*B and B*)
(7) A film extra with a natural beard. (*B and B*)
(8) A woman's pubic hair.

BEARD BAG A bag worn over the beard at night for protection. 16th/18th century. (*Dulaure*).See also Beard case.

BEARD BASIN A flat basin of earthenware, pewter, faience or silver, with a hollow for the chin, used during shaving to hold the whisker-impregnated lather. See also Barber's basin. 16th/18th century.

BEARD BRUSH In the 16th/17th century it was customary to carry a brush for the arrangement of the beard hairs when disordered. 'His beard-brush ever in his hand, for if he vouchesafe you a word in complement he straight doth turne his head and under colour of spitting, brushes his beard into order again.' (*The Wizard*, a play of 1640. So recorded by Nares but I have not identified this play. JSC)
'I like this beard-brush, but that the haire is too stiff.' (*Dekker, 1631*)

BEARD CASE A case or cover made of pasteboard used to put over the beard at night to protect it from rumpling and preserve its form. 17th/18th century. (*Repton*)

BEARD CLIPPER (1) A barber. 15th century. Facetious usage. (*Durfey*)

(2) A small clipper with finger and thumb grips similar to those of scissors. (O G *Cat.* 1901)

BEARD COMB A small comb for the beard, often carried on the person. Early 17th century. See also Beard brush. (*Heywood; Holme*)

BEARDED, THE (1) Socrates (*c* 468–399 BC)

(2) Constantine IV (d 685)

(3) Geoffrey of Boulogne (1061–1100)

(4) George, Duke of Saxony (1471–1539)

(5) Bouchard of the House of Montmorency.

(6) George Killingworth at the court of Ivan The Terrible of Russia whose beard, recorded Hakluyt (*Voyages 1599–1600*), was 5′ 2″ long, yellow, thick and broad.

BEARDED APHRODITE, THE A bearded goddess of Cyprus. (*Larousse*)

BEARDED CHILD A correspondent of *Notes and Queries*, June 1860, records the case of a boy of about three years of age with a little beard growing under his chin.

BEARDED, DEITY, THE Bacchus, the God of Wine. (*Strabo*)

BEARDED KING, THE Baldwin IV, Earl of Flanders; also called Handsome Beard (1160–1186). (*Brewer*)

BEARDED LADY, THE A searchlight having diffused beams. Slang, 1939. (*Partridge*)

BEARDED MARY A girl, seen by Montaigne on his journey to Italy, who up to the age of 22 was thought to be a girl, but turned out to be a boy. (*Diary of Montaigne's Journey to Italy* in 1580 and 1581)

BEARDED MASTER, THE Socrates was called this by Persius, the Roman poet (BC 468–399).

BEARDEDNESS A bearded condition.

BEARDED ONES The Spaniards thus called by the Incas of Peru.

BEARDED VIRGIN Antonia Helena. (*Bulwer*)

BEARDED WOMAN, THE Josephine Clotullia, exhibited in New York, 1853. (*Wells*)

BEARDED WOMAN OF DRESDEN In 1732 there lived at Dresden a bearded virgin. Her beard grew from each side of her chin, was three inches long, and of snowy whiteness. She cut it at first every month, then every fortnight, afterwards twice in the week. On her lip was a moustache of short black hair. (*Home Companion*, 1853)

BEARDED WOMEN St Vuilgefortis or Wilgefortis. Her day in the calendar is 20th July (*Southey*); St Paula, a Spanish Saint; Bartel Graetje of Stuttgart, b 1562; Mlle Bois de Chêne, b Geneva 1834; Julia Pastrana, a Mexican, d 1862 (*Brewer, PF*); Ursula Dyan 1668 (*Pepys*); Augustina Barbara, 17th century. (*Reynolds*); Antonia Helena, b in archbishopric of Liege (*Bulwer*); Margaret, Governess of the Netherlands, had a long, stiff beard; Phoetusa, wife of Pythias of Abdera; Hamysia, wife of Gorgippus of Thasos (*Hippocrates*); see also *Hoyerus, Laurence, Joch* and *Procter*.

BEARDIE (1) A man with a beard or long hair. Australian slang, 20th century. (*Partridge*)

(2) An Australian nickname for the Christian Israelites, followers of John Wroe.

(3) American nickname for a Jewish convert to christianity. 19th century. (*Franklyn*)

BEARD JAMMER A whoremonger. American slang. (*B and B*)

BEARD LICENCE A copper disc carried by a beard wearer in Russia to show that he had paid the beard tax imposed by Peter the Great in 1698. (*Corson*)

BEARD OF THE PROPHET The prophet Mahomet, whose beard was hennaed a red colour, and by whose beard millions swore their oaths, required his followers to wear beards in order to distinguish them form the shaven idolaters.

BEARD PRESS A wooden apparatus to press the beard during sleep. 16th/17th century. 'Anights he puts it in a presse, made of two thin trenchers . . . that it may come forth the next morning with even corners, narrow above, and broad beneath.' (*Bulwer*)

BEARD PRODUCER A preparation to encourage the growth of the beard, *cf* Hair restorer. Many beard producers were manufactured and sold in the 19th century, most of them completely useless.

BEARDS Sepals of apple blossoms. Devon usage. ((*Gregory*))

BEARD STYLES See under their distinctive names.

BEARD TAX Under Czar Peter the Great the Russians had to pay 100 roubles for the privilege of wearing a beard, or lose their heads.

BEARD TREE (*Corylus Arellana*). The fiberd tree. (*B and H*)

BEARD WAX A scented pomade for dressing the beard.

BEARD WITH A HAIR CUT A vandyke beard. Slang American usage, 20th century. (*B and B*)

BEAR'S GREASE (1) This unguent or dressing for the hair and head had a long period of popularity. As early as 1562 William Bulleyn, in his *Booke of Simples* wrote: 'The beare is a beaste whose flesh is good for mankynd; his fat is good, with laudanum, to make an ointment to heale balde-headed men to receive the hayre agayne'. Its use continued as a dressing for the hair until the late 19th century. Two varieties were used; one of the consistence of thick olive oil, which was obtained by boiling the fat about the caul and intestines of the animal, the other was much harder and in appearance resembled hard honey and was obtained from about the kidneys. Both sorts before perfuming, had a rank, rancid smell. In the 19th century rancid lard was sold for bears grease. (*Francis*) 'Lewis Hendrie, Comb-Maker in Ordinary to their Majesties . . . of Shug Lane, Golden Square . . . has just had a very large Fat Bear killed, and such as please to have any of the grease will either call or send their servants to see it cutt off the animal.' (*The Morning Herald*, 13 Dec 1787). 'Bears grease' was concocted without the genuine grease of the bear. A popular 19th century formula was:

Huile de Rose	
Huile de Fleur d'orange	
Huile de Acacia	of each ½ lb
Huile de Tubereus and	
Huile de Jasmin	
Almond oil	10 lb
Lard	12 lb
Acacia pomade	2 lb
Otto of bergamot	4 oz
Otto of cloves	2 oz

Melt the solid greases and oils together by a water-bath then add the ottos. (*Piesse*)   *243, 244*

(2) Mud peat. Lincolnshire usage. From its similarity in appearance to the hair pomade. (*Arkell*)

BEATLE BOB Bobbed hair style with a long, heavy fringe, named after The Beatles (see Beatle cut).

BEATLE CUT Hair style for men in which the hair is worn long and combed over the forehead. So named from a 'Pop' singing quartette whose hair is cut in this manner. They originated in the Liverpool area and the name Beatle is derived from an amalgamation of Beat and Bootle, giving Beatle, 1963.

BEATNIK STYLE Long hair without artificial curl or wave, worn by young people of both sexes, the hair often being in a dirty, unkempt or tousled condition, but not necessarily so. Beatniks can be sub-divided into several categories, two of which are the clean and the unclean.

BEATRICE CHIGNON A solid dressed chignon composed of a long coiled plait. (*Creer*) 227

BEATRICE D'EST COIFFURE A 15th century hairdress in the style of that worn by Beatrice d'Esté, the duchess of Ferrare. Its feature was the long fouriaux coiffure.

BEAU A dandy; a handsome man.

BEAU CATCHER A curl. American slang. (*B and B*)

BEAUMONT See A la Beaumont.

BEAU PERUKE 18th century wig style.

BEAUTICIAN A practitioner of beauty culture, *qv*.

BEAUTISTRY Beauty culture. The science and art of making beautiful. American usage.

BEAUTY BOXES Small and medium sized boxes of silver, horn, leather or other suitable material, carried by ladies of the past and of the present, in which are stored the aids to beauty of a woman including powder, lipstick, rouge, nail file, scissors, curlers, combs and many other accessories of a similar nature.

BEAUTY CAP See Sleeping net.

BEAUTY CULTURE The culture of beauty by treatment designed to improve the hair, face and nails of the hands. See also Cosmetology.

BEAUTY PARLOR See Beauty parlour.

BEAUTY PARLOUR A saloon, room or other place where the culture of feminine beauty is professionally practised, including hairdressing and make-up of the face. American spelling Parlor.

BEAUTY SHOP See Beauty parlour.

BEAUTY SHOPPE See Beauty shop. The spelling shoppe and sometimes shoppee is a gimmick derived from an imaginary archaic spelling of the word shop. American usage.

BEAUTY TREATMENT Any treatment designed to improve the beauty of a woman, although in recent years facilities for males have also been provided by a few enterprising hair and beauty establishments.

BEAUTYRAMA Extravaganza of beauty. A beauty shop. American usage.

BEAVER (1) A film extra with a natural beard. American slang (*B and B*) By extension any man with a beard, and the beard itself.
(2) A false beard. American slang. (*B and B*))
(3) A bearded man, and hence an unmannerly street-call of 'beaver' by young urchins directed against bearded men, *c* 1922. This name beaver had been applied to a bearded man since before 1910. (*Richardson*)
(4) A game in which points were scored by spotting beards and shouting 'beaver'. Popularized by P B Wyndham Lewis in his Beachcomber column in the Daily Express *c* 1921. An ordinary beaver scored 10, a King beaver (*Bushy*) 50, etc.

BEAVER'S TAIL A banging chignon, *qv*, 1865. (*Leech, J, Pictures of Life and Character*, 4th series, 1865)

BEBE SCALPETTE A small scalpette.

BECHONNER To curl the hair (Fr) (*Creer*)

BEDFORD CROP Unpowdered short-hair style popularized by the Duke of Bedford and some of his associates in 1795 to avoid the hair-powder tax, *qv*. See also Crop cut. (*The Times*, 14 April 1795)

BEDFORD CURL See Bedford crop.

BEDFORD LEVEL The same as Bedford Crop, *qv*. See also Crop cut.

BEEHIVE A high beehive-shaped coiffure for women. Dressed by vigorous back-combing and held in position by a liberal application of lacquer, also dressed over a wire or plastic frame. Popular 1959–1963. 273

BEEHIVE HAIRDRESS See Beehive.

BEEHIVE-TOPPED HEADDRESS See Beehive.

BEESWAX A substance obtained from the honeycomb of the bee. Soluble in benzene, carbon disulphide, chloroform and ether. Used in hair creams and hair dressings.

BEETLE BROWS Prominent or shaggy eyebrows. (*Brewer*)
Petulas: What is she beetle browed?
Licio: Thou has a beetle head, I say the brow of a beetle, a little flie, whose brow is as blacke as velvet. (*Lyly*, 1592) 102D

BELD Bald, without hair. Scottish word. (*Henderson*)

BELGIAN HONE Imported from Belgium: a deposit of silt solidified on natural slate, yellow in colour and a very fine surface when cut and polished. Cut to size with slate as base. Where the deposit was thick, the stone was cut to size and cemented on slate. Highly sought for quality by barbers for setting razors. Classified in three qualities:- fast cutting, medium and slow; the fast for getting good edge, slow or fine for finishing the edge for a smooth edge. The lubricant commonly used was Neats-Foot oil, soap lather and 'spit'.

BELGRAVE A beard style of the early 20th century. 469

BELLARMINE BEARD A medium length, square-cut beard with flowing moustache, similar to that worn by Cardinal Bellarmine (1542–1621) and named after him. 16/17th century. See also Greybeard jug.

BELLE A reigning female beauty.

BELLE FERRONNIERE, LA A woman's hair style of the 15th century as depicted in the portrait La Belle Ferronnière by Leonardo da Vinci in which the subject is wearing round her forehead a ferronnière (a chain secured by a single jewel). Leonardo's portrait was not La Belle Ferronnière who was a favourite of François 1er (1494–1547)346

BELLE POULE See A la Belle Poule.

BELL ROPE A hanging curl. American slang. (*B and B*)

BELL WEFT See fly weft, so called from its similarity to the shape of a bell when the woven hair is seen from the end of the weft. (*Symonds*)

BELLY BRUSH The hair on a man's belly. Air Force slang. (*Symonds*)

BELLY MAT The hair on a man's belly. Air Force slang. (*Symonds*)

BELLY THATCH The hair on a man's belly. Air Force slang. (*Symonds*)

BELT-STROP A 3″ wide length of leather on which razors were stropped. There was a metal ring at one end to secure the strop to a fixing point and a leather handle at the other end which was held in the left hand. The strop was held taut, and the right hand held and stropped the razor.

BELZONI, GIOVANNI BATTISTA (1788–1823) Egyptologist, worked as a lather boy in his father's shop at Padua.

BENCH The worktable, also called the board; hence board-work for the manufacture of artificial heads of hair. 86

BENCH-BOTTLE An undecorated, large bottle for use by barbers in the saloon. American usage. (*Smith*)

BENJAMIN WATER Benzoin water.

BENT COMB A comb of horn or shell shaped to fit the contour of the head. 18th century. (*Earle*)

BENZENE Benzol C_6H_6, a clear, colourless, highly flammable liquid. Poisonous. Used in dyes, lacquers and as a solvent for waxes, resins, oils, etc.

BENZINE Petroleum Benzine; Petroleum Ether. A clear, colourless, volatile, highly flammable liquid, used as a solvent for oils, fats and waxes in perfumery and cosmetic industries.

BENZINE SHAMPOO A shampoo that was popular in the 1920s, but is dangerous and its use has been discontinued. It consisted of pouring benzine over the hair and squeezing.

BENZOIN Gum Benzoin or Benjamin. A balsamic resin from styrax benzoin used in hair lacquers and hair lotions.

BEPERIWIGGED Wearing a wig. (*Tuke*, 1616)

BERD A beard. (*Levens*, 1570)

BERENICE'S HAIR The constellation Coma Berenices.

BERGAMOT HAIR POWDER A starch hair powder perfumed with bergamot. 18/19th century. (*Lillie*)

BERGAMOT OIL A volatile oil expressed from the rind of fresh fruit of citrus aurantium, used in perfumery for hair oils and pomades. (*Merck*)

BERGER A plain, small lock, à la shepherdesse; turned up with a puff, 1690. (*Evelyn*)

BERGMANN'S BEARD-PRODUCING TINCTURE A 19/20th century 'secret' preparation consisting of an alcoholic extract of tree bark, scented with a little oil of rosemary and thyme. (*Koller*)

BERGMANN'S ICE POMADE A 19/20th century 'secret' preparation for curling hair. It was ordinary pomade, *qv*. (*Koller*)

BERTHA FRIZETTE Stems made with straight hair of medium thickness, about 17″ long and used with the Berthe or Bertha headdress from 1866. See also Frizette. (*Creer*)

BERTHE COIFFURE A woman's hair style of 1866. (*Bysterveld*, p 79)   323

BERTHE PLAIT Consists of three plicatura stems secured to a comb, the stems being covered with 2 oz or more, as required, of 20″ hair.

BERZELIUS'S HAIR DYE A 19th century preparation consisting of: nitrate of silver 1 oz, slaked lime 2 oz, and a little oil or pomade to prevent blackening of the skin. (*Dussauce*)

BESOME-BEARD A coarse, ragged beard. From 17th century. 'A dapper Spaniard with a kind of besome beard, and a voice not unlike the yapping of a frysting cur.' (*Querodo*, 1667)

BESSARION'S BEARD Bessarion, a convert from the Eastern Church to the Western Church in the 15th century, insisted upon retaining his fine oriental beard when he became a Cardinal. (*Reynolds*)

BEST WIGGED PRINCE IN CHRISTENDOM The guardian, uncle-in-law and first cousin of the Duke of Brunswick, who was given this name. (*Brewer*)

BETA KERATIN The stretched form of the protein of human hair. See also Alpha keratin. (*Savill*)

BEVEL CUT See Bevelled cut.

BEVEL CUTTING The same as graduation cutting, *qv*.

BEVELLED CUT (Bevel cut) Hair cut so that the cut ends lie in a bevelled plane. The graduated neck-line of a man's short hair style is bevelled.

BEVER BRUSH See Brush.

BEWIGGED Wearing a wig.

BIAS BANG (1) A bang or fringe with one side longer than the other.
(2) A bang or fringe of variable length.

BIAS BOB A bob with variable lengths of hair; for instance longer at the back than at the sides. See also Bias bang.

BIAS CUT The cutting of hair asymmetrically. (*WO*, 10.10.64)

BIAS SHAPING Shaping for an asymmetrical style. (*Reno*)

BIBLICAL WAVE A long, waved hair style for men. American usage. 1964.

BICHLORIDE OF MERCURY Is used at 0.1% as a germicide. Poisonous and an irritant.

BIEDERMEIER COIFFURE A woman's hair style with clusters of curls, circa 1830. The term Biedermeier was applied to many other objects that caught the popular fancy, such as clothing, hats, etc. (*Wall*)

BIFID Divided by a cleft.

BIG COMB See Rake.

BIGODE See Bigoudi, which is the preferred spelling.

BIGOTE A moustache. Early 17th century. (From Spanish)

BIGOTELLE (Fr) A leather case to protect the dressed moustache during the night. (*Dictionnaire de l'Academie*)

BIGOUDI (1) a baked clay, wooden or, rarely, a glass curler upon which straight hair is wound and then boiled to produce frisure forcée for wig-making. The diameter of the curler is greater at the ends than at the centre to compensate for the greater thickness at the centre when wound, due to the use of tapered hair. Bigoudis of bamboo, mahogany, boxwood, clay pipe stems, baked clay, and glass were in the collection of croquignole curlers used by John Stevens of Bristol in the 1860s. The glass bigoudis were used for curling white hair to prevent discolouration. See also Bilboquet and roulette.   88 (4.5.6), 241
(2) A wooden curling stick tapered at both ends.   231

BIG WHISKER, THE A beard. American usage.

BIGWIG A magnate or person of importance. From the large wigs worn in the 17th and 18th century by men of fashion and importance. Also used as a term of derision for an officious person.

BIKINI COMB A tail comb with ½″ long teeth used for back-combing the hair. 20th century.

BILBOQUET A hair curler of pipe clay used to prepare curled hair for wigs. See also roulette and bigoudi. 17th/18th century. (*Fairholt*)   88 (4.5.6)

BILLIARD BALL A bald head. Slang.

BILLIES Full medium length chin whiskers.

BILLY GOATEE A goatee beard. Slang. (*B and B*)

BILLY WHISKERS See Billies.

BINARY Made of two parts.

BIND (1) See Bind ribbon.
(2) Subs. The outer edge of a wig or transformation.
(3) Verb. To tie, fasten or attach; to wreathe the head with.
(4) See Binder (1).

BINDER (1) A cord, tape, rubber band or other suitable material for securing a tress or strand of hair.   299
(2) A substance that has the power of causing the hair to retain its set position. An agglutinant, *qv*.

BINDING The galloon or ribbon to which the wig net is sewn and which gives the wig its shape.

BIND RIBBON (1) the ribbon that encircles the circumference of the head in the wig foundation and except at four points (above each ear, and above both sides of the forehead, where it is contiguous) is within the contour or outer-edge ribbon. This is the ribbon that 'binds' the wig to the head. Also called: circumference band, circumference bind, the bind, bind galloon, circumference galloon, circumference ribbon and galloon bind.
(2) The ribbon forming the outer edge of a wig or transformation is sometimes, but incorrectly, called the bind ribbon.

BIND-SPRING The tension spring in the neck of a wig or transformation. In a semi-transformation the tension-spring is within the short ribbon.

BINET Hairdresser of Louis XIV of France.

BINETTE A small, circular receptacle of plastic or metal for waste hair and other saloon debris.

BINGLE A short hair style for women, *c* 1929. It followed the shingle and was a little longer.

BIRD'S NEST (1) A pompous, overdressed hairdo; a full, heavy coiffure. Slang.

(2) A hairdress consisting of a long, uncombed, untidy, bedraggled mat of hair, often in an insalubrious condition, worn by beatniks, both male and female. From c 1960.

BISCUIT A flat, circular dressing of a coiled strand of hair. When dressed over the ears also called an earphone, qv.

BISHOP'S WIG A physical bob worn by bishops of the English Church. The foretop was sometimes dressed 2″ or 3″ high. Wigs were worn by Bishops in the House of Lords until 1830, when Blomfield, Bishop of London, obtained the permission of William IV for the episcopal bench to discontinue the practice. Archbishop Summer appears wigged in the picture in Windsor Castle by John Phillip of the marriage of the Princess Royal in 1858. At the age of 71 he officiated at the Great Exhibition in his wig. (*Illus Lon News*) 256

BISMUTH Used to whiten yellowed white hair.

BIZARRE Odd, fantastic. (*Creer*)

BLACKBEARD THE PIRATE Thatch a 17th century pirate. (*Johnston, Lives of the Pirates*)

BLACK HAIR In the classical theatre of Greece and Rome it symbolized the tyrant. (*Haigh*)

BLACK HAIR DYE An early 19th century recipe to turn hair black: 1 lb bruised gall nuts, boil in olive oil till soft, dry, reduce to a fine powder, mix with equal parts willow charcoal and common salt. Add small quantity of lemon and orange peel dried and reduce to powder. Boil in 12 pounds of water until the sediment is the consistency of black salve. (*Toilette*, 1832)

BLACK HAIR-POWDER An 18th/19th century recipe: 4 lb fine starch powder made into paste with 1 pint blackest Japan ink. Dry, grind and sift. Mix this with Japan ink three times, drying as before, then add 1 lb ivory black. (*Lillie*)

BLACK-LEAD COMB See Lead comb.

BLACK MIRROR A black convex glass which has the power of reflecting a scene in miniature, but with little detail or colour. 17th to 18th century.

BLACK PERSIAN HENNA A mixture of Indigo and Persian Henna producing dark brown hues.

BLACK POMATUM Made from pomatum (common), qv, with the addition of yellow wax melted together with ivory black. (*Lillie*)

BLACK RIDING WIG An 18th century wig, fashionable in Queen Anne's reign.

BLACK SCRATCH A man's wig style of the 18th century. See Scratch wig.

BLACK SCURF See Seborrhoea nigricans. (*Wheeler*)

BLACK SOAP Made from Castile soap and ivory black. 18/19th century cure for crab lice. (*Lillie*)

BLACK WIG Traditionally worn on the stage by actors taking the part of a murderer or equally villainous character. (*Stewart*)

BLADED COMB A comb with a cutting blade attached. When the comb is drawn through the hair it is cut by the blade.

BLANC French word for white.

BLANC CHIMIQUE (Chemical white) Chemically bleached white hair.

BLANCH Make white by removing colour cf Bleach. 'She has now had her blond hair blanched.'

BLANCHING Bleaching. A word used in the 19th century when preparing hair for wigmaking.

BLANKET STITCH See Stitching.

BLAZE, BISHOP See Woollen wig.

BLEACH (1) Verb: to lighten or decolour.

(2) A substance that will lighten the colour of another substance. By the 19th century chlorine, sulphurous acid, bisulphide of magnesia, lime and hydrogen peroxide had all been used to bleach hair. Hydrogen peroxide is now the only one of these chemicals that is still widely used. Peroxide.

BLEACH BATH A preparation of liquid bleach in which hair is immersed to bleach or lighten it.

BLEACH PACK Bleach mixed with a powder carrier to prevent running.

BLEACH RINSE A hair rinse containing bleach; see also Colour rinse and Henna rinse.

BLEACH SHAMPOO A soap shampoo in which is incorporated hydrogen peroxide to the required strength and a few drops of ammonium hydroxide.

BLEACHING The process of lightening hair on or off the head by means of exposure to sunlight or suitable chemicals. From the 17th to 19th centuries the following methods were used:

(1) Firstly the hair way washed in strong, warm pearlash water to deprive it of all grease. It was then spread upon the grass in the open for several days to expose it to dew and sun. This natural bleaching was certainly the earliest method used and hair treated in this way was called field hair.

(2) The hair was soaked in pearlash water and then in a solution of bleaching liquid, either chloride of lime or chloride of potassium.

(3) After a partial bleaching by Nos 1 or 2, the hair was suspended in tufts or loosely in a box containing burning sulphur, the sulphur dioxide acting upon the hair as a bleaching agent. (*Francis*). From 1867 hydrogen peroxide in conjunction with ammonium hydroxide has been the safest and most satisfactory method of bleaching hair. See Hydrogen peroxide. 'Strong German washes bleach and redden too pronounces.' (*Martial, Epigram XIV*). 'Voluptuous harlottes that make theyr heyre to appere at theyr browes, yalowe as fine golde made in little tresses for to drawe yonge folk to theyr love.' (*John Skelton, Book of Three Fooles*, early 16th century)

Stukeley, writing in 1725, gives the following methods of lightening hair as practised by the periwig makers in his day:

(1) Frequent washings with Lixivia.

(2) Exposure to the sun.

(3) Application of Aqua Fortis.

(4) Suffumigation of sulphur.

BLEEDING The tendency of poor hair dyes to wash out in water.

BLENDING (1) Cutting the hair by tapering or graduating, qv, so that no line of demarcation is apparent.

(2) Mixing hair for postiches.

(3) Graduating colour to avoid lines of demarcation during retouching. (*Trusty*)

(4) Application of a dye to faded hair to produce a uniform colour.

BLINKERS A 19th century fashion in which the hair was brought down the sides of the face. (*Cooper*) 274

BLIZZARD HEAD A blonde woman. American slang. (*B and B*)

BLO-BRUSH A hair brush with holes in the pad through which warm air is blown to facilitate the drying of wet hair whilst the hair is being brushed.

BLO-COMB A comb with holes in the teeth through which warm air is blown. See Blo-brush.

BLOCK A dummy head. (1) Wooden mounting block on which are made wigs and other postiches.

110, 111, 113–117

(2) Malleable block, cork-stuffed and covered with material on which to dress wigs and other postiches.

182, 183, 185–187

(3) Display block of china, wax, papier mâché or other suitable material for the display of wigs.

BLOCKED WIG A wig that has been secured to a malleable block preparatory to setting and dressing.

BLOCK HOLDER A metal or wooden clamp with an adjustable peg upon which the block sits and can be moved and held in any desired position. Also a padded container in which the block is held for knotting. *90(7), 95*

BLOCKING (1) Dividing the hair on the head into convenient rectangular divisions for winding on curlers preparatory to processing it for a permanent curl. See also Sectioning. (*Wall*)

(2) Positioning a wig on a malleable block preparatory to setting and dressing it.

BLOCKING OIL An oil to protect the remaining curl on the end lengths of hair during a re-wave.

BLOCK PADDING See Padded block.

BLOCK PEG A wooden peg for fixing a wig block to the work bench.

BLOCK POINT Thin, headless nail about ¾″ long to tack galloons, etc, in position on the wooden block preparatory to constructing the mount in wig-making. When the foundation is constructed the block points secure the bracing cottons which hold the foundation in position on the block during the hair-knotting process.

BLOCK WITH HAIR See Practice block.

BLONDE, BLOND (1) Adj. Very fair in colour, light auburn-coloured, in reference to a woman but blond when connected with a man.

(2) Noun. A fair-haired female usually, if naturally a blonde-haired person, with fair skin and blue eyes. Women with blonde hair enjoyed a great vogue for a few years in the 1920s. Anita Loos's novel *Gentlemen Prefer Blondes* undoubtedly encouraged this fashion in women's hair colour. 'It is impossible for a *Blond* to approach a *Brunette* in perfection of Beauty', 1724. (*Wheatley*, p. 63). See also Peroxide blonde.

BLONDE BOMBSHELL, THE Jean Harlow, the American Film actress.

BLONDE JOB (1) A fair-haired girl.

(2) A hair bleaching assignment.

BLONDE MENACE A blonde woman. Slang. (*B and B*)

BLONDE ON BLONDE A lighter blonde on the surface of a blonde hairdress giving the effect of a blonde head, sun-bleached.

BLONDE-TIPPING Bleaching the tips (½″ to 2″) of small wisps of hair.

BLONDETTE A blonde woman. Slang. (*B and B*)

BLONDIE A blonde woman. Slang. (*B and B*)

BLONDING (1) Bleaching.

(2) Lightening the hair in preparation for the application of a toning shade.

BLOND WASH A shampoo incorporating a bleach, usually hydrogen peroxide.

BLOOD'S SKULL COVERING Facetious name for a scratch wig, *qv*, 18th century. (*LC March 1972; Once a Week*, 3 Sept 1864)

BLOOM The shine and radiance of clean, healthy, natural hair.

BLOUSE See Winding blouse

BLOUSE ROLL Hair worn in a loose roll around the front of the hairdress, 1898. American usage. (*Corson*)

BLOUZE A woman with hair or head-dress loose, or decorated with vulgar finery. (*Holloway*)

BLO-WAVE See Blow waving.

BLOWCOMB A comb so constructed that warm air can be blown through or over the comb's teeth. Used to dry, form and wave hair. 20th century.

BLOW SET The process of setting the hair in a style whilst combing and shaping it with a comb and drying it with a hand-dryer without the use of a setting net. See also Blow waving.

BLOW STYLING See Blow set.

BLOW WAVING The setting of waves in the hair by means of a comb and a hand-held hair drier or trunk drier with a flattened or round nozzle by which the wave is shaped and blow-dried into position. Fan waving is the usual American term for the English 'blow waving'. First used about 1900 after the invention of the gas heated, electrically blown, pedestal hair dryer. Before the invention of an apparatus that would expel hot hair through a nozzle, blow waving was impossible.

BLOWZED Disordered in hair or dress. 18/19th century.

BLUEBEARD (La Barbe-Bleue) (1) The blue bearded chevalier, Raoul, in the Contes of Charles Perrault, 1697. (*Brewer*) Jacques Offenbach's operetta Barbe-Bleue (1866) was a burlesque based on the Bluebeard theme. The same theme was employed by Bela Bartok in his opera *Duke Bluebeard's Castle* (1911) – libretto by Bela Balasy (*Benet*)

(2) Nickname of the dissolute Gilles de Rais (1404–40).

(3) Landru the French murderer.

BLUEING The addition of a weak blue rinse to white, grey, fair or platinum blonde hair in order (a) to eliminate yellowness, or (b) using stronger solutions of blue, to tint the hair to any required degree of blueness.

BLUEING RINSE See Blue rinse.

BLUE RINSE A hair rinse containing blue colouring matter used to give blue tints to white, grey or blonde hair; also in weaker solutions employed to drab yellowing in white or grey hair. Also used to drab down brassy blonde hair.

BLUNT CUT Subs. American term. See Club cut.

BLUNT FRINGE See Bang.

BLUNTING American usage meaning clubbing or bobbing, *qv*. (*Trusty*)

BOARD The work-table or bench at which the wigmaker sits when making wigs and other forms of postiche.

BOARDMAN (also Boardsman) A person of the male sex who works at the bench making wigs and other forms of postiche. The wig dresser is always known as a posticheur.

BOARDWOMAN A female boardworker, *qv*.

BOARDWORK Work performed at the board or bench for the production of wigs and similar forms of hair-work.

BOARDWORKER A person who works in hair off the head at the bench or board. See also Boardman.

BOB (1) A short hair style introduced and popularised by Irene Castle, the dancer, 1914. The bobbed style is one of the simplest and oldest of all hair fashions for men. From before the Roman period and throughout the Middle ages to after 1800 this style was commonly worn by sections of the community.

(2) A girl with bobbed hair. Slang. (*B and B*)

(3) Verb. To club cut a head of hair so that the free ends hang above the shoulders.

(4) The scalp area over the ears. Birmingham usage. Possibly derived from bob-ear-ring. (*Symonds*)

BOBBED HAIR (1) Woman's short cut hair style. This mode had been accepted in New York by March 1915. See Bob (*A H April 1915*)

(2) a head of hair cut straight across at the neck. *193*

BOBBED WIG A short haired wig dressed in the style of the early 20th century bob cut. See Bob.

BOBBIN CURLER A short round curler used for the temporary or permanent curling of hair. (*H W J*, 8.3.62)

BOBBING The cutting of long hair to the short bobbed hair style. See Bob (*Trusty*)

BOBBY A girl with bobbed hair. Slang. (*B and B*)

BOBBY CHARLTON Name of a man's hair style in which a fringe of long hair from the periphery of the skull is combed over a bald crown. Named after the renowned soccer footballer of the 1960s.

BOBBY PIN A hair grip of 2″ to 3″ in length consisting of a thin, flat length of metal or plastic bent in the middle so that both free ends are adjacent. (American usage). In England this accessory is usually referred to as a hair grip, or by the proprietary name, Kirbigrip.

BOB CURL The curl formed by rolling a small section of hair with curling irons from the points towards the roots.

BOB MAJOR A man's wig style of the 18th century.

BOB PIN See Bobby pin.

BOB TAIL 18th century. American wig style. (*Earle*)

BOB WIG A man's 17/18th century periwig with the bottom hair turned up into short curls or bobs. The long bob covered the whole of the back of the neck. The short bob reached to the top of the neck. First recorded in 1684. Much worn by tradesman. 'I cut off my hair and procured a brown bob periwig of Wilding of the same colour, with a single row of curls just round the bottom, which I wore very nicely combed and without powder.' (*Creer*)

BODKIN (1) A hair-pin (*Lyly*, 1592). '. . . with her bodkin curls her hair.' (*Dekker, The Honest Whore* pt 1 1604, pt 2. 1630). Originally a dagger, later a hair-peg and finally a hairpin.
Randle Holme gives a 17th century description as follows: 'The Bodkin is a thing useful for women to bind up their haire with and aboute, they are usually made of silver and gold, the inferiour have them of Brasse, but the meanest content themselves with a scewer or sharp pointed stick'. Holme depicts what he describes as the new fashion and the old. 'The new fashion called an Haire combe (because it first readieth the haire by its wide teeth) or a single tooth combe, or back combe, or Peruwick combe, being principally used by Peruwick Makers. This replaces the bodkin.' (2) A kind of coarse needle made of tortoise-shell, ivory, bone or metal with an eye sufficiently large (an oval ¾″ × 1″) to contain the hair of a normal single spill tail, used to dress complicated chignons. 18/19th century.

BODKIN BEARD Small, sharp and pointed, the same as the stiletto beard, *qv.* Bodkin beard referred to by poet Skelton in 1529. The name and style had a very long life.
189 100(21, 22 etc)

BODY To put body into hair means to stiffen and coarsen it either by coating the hair shaft with a suitable substance, or applying a substance that can be absorbed by the hair.

BODY COLOUR A pigment which possesses 'body' or opacity in contrast with pigments that are transparent.

BODY CURL A large softly formed curl, the result of a permanent wave by which so-called 'body' is put into the hair. American usage. (*A H* 1964). See also Body wave.

BODY PERM See Body wave.

BODY WAVE A curling process that is claimed to put 'body' into the hair and make it more suitable for bouffant styles. The word is a gimmick word, *qv.*

BOIS DE CHENE, MLLE A Frenchwoman exhibited in London in 1852–53 had a profuse head of hair, a strong black beard, large whiskers and thick hair on her arms and legs.

BOLOGNA WASH-BALLS Made of Castile soap, honey water, cassia lignum and gum labdanum. 19th century.

(*Lillie*)

BOLSTER BANG The same as a rolled bang, *qv.* (*Morris*)

BOLTING CLOTH A stiff, transparent fabric made of silk on hand looms, mostly in Switzerland. 24 different meshes from 0000 (the coarsest) to 25 (the finest) which has 200 meshes to the linear inch. Used for foundations of certain types of wigs and toupees. Also used for sifting flour.

BOMBAGE Subs. (1) Rounded fullness of a head of hair, achieved by backcombing or frizzing.
(2) A hair style for men, 20th century.

BOMBAGE CURLING Hot-iron curling or setting a head of hair on small curlers preparatory to combing it through to produce a bombage effect.

BOMBE Bulging. 'Hair dressed bombe,' 1812.

BOMING Long hair hanging down. Somerset usage. (*Williams*) She d'a wear her hair boming.'

BONE See Wig bone

BONE COMB A hair comb of animal bone, 'made of the shank bones of horses and other large beasts'. 17th century. (*Holme*). Used when singeing was practised as the Vulcanite comb was flammable.

BONES AND HAIR Nautical rhyming slang for Buenos Aires. *c* 1900. (*Partridge*)

BONNET COMB A two-pronged horn or tortoiseshell, etc, comb used to secure a bonnet on the head. (*OG* Cat, 1901)

BONNET HAIR DRYER An electrically motivated hair dryer with a bonnet-shaped hood to cover the head at a distance of about 2″ from the whole inner surface. Similar to a hood dryer. The original bonnet hair dryers were motivated by electricity and heated by gas. Such a dryer was in use in Bristol until 1920.

BONNET HEAD-DRESS A woman's hair style of 1866. (*Bysterveld* p. 89)

BONNET STYLE See Bonnet shaped hairdress.

BONNET SHAPED HAIRDRESS A hair style that resembles in contour a 19/20th century baby's bonnet. See also Cap-shaped hairdress.

BONNET WIG An 18th century wig style.   *91(1,2)*

BON TON Good manners.

BOOGIE HAIR STYLE A style for men in which the hair is combed forward from the crown and turned back in a roll over the forehead to produce what is called a scroll effect. American origin. (*Trusty*)   *104D*

BOOMERANG COMB A setting/dressing comb shaped like a boomerang with the teeth on the convex side of the spine.

BOOSTER An apparatus or chemical that accelerates a process or action in dyeing, bleaching or permanent curling. The same as an accelerator.

BOOTH Small compartment in a room or shop in which clients can be privately treated. USA (*K-C*). Called a cubicle in England.

BOOTH STAND See Work stand.

BORDER (OF HAIR) Subs 1 to 4. (1) Hair worn around the edge of the hair line of the head 16–20th century.
(2) A plait or braid of hair worn around the front of the head from temple to temple. (*Procter*) Women 'frizle and lay out their hayre in borders' 1600. (*Vaughan*) 'the graines arranged spikewise and as if they were plaited and braided like a border of haire'. (Holland's *Pliny*, 1601) 'John Mullier, barber, in Northampton, left off his imployment of borders and Perriwig-Making'. (*A Testimony against Perriwigs*, 1677).
(3) Locks to cover the ears and neck. They were fixed to a cap, having no head of hair, 17th century. (*Holme*)
(4) A front of hair, waved or curled. 19th/20th century.
(5) Verb. To broider, to braid. 'The hair . . . had been coloured, pleated and bordered.' 1585 (*Sandys*)

BOREAS (The North Wind) Depicted by the ancients in art as an old man with hair and beard covered in snow or hoar frost. (*Salmon*)

BORGIA, LUCREZIA See Lucrezia Borgia's hair.

BORIERE A tapered, metal hair curler. SW England usage.

BORODOVAIA A copper disc with a bearded head on one side. Used in Russia in the 18th century as a receipt for payment of the beard tax. (*Reynolds*)

BORREL An attire or dress for the head. 17th century. (*Phillips*)

BORRELLI, MARIO Catholic priest, born Naples, Italy, 1922, founder of the House of Urchins there. At eight years of age he worked in a Naples barber's shop.

BORROWED LOCKS A peruke or wig. (*Howell*, 1660)

BOSCO Fold of loose skin hanging from beneath the chin. 'The boscos and suboscos (I mean) the dulapes and the fleshy part of the face.' (*Gayton*, 1654)

BOSKY Bearded. West of England slang.

BOSS (1) A caul to enclose the coils of plaited hair worn on both sides of the head. Late 13th century to late 14th century.
(2) A puff-cushion. Used for dressing puff curls and other small postiches. Birmingham usage. (*Symonds*)

BOSTON NECKLINE The back contour of a man's hair style in which the neck hair is cut high to a straight line across the neck, which is shaved. Originating in America early in the 20th century (before 1914). It has subsequently been variously interpreted by the English barber.

BOTANIC OIL A proprietary lotion for growing hair and dyeing red hair to brown or black. Made by J Middlewood, Liverpool, *c* 1814. (*Printed Broadside*)

BOTANIC WATER A preparation prepared and sold by Ross and Sons, 119 Bishopsgate Street Within, London, Peruque Makers, for cleansing and stimulating the growth of hair. (*Thackeray*)

BOTTICELLI STYLE From the hair style depicted on women in his painting 'Spring' by Sandro Botticelli (*c* 1447–1510), Italian artist of the Florentine Renaissance. *250*

BOTTLE BABY An artificial blonde. Slang. (*B and B*)

BOTTLE BLONDE An artificial blonde whose blondness comes out of a bottle of peroxide of hydrogen. Slang.

BOTTOM LOCK The side lock on a peruke that hangs down on the shoulders and back. 17th century (*Holme*)

BOUCLE A curl, or ringlet. French word. (*Creer*)

BOUCLER French word, to curl hair. (*Creer*)

BOUCLE REPENTIR A hanging ringlet of hair. (*Menard*)

BOUCLES CASCADEUSES Long, flowing, curled and wavy hair. Literally waterfall curls. (*Creer*)

BOUCLES RENVERSEES See Reversed curls.

BOUCLET The frame used in the 18th century to dress the high hair styles over. (*McColl*)

BOUDICCA (Boadicea) Queen of the Iceni, had long, flowing hair reaching to the middle of her back, according to Dio Cassius.

BOUDIN A long curl. (*Creer*)

BOUDOIR Lady's private room. (*Creer*)

BOUDOIR HELMET A decorated hair net of silk or other suitable material for wear by a woman in the boudoir to keep her hair in position during her toilet activity.

BOUE A wig style similar to a goat's beard; also called Goatee.

BOUFFANCE The condition of fullness or puffiness in relation to a hairdress. (*AH* 1963)

BOUFFANT A 19th century French word used to denote a puffed out part of a dress. Re-used in 1958 to describe and name a puffed, short hair style popularised by Princess Margaret, still commonly worn in 1965. (*Creer*)

BOUFFON Group of loose curls or waves hanging over the ears to the side of the chin; also called a Spaniel ear. 17th century.

BOULANGER A beard style (*Gents Academy*).

BOUNCE Hair that is dressed in a loose, full, resilient style said to have bounce. (From *c* 1960)

BOUQUET Bunch of feathers, flowers, etc, often constructed with coloured hair. (*Creer*)

BOURBON-LOCK A love lock.

BOURGEOISE COIFFURE A woman's 18th century hair style. (*Uzanne*)

BOURGOIGNE The first part of the dress for the head next to the hair. (*Evelyn*)

BOURRELET A crescent shaped, decorative pad worn in the hair by women. 17th century. French. (*Corson*)

BOURSE The bag appended to a wig. (*Fairholt*) 'Your bourse seems to be as well fashioned as those that are made by the dresser for the King's pages.' (*The Rival Modes*, 1727)

BOUTIQUE A small privately owned shop offering specialized personal service and/or good quality goods.

BOWER CURL A curl forming three quarters of a circle only.

BOWSER (1) A pubic hair-piece. London usage, 19th century.
(2) A ring shaped bun pad of crêped hair. Slang.

BOWSPRIT FENDER A man's pubic hair. Air Force slang. (*Symonds*)

BOX-CAR MOUSTACHE An American moustache style. (*Trusty*) *101H*

BOX COMB A hair comb made of box tree wood. 17th century. (*Holme*)

BOX-CRIMPING IRON See Crimping iron.

BOX IRON See Crimping iron.

BOX-WAVING IRON See Crimping iron.

BOX WOOD Used from Graeco-Roman period until 19th century for hair combs.

BOY HEADED A girl's hair cut short like a boy. 1850. (*Companion*)

BOYISH BOB A short, rounded hair style for women resembling a man's hair cut but the hair is left longer. Popular in the 1920s.

BRACE Cotton or silk threads from the galloon at the point where the block point holds it, to another block point both outside and inside the area of the wig foundation for the purpose of holding the foundation in position on the block and thus enabling the wigmaker to knot hair on the net foundation.

BRACING The positioning of the braces. See Brace.

BRACING COTTONS OR SILKS The cottons or silks used to brace or anchor the foundation of a postiche in position on the block.

BRAID subs. (1) A plait of human hair; a plaited three spill switch of hair. 'Braydes of a woman's heer.' (*Palsgrave*), 1530. In the 19th century also applied to the flat bands of hair worn by women over the side of the face, as in the early portraits of Queen Victoria.
(2) A woven string, cord or other suitable material used for tying the hair, or forming a mount to use in a dressing. *138*

BRAID Verb. (1) To plait, intertwine or twist the hair in and out. 1530 'I broyde heere; or lace, or such lyke.' (*Palsgrave*)
'Hire yelwe heer was browdid in a tress
Behynde hire back a yerde long, I guess.' (*Chaucer*)
(2) To bind or confine the hair with a ribbon or braid. 'Yet ne'er again to braid her hair.' (*Scott, Lady of the Lake*, 1810). 'With roseate wreaths they braid the glossy hair.' (*Southey, Triumph of Women*, 1793)

BRAID-COMB A long-toothed hair comb to secure braided hair in a hairdress.

BRAIDING PIN A type of needle of bone, ivory, metal or other suitable substance, with a very large eye through which a strand of hair could be threaded and then interwoven into the coiffure as required. Needle lengths varied from 3″ to 15″. 18/19th century. (*Thornbury*)

BRAMBLE (*Rubus Fructicosus*) A hair dye was made by boiling the leaves of the bramble in strong lye. It imparted a permanent soft black colour to the hair. (*Fernie*)

BRAN Used for cleaning the hair by sprinkling it on, massaging it in and brushing it out. 17/19th century. (*Toilette*)

BRANNY TETTER Scurf. (*Wheeler*)

BRASS BASIN A 16th century term for a barber, in allusion to the brass basin used in the barber's shop.

BRAVADO FASHION 16th century hair style for men. (*Stubbes*)

BRAZILIAN PLAIT A plait made of dried fig grass from S America or West Indies.

BRAZILIAN TONSURE In the 17th century some of the men of Brazil shaved the forefront of their heads. (*Bulwer*)
102E

BRAZIL WAX See Carnauba wax.

BRAZIL WOOD Formerly used in hair dyes.

BREAKAGE A hair condition in which the hair readily breaks off. It is usually caused by excessive bleaching or dyeing, harsh permanent waving lotions, over-strong shampoos, too hot curling irons or even long exposure to strong sunlight.

BREAKING-POINT OF HAIR The force required in a direct pull to break a single hair.

BREAKWATER American usage. A very small beard on the tip of the chin similar to that worn by Benjamin Disraeli, the English Prime Minister.

BREE Eyebrow, 16/17th century. (*Fry*)

BRESSANT, LA A hair style for a man. (*Alexandre*)

BRICK TOP Auburn haired. American slang. (*B and B*)

BRIGADIER WIG Similar to the Major wig, *qv*. A style with a double corkscrew queue or tail tied with a bow at the nape of the neck, worn by military men and those affecting a military appearance in the second half of the 18th century. (*Garsault*)
91 (14, 15)

BRIGHT RINSE Two volume hydrogen peroxide used as a rinse after a shampoo to slightly bleach or 'lighten' the hair. (*Wilson*)

BRIGHT SHAMPOO See Brightening shampoo.

BRIGHTENING SHAMPOO A soap shampoo containing a quantity of hydrogen peroxide, used to cleanse and lighten the colour of the hair in the single process of the shampoo. (*Rohrer*)

BRILLIANTINE (liquid) An oily type dressing for the hair and beard. In Biblical days reference was made to the anointing of heads with perfumed oil. Three 19th century formulae were:
(1) A solution of 1 part Castor oil in 4 parts of Eau de Cologne. (*Creer*)
(2) Castor oil 1 oz; esprit de rose 1 oz; spirits of wine 2 oz; and a few drops of saffron to colour.
(3) Glycerine 8 lb, extract of jasmine 2 quarts. (*Atkinson*)
Light mineral oil, coloured and perfumed to taste, is the simplest and commonest type of brilliantine in the 20th century.

BRILLIANTINE (for the beard) A 19th century formula was: Castor oil 7 parts; almond oil 50 parts; glycerin 22 parts; Jockey Club extract 2½ parts and white spirit 125 parts. (*Koller*)

BRILLIANTINE (solid) Vegetable or mineral oils which have been stiffened to the required consistency with the aid of suitable waxes. The term is nearly synonymous with pomade although pomade is usually of a softer consistency. (*Sagarin*)

BRILLIANTINE TRAY A small metal or pottery tray on which brilliantine and other bottles were kept.

BRINDED Burnt; the different shades produced by the action of singeing; marked with streaks. (*Toone*)

BRIOCHE Woman's hair style 1962. Long loose bob with large bun on crown. Named after brioche, a kind of cake, whose shape the style resembles.
271

BRIOCHE LOOK See Brioche. Made fashionable by Jacqueline Kennedy (1962), wife of the late American President. (Photo *Sunday Telegraph*, 15 April, 1962)

BRISTLE (1) Subs. Short stiff hairs from a hog's back or other animal used in hairbrushes and bristle roller hair curlers.
(2) Man's short-cropped beard.
(3) Verb. To be thickly set with hair.
(4) Verb. (Hair) To stand on end with fright.

BRISTLE ROLLER A large diameter hair curler covered with bristles to facilitate the winding of the hair, *c* 1950.

BRISTLES The Beard. Slang. American usage. (*B and B*)

BRISTOL SOAP A good type of tallow soap made in Bristol, 19th century. (*Lillie*)

BRISTOL STYLE (1) A neat and tidy hair style. West of England usage 20th century. Derived from the 17/18th century saying 'ship-shape and Bristol fashion', ie in good order.
(2) A fantasy hair style incorporating a ship.

BRITISH BEARD Heavy, long moustaches on the upper lip hanging down either side of the chin, all the rest of the face being bare. 17th century. (*Holme*)

BRITISH HAIRDRESSERS' BENEVOLENT & PROVIDENT INSTITUTION Founded 1831 for the purpose of affording relief to distressed members and their widows.

BRITONS The ancient Britons were described by Julius Caesar as wearing long hair and flowing moustaches, although they shaved their chins. (*Stukeley*)

BROAD BEARD Cathedral beard, *qv*. Patriarchal Beard, *qv*.

BROBDINGNAG-HAIRDRESS A monstrously large coiffure. Derived from Swift's *Gullivers Travels*, 1726, where Brobdingnag was a country of enormous giants.

BROID Variant of braid. To plait. 'Hir yelow heer was broyded in a tresse.' (*Chaucer*, 14th century)

BROIDED Plaited. 'Not with broided hair, or gold, or pearls, or costly array;' (1 *Timothy*, ch 2 v 9)

BROKEN COLOUR Variation of colour produced by the presence of another colour or colours on the head which affects and is affected by a colour or colours in proximity.

BROKEN CURL A mixture of curl, curve and part wave. 'She had a flouncy looking head of broken curl.'

BROKEN POMPADOUR See Semi-Pompadour.

BROMIDROSIS CAPITIS A condition of the hair or beard which is characterised by fetid perspiration or an exhalation of disagreeable odours from the hair. (*Wheeler*)

BROMINE SOAP See Medicated soap.

BRONZING The application of a bronze-coloured covering to the head hair, usually sprayed on and readily removable by shampooing.

BROW HAIR See Full front.

BROWNETTE (1) A brunette. Slang. (*B and B*)
(2) A head of hair intermediate in colour between blonde and brunette.

BROWN GEORGE A man's brown wig resembling a loaf of bread. Worn by Sir Clowdisley Shovell (1650–1707), see monument to him in Westminster Abbey; also worn by Thomas Dawson, Viscount of Cremorne. This wig was also called a Sir Clowdisley Shovell, *qv*.

BROWN HAIR-POWDER Mixture of umber and black hair powder with honey water remains, 18/19th century. (*Lillie*)

BROWN POMATUM As black pomatum but coloured with fine damask powder instead of ivory black. 18/19th century. (*Lillie*)

BRUGIER'S TOLMA A 19/20th century 'secret' hair 'preservative' was a rose-coloured liquid, that consisted of 1 part ordinary glycerine, 10 parts of water, and a little sulphur in suspension. (*Koller*)

BRUHL Count Bruhl of Saxony formed a wig museum in which was represented chronologically arranged, every variety of beard from the time of Aaron to the Count's own days. (*Doran p 162*)

BRUN French word for brown.

BRUNETTE A brown-haired person, especially a woman. A diminutive form from the French brun, brown.

BRUSH Subs. (1) An implement of bristle, wire, plastic, hair or other suitable material set in wood or rubber, for brushing hair, applying hair dye or bleach, etc. 'A square brush, or a bristle brush, the finest sort of them is made of horse-hair from its mane or tail. They are generally termed Buffet or Bever brushes.' 17th century. (*Holme*). In Mechis' *Catalogue of Cutlery* (4 Leadenhall St, London), 1840, the following brushes for use on hair are listed: hair brush, patent hair brush, taper shaving brushes of pig, camel, badger and horse-hair, curl brushes.
(2) A head of hair, 18/20th century.
(3) 18th century wig style. (*London Magazine*)
(4) Pubic hair of a man. 18th century Slang. (*Button*)
(5) The beard. American slang. (*B and B*)
(6) The short, curled feather on top of a man's dressed head. 1782 (*Stewart*). See also Drawing brush.

BRUSH AND COMB BAG A small fabric bag for carrying a brush and comb.

BRUSH-BACK WIG A man's wig in which the hair is brushed back in a pompadour style, *qv*.

BRUSH COMB A hybrid implement between a brush and a comb, with 2 or 3 rows of slightly flexible plastic teeth. 1950s.

BRUSH CURL A curl formed by brushing the hair from the roots spirally around the index finger of the left hand.

BRUSH CURLER See Brush roller.

BRUSH CURLING See Brush curl.

BRUSH CUT A hair style for men in which the hair is cut short at the back and sides and the longer hair at the top and front is combed up like the standing hair of a brush. A popular style in America, England and in France as 'La brosse' in the 1950s. (*Trusty*)

BRUSH GRIP ROLLER See Brush roller.

BRUSHOUT (1) Subs. The arrangement of the curled hair on a head by brushing, combing and positioning it after the hair has been removed from the rollers or curlers in preparation for the final arrangement of the tresses by the fingers, tailcomb or steel needle. From *c* 1930. (*cf Combout*)
(2) Verb. To brush through the set and dried hairdress preparatory to the final arrangement of the tresses. (*cf Combout*)

BRUSH PEDLAR A film extra with a natural beard. American slang. (*B and B*)

BRUSH ROLLER A circular hair curler constructed from a spiral spring covered with spikey bristles for ease of winding. Also called bristle, spikey or hedgehog roller.

BRUSH TOP A man's short haircut. The top cut short and flat, the hair standing erect. Similar to flat top, *qv*.

BRUSH WAVE (also Brushwave) A wave that is set in the hair by means of brushing and the fingers after the hair of the head has been curled on large diameter or jumbo curlers.

BRUSH WEIGHT A heavy piece of metal, usually lead or iron, often an old weight or flat-iron, used to hold the upper brush in position on the lower brush preparatory to drawing off hair from between the drawing brushes.

BRUSH WIG An 18th century wig style for men commonly worn by Judges. Lord Eldon, when made Chief Justice of the Common Pleas, objected to wearing the coventional powdered brush wig, but George III would not permit its abandonment by judges.

BRUTUS STYLE or BRUTUS HEAD A short cut head of hair of untidy appearance of frizzed, affected at first by the French Revolutionaries in the 18th century when the ideal was the incorruptible Roman. (*Manuel Alvarez Espriella, Letter from England*, 1807; also *Weekley*)

BRUTUS WIG A brown unpowdered wig of untidy appearance, 1790–1825. Originally from the Brutus hair style of the 18th century. *qv*.

BUBBLE CURL A thin, light-weight curl of small or medium diameter and narrow width, dressed loosely, airily, bubbly.

BUBBLE RINSE A colour rinse incorporated in a shampoo.

BUBBLES HAIR STYLE A popular style for young women *c* 1890 and for children, earlier and later. Short hair was dressed in curls all over the head. The Pears Soap advertisement (late 19th century) after Millais' picture in which appeared a child with a bubble hair style blowing bubbles, probably gave the name to the style.

BUCHLIGEN'S HAIR PRESERVATIVE A 19/20th century 'secret' preparation, consisting of a mixture of arnica tincture 10 parts; glycerine 5 parts; water 60 parts; and alcohol 10 parts. (*Koller*)

BUCKLE (1) Verb. To curl or bend. *cf Boucle* (French) curl.
(2) Subs. An 18th century man's curled wig style.
(3) Subs. A curl. *218*
(4) Subs. Bent-back points of a strand of hair in a curling process.
(5) Verb. To bend-back the points of a strand of hair in a curling process.

BUCKLE CHAIN 18th century wig style. See Chain Buckle.

BUCKLE SWATHE A waved swathe of hair.

BUCKLED WIG Curled wig. 18/19th century.

BUCKLE WIG See Buckle.

BUCKLING See Buckle.

BUCKLING COMB A dressing comb used during the hair curling process. 1763. (*Earle*)

BUCKRAM A strong, coarse, stiffened linen cloth used to cover malleable blocks upon which wigs, etc, are dressed. (*Drapers' Dicy*)

BUDDHIST-SHAVEN-HEAD Symbolizes Buddha's renunciation of worldly wealth.

BUFFER CURL See Barrel spring curl.

BUFFET BRUSH A hairbrush bristled with horsehair. 17th century. (*Holme*)

BUGLES Long, slender, glass beads used to ornament the high hairdress of the 18th century. (*Tatler and Fairholt*)

BULBOUS Like a bulb; a nearly spherical object.

BULLDOG SCALP Cutis Verticis Gyrata, popular name for a condition in which the skin of the vertex appears to be in folds. It is rare, congenital or acquired.

BULLET HEAD MOUSTACHE A moustache curled at the ends near the corners of the mouth.

BULLHEAD COIFFURE See Taure.

BUMPING See Barrelling.

BUN A tight gathering of hair at the back of the head, usually effected by coiling the twisted or plaited hair, or by dressing the hair over a bun pad.

BUNCH Strands of hair clustered together.

BUNCH HAIR See Pubic hair.

BUN FOUNDATION See Bun pad.

BUNKER HILL An 18th century high dressed American wig style for women. Inspired by the battle of Bunker Hill. *378*

BUN NET A small purse-like net of human hair used to encase the dressed bun of hair at the back of the head.

BUN PAD A small pad over which the hair can be dressed to produce the familiar hair bun.

BUN PENNY A bronze coin of Queen Victoria's reign, so-called because of the bun hair style of the young queen.

BUN RING A small ring of crepe hair through which the hair is drawn to form a bun dressing.

BUNTY FRINGE A pair of small, flat half curls, one on each side of the forehead, turning towards the centre of the forehead. Popularised by and named after Bunty Biggar, a character played by Miss Kate Moffat in the play *Bunty Pulls the Strings* by Graham Moffat, produced at the Playhouse Theatre 4 July 1911 and at the Haymarket Theatre 18 July 1911. (*Play Pictorial* No 122, Vol XX)

BURCHIELLO, DOMINICO DA GIOVANNI (b Florence 1404, d Rome 1449). An Italian poet but a barber by trade. He wrote humorous, satirical verses, many of which were directed against the Medici. He was compelled to flee Florence and died in poverty.

BURD A beard.

BURGUNDY-PITCH The resinous juice of the spruce fir used for the removal of superfluous hair, from before 1700 to early 20th century. (*Lady's Magazine*, Dec 1759) The resin was spread on a square of cloth or soft leather and pressed on the unwanted hair then quickly plucked away from the skin with the hair attached.

BURNSIDE A beard style popularized by General Burnside. It consisted of a moustache, whiskers and the chin clean shaven. Burnsides (called sideburns in England) also used to denote long side whiskers, *c* 1875. American usage. (*Webster*)

BUSBY (1) A large, bushy wig, *c* 1765 +. MacArdell's print of Lord Anson after the painting by Sir Joshua Reynolds depicts an early, possibly the earliest, example of the busby. This style was also worn by Dr Samuel Johnson (1709–1784). Lord Monboddo (1714–1799) and the Rev George Whitefield (1714–1770) in their later years. (*Smith*) It has been suggested that the word originated from the famous Head-Master of Westminster School, Dr Busby (1606–1695), who is said to have worn a wig of this type. However that may be, certain it is that the word was applied to pubic hair (see 2 below) and popularly understood as such before 1723.

(2) The pubic hair of a woman. 18th century slang. 'And shoul'd you, with Hunter, go a-sporting in Busby . . .' 1723 (*Button*)

(3) A beehive hairdress of women, 1959–1970.

BUSH (1) The beard. Slang, American usage.

(2) A wig.

(3) Vernacular term for a thick, untidy head of hair. (*B and B*)

(4) Pubic hair.

BUSH BEARD A thick, full beard; medium to long.

BUSHES A false beard. (*B and B*)

BUSH WIG 18th century wig style.

BUSHY See Bush wig.

BUSHY, THE A 20th century hair style for men.

BUSK To dress, adorn. 14th century to 19th century.

BUSKER A ladies' hairdresser, 16th century. 'The fynest dresser of a woman's head or heare.' 1568. (*Chalmer*)

BUSTER BROWN BOB American usage. A long bobbed, straight hair style with middle parting and a fringe, worn by boys and girls from *c* 1904 onwards and popularised by a coloured strip cartoon in The New York Herald, in which the character, Buster Brown, regularly appeared in this hair style. (*Rohrer and NYH* April, 1904) *264*

BUSTLE-BACK COIFFURE A hair style in which the back hair is dressed to stand out from the head. Expression derived from the Victorian bustle.

BUTCH CUT or STYLE A hair style for men in which the hair is cut very short. Derived from butcher and, in the shortened form, Butch – a popular American nickname indicating strength and virility, butchers usually being fat, strong men.

BUTCHER Verb. To ruin a head of hair by bad hairdressing. 'That new assistant had butchered my hair.'

BUTCH RAKE A flat metal attachment for hair clippers which facilitates the cutting of a Butch style for men, *qv*. (*Jones*)

BUTLER PARTING A middle parting extending from the forehead to the nape. (*Hairdressing Illustrated*, Vol 4, No 1, 1926)

BUTTERFLY COMB Boomerang comb, *qv*.

BUTTERFLY CURL CLIP See Pincurl cage clip.

BUTTERFLY FRINGE A light divided fringe of two half circles of curl symetrically positioned with a spherical gap in the middle of the forehead.

BUTTERFLY HEAD-DRESS A woman's hair style of *c* 1460 in which the horns of the horned head-dress, *qv*, were extended by a wide frame and over which a kerchief was arranged with the back edge floating out behind. (*Gardiner*)

BUTTONHOLE STITCH See Stitching.

BUTTONHOLING The making of a buttonhole.

BUTTON MOUSTACHE See Charlie Chaplin.

BUZFUZ, SERJEANT A character in Dickens's *Pickwick Papers*, 1837. Name derived from a combination of Buzz, a wig, and Fuzz.

BUZZ A frizzled, bushy wig, *c* 1800. See also Buzz wig and Busby. (*Smith, J T*)

BUZZ WIG The same as Busby, *qv*, for which it was an alternative name.

BYRLET Tyring for the hair. A padded roll of material for a woman's head; a hood. (*Levens*, 1570)

BYRON, LORD See Lucrezia Borgia.

BYZANTINE SNAIL A snail-shaped twist of hair worn on top of the head. It formed a constituent part of a hair style of women of the Byzantine Empire (395–1453).

BYZANTINE STYLE Art forms, including hair styles, of the Eastern Roman Empire, 5/15th century.

C

CABINET DE TOILETTE (Fr) Dressing room. (*Creer*)

CABLE COIL A cable twist, dressed in a coil formation.

CABLE PLAIT A thick plait. Take three thick strands of hair of equal size, place one in the centre; take the left hand strand and lift it under the centre one, and over it and back to its own place; take the right hand strand and lift that under the centre one and over it, and back to its place; work on thus alternately to the end. (*Ladies' Companion* 1851, and *Elegant Arts*)

CABLE TWIST (1) A thick single stem switch that is dressed in a twist, either clockwise or anti-clockwise, according to requirements. (*Creer*)
(2) A thick switch formed from a twisted two-spill switch or two twisted single-spill switches. *420*

CABRIOLE A hair ornament in the form of a carriage, 1756. Also spelt Capriole. (*Connoisseur*)

CABRIOLET See A la cabriolet.

CACAO BUTTER (Cocoa butter) A fatty substance obtained from the cacao nut and used in the manufacture of pomades, etc.

CACHE-FOLIES An early 19th century name for a wig. In 1793, after the French Revolution, a very short hair style (cut to an inch or two from the scalp) became popular for women. The vogue did not last long and many women wore natural looking wigs, called Cache-Folies, to cover their growing hair. (*Creer*)

CACHEPEIGNE or CACHE PEIGNE Bunch of curls on a comb; a hidden comb. (*Creer and B and SP*, 41) *329, 430*

CACTUS See Hair dye.

CADAVER HAIR Hair from dead bodies. At one time (16/18th century) used in the manufacture of wigs. 'Thatch your poor thin roofs with burdens of the dead: some that were hanged. No matter: wear them, betray them.' (*Shakespeare*). See also False hair (1).

CADENETTE also CADANETTE and CADANET A hair queue worn at the neck of a powdered wig. See also Cadanette wig. (*Creer*)

CADENETTE WIG A man's 18th century powdered wig with two plaited hair queues worn at the neck. This coiffure was brought into fashion in France in the time of Louis XIII by Honore d'Albret, brother of the Duke de Luynes, the Lord of Cadanet. (*Bracher*). See also Cadanette.

CADIZ BEARD A medium length, pointed beard, probably derived from a Spanish style and similar to a 16th century *pic-a-devant*, *qv*.

CADOGAN Knot of hair worn on the nape of the neck. This was the queue worn by Macaronis in the 18th century *qv*. See also Cadogan wig.

CADOGAN WIG Also called Club wig. This style appeared in the 1760s. The queue, broad and straight, was folded back on itself and tied around its middle. Probably named after Charles, second Baron Cadogan (1691–1776).

CADS BEARD Probably a corruption of Cadiz Beard, 16th century.

CAESAR The name Caesar derived from Caesaries denoting a thick head of hair.

CAESAR CUT A man's hair style; cut tapered, dressed forward onto the forehead as was the hair of Julius Caesar, the Roman Emperor. Popularised by the film Cleopatra in 1962/3. *102L*

CAESARIES Particularly head hair of a man. See Hair nomenclature.

CAESAR STYLE See Caesar cut. 1962/3.

CAGE A wire or plastic shape with or without hair attached for incorporation as a constituent element in a hairdress. See also Chignon cage.

CAGE CLIP See Pincurl cage clip.

CAIN-COLOURED HAIR The reputed colour of the hair of Cain, whose beard, traditionally, was reddish-yellow as was that of Judas Iscariot. 'A little yellow Beard; a Caine-coloured Beard.' (*Shakespeare, Merry Wives of Windsor*)

CALAMIST One having his hair turning upward: 17th century. From Calamistrum – Roman hair-curling irons. (*Cockeram*)

CALAMISTE A slave who combed and curled hair. (*Forbes*)

CALAMISTRATE Verb. To curl, crimp or frizzle the hair. 17th century. (*Burton*, 1621)

CALAMISTRATION The process of curling. 17th century. (*Burton*)

CALAMISTRUM Roman hair-curling irons.

CALASH A large collapsible hood of silk made on a frame of wire, to wear over the high, powdered coiffures of the 18th century.

CALCIUM THIOGLYCOLLATE An ingredient of some depilatories. Experiments have shown that solutions containing less than 8% of purified thioglycollate apparently do not induce primary skin irritation. (*Sagarin*)

CALEMBUC (Calumbuc, calambac, etc). Comb. A comb for combing the hair made from an aromatic wood grown in the East Indies. It imparted a very fragrant scent to the hair. Calambac is an eastern name of aloeswood or eagles-wood. Produced from *Aquilaria Agallocha*. (*Evelyn*, 1690)

CALEMBUS COMB Metal comb; a rake *qv* made of pewter (*Chalmers*).
'Calembus combs in pulvil case
To set and trim the hair and face.' (*Evelyn, Mundus Muliebris*, 1690)

CALF LICK Hair which does not lie in the same direction as the remainder (Craven district) so called because it looks as if it has been licked by a calf. (*Holloway*) See Cowlick.

CALGON Sodium hexametaphosphate, a water softener.

CALIFORNIA CUT See Flat-top crew cut.

CALLOW Bald, unfledged. (*Bardsley*)

CALORIE Unit of quantity of heat; amount of heat required to raise one gram of water 1°C.

CALOT (1) A small cap-shaped postiche foundation. 19/early 20th century.
(2) The cap-like foundation for a chignon.
(3) A cap-shaped hair frame.

CALVA SUPERCILIUM Absence of eyebrow. (*Wheeler*)

CALVES-TAIL WIG Wigs made of calves' tails. 'He will make perukes of calves tails, which he engages will last a long time. This kind indeed (as there is very little profit to be had by them) he only makes to oblige the fathers of such young gentlemen who honour him with their custom.' (*London Magazine*, 1764)

CALVITIES Baldness.

CALVUS Bald. (*Wheeler*)

CALVUS, GAIUS LICINIUS Roman orator and poet. The name means bald pate.

CAMBERWELL FRINGE A short, narrow beard, running round the face, worn by farmers in the 19th century. (*Thompson*, p 99)

CANE-COLOURED BEARD (*sic*) Held in detestation as, by tradition, this was the colour (reddish yellow) of Judas Iscariot's beard. See Cain-coloured hair.

CANITICS (1) A branch of science which treats the disease known as canities or grey hair. (*Wall*). An American word first commonly used in England in the early 1920s.
(2) The art and science of hair dyeing especially white or grey hair.

CANITIES Loss of pigment in growing hair resulting in whiteness.

CANATIST A person who dyes white or grey hair.

CANNON CURL A long croquignole curl; a long barrel-spring curl. A long curl rolled up close to the head and left open in the middle and fixed horizontally.
'John Howard . . . with cannon curls,' (*Dobson, Later Essays* p 71)

CANTHARIDES *Cantharis Vesicatoria*. Also called Spanish fly, blistering beetle. At one time it was used in the preparation of hair restorers. Highly irritant. Ingestion or absorption from skin or mucous membranes may produce severe gastroenteritis, spermatorrhea, priapism collapse and death. In England it is no longer legal for preparations of Cantharides to be made except by qualified chemists and doctors.

CANTON STROP See Cowvan's canton strop.

CANVAS Strong unbleached cloth of hemp or flax; sometimes used to cover malleable blocks.

CANVAS HEAD A malleable block.

CANVAS STROP Usually made of linen or silk. See Strop.

CAP (1) A plastic, paper or waterproof cover to envelop the hair and head in a dyeing or bleaching process and accelerate the development by the retention of the head's heat.
(2) Wig cap, *qv*.

CAP CURLS Curls mounted on a cap frame and worn at the back of the head. *c* 1910.

CAP CUT A short hair style cut in the general form of a cap and dressed close to the head.

CAPE The protective covering placed around the client's shoulders to prevent hair or liquids falling upon the clothing. A dye cape is usually made of a non-absorbent material such as rubber or plastic.

CAPE MARTEAU A very large marteau worn as a cape of hair hanging from the back of the head. See Comb marteau. (*Symonds*)

CAPILLACEOUS Resembling hair.

CAPILLAMENT (1) A hair-like fibre or filament.
(2) A wig. 'How many bad women do you think have laid their heads together to complete that mane of yours? I'll warrant you now you are as proud of your fine capillament as a morrice-dancer is of his bells, . . .' (*The Weekly Comedy*, 1690)

CAPILLAR Hair-like or pertaining to hair.

CAPILLARINE HAIR RESTORER A 19/20th century 'secret' preparation of absolute alcohol, onion juice, French brandy, Peruvian balsam, burdock-root oil and juniper-berry oil, with an addition of fat or tallow. Probably as many 'baldheaded' drank this concoction as applied it to their scalps. (*Koller*)

CAPILLARIS ARBOR 'Tree of Hair.' Recorded by Sextus Festus as the repository for the ceremonially shaven first beards of Rome's young men.

CAPILLARY (1) Subs. Anything resembling a hair.
(2) Adj. Pertaining to or concerned with hair.
(3) Adj. Hair-like.
(4) Adj. Having a minute hair-like internal diameter, eg capillary tube.

CAPILLARY ARTIST A hairdresser. (*Chambers' Journal*, Nov 1866)

CAPILLATE Adj. Furnished with hair.

CAPILLATION Condition of being hairy.

CAPILLATURE (1) The hair of the head.
(2) A frizzling of the hair.

CAPILLIFORM Hair shaped.

CAPILLOSE Adj. Hairy.

CAPILLUS (1) A head hair.
(2) Hair of the head. See Hair nomenclature.

CAPILLUSTRA Hair lustre.

CAPILONI The hairy ones. Italian name for English beatniks. (1966 BBC)

CAPLESS WIG A wig of wefts sewn on an open meshwork foundation which usually consists of narrow stretch tapes or other suitable elasticized material.

CAP NET A hair net in the form of a cap, usually manufactured from oriental hair. (*Ingerid*)

CAPOUL, LA A man's hair style. (*Alexandre*)

CAPPING-LEATHER Kid leather used for capping the ends of positional springs in a postiche.

CAPRICIEUSE COIFFURE A woman's hair style of 1867. (*Le Moniteur de la Coiffure*, 10 May, 1867)

CAPRIOLE See Cabriole.

CAP SHAPE A short hair style dressed close to the head.

CAPTAIN An English moustache style. 20th century. (*Foan*) *101, 4*

CAPTAIN KETTLE BEARD A short, pointed beard named after the hero of C J Cutcliffe Hyne adventure stories, 1898.

CAP WIG 18th century man's wig style. (*Garsault*)

CARACALLA CUT A short cut for women, the hair worn in flattened sausage-shaped curls. Early 19th century. (*Walker*)

CARACALLA WIG Woman's black wig, *c* 1798, dressed in flat-sausage-shaped curls. From headdress of Roman Emperor of that name (ad 188–217) which appeared on his coins.

CARBOLIC ACID Phenol, C_6H_5OH. Used as a general disinfectant. Poisonous and caustic.

CARBONATE OF SODA See Sodium carbonate.

CARBON TETRACHLORIDE CCL_4. A colourless, clear, non-inflammable, heavy liquid with a characteristic odour. Used for cleaning postiche and sometimes for 'dry' cleaning hair on the head, but the utmost care is necessary owing to its possible danger. Special caution – it may form phosgene gas if used to put out electrical fires. Use only with adequate ventilation and with the door open for instant exit. (*Merck*)

CARCANET Bands of jewels entwined in women's hair. A sort of necklace set with jewels used for a hair ornament; also Carkenet and Carkant. 16/17th century. In 15th century applied to necklaces. (*Fairholt*, also *Smith*)

CARD A steel-toothed instrument for disentangling hair and laying parallel the individual hairs in the strand preparatory to mixing, weaving or knotting, etc. *88 (2–11)*

CARDING the disentangling of hair by drawing it through a card.

CARICATURE HAIR STYLE A satirical representation of a hair style of any person by a ridiculous over-emphasis of its characteristic features.

CARLOVINGIAN HAIR STYLE A hair style of the period of the second French dynasty founded by Charlemagne (751–787).

CARMAN'S KNOT The *noeud de charretier* of the French. The neckcloth knot of the carman or carter who drove the horses of the 19th century. Both twists and coils of hair were dressed in the form of a carman's knot.

CARNAUBA WAX A hard wax from *copernicia cerifera* used in cosmetics and in the manufacture of wax models for the display of postiches. (*PPB*)

CAROLINGIAN See Carlovingian.

CARPET KNIGHT A man whose main interest was the appearance of his peruke in preference to the affairs of life. *George Savile, Some Cautions Offered . . .* 1695 Marquis of Halifax. (*Wing No H 322*)

CARPET-THREAD Used for weaving hair on in the manufacture of crêpe hair.

CARRAGEEN See Irish moss.

CARRIER A substance used to carry the active ingredient, such as Kaolin which carries the hydrogen peroxide in a bleaching treatment.

CARROT COLOUR Auburn.

CARROT HEAD A red-haired person. Slang. (*B and B*)

CARROT PAD A cone-shaped frizzett or pad of crepe hair.

CARROT TOP A red-haired person. Slang. (*B and B*)

CARROTS Red or auburn hair. Slang. 18th/20th century. (*Grose*)

CARROTTY PATED Red haired. Slang. (*Grose*)

CARROTTY POLL 18th century man's red coloured theatrical wig. (*Ency Brit*)

CARVED PIN CURL A hand-formed curl, not fluffy or light in appearance – similar to a sculpted pin curl.

CASCADE (1) A loose fall of hair.

(2) A postiche piece dressed in a style as (1).

CASCADE CURL A large diameter stand-up curl, *qv*.

CASCADE WIG A long flowing man's wig. 18th century.

CASHEW DYE A hair dye consisting of the fluid between the kernel and the shell of the fruit of *anarcardium occidentale*. Every shade of brown to black may be produced by it. (*Cooley*)

CASQUE, THE A woman's hair style of 1830 in which all the hair was combed together and tied up at the very top of the head like that of a Chinese woman and there raised in bows or plaits over wire or whalebone foundations into a kind of reversed pyramid. (*Ladies' Companion*, 1851.)

CASQUE (1) A foundation to dress the hair over.

(2) A helmet-shaped arrangement of the hair.

CASQUE A LA CLORINDE A late 18th century hair style for a woman. (*Villermont*) 223

CASSIA-LIGNUM An aromatic bark from Ceylon and other tropical islands, used in perfumery. (*Lillie*)

CAST See Plaster cast.

CASTILE SOAP A soap prepared from olive oil and soda, with a hard, close grain containing but little water in combination and coloured by protosulphate of iron. (*Piesse*)

CASTING BOTTLE A bottle for sprinkling perfumed water, formerly used by barbers to annoint the hair and beard of their customers. (*Toone*)

'Now as sweet and neat as a barber's casting bottle.' (*History of Antonio and Mellida*, 1602. See also *John Ford, The Fancies, Chast and Noble*, 1638 for other references.)

CASTLE CLIP A bobbed hair style *c* 1915 popularised by Irene Castle, the dancer. (*AH* 1915)

CASTLE LOCKS A high headdress. (*Rev John Logan, Poems* 2nd ed, 1782)

CASTLE SOAP A soap made from tallow, 19th century. (*Lillie*) 'There'l be no need of castle-soap.' (*Ovidius Exulans*, 1673. *Wing* 0.699)

CASTOR OIL A fixed oil, *qv*. Unsatisfactory for use on the hair in pure form as it becomes sticky and rancid.

CASUAL CURL A loose, irregularly shaped curl.

CASUAL STYLE A hair style of studied untidiness. Informal, haphazard, unlaboured.

CATAGAN A chignon of plaits or ringlet curls tied with a ribbon; 1870/75. See Cadogan from which catagan was originally derived.

CATAGAN HEAD DRESS Woman's style, late 19th century. Plaited hair at back was turned up and secured with a ribbon. Commonly worn by schoolgirls until *c* 1928, when short hair, the shingle and bob, largely replaced it.

CATAGAN NET A hair-net to enclose and secure the catagan. 19th century.

CATAGEN The state of changing from growth to a period of rest in a hair follicle.

CATECHU An astringent substance with tannin from the bark or part of certain fruits of eastern plants. Used in hair dyes in the 18/19th centuries.

CATHEDRAL BEARD A long beard, very broad at the bottom, spreading like the tail of a fish, worn by Bishops and dignitaries of the Church. Mid 16th to 17th century. (*Holme*)

CATHERINE DE MEDICI COIFFURE (1519–1589) Daughter of Lorenzo de Medici and Queen (1533) of Henry II of France. A hairdress in the style worn by her.

CATHERINE THE GREAT COIFFURE A hairdress in the style worn by this Empress of Russia (Catherine II), b 1729, d 1796, her reign was marked by increased contact with the west. At this period French culture and fashions were predominant in Europe.

CATOGAN (1) Club of hair in powdered hairdress. 18th century. See Cadogan.

(2) Club of hair. 19th century. 388

CATOGAN CHIGNON A twist with a four-strand plait and ribbon bow. (*Creer*) 419(2)

CATOGAN PLAIT COIFFURE A late 19th century hair style for women in which the catogan plait is featured. (*Mallemont*)

CATOGAN TRAVELLING HEADDRESS A 19th century hair style for women similar to the catogan plait coiffure, not easily disarrayed and suitable for a woman who was to make a journey.

CATOGAN-WIG A man's wig with a wide queue that was folded back on itself and secured with a black ribbon. Also called Club wig. Late 18th century. 92(5.6)

CATTLE-MARKER A pair of small, curved scissors used for cutting ownership marks in the hair of cattle and recently (since *c* 1945) used by some hairdressers for haircutting, especially hair tapering.

CAUCASIAN HAIR See European hair.

CAUL (CAWL) (1) In the medieval period a net of gold or other thread which was used to confine the hair of noble ladies. Also a small cap for covering the head like a skull cap.

'Let se, which is the proudest of hem alle,
That werith on a coverchief or a calle.'
(*Chaucer, Wife of Bath's Tale*, 1388)

'A caul to cover the haire of the head withall, as maydens use.' (*William Clerk, A Little Dictionarie for Children*, ed 1622)

'Her head with ringlets of her hair is crowned,
And in a golden caul the curls are bound.'
(*Dryden, Virgil*, 1697)

Also called crestine, creton, crespine and crespinette.

(2) A cap-shaped wig net of soft, supple open weave, used for the crown area of a wig. 19/20th century. See also Caul net.

(3) The plain part at the back of a woman's cap.

(4) The membrane enclosing the foetus, a part of which is sometimes found on the child's head. This was believed to be a good omen and a charm against drowning.

CAUL CAP A kind of net skull cap with a draw string in the centre for adjustment to incorporate in a wig and cover the crown area of the head.

CAULIFLOWER WIG A white, close curled, bob wig of short hair commonly worn by the dignified clergy and physicians in the 18th century and from late 18th century to early 19th century by coachmen. (*London Mag*, 1753, *Grose*) 258

CAUL NET The soft net of silk or other suitable material used for the crowns of wigs. Late 17th to 20th century. 'To the foretop of his wig . . . down to the very net work named the caul.' (*Dr John Wolcot, Peter Pindar*, 1786)

CAUSTIC POTASH Potassium hydroxide, KOH.

CAUSTIC SODA Sodium hydroxide, NaOH.

CAVALIER A long, curled lock of hair. 17/18th century.

CAVALIERE See A la Cavaliere.

CAXON WIG Called Caxton originally and until after 1725. So named after a murderer who disguised himself in a wig but was hanged and exposed on the gibbet near Caxton, a market town in Cambridgeshire. Hence arose the name Caxton for a weather-beaten wig, which was the word's original connotation. (*Stukeley MS*, 1725). The term was later applied to a kind of tie wig worn chiefly by professional men. A big Cauliflower wig, *qv*. See Woty's poem *The Caxon*, 1760. Even later the word was used as a synonym for wig. (*Brewer*). In Sir Walter Scott's *The Antiquary*, 1816, the name of the wig-dresser is Caxon.

CAXTON See Caxon.

C-CURL (1) A pin curl formed flat on the head in a clockwise direction. (*Morris*)

(2) A semi-circular or crescent curl, *qv*.

CC CURL A pin curl that is formed flat on the head in a counter or anti-clockwise direction. (*Morris*)

CERTIFIED COLOUR a safe, temporary colour that coats the hair and can be removed by shampooing. American usage.

CHAFER (1) A vessel for heating water, 14th century and later.

(2) A portable grate; a chafing dish. From 15th century (*Procter*, p 203)

CHAFING DISH A vessel with burning charcoal inside used in 15/17th century for heating curling tongs. Also used for keeping warm, articles such as dishes placed on it. (*Procter* p 203)

CHAIN BUCKLE A curled wig worn by men in the mid-18th century (*London Mag*). See En-chaine.

CHAIN-PLAIT Take four small strands of hair, plait with only three of them, weaving them over and under the fourth, which serves to draw the chain up, in the way in which a plait of three is usually worked. Taking first the left hand outside strand and working it under one and over the next until it takes the place of the right outside strand, which in its turn is worked to the left side and so on, alternately, always retaining one strand unmoved in the middle. (*Ladies' Companion*, 1851. *Elegant Arts*.)

CHAIN STITCH See Stitching.

CHAMOIS LEATHER Pliable leather made from sheep, goat or deer hide. Used in boardwork for covering ends of flat springs, etc.

CHAMOMILE SHAMPOO A soft soap shampoo or shampoo in powder form incorporating chamomile, an aromatic creeping plant with daisy-like flowers, extracts of which are used as a tonic, as chamomile tea and as a hair wash.

CHAMPAGNE A notable French hairdresser of the mid 17th century, who displayed a genius for creating new styles. He was hairdresser to Princess Marie de Gonzague and Queen Christine of Sweden. (*Villermont*)

CHANCELLOR A wig worn by men in the 18th century. (*London Mag*)

CHAPLET (1) A wreath of flowers, ribbons, jewels, etc, for the head.

(2) A wreath of curls or worked hair worn around the head.

CHARACTER-WIG A theatrical wig personating the character being played by the actor.

CHARLES THE BALD Charles II, Emperor of Germany, born 823, d 877.

CHARLESTON-CUT Short bobbed hair style dressed in waves, c 1925.

CHARLEY, A (1) 19th century slang term for the Imperial Tuft, a small beard confined to the chin. Also called a Royal (19th century) and a Mouche (19th century).

(2) A small moustache as worn by Charles Chaplin, the film star. See also Charlie.

(3) A film extra with a moustache. American slang. (*B and B*)

CHARLIE A small moustache, as worn by Charlie Chaplin. See also Charlie Chaplin moustache.

CHARLIE CHAPLIN MOUSTACHE A small toothbrush moustache worn and made famous by Charlie Chaplin, the 20th century film comedian.   *101F*

CHARLOTTE CORDAY A hair style worn by the French woman Marie Charlotte Corday d'Armans (1768–1793), the slayer of Marat.

CHASE-ME-CHARLIE A kiss curl.

CHASSEUR See Au chasseur.

CHATAIN Chestnut or nut brown colour.

CHATELAINE Castellan lady; name given to the 'berthes' or large plaits. (*Creer*)

CHATTER, V. To rapidly and continuously open and close the Marcel waving irons when forming the crest of a wave.

CHATTERING The rapid and continuous opening and closing of the Marcel waving irons when forming the crest of a wave.

CHAUVE French for bald.

CHEATING IRONS See Revolving sleeve.

CHEEK-WAVE A wave that overlies a part of the cheek, *cf*, Forehead wave.

CHEESE CUT A haircut in which all the hair is cut off and the head shaved. See also Kojak cut. 19th century.

CHEMICAL BLONDE A woman with artificially bleached hair. Slang. (*B and B*)

CHEMICAL BREAKAGE Damage to hair from chemicals used in dyeing, bleaching or permanent curling, resulting in hair breakage.

CHEMICAL RAZOR A depilatory.

CHEMISE A teenage hair style of 1962 in which the hair is allowed to hang loosely. Name probably derived from the then prevalent habit of girls wearing men's shirts and allowing them to hang loosely over their slacks or trousers.

CHENILLE HAIRNET A large-mesh net of chenille for decoratively covering the hair. Popular in the Victorian period. (*The Ladies' Treasury*, 1859)

CHERUB A short hair style based on the bingle, with soft waves and sculptured curls forming a halo at the back and sides. From Spring 1932.

CHERUB LOOK A hairdo of loose curl. 20th century.

CHESTER, THE English hair style for men (*Foan*)

CHESTEN Chestnut colour. 'Faire aburne or chesten colour,' 1576.

CHEST MAT (1) A man's chest hair.

(2) A chest wig. Slang. 1920s.

CHESTNUT (chesnut) colour. Since 17th century the colour of a chestnut, deep reddish brown; but originally the colour of a newly husked chestnut, light reddish brown. 'Faire aburne or chesten (chestnut) colour,' 1576.

CHEST WIG A light-weight wig worked on a hair net foundation, for disguising the bare chests of men to increase their appearance of virility when exposed for bathing or sunning at the seaside. One advertisement in the 1920s read: 'Be a real he-man, wear a Tarzan chest wig'.

CHEVALIER A hairdresser. (*Hone, W, Year Book*, 1832; *Column*, 1509)

CHEVELER A wig. (*Fairholt*)

CHEVELU French word meaning 'hairy'.

CHEVELURE French word for a head of hair.

CHEVELURE EN PORC-EPIC See Porcupine hairdress.

CHEVEU (pl cheveux) The French word for hair.

CHEVRON BANG A fringe that is cut to a point. American usage.

CHEVRON MOUSTACHE A moustache extending beyond the corners of the lips, wide in the centre and narrower towards the ends. (*Trusty*)   *101D*

CHEVRON NECK CUT A V-shaped neck line. (*Trusty*)

CHIEN COUCHANT Woman's coiffure. 18th century
369

CHIFFON A thin gauze used in certain postiche foundations.

CHIFFONIER HAIR Waste hair collected by the chiffonier (the French equivalent of the rag and bone man) from garbage heaps, where it had been consigned as combings amongst the household rubbish. See also Waste air. (*Creer*)

CHIGNON (1) A large bunch or coil of hair worn at the back of the head or nape of the neck and often dressed over a pad. (2) An artificial back hair piece of no particular shape or size. (*Creer*)   *144(5, 6), 333, 334*

CHIGNON A DEUX TRESSES An 18th century hair style for women. (*Uzanne*)

CHIGNON ALOPECIA *Alopecia compressio* in the posterior region of the vertex or back of the head.

CHIGNON BALDNESS See *Alopecia compressio*.

CHIGNON BLOCK A malleable block on which chignons are dressed.

CHIGNON CAGE Usually a hemispherical wire shape covered in mohair, used as a foundation for a chignon hairdress. These cages were made in different sizes and shapes. 19th century.

CHIGNON CUSHION A rounded, cloth-covered (usually velvet) cushion, flattened at the top and bottom and filled with compressed hair or other suitable material, on which chignons and other pieces of small postiche may be dressed.

CHIGNONED Wearing a chignon.

CHIGNON EN CROIX DE CHEVALIER 18th century hair style for women. (*Uzanne*)   *370*

CHIGNON EN QU'ES-ACO 18th century hair style for women. (*Uzanne*)   *375*

CHIGNONETTE A small postiche chignon.

CHIGNON FLOTTANT 18th century term for one or more loops of hair hanging down the back of the head to the neck.

CHIGNON FUNGUS A fungus which was supposed to have commonly been found on women's chignons in the 1860s; but whatever this fungus may have been it had nothing to do with chignons as such. Nevertheless the Chignon Fungus scare was used in the attack on the fashion of chignons which was described as unhygienic. (*Creer and Beigel*)

CHIGNON KNOT A knot of hair, such as a gordian knot, Grecian knot, etc, worn as a chignon. (*Creer*)

CHIGNON MARTEAU A marteau of hair suitable for dressing as a chignon. (*Creer*)

CHIGNON NET A net to enclose a chignon.

CHIGNON NORMAND A full chignon of smooth folded hair, after a style worn by the peasants of Normandy in the 19th century   *334*

CHIGNON NOUE 18th century hair style for women. (*Uzanne*)   *373*

CHIGNON PERON A knotted semi-circular postiche strip for wear at the nape to transform a shingle into a long-hair dressing. (*Hairdressing*, Sept 1925)

CHIGNON QUADRILLE A woman's topknot constructed with long hair. (*Taylor Briggs*). With this exception, every other use of the word chignon refers to a coil, lump or dressing of hair on the back of the head. The word is a French export and still has its original meaning – nape of the neck – in France. This chignon has 'quadrilled' from its expected position to the supreme point of dominance usually occupied by the topknot.

CHIGNON RECAMIER Early 19th century hair style for women. Named after the style of chignon worn by Madame Recamier (1777–1849), famous leader of French society.

(*Coiffure Européen*, 1876)

CHIGNON UNIVERSEL Made of straight and creoled hair on a comb and worn to make good a deficiency in the back hair. (*Creer*)

CHILD'S HAIRCUTTING CHAIR A small-seat, high-legged, revolving chair (or an ordinary high chair with footrest) for the use of children when having their hair cut. 19/20th century.

CHINA CLAY See Kaolin.

CHINA HAIR Pubic hair. Hair as exposed to the china chamber pot. 'How often have these novices with their downy chins, and a few *china* hairs, been crowned acteon-like, with spacious horns . . .' (*Wiltoringold*, 1742)

CHIN ARMOUR A false beard. Slang. American usage. (*B and B.*)

CHINA WATER A 19th century hair-dye consisting of nitrate of silver 1 oz, hydrated lime 4 oz dissolved in water.

CHINCHILLAS The beard. Slang. American usage. (*B and B*)

CHIN CURTAIN BEARD American usage. See Collier (*Trusty*)   *97A*

CHINESE HAIR A dark, coarse type of human hair from Chinese and other oriental heads, imported into England for the manufacture of theatrical wigs and cheap fashion-wear wigs. Inferior to European hair for necessity wigs or best quality fashion wigs.

CHINESE RAZOR SHARPENER The same as Cowvan's Canton Strop, *qv*.

CHINESE STYLE (1) A coiffure style dressed in large curves.
(2) The hair combed towards the crown, away from the forehead, cheeks and neck and dressed to that basic conception was known as the Chinese style or à la Chinoise, in the mid-Victorian period.   *327*

CHINESE WASH A dangerous solution of silver used in the 18th/19th century to dye hair. Instances are recorded of persons being reduced to frenzy after the application of this dye to their hair. (*Toilette*, 1832)

CHINESE WIG A wig with a pigtail imitating the hair-styles of the Chinese in the 18th century. Theatrical use.

CHINOIS Chinese. (*Fr*)

CHINONG – Chignon, *qv*. The form used by Stewart in 1782.

CHIN PUFF Small beard on chin tip. American usage. (*Trusty*)

CHIN SCRAPER A barber. 18th century. (*The Barber's Wedding*)

CHIN WHELK See *Tinea sycosis*. (*Wheeler*)

CHIN WIG A false beard. 18th century. (*Dulaure*)

CHIRURGICAL TIE See Physical tie. 18th century.

CHIVE, TO To shave. Slang. American usage. (*B and B*)

CHIZZELLED WIG A short cut wig. Probably similar to cauliflower wig, *qv*. 'White chizzel'd wig.' (Short account of the new pantomine *Omai* by John O'Keefe, 1785)

CHLOE HAIRDRESS A woman's style of 1866. The top waved and curled, some bunch ringlets winding amongst the hair at the back. The bandelettes arranged as shown in the figure.   *337(5)*

CHLORHEXIDINE $C_{22}H_{30}Cl_5N_{10}$ Used in a 1% aqueous solution to disinfect hair for use in boardwork.

CHOISY See A la Choisy.

CHOLESTEROL $C_{27}H_{46}O$ Principal sterol of the higher animals. Prepared commercially from spinal cord of cattle and from wool grease. Used in hair creams, lotions, conditioners and hair waving preparations.

CHONGO Hair tied into a bundle or club at the nape of the neck of Pueblo Indian. Colorado, USA.

CHOUX The round bun or bundle of hair worn at the back of the head, resembling a cabbage. A chignon. (*Fairholt*)

CHRISTIAN DIOR Verb. To dress hair, body and extremities in a most fashionable and exclusive style. 'Christian Dior me,' 1978. After the world famous French couturier, Christian Dior.

CHRIST'S CUT The beard cut round like 'halfe of a Holland cheese'. 16th century. (*Greene, a quip for an upstart courtier,* 1592)

CHRIST'S HAIR Hart's tongue fern. Guernsey usage.

CHRISTY WAVECUT The American, Kenneth A. Christy, introduced his method of wave cutting to England in 1938. See Wavecutting. (*Daily Herald,* 1 Sept 1938)

CHUFF HEADED Having a big, fat, hairy head. 16th century.

CHUFFY Puffed-out hair. Used in this sense on BBC Aug 1967. 'Her frizzed hair gave her head a chuffy appearance.'

CHURCH HAIR Hair purchased from European nunneries, used for postiches.

CIBBER, COLLEY (1671–1757) The English actor and dramatist had a wig of such noble proportions for one of his theatrical parts that it was brought upon the stage in a sedan chair by the chairmen. (*Creer*)

CICATRICIAL BALDNESS Baldness caused by scarring. (*Lubowe*)

CILEX Haircloth. Latin word. Medieval English usage. (*Fisher*)

CILICIOUS Belonging to hair cloth. (*Glosso*)

CILIUM (Latin) Eyelash, plural cilia.

CINCINNI The hair hanging behind the ears. See Hair nomenclature.

CINIFLONES The Roman slaves who dressed their mistresses' hair.

CINQUEFOIL A five lobed grouping of hair.

CIRCASSIAN PLAIT See Plait.

CIRCASSIENE A Grecian hair plait. (*Creer*)

CIRCINATION (Subs.) A circling or turning round.

CIRCULAR BEARD A style in which the outline of the beard forms three parts of a circle. 99(13)

CIRCULAR BRUSH A brush with its bristles encircling the spine of the brush. Also called blow-wave brush, *qv*.

CIRCULAR PAD A hair pad made of crepe hair in a circular form. Larger than a ring pad.

CIRCUMFERENCE BAND Bind ribbon, *qv*.

CIRCUMFERENCE RIBBON The same as bind ribbon, *qv*.

CIREE Waxed. 'A moustache cirée.' (*J Ashby Sterry, The Shuttlecock Papers,* 1873)

CIRE A MOUSTACHE Moustache wax, *qv*.

CISSERS Scissors. (*Levens,* 1570)

CITIZENS' SUNDAY BUCKLE An 18th century man's wig that had several tiers of curls around the back and sides. Facetious name for a long bob wig. Also called Bob-Major, *qv*. (*L C March,* 1762)

CITRIC ACID (Anhydrous Ch_8O_7) Used in depilatories, hair rinses and hair curling and colouring preparations. Its commonest hairdressing use is as a hair rinse. 3%–5% acid to 97%–95% water dilution. Non-toxic in usual doses. (*Sagarin*)

CITRONELLA (*Andropogonis nardi*) The oil from lemon grasses of Ceylon and Java, used for perfuming shampoos. (*Verrill*)

CITRONELLE See Citronella.

CIVET A substance once used in perfumery. It is a secretion of the *Viverra Civetta* or civet cat and is formed in a large double glandular receptacle between the anus and the pudendum of the animal. In its pure state civet has, to most

people, a disgusting odour but when diluted to an infinitesimal proportion its odour is most agreeable. (*Plesse*)
'He rubs himself with civet.' (*Shakespeare, Much Ado,* iii. 2)
'Lady, I would descend to kiss thy hand
But that 'tis gloved, and civet makes me sick.' (*Massinger,* 17th century)

CIVET CAT A dandy, 18th century. Because of their use of civet, a musk-like perfume obtained from the civet cat. (*Pope, Epilogue to the Satires*)

CIVET HAIR POWDER A starch hair powder, scented with civet. 18/19th century. (*Lillie*)

CLAMP See Curling clamp.

CLARA-BOW STYLE Similar to the Crimp (3), *qv*. Clara Bow was a famous film actress of the 1920s.

CLARK GABLE MOUSTACHE A neat thin line moustache similar to that worn by the American film star, Clark Gable from the 1930s.

CLASSICAL HAIR STYLE (1) A Greek or Roman style.
(2) A hair style of any period that portrays the characteristic qualities of Greek and Roman art, such as simplicity, discipline, order, restraint, objectivity, harmony, proportion, etc. The opposite to the Romantic hair style, *qv*.

CLASSICAL POSTICHE A phrase coined by A. Mallemont *c* 1896 to include the following artificial additions of hair for the head: tails or switches, plaits, curls, marteaux, pincurls, frizettes, chignons, knotted fringes, transformations and wigs.

CLASSING The separations of turned and drawn waste hair, *qv* into three length groups: (A). The longest for plaits; (B). Middle lengths for chignons and (C). Short for men's wigs. (*Creer*)

CLASTOTHRIX See *Trichorrhexis nodosa*.

CLAWING See Claw out.

CLAW OUT, TO Using the initial tooth of a comb or rake to disentangle hair is called 'clawing out the tangle'.

CLEAN CUTTING Cutting without slithering or tapering. Club cutting is achieved by this method.

CLEANING This word refers to the cleansing of postiches. It is not used in connection with the growing hair. See Shampoo.

CLEANING POSTICHES The cleansing of wigs and other postiches by means of spirit, petrol (gasoline) purified and without additives, and, with great care, carbon tetrachloride, *qv*. Raw, unworked hair is cleansed in soap solutions which are unsuitable for worked hair as they would cause loosening of the anchored hair and tangling.

CLEANING SOLUTION (for wigs) Pure petrol; solvent SBP 1–6; carbon tetrachloride (not recommended).

CLEANSING HAIR See Shampoo.

CLEAVAGE The cleft, split or division in a coiffure. See also parting.

CLEO BANDEAU An almost straight front of hair, the ends usually being dressed in curls or a low chignon at the middle back part of the head. 385

CLEOPATRA LOOK A woman's hair style of Egyptian origin popularised by the actress Elizabeth Taylor in the title part of the film *Cleopatra*. From 1962.

CLERGYMAN'S BOB See Long bob. (*KP,* May 1739)

CLERICAL WIG See Long bob.

CLIP (1) Any metal or plastic appliance for the hair which secures it in position, by tightly gripping the hair.
(2) VT. To cut hair with a clipper.
(3) VT. To club-cut hair with scissors.

CLIP MARK A noticeable indentation in a curl caused by the pressure of a metal clip during the drying of the hair.

CLIP-ON HEADBAND A semi-circular, resilient, decorated headband of metal or plastic, which clips over the top or front of the head. They are sometimes covered with worked curls. When undecorated they are often called Alice bands.

CLIPPER (1) An instrument for clipping the hair, consisting of a moveable plate with serrations, which moves laterally across a serrated fixed plate, cutting the hair between the serrations at the points of contact. See also Hand clipper and Electric clipper.
Number:
0000 cuts hair nearly as close as shaving
000 cuts hair 1/100″ in length
00 cuts hair 1/64″ in length
0 cuts hair 1/32″ in length
0A cuts hair 3/64″ in length
1 cuts hair ⅛″ in length
2 cuts hair ¼″ in length. (*Hovenden*)
(2) A barber. 15th century.

CLIPPING (1) The removal of neck hair, etc. by means of the hand clippers.
(2) Cutting off the tips of the hairs by the use of scissors.

CLIPPING COMB the same as Neck-comb, *qv*.

CLIPPINGS The hair ends that have been cut or clipped off the head.

CLITPOLE A head of frizzed, curled or tangled hair. Dorset and Somerset usage. (*Barnes*)

CLITTY Tangled. Dorset, Somerset. 'Her hair be all clitty.' (*Barnes*)

CLOCK-SPRING Positional spring, *qv*.

CLOCK-SPRING CURL A curl in which the diameter of the inside curled hair is smaller than the diameter of the curled hair on the outside of the curl. 199

CLOCKWISE Going in the direction of the movement of the hands of a clock.

CLOSED CURL A clock-spring curl, *qv*.

CLOSE PLAIT Three or more strands of hair firmly and evenly interlaced to form the plait.

CLOSE SHAVING A double shave or twice over in which the second shave is given against the growth of the beard. It is an undesirable practice on many faces and can cause considerable skin irritation and even eruptions.

CLOSE WEFT See Once-in weft.

CLOSE WORK Working a drawn-through parting.

CLOUDY A woman's hair style of Victorian times in which the hair was dressed to a middle parting with loose, bedraggled, waved tresses hanging like hound's ears on each side of the head, and a chignon at the back. (*HTATH*)

CLOVE Cloves are sometimes added to a henna paste to give a deeper shade; also used in some toilet preparations for men to give a 'manly' tang. The clove is the dried flower bud of *Eugenia Aromatica*, a tropical tree of the Myrtle family. (*Van Dean*)

CLUB Verb. To cut hair straight across. See also Club cutting.

CLUBBED ENDS The ends or points of the hair that are club cut.

CLUBBING (1) Club cutting. The cutting of hair straight across so that all cut hair between the scissor blades and the scalp are of equal length.
(2) In boardwork, drawing-off hair in such a way that the drawn-off ends of the hair (points or roots) lie in the same plane.

CLUBBING KNIFE A drawing knife.

CLUB CUT See Club cutting.

CLUB CUTTING Cutting hair straight across so that all cut hair between the scissor blades and the head are the same length, *cf* Taper cutting.

CLUB WIG The same as a Catogan wig, *qv*.

CLUMP See Club.

CLUMPING (1) Cutting en masse; club cutting. (*Foan*)
(2) See Clumps.

CLUMPS (Pinching irons) A pair of iron forceps with discoid ends, used when heated, in a process called clumping that consisted of heating between paper the curled hair of the head. See also Curl paper and Papillotage. (*The Journal of the British Archaeological Association*, 1876)

CLUMPY HAIR Thick, clubbed hair. West country usage.

CLUSTER (1) Short lengths of hair mounted in a small frame, worn to give height to the crown.
(2) A group of curls.

COACHMAN'S CURLY A long haired, curled wig 'coming entirely over the shoulder'. 18/early 19th century. (*Spirit of the Public Journals*, 1824)

COALMIN A Celtic woman's name meaning 'soft haired'. (*Long*)

COAL TAR COLOURS Colours obtained by the distillation and chemical treatment of coal tar, a product of coal during the manufacture of coal gas.

COARSE WIG NET See Caul net.

COATING See Colour coating and Coating dye.

COATING DYE A hair dye that does not penetrate the hair shaft, but adheres to the outer face of the hair cuticle, coating it.

COCKADE A stand-up hair decoration of ribbon, flowers, etc.

COCKATOO A young child's style in which the young growth of hair is brushed into a ridge in the centre of the head.

COCKERNONY (Scot) The gathering of a woman's hair, when it is wrapped or snooded up with a band or snood. (*Ramsay*)

COCKES BEARD A little beard. 16th/17th century. (*Percival*)

COCKLE-CURL A small curl like a Snail curl, *qv*. 16th/17th century. 'Instant she sped to curl the cockles of her new-bought head.' (*Du Bartas*)

COCKLE SHELL A single stem tail coiled into a cockle shell shape.

COCKLESHELL COIFFURE A short hair style which followed the Eton crop. Popular in 1927. (*Daily News*)

COCKSCOMB, COCK'S COMB or COXCOMB (1) A back-combed, high dressed, elongated curl or half curl forming a feature at the front of coiffure. Name derived from the cock's comb or crest. Popular in the 1920s.
(2) A ludicrous appellation for the head.
(3) Man's hair style, 1920s 261

COCKTAIL BANG A curl shaped like the letter J, dressed on the forehead. Slang. American usage (*B and B*)

COCKTAIL SHAMPOO (1) A temporary colour toner incorporated in a shampoo. American usage.
(2) A mixture of different shampoos and ingredients, such as chamomile and olive oil, or pine tar and hydrogen peroxide, etc.

COCKTAIL STYLE A hair style suitable for wear at a cocktail party.

COCOA BUTTER (Cacao butter) A fatty substance obtained from the cacao nut. It is used for making pomades. Also called lactine pomade in the 18th century. (*Brodie, Price List*, 1890)

COCONUT BOB A popular short bobbed hair style for women, 1926, in which the hair was cut short with a thick fringe and no parting. 410

COCONUT OIL Copra oil. Expressed oil from the kernels of *cocos nucifera*, Latin: *Palmae*. Used in the manufacture of shampoo, soap and hair dressing.

COCUS COMB A comb made of cocus wood (*Brya Ebenus*), a small tree from the West Indies, also called Jamaica ebony, 1688. (*Holme*)

COHESIVE SET A hair set in which is used a strong setting lotion to hold the hair firmly in position; in which the hairs are sticking together.

COIF Substantive (1) A close-fitting cap or skull cap;
(2) An ecclesiastical headdress;
(3) A white cap worn by a lawyer;
(4) The inner lining of a helmet;
(5) A coiffure or headdress, since *c* 1950. 'A shining new coif.' (WO 10 October 1964)
(6) The head hair especially the forelock or top hair, 17th century. From coif, a close-fitting cap. This usage does not appear in the *OED*. 'Else, sure as he was void of life, Sybil had pull'd him by the coife.' (*John Phillips, Maronides* 1672)
(7) An English hair style for men.   *104A*

COIF Verb. To dress or arrange the hair of the head. 'The soubrette who sells you a cigar is coiffed as for a ball.' (*Willis Pencillings* 11, LX11, 174, 1835)

COIFFAGE A hair-dress, the styled and dressed hair.

COIFFE (1) Subs. A headdress. See Coif.
(2) Verb. Fr. Having the head dressed.
Coiffé d'une peruque = wearing a wig.

COIFFER Fr. To dress hair.

COIFFER STE CATHERINE To be 25 years of age and still unmarried.

COIFFEUR A male hairdresser.

COIFFEUR DE DAMES A male ladies' hairdresser. *Coiffeuse de Dames* – a female ladies' hairdresser.

COIFFEUR D'HOMMES Barber or male gentlemen's hairdresser. *Coiffeuse d'hommes* – a female gentlemen's hairdresser.

COIFFEUR POSTICHEUR A hairdresser wigmaker.

COIFFEUSE A female hairdresser.

COIFFURE A headdress. 1631.

COIFFURE A LOGE DE L'OPERA A high hairdress designed for Marie Antoinoinette, Queen of France. It was 'composed of numberless plumes, waving at the top of a hair tower'. (*Guernsey Magazine*, October 1884)

COIFFURE BONNET A light-weight bonnet type covering for a dressed head of hair to hold it in position and protect it from wind or other disarranging factors.

COIFFURE BOURGEOISE 18th century hair style for women. (*Uzanne*)

COIFFURE BOURGEOISE PETITE MALTRESSE 18th century hair style for women. (*Uzanne*)

COIFFURE CUT OUT A photographic mask of hair.

COIFFUREDOM The world of the hairdresser. American usage. (*Hairdo* Jan, 1965 NY)

COIFFURE EN BANDEAU A hairdress in which the front section is dressed flat in waves at right angles to the forehead. (*Mallemont*)

COIFFURE EN COLISEE 18th century hair style for women. (*Uzanne*)

COIFFURE EN CROCHETS 18th century hair style for women. (*Uzanne*)

COIFFURE EN POIRE A pear-shaped hair style.

COIFFURE HURLUBERLU See Hurluberlu.

COIFFURE PUFF A hair style in which the front hair is dressed puffed with curls. (*Mallemont*)

COIFFURISTE A woman who dresses hair. A made word derived from the anglicised French word coiffure – the way one's hair is dressed. 20th century. (*Wykes-Joyce*)

COIL A twisted tress of hair, arranged in concentric circles.

COILED CHIGNON A chignon dressed in a coil, *qv*.   *197*

COILED TORSADE A coil composed of a one or two-stem twisted switch.

COIL FRAME A semi-spherical, circular or oval frame, constructed of wire and mohair, with a hole in the middle of the circular type, and near the top of the oval type. The hair was drawn through the hole and the frame secured to the head hair. The drawn-through tail was then dressed over the frame in a coil.

COIL SPRING Tension spring, *qv*.

COIL OF HAIR See Coil.

COLD PERMANENT WAVE The transformation of straight hair to curled hair by means of chemicals without the application of heat. Some of these chemicals can be dangerous if not correctly used and even accidental death has resulted in their use during the process of permanent waving. (See *Journal of the American Medical Association*, Vol 116, No. 14, also *Wickenden*)

COLD WAVE See Cold permanent wave.

COLD WAVING See Cold permanent wave.

COLD WAVING SOLUTION The chemicals used to produce a cold permanent wave, *qv*. Modern formulae are based on thioglycolates. A formula suggested by Keithler is as follows: Thioglycolic acid (75%) 18.6 g; Ammonia (28%) 18.0 cc; Wetting agent 0.2g; Distilled water 200.0 cc. (*Sagarin*)

COLEMAN MOUSTACHE See Ronald Coleman moustache.   *101Z*

COLETA CURL A half curl, like the J-shaped decoration on the matador's hat. (*Hairdo*, January 1965)

COLIGNY, GASPARD de (1519-72) French Admiral and Huguenot leader who carried his toothpick in his beard. In the 16th century the beard was commonly used for this purpose.

COLLIER BEARD Beard style comprising a fringe of whiskers, but leaving the lips clean shaven. Also called Farmer Giles.

COLLIWOG A wig hat of synthetic hair, 1962.

COLLODION A solution of 4 g, pyroxylin (chiefly nitrocellulose) in 100 ml of a mixture of 1 vol alcohol and 3 vols ether. It contains approximately 70% ether and 24% absolute alcohol by volume. A clear, syrupy liquid which, when exposed in thin layers, evaporates and leaves a tough, colourless film. Flammable. Used to cover the dye patch in the application of dye to the skin to test the subject's reaction.

COLLODIUM See Collodion.

COLLOID A substance of a non-crystalline semi-solid kind, suspended or dispersed in a suitable medium, eg gelatine and starch.

COLLOIDAL BLEACH A chemical substance of non-crystalline semi-solid type in suspension or dispersed in a medium.

COLLOIDAL SETTING-LOTION Of a semi-solid, non-crystalline kind dispersed or suspended in a suitable medium, eg starch in water. In consistency it may be thick or thin.

COLOGNE WATER See Eau de Cologne.

COLOMBIAN HAIR DYE (also called Argentine hair dye, etc) A 19th century hair dye consisting of: Hydrosulphuret of ammonia 1 oz; solution of potash 3 drachms; distilled water 1 oz. This solution was applied to the hair for 15 minutes, then a solution of nitrate of silver 1 drachm in distilled water, 2 oz was brushed in until the required shade was effected. (*Enquire Within*)

COLOUR A particular hue, one or any mixture of the constituents into which light decomposes as in the spectrum. Colour possesses three qualities: (1) Hue, ie the actual colour, such as brown or red, (2) Chroma which is the relative intensity of the colour, such as brilliant red or dull brown, and (3) Value, the modification of the colour by distance, light, etc.

COLOURANT See Dye (2).

COLOUR APPLICATION The application of a dye, tint or bleach to the hair of the head.

COLOUR BATH A preparation of liquid dye in which hair is immersed to dye or tint it. See Dyeing.

COLOUR BLEACH A process of changing the colour of hair by a preparation that bleaches and effects a colour change in one application.

COLOUR BLENDING (1) Combining different ingredients in order to produce the dye colour required.
(2) The process of securing a uniform colour throughout a strand or head of hair.

COLOUR BUILDER A filler, *qv*, used to provide a base on over-porous hair so that it can be effectively and evenly coloured by a dye.

COLOUR COATING A method of colouring hair by covering the surface of it with colour by means of a rinse, spray or other suitable application. Henna is an example of a coating dye.

COLOUR COMB Tail comb with a small absorbent sponge on the end of the tail.

COLOUR CREAM A hair dye incorporated in a cream.

COLOUR DEVELOPMENT The chemical and physical change which takes place in or on the hair shaft after the application of a dye.

COLOURED RINSE See Colour rinse. In English usage, colour or color (American spelling) should be preferred to coloured or colored rinse. A coloured rinse means that the rinse is coloured, but not that it will impart colour to the hair. Whereas a colour rinse means a rinse that will colour hair although the rinse itself could be colourless.

COLOURED STIFFENER Coloured lacquer.

COLOUR FOAM See Colour rinse.

COLOUR GRADING Colouring with tints passing into each other.

COLOURING That part of the hairdresser's art by which the hair receives its induced complexion together with lights and shadows. See also Dyeing.

COLOURING RINSE See Colour rinse.

COLOURING SHAMPOO See Colour shampoo.

COLOUR MIXING The mixing or blending of two or more shades in order to produce another desired shade.

COLOUR OIL BLEACH A process of changing the colour of hair by a preparation containing oil, dye and peroxide of hydrogen that bleaches and effects a colour change in one application.

COLOUR PACK A dye preparation in the form of a cream that after being applied to the hair is covered with a plastic dye hood to speed the development of the colour.

COLOUR REDUCER A preparation that will remove dye which has been applied to the hair.

COLOUR REDUCTION The removal of dye or colouring matter which has been applied previously to the hair.

COLOUR REMOVER (1) A preparation that will remove colour or dye from the head.
(2) A bleach.

COLOUR RESTORER A euphemism for a hair dye.

COLOUR RINSE (1) A water-borne temporary colour wash applied to hair and adhering only to the outside cuticle after shampooing or in the final shampoo rinse. From 1920s.
(2) Another type of 'colour rinse' will effect a slight but permanent change in the hair colour. Strictly this variety is a mild dye unlike the easily removable, temporary tint of (1)

above. With this second type it is essential to test the subject's susceptibility to dermatitis by means of a skin test. Since the second World War both types of colour rinse have been widely and successfully marketed directly to the public; but expert hairdressers were using both in their saloons as early as the 1920s.

COLOUR SHAMPOO A shampoo in which is incorporated colouring matter that will give slight added colour to the hair. See also Colour rinse.

COLOUR SPRAY The application of colour by means of a spray.

COLOUR TEST (1) Testing the developing of a colour by washing a part of a small strand of the dyed hair and viewing the development of the dye.
(2) Testing colour on a small strand of hair to observe its reaction and the development of the colour before committing the whole head to a colour treatment or dye. See also Strand test.

COLOUR TESTING See Colour test.

COLOUR TONE The colour quality or chroma. See Colour.

COLOUR TONER A weak tint used on bleached hair to impart a delicate shade. Example: Strawberry blonde.

COLOUR USAGE The use of dyes, tints, colour washes and bleaches on hair.

COMA (1) The hair of the head, particularly the head hair of a woman.
(2) A brush of hair. (*Bailey*). See Hair nomenclature.

COMACHROME This 19/20th century 'secret' black hair dye was a solution of silver nitrate with pyrogallic acid. (*Koller*)

COMATE Hairy; having long hair. 'How comate, crinite, caudate stars are fram'd.' (*Fairfax, Tasso*)

COMB (1) Subs. A toothed strip of plastic, bone, horn, tortoiseshell, vulcanite, ivory, wood, metal, etc, for disentangling, arranging, confining, or positioning the hair. A comb 'is a thing by which the hair of the head is layed smooth and streight and kept from growing into knotts and arslocks'. (*Holme*)

A 17th century description of 'the parts of a combe: The end teeth; the middle, the sides; the small teeth; the wide teeth, the back, having teeth on one side; round teeth having the teeth round and stiffe; flat teeth the teeth slender and thine (fine). Bastard teeth hath close teeth; open teeth, teeth wide asunder.

'Sorts of comb: The Horse or Mane Comb, a strong wood comb with a thick back. The wiske combe, have teeth on one side, and are wide and slender. The back tooth comb, having teeth but on one side. The beard comb, a small sort of comb, almost 4″ square. The double comb, two combs, one clasped into the other. The Merkin comb. The Peruwick comb, having round open and strong teeth. The small tooth comb, having teeth on both sides, one side wider than the other.

'Of what combs are generally made: Wood combs, made of light and closed wood as black thorn; Box combs, made of Box tree; Horn combs, made of oxe and cows horns, Ivory combs, made of elephants teeth, Bone combs, made of the shank bones of horses and other large beasts; Tortois combs, made of the sea and land tortois shell, the counterfeit combs of this sort are Horn stained with tortois shell colours; Cocus combs, made of cocus wood. Lead combs, used by such as have red hair, to make it of another colour.' 17th century (*Holme*).

'The combe is a necessary instrument for trimming of the head and seemeth (as touching the forms thereof) to have been devised by imitation of the back-bone of a fish: and serveth not onely for cleansing the head from danderuffe and other superfluities; but is of most use with women for shedding and trimming their haire and head-tires, wherein some of them bestow more labor for the adorning of them than their whole bodie is worth.' (*Guillim* p. 29)

'The various combs for various uses;
Fill'd up with dirt so clolely fixt,
No brush cou'd force a way betwixt;
A paste of composition rare,
Sweat, dandruff, powder, lead and hair.' (*Swift, The Lady's Dressing-Room*, 1730)

In Mechi's catalogue *c* 1840 the following types of comb are listed as being made by his workmen and offered for sale: Dressing, pocket, and tail combs in tortoiseshell, stained horn, and variegated horn. See also Tail comb, Rake, Dressing comb, Lady's comb, Setting comb, Cutting comb, Dust comb, Flea comb, Baby's comb, Double comb, Brushcomb, Tapered comb, Bladed comb, Pocket comb, Beard comb, Merkin comb*109, 136, 230, 242, 246*

(2) A toothed implement made of similar materials to (1) above. Used for holding the dressed hair in position and serving the same purpose as the hair pin. Many of this type of comb are ornamented. 'Ivorine Combe' listed as early as 1602. (*Clerk*) *135*

Tortoiseshell, Ivory, horn and buffalo horn fancy combs offered for sale in 1851 by W Pauly, A Moulton, and W H Brown of New York. (*Belden*)

See also Back comb, Side comb, Ornamental comb.

(3) Verb. To draw a comb through the hair.

(4) To beat on the head. Slang.

(5) A crest, ridge or protrusion of hair: a cockscomb. 'His beard . . . that comb of hair.' (*Lorna Doone*)

COMB BRUSH (1) A hairbrush with bristles of irregular lengths. They penetrate the hair better than brushes with bristles of equal lengths. (*The Ladies Treasury* 1859)

(2) A small, round, stiff brush used to clean between the teeth of hair combs. (*Diderot, and the Family Economist*, 1859)

COMB CLEANER (1) A strip of crinkled horse hairs secured at both ends. To use, one end of the strip is secured to an anchorage, the other end held in the hand and the comb teeth pushed into the strip and rapidly pushed backwards and forwards.

(2) A small stiff-bristled brush.

COMBINATION HONE Two types of hone incorporated back to back in a single unit, eg a carborundum and a swaty.

COMBING The action of drawing a comb through the hair to disentangle or arrange it.

COMBING CLOTH A hairdressing gown worn over the body to protect the clothes whilst the hair is receiving attention. 17/18th century. (*Boyer*)

COMBING OUT See Comb-out.

COMBINGS Mixed and matted hair combed from the head when women's hair was worn long. It was disentangled (got out), turned, *qv*, cleansed and classed (see Classing) preparatory to use in hair work. Women commonly collected their own combings and when they had sufficient took them to the wigmaker to be made into a switch or chignon. They were then still wearing their own hair!! (*Creer*)

Combings were also sold by women to hairdressers who cleaned them and then sold them to the wigmaker. 18th century to early 20th century.

COMBINGS CUP A hair tidy of porcelain or pottery for the reception of combings. Also called a hair-tidy.

COMBINGS JAR A large glazed, earthenware jar in which hair combings are sterilized before use for postiche.

COMBINGS HAIR Hair prepared for the wigmaker from combings.

COMBMAKERS, GUILD OF The earliest mention appears to be of a guild at Nürnberg in 1592. (*Yeats*)

COMB MARTEAU A large type of marteau mounted on a comb or slide. (*Symonds*)

COMB OUT (1) Subs. The act of combing the hair after setting and drying. 'The comb-out is not to be hurried.'

(2) Subs. The act of combing a head of hair as a preliminary to any further attention such as shampoo or haircut.

(3) Verb. To comb through the set and dried hairdress preparatory to the final arrangement of the tresses *cf* Brushout.

(4) Verb. To comb a head of hair.

COMBOUT American form. See Comb Out.

COMB QUEEN A self-conscious, compulsive, self-comber. A female addicted to continuous combing of her locks in public and brandishing her comb as a queenly staff of office.

COMB SLIP-ON A hairpiece attached to a comb.

COMB SPRAY A method of spraying an in-pli postiche by dipping the fine teeth of the dressing comb in water, holding the comb near the hair and running the thumb down the teeth. As the wet teeth return to their normal position they flick off the water onto the hair in a fine spray.

COMB TUFT A comb with hair attached for fixing to the temples or forehead to augment the natural hair of a woman. (*Walker*, 1837)

COMB WIG (COMB WIGG) Barber, 17/18th century term, facetious usage. (*D'Urfey*)

COMEDY HEAD 18th century man's theatrical wig style of a humorous appearance. (*Stewart*)

COMET 18th century man's wig style. (*London Magazine*)

COME-UP Verb. To develop. 'The colour has come-up too quickly.' Slang, 20th century.

COMFORTABLE-TEMPERATURE The temperature of the liquid that is acceptable to a client when being shampooed, rinsed, etc. Tastes differ, but a temperature between 35°C and 50°C is acceptable to the majority of clients.

COMMA CURL A flat partial curl, shaped like a printer's comma.

COMMA TAIL A loose hanging curl in the shape of a printed comma.

COMMETTE See A La Commette.

COMMODE A frame of wire, covered with silk 'on which the whole head-attire is adjusted at once upon a bust, or property of wood carved upon the breasts, like that which perruque-makers set upon their stalls'. 17th century. (*Evelyn*)

COMMON CUT 16th century hair style for men. Probably what would be called a bob cut to-day (1965). (*Stubbes*)

COMMON GREY 18th century man's theatrical wig style. (*Encyl Brit*)

COMPASS In the 18th century a graduated compass was used when haircutting, to aid the creation of the hair style and get its proportions correct. (*Legros*)

COMPATIBILITY TEST (1) A test used on a small strand of hair before a dye, bleach or permanent wave, to ensure that the chemicals used are compatible with the chemical composition of the previously treated hair will not cause it damage, and will produce the desired result in colour or curl.

(2) A skin test to determine the subject's reaction to a chemical used in dyeing or permanent waving. The same as Skin test, *qv*.

COMPLEMENTARY COLOURS Those colours that display the maximum of contrast in the colour spectrum, such as red opposite to green; and, when mixed, neutralize each other, producing shades of grey.

COMPOSITE COLOUR A colour produced by the mixture of two or more hues. For example: in the preparation of hair for postiches the mixing of light and dark brown hair to produce mid-brown.

COMPOSITION The organisation or arrangement of the hair in a hairdress by its manipulation into the desired form.

COMPOSITION MODEL An artificial bust for the display of wigs or other postiches.

COMPOUND HENNA See Henna.

CONCAVE With an outline curved like the interior of a circular object.

CONCAVE BRUSH A hair brush with the bristles set in a concave wooden base to conform to the shape of the head's surface. (*Walker*, 1837)

CONCAVE CHEEK WAVE A wave on the cheek, whose trough is pointing towards the ear.

CONCAVE RAZOR See Hollow-ground razor.

CONCAVE STROP Also called French strop. A rigid strop with a handle and two concave stropping surfaces, one of which is lined with leather, the other being of hard wood. (*Foan*)

CONCAVING The action of grinding the sides of razor blades to a concave shape.

CONCENTRATE A preparation that needs dilution before use.

CONCENTRE Fr. Concentrated.

CONDITIONER See Hair conditioner.

CONDITIONING CREAM Cream composed of chemicals that will improve the condition of the hair. They often contain lanolin or cholesterol. A published formula includes: Stearic acid, double pressed 11.2%, lanolin 1.4%, Cetyl alcohol 0.3%, Mineral oil 60/70 16.8%, Petrolatum, white 11.2%, water 56.2%, Preservative 0½1%, Perfume, QS.

CONDITIONING SHAMPOO A shampoo containing additives that will improve the condition of hair needing such attention.

CONE A wire or plastic conical shape over which the hair can be dressed for wear on the head. See Cage.

CONECTI, THOMAS A monk who preached against the high, extravagant, horned head-dresses of the women of his period. 15th century (*Speight*)

CONE HEADDRESS A high hair style worn by men of the Mashakulumbwe (Barotse) people of Northern Rhodesia. The hair was allowed to grow and built up with added hair around a sliver of Gemsbuck (*oryx gazella*) worn to a height of 4 ft or over. It was regarded as a visible and recognisable sign of masculine virility. The wearers were known as cone men. (Photo, Rev C. F. Pickering, 1895, from his ms diary) *250*

CONFIDANT A small curl near the ear, 17th century. (*Evelyn*)

CONGENITAL A condition prevailing from birth.

CONGENITAL ATRICHOSIS or ATRICHIA See *Atrichia congenita*.

CONGENITAL CALVITIES Hairless from birth. (*Wheeler*)

CONJOINED EYE-BROWS Regarded by the ancients as beautiful. Ovid records that Roman ladies painted the interval between the eyebrows, that they might appear to form but one. The same taste prevailed among the Arabs. (*Toilette*, 1832)

CONQUERANT See A La Conquérant.

CONSERVATIVE HAIR STYLE A coiffure restrained in its design.

CONSORT An English moustache style of the 19th century. Popular in the 1930s. (*Foan*)   *101T*

CONSTRUCTIVISM The construction of hair styles by the use of added substances such as wire, plastic, bone, etc.

CONTACT-SPRING See Positional spring.

CONTACT TIME The length of time a bleach or dye is allowed to remain in contact with the hair before removal by shampooing or rinsing.

CONTINENTAL HAIR STYLIST (1) A hairdresser from the continent of Europe, or at least reputedly from that continent.

(2) A hairdresser of English or any other European nationality who offers a service which includes fashionable hair styles from Europe.

CONTOUR The outline or boundary of a hair style. The external line enclosing form. It will have innumerable variations of shape depending upon the viewpoint of the observer.

CONTOUR BOB A bobbed head of hair so cut that it reveals the head's shape. 20th century.

CONTOUR CUTTING Hair cutting planned to produce a desired contour of the head.

CONTOUR GALLOON The galloon in a wig foundation that follows the contour of the hair-line. Also called outer-galloon and outline galloon.

CONTOUR HAIR STYLING A form of hair styling in which attention and emphasis is given to the contour of the dressed head as opposed to emphasis on detail such as whisps of loose curl or feathered ends, etc.

CONTOUR PERM A permanent wave that produces only a slight change in the hair's structure and enables very large diameter waves or curls to be set.

CONTOUR-RIBBON See Contour galloon.

CONTOUR WAVING Waving hair to reveal the head's shape.

CONTRA CURLING See Reverse curling.

CONTROL DRESSING A preparation of cream, oil, emulsion or other substance that can be used to hold hair in position.

CONVERGENT CURLS Curls rolled towards each other.

CONVERGING PLAITS Two plaits whose ends are plaited together forming a single plait; ie the ends of the two plaits terminate in a single plait. A common hairstyle among the women of Oaxaca, Mexico.

CONVERTIBLE A hair style that can be readily adapted to form another style without re-setting.

CONVERTIBLE CUT A haircut suitable for several different styles. (USA)

CONVERTIBLE PARTING The parting of a postiche so constructed that it (the parting) can have its positon altered to meet the needs of hair-style change.

CONVERTIBLE TOP American slang term for a wig. (*Berrey*)

CONVEX Curved like the outside of a sphere. The opposite to concave.

CONVEX CHEEK WAVE A wave, the trough of which points towards the cheek.

CONVICT CROP A very short hair style for men. Named after the short cut hair of English convicts.

CONY WOOL The pubic hair of a woman. 18th century slang. (*Button*)

COOKIE DUSTER A moustache, slang. American usage. (*B and B*)

COOKIE HAIRSTYLE Any modern with-it style for a young woman. 1950s

COOLAULIN A celtic woman's name meaning 'beautiful hair'. (*Long*)

COOL COLOUR A colour, such as blue or green, which is opposed to a warm colour such as red or yellow.

COP A tall headdress. (*OED*)

COPERNICIA CERIFERA Carnauba wax, *qv*.

COPPED CROWN'D A conical shaped head. 17th century. (*Comenius*)

COQUE (1) A smooth loop or bow of hair, worn erect. See Croisat's 1830 Coiffure for example. *335*
(2) A topknot.

COQUE D'APPOLLON See Apollo bow.

COQUET, THE A woman's hair style of 1865. (*Bysterveld* p 66)

CORDED BUCKLE 18th century man's wig style. (*London Magazine*)

CORDED WOLF'S PAW Man's 18th century wig style. (*Lon Mag*)

CORDELIENE Fr. Cord-like.

CORD LOOP PINCURL A pincurl with a small cord loop at the root ends to facilitate fixing to the head hair.

CORIUM The vascular layer beneath the epidermis.

CORK BOB 18th century wig style. See Cork wig.
'By the cork bob, that sits so snug and tight,
Whose light formation wraps a head as light;
Worn by each Jemmy of a country town,
To make him look more clever than the clown!' (*The Wig*, 1765)

CORK MOUSTACHE A moustache marked on the upper lip by means of burnt cork. For theatrical use.

CORK WIG A very light-weight wig.
'John Light, peruke maker, has brought to great perfection the best method of making cork wigs, either smooth or in curls and also cork bag-wigs in the neatest manner.' (*Salisbury Journal*, 1763)

CORKSCREW See Corkscrew curl.

CORKSCREW CURL A hanging curl shaped like a corkscrew. Also called Drop curl and Spiral curl, *qv*. *325*

CORNER PLAIT A very small plait (plaitlette) in the neck, behind one ear. 1982.

CORNET (1) 'The upper pinner dangling about the cheeks like a hound's ears.' 17th century. (*Evelyn*)
(2) A coiffure dressed to a high point like a dunce's cap. (*Creer*)

CORNEUM The top, horny layer of the epidermis.

CORNISH HAIR Coarse sheep's wool. (*Childrey, J, Britania Baconica*, 1661)

CORNUA HUMANA Human horns. Hard projections from the skin of the head and sometimes on other parts of the body. (*Wheeler*)

CORONAL PLAIT An encircling plait, worn like a garland. (*Elegant* Arts)

CORONATION CIRCLET Curls worked on a circle of galloon-covered clock spring, and dressed in curls, *c* 1910.

CORONATION TRANSFORMATION A postiche of natural wavy hair styled and introduced by Nicol, the London hairdresser in 1902 to celebrate the coronation of Edward VII.

CORONET (1) A small decorated crown to adorn the head. A fillet of precious materials.
(2) A hair style in which a coronet is featured. 20th century.

CORONET OF CURLS A coronet composed of either small curls, *qv*, or small puff curls, *qv*.

CORONET PLAIT A plait of hair dressed in the form of a coronet. (*Creer*, p 34) *419(1)*

CORRUGATE Verb. To mark with furrows and ridges, as is corrugated iron.

CORRUGATION Subs. A groove and ridge. See also Corrugate. Crêped hair is corrugated. The effect is also produced by crimping irons.

CORSINA A character in *Princess Fairstar*, a fairy tale by Contesse d'Aulnoy, published 1682. Every three days when she combed the hair of Fairstar and her two brothers, 'a great many valuable jewels were combed out, which she sold at the nearest town'.

CORTEX The inner or middle layer of the hair shaft, formed of elongated cells which contain the pigment which gives the hair its colour.

CORYMBUS (Corymbos) (1) A chaplet of leaves and cluster of ivy worn as a festive ornament by the Romans.
(2) An Athenian mode of dressing the hair of men; worn short and radiating from a circle at the crown, the crown hair dressed in two upright, flowing, curly tresses. (*Mee*)
(3) A helmet shaped headdress for women. Roman period. (*Mallemont*)

COSMAS and DAMIAN (Saints) Twin brothers and Patron Saints of Barbers. Symbol in art: phial and box of unguent. They were probably Arabians and were beheaded during the Diocletion persecution *c* AD 303.

COSMETIC A preparation, externally applied, to beautify the skin, hair or complexion. Any substance used for the purpose of cleansing, beautifying or altering the human appearance. See Cosmetologist.

COSMETIC BRUSH A small brush used to apply or remove a cosmetic. See also Powder brush.

COSMETIC FIXATEUR A dressing for the hair, beard and moustache.

COSMETICIAN One skilled in the art of cosmetology.

COSMETIQUE Fr. Cosmetic, *qv*.

COSMETOLOGIST One whose business is to beautify hair, skin or complexion. American usage. (From Greek *Kosmetikos*: Adornment).

COSMETOLOGY The art that is concerned with beautifying hair, skin and complexion. the art and science of beauty culture.

COSTUME WIG (1) A wig worn as part of the costume, such as that of a Judge, Barrister or Speaker of the House of Commons; also a theatrical wig used to complete the costume of a character.
(2) A fashionable wig worn by a woman whose own hair for some reason cannot readily be dressed to the style and in the colour required, *cf* Wig of necessity, worn to repair a deficiency of nature.

COTELETTES The same as mutton chop whiskers, *qv*.

COTMAN, JOHN SELL (1782–1842) Son of a hairdresser.

COTONNE Fr. Woolly (of hair).

COTTAGE LOAF A woman's hair style *c* 1960, the general contour of which resembles the old-fashioned cottage loaf, in which one globular form rests on a larger globular base. 20th century.

COTTER A hair tangle. Midland and North country usage.

COTTON WOOL HOLDERS A container of glass, china, metal for accommodating cotton wool.

COUNT A man's hair style popularized in the 1920s by Paul Glaus of the London Gentleman's Hairdressing Academy.

COUNTER CLOCKWISE The same as anti-clockwise, *qv*.

COUNTERFEIT CALVINIST Abusive term used by Quakers of wig wearers. (*Nare*)

COUNTESS OF JERSEY Hair style for women in which the hair is dressed to a parting in loose drop curls of irregular lengths.

COUNTESS OF POURTALES KNOT *216F*

COUNTRY CUT An indifferent haircut, so called because the country barber in England was often a farm labourer also and his barbering skill left something to be desired. See also Cut of the Country.

COUNT SAXE'S MODE 18th century man's wig style. (*London Mag*)

COURT COIFFURE Regulations regarding the wearing of plumes in court coiffures changed about 1911. The requirements were more strictly enforced and three plumes were obligatory. They were of regulation length and pure white. The centre feather was a little longer than the two on either side of it which were of identical length to each other. Previous to the new regulations the plume had been inserted in the hair at the centre of the back dressing and allowed to droop forward or to the side in a natural manner. The new rules decreed that the feathers should be inserted in the same position, but, when fixed were to be inclined towards the left, tilting slightly over the left side of the head. The veil was fixed below the feathers and rested in loose folds over the back dressing. It was secured by fine hairpins. (*Nicol*) See also Court headdress.

COURT CUT A man's 16th century hair style. (*Stubbes*)

COURT HAIRDRESSER Originally one employed at a Royal Palace to dress hair. Today and since the 19th century a term legitimately used by a skilled hairdresser who actually specializes in dressing the hair of ladies or gentlemen attached to the Royal Court or the hair of those who are presented at Court. By an extension of meaning the term is sometimes used by those who have the ability to dress hair suitably for court occasions but whose headdresses have never been to Court. By a further stretch of meaning the term is employed misleadingly by some who have neither the skill to dress suitably, and never have dressed the hair of anyone who has got within the outer railings of Buckingham Palace.

COURT HEADDRESS A formal hair style with or without plumes or other decoration suitable for wear at a Royal Court.

COURT WIG A wig, made of white or grey hair, and suitably dressed for the wearer to appear at a Royal Court. 17/20th century.

COVERAGE The cover or overlay provided by a hair dye. One can speak of good or bad coverage.

COVERED FRAME A frame of wire covered with crepe hair, worn on the head and used to give bulk to hair dressed on or over it.

COVERED HAIRPIN A hairpin covered in silk to match the hair.

COVERING A front, semi-transformation, transformation, half wig, three-quarter wig, wig, toupee, etc. (*Illustrated London News*, 6 August 1892)

COVERING POWER The cover or overlay provided by a hair dye. See Coverage.

COVER-UP POSTICHE A postiche, the use of which is primarily for covering bald or balding patches, and not for decorative purposes.

COWLICK A tuft of hair (usually at the front of the head) that grows in such a way that it looks as if it has been licked by a cow.

COWL See Head cowl.

COWN CURLS A cluster of curls mounted on a small flexible foundation which could be worn pinned to the wearer's own hair. (*The Gentlewoman*, 7 Jan 1911, p IX)

COWVAN'S CANTON STROP A four sided razor strop with faces suitable for grinding, setting, stropping and finishing the razor. Made by B and S Cowvan, 164 Fenchurch St, London, *c* 1840. (Adv)

COXCOMB See Cockscomb.

COX'S BOHEMIAN BALSAM OF TOKAY The celebrated mixture for human hair, sold by barber Cox in Thackeray's *Cox's Diary*. (*Micellanies*, Vol. 1, 1855)

CRAB-TREE COMB A cudgel. Slang, 16th century.

CRADLE CAP A yellow crust sometimes found on infants' scalps. (*Cocroft*)

CRAMP CURL (1) A curl formed by gripping a hair firmly between the thumb nail and flesh of the first finger and drawing them smartly down the hair shaft. This contracts the longitudinal section of the hair and expands the opposite longitudinal section, causing the hair to curl tightly. The curl is only temporary however and is of no practical use except for demonstration purposes.
(2) A twisted curl in which the hair is first twisted before shaping into a curl.

CRANIUM The skull.

CRAPAUD The bag, 'bourse', or purse in which the queue was enclosed. See Bagwig. Fr crapaud: a toad.

CRAPE The English spelling of the French crêpe, but the French form is more commonly used in hairwork circles in England.

CRAPE HAIR See Crêpe hair.

CRAPING See Crêpeing.

CRATES Whiskers. 16th century '. . . whether he will have his crates cut low like a juniper bush'? (*Green*, 1592)

CRAVAT BOW See Apollo bow.

CREAM BLEACH A bleach for the hair in the form of a cream, such as hydrogen perioxide mixed with magnesium carbonate and sodium perborate.

CREAM SHAMPOO Any shampoo that has the appearance of a cream is loosely called by this term. It is indicative only of the shampoo's consistency and has no reference to its ingredients.

CREAM TINT A hair dye used with a suitable cream as a carrier to prevent running.

CREEPER A louse. An early name for head lice, a common infection until the 20th century. Now rare. (*Percy*, ii 151/68)

CREEPING OXIDATION The slight development of colour or bleach that can occur after surplus oxidation dye or bleach has been removed from the hair by shampooing.

CREME (Fr.) Cream. The use of the French word *Creme* for cream is a modern affectation.

CREME DE MAUVE See Hair gloss.

CREOLAGE (1) Hair frizz. (*Menard*)
(2) a quantity of creôled hair.

CREOLE Subs. (1) Hair that has been tightly plaited and steeped in boiling water for 5 minutes or so, thus producing a series of uniform undulations along the hair shaft. (*Sutton*) A similar result can be obtained by crimping with the box crimping iron or tightly plaiting the hair and pinching with hot pinching irons.
(2) Crêped long hair as for the 'chignon universel'. (*Creer*) Verb.
(3) To crimp or kink temporarily in order to produce fullness.

CREOLED HAIR Hair that has been creoled, *qv*.

CREOLING IRONS Irons with corrugations for creoling hair, similar to crimping irons.

CREOSOTE SOAP See Medicated soap.

CREPE (1) Subs. Hair that has been permanently kinked by means of weaving on strings and boiling.
(2) Verb. To crimp or kink woven hair by boiling in water. To permanently crimp hair. See also Crêpe hair.
(3) Short artificial beard. Slang American usage. (*B and B*)

CREPE BOUFFANT A puffy bunch of crêpe secured to a comb and used to give fullness to a part of a dressing.

CREPE FIBRE Fibre tightly plaited on string to form a sort of rope which is then suitably processed by boiling in an alkaline solution.

CREPE HAIR See Crêpe. Also Crape Hair, crape being the Anglicised form in use since late 18th century. Both forms of the word are currently used in England but the French form is the most usual.

CREPE PAD A pad constructed of crêped hair for dressing the hair over.

CREPER (Fr) To crisp, frizzle or crimp.

CREPE ROPE Lengths of woven and baked crêpe hair on the carpet thread or coarse twine as woven and not yet loosened for use.

CREPE WEFT Strands of hair woven from the points to roots on carpet thread preparatory to boiling the weft to make crêpe hair. Figure-of-eight weft.

CREPE WOOL Crêped hair, unworked, teazed out into a loose woolly pad.

CREPING (1) Weaving and boiling hair to transform it into crêpe hair.
(2) Crimping.

CREPON (1) Subs. A front of hair worked on a crêpe pad and dressed in pompadour style to give fullness to the finished dressing. *306*
(2) Subs. Crisped, frizzled or woolly pad. (*Creer*)

CRESCENT Subs. A convexo-concave shaped hair ornament. 18/20th century 'An epigram on a certain lady's coming into the room at Bath, with a diamond crescent in her hair', 1768.
'Chaste Dian's crescent on her front displayed.
Behold! the wife proclaims herself a maid!'
(*NFH* Vol 1 p 10)

CRESCENT CURL A half curl, a C-shaped curl, a semicircular curl; a strand of curled or curly hair too short to permit a complete circination of the potential curl.

CRESCENTIC Crescent shaped.

CRESCENTIFORM CURL See Crescent curl.

CRESPINE A jewelled net for enclosing the hair on the head; 15th century. The hair was bunched up at the sides over the ears and held in position by a band over the forehead or, in the case of aristocrats, by a coronet or crown. (*Gardner*)

CRESPINETTE A coarse net of silk and sometimes fine metal filaments for covering the hair.

CREST CURL See Ridge curl.

CREVE-COEURS Heart breakers. Two small curled locks at the nape of the neck. 17th century.

CREW CUT Man's short cut hair style, origin USA. Similar to that formerly worn in the German Army. *104C*

CRICKE A louse. See also Creeper. (*Percy*, ii, 323/12)

CRIMP (1) Verb. To frizz or corrugate hair with hot crimping irons.
(2) Subs. Frizzed or corrugated hair.
(3) A woman's short, tousled hair style introduced by Vidal Sassoon in August 1967. The hair was crimped and stood out from the head. 'Geometric cut permed and then left crimpily unset.' See also Crimping.

CRIMPER A hairdresser. Slang, *c* 1920s to date.

CRIMPERS See Crimping irons.

CRIMPING Crisping or frizzing or corrugating the hair by means of crimping irons or hot pressing irons on plaited hair. (*Creer: Sutton*) A 19th century country method was as follows: The plaited lock, growing on the head, was laid on a table and a hot smoothing iron or flat iron placed on the plaited lock. Pronounced as 'awkward but efficient', in 1874. (SDP.)

CRIMPING IRONS An iron for crimping hair. There are two types:
(1) The box crimping iron. This comprises two rectangular blocks of iron so corrugated on one face that the convex corrugations of one block fit into the concave corrugations

of the other. The blocks of iron have handles. *448*
(2) Pronged crimping iron. This has two, three or four tines or prongs on one head, and three, four or five tines or prongs on the other head. When the tines are closed they pass each other. See also Pinching iron and Pressing iron.
416, 449

CRIMPING PIN A metal pin of small diameter which when heated had hair wound around it to produce a frizz. 18/19th century.

CRIMPLE, TO To crimp or crinkle (hair).

CRINES The hair at the back of the head. See Hair nomenclature.

CRINETUM Cord made of hair. Medieval usage. (*Fisher*)

CRINGLE A short hair style based on the shingle, but having the hair cut relatively shorter on the top and sides and left longer on the neck than the classic shingle. 1932.

CRINGLOW Wigmaker to Louis XIV, King of France.

CRINICULTURAL Pertaining to the culture of the hair.

CRINICULTURE Hair culture.

CRINIFEROUS Bearing hair.

CRINIFEROUS BUGBEAR 17/18th century slang for hairy parts of a whore, bugbear being an object of dread and criniferous meaning hairy. 'She could not stop but she must fright the standers by with the terrible appearance of her criniferous bugbear.' (*Ward* p 82)

CRINIGEROUS Hairy; wearing hair.

CRINIPAROUS Hair producing.

CRINITE Hairy.

CRINITIFRATRES The hairy brothers, a religious order. (*Prynne*, *Histrio-Mastix* p 202, 1633)

CRINITORY Hairy; having the nature of hair.

CRINIVOROUS Hair devouring.

CRINKLE (1) A corrugation.
(2) To corrugate or crimp the hair.

CRINKLED HAIR Hair that is wrinkled, twisted or corrugated.

CRINOLINE WEFT See Fly weft. So called from its similarity to a crinoline when the weft is seen from the end.

CRINOSITY Hairiness.

CRIP Verb. To clip hair. Somerset usage. (*Williams and Jones*)

CRIPSING IRON A curling tong. Somerset usage. A variation of Crisping iron, *qv*. 'She be going to cripsy her hair with this cripsing iron.'

CRIPSY To curl tightly or frizz with a cripsing iron. Somerset usage. A deviation of crisp.

CRISP or CRISPE (1) Adj. Curled or curly.
(2) Subs. A curl.
(3) Verb. To curl tightly, 17/20th century. To frizzle. (*Phillips*). (From Latin *crispus*: curled). 'A pinn to crispe the hayre with.' 1602. (*Clerk*)

CRISPED HAIR (1) Hair lying in a wave. 17th century. (*Holme*)
(2) Curled hair.
(3) Frizzed hair.

CRISPING IRON Curling iron, before 1616. 'For never powder, not the crisping iron
Shall touch these dangling locks.' (*B and F The Queen of Corinth*, IV. 1)
A curling or crimping iron used to tightly curl or crimp hair. 16/18th century. Later called a Crimping iron. Randle Holme in 1688 described this implement thus: 'In former times these were much used to curl the side locks of a man's head, but now (1688) wholly cast aside as useless; it openeth and shutteth like the forceps, only the blades are broad and square, being cut within the mouth with teeth curled and

crisped, one tooth striking within another.' A similar tool to the box crimping-iron of the 18/20th century.

CRISPING PIN Curling iron, 16/18th century. 'To crispe and courle the haire with an yron pinne (*capillis torquere ferro vel calamistro.*' *Ovid*) (*Baret* 1580)

CRISPUS A Roman emperor. The name means curl-pate. (*Fitzpatrick*)

CROCKET A large roll of hair worn by both sexes in the 14th century. 'They kembe their crockettes with crystal' combs? (*Chaucer, Plowman's Tale*)

CROCUS COMB A comb made of crocus wood.

CRONGEE Welsh name for man's short haircut.

CROP (1) Subs. Short cut hair. 'For dead is custom, 'mid the world of crops.' (*Pindar, Hair Powder*, 1790) Such was the universal disquiet at the 19th century powder tax that thousands of men sacrificed their curls.
(2) Verb. To cut short. 'I will crop his hair.'
(3) Adj. Short. 'Crop curl is used for men's wigs.'
(4) Subs. A growth of beard. Slang. American usage. (*B and B*)

CROP BEARD A short cut beard, 17/18th century. 'The young crop-bearded courtiers laughed . . . his old fashioned phyz.' (*Dulaure*)

CROP CLUB A gentleman's club formed in 1795 as a protest against the guinea wig powder tax introduced in that year. Members had to have their hair cropped and unpowdered. The new cut was called the Bedford level, the Duke of Bedford being one of the first to discard the wig and affect a cropped hair style. (*The Times*, 14 April 1795)

CROP COMB See Bladed comb.

CROP CURL A half curl on short hair. Used in the manufacture of men's wigs. See Crop hair.

CROP CUT (1) A short cut style for women.
(2) A very short haircut for men.
(3) A man's short hair style introduced to evade the Powder tax. See Crop club.

CROP EARED Having the hair cut short revealing the ears. 17th century.

CROP EARS A Roundhead, *qv*, whose cropped hair revealed the ears in contradistinction to the Royalists whose long hair covered the ears. 17th century.

CROP HAIR Short hair with a very slight turn, curled on large diameter bigoudis, used for men's wigs. (*Creer*)

CROPPED WIG A close-cut wig.

CROPPERS Fine clippers. (*Symonds*)

CROPPIE One who has had his hair cut in prison. Slang, 19th century. (Quaritch)

CROPPING SCISSORS Large hair-cutting scissors, *cf* Tapering scissors, which have small short blades.

CROPPY Members of the society, *The United Men of Ireland*, in USA, were so called on account of their short cropped hair. 19th century. (*Hall*)

CROP-RINGLET WIG A wig made with crop hair dressed in curls. (*Brodie, Price List*, 1890)

CROP-SCRATCH WIG Short natural wig. See also Scratch wig.

CROP WEFT See Thrice-in-Weft.

CROP WIG A man's wig made of crop hair.

CROQ A shortened and commonly used form for Croquinole, *qv*.

CROQUIGNOLE (1) Subs. Hair that has been wound round a curler from the points towards the roots and baked to produce a permanent curl. 'Croquignole is used for wigs.'

CROQUIGNOLE HAIR Hair that has been permanently curled by means of the croquignole winding method.

CROQUIGNOLE IRON WAVE Similar to Croquignole Marcel waving, *qv*.

CROQUIGNOLE MARCEL WAVING The hair is curled in croquignole fashion with the Marcel waving irons and then combed and brushed into waves and curls as desired. (*Thomas*)

CROQUIGNOLE MARCELLING The same as croquignole marcel waving, *qv*.

CROQUIGNOLE WIND A method of flat winding a strand of hair on a curler from the points towards the roots by overlapping each succeeding circination. The curler used is of smaller diameter in the centre than at its ends. (*Smith*)

CROQ WINDING Croquignole winding. Hair wound on a curler from the points to the roots, *cf* Spiral winding.

CROSSBAR KNOTTING Hair knotted in every hole in every direction.

CROSS KNOTTING Also called stagger or staggered knotting. One row knotted to the right, the next row knotted to the left, *ad lib*. This type of knotting is used when the hair style requires the hair to stand away from the foundation and not lie flat.

CROSS-OVER BEARD A beard used by an actor who doubles in a part. (*B and B*)

CROSS PARTING A parting of the hair made across the head or part of the head, from the left side to the right side, or vice versa. See also Transverse parting.

CROSS SHADE Hair lying across the forehead, with a silk thread in the middle of it. 17th century. (*Holme*)

CROSS STITCH See Stitching.

CROTCHET An artistic fanciful device used as a hair ornament, 16th century. See Crotchet of diamonds.

CROTCHET OF DIAMONDS A fanciful artistic device ornamented with diamonds in the form of twigs or a spray, used in the hair as an ornament. 16th century. 'Like to the sticking a crotchet of diamonds in a well-dress'd lady's hair.' 1724 (*Whatley*)

CROTON OIL SOAP See medicated soap.

CROWN (1) The hair at the turn of the crown of a peruke or head. 17th century. (*Holme*)
(2) A separately worked crown piece for sewing into a wig.
(3) A circular dressing on top of, or at the back of, the head.
(4) A small postiche for wear at the crown of the head.

CROWN AND PARTING A kind of toupet for a woman. Late 19th century. (*Adv*)

CROWN BOMBAGE Fullness in a hairdress at the crown of the head.

CROWN CAP Toupée for the crown area of the head. (*Stevens, Ms*, 1896)

CROWN CURLS A bunch of light curls for wear on top of the head.

CROWN HAIR Hair, the roots of which have their origin at the crown of the head.

CROWN PIECE A postiche patch for wear on the crown of the head.

CROWN WIG A toupet.

CROWT To curl up. (*Percy Ballads*, ii, 308/114)

CRUCHES Small curls arranged on the forehead. 17th century. (*Evelyn*)   356, 360

CRUCIFORM Shaped like a cross.

CRUDE HAIR Untreated natural hair.

CRUTCH (1) 18th century man's wig style. (*Lon Mag*)
(2) (of scissors) The cutting part of the scissor blades nearest the pivot.
(3) See En-beguille.

CRYMPAN Curl (*AS*)

CUBE CUT A woman's short hair style of the 1930s.   412

CUBICLE A small compartment in a room or shop in which clients can be privately treated. In England all ladies' hairdressing saloons were separate rooms or were divided into cubicles until *c* 1930, when the open saloon, similar to the barber's saloon, started to be fashionable and has now (1965) become the usual accommodation for ladies seeking attention to their hair.

CUE See Queue.

CUE-PERUKE See Queue peruke.

CUE WIG See Queue wig.

CULBUTE A flat chignon composed of an encircling plait. 17th century. (*Villermont*)   *364*

CUP-HANDLE CURL A Stand-up curl, *qv*, shaped like a cup handle, *c* 1960. Also called a Bow curl.

CUPID or CUPIDO The celebrated god of love. This name has been incorporated in many hair style appellations but the styles were of such a transitory nature that it is impracticable to enumerate them.

CUPOLA A grouping of curls, or bunching of hair, on the top of the head; eg a cupola of curls, *cf* Top-knot. 20th century.

CUPOLA COIFFURE A dome-shaped hairdress.

CUPPEE A kind of pinner. (*Evelyn*)

CUPPING Bleeding a person by means of a cupping glass. This was once part of the barber's services.

CUPPING GLASS A glass container into which the blood ran during the operation of cupping, *qv*.

CURD Calcium soap scum.

CURDLE Subs. A curl of hair. Dorset, Somerset and Wilts usage. (*Barnes; Dartnell*).
Verb. To curl hair.

CURD SOAP A nearly neutral soap of pure soda and fine tallow. (*Piesse*)

CURL (1) Subs. A ringlet of hair; a spiral lock of hair; a group of propinquant hairs describing a circle. A curl may be wide or narrow. When very wide it is usually called a roll, when narrow a ribbon curl, or when very narrow a tendril or a filament curl. These descriptions have no reference to the diameter of the curl, but only to the width of hair forming the circle of curl. The diameter of a curl may vary from small to large.
(2) Verb. To form curls, 1530. 'To crispe and courle the haire.' 1580 (*Baret*). For various types of curl and methods of forming see – Buckle, Clock-spring curl, Barrel-spring curl, Croquignole, Ringlet, Tendril, Filament, etc.

CURL BAND A band or ribbon with false curls attached which can be slipped over the head hair, *c* 1890.

CURL CLIP A metal or plastic clip closed by a small spring that holds a wound curl in position.

CURL CLUSTER A group of curly tresses.

CURL COMB A comb with a pointed handle. See Tail comb. (*Walker*, 1837)

CURL CUT A short, tapered haircut that will reveal the full strength of the hair's curl.

CURLE AND FRISE 'When the hair is neither curle nor frise, but both or between both.' 17th century. (*Holme*)

CURLED BOB A man's short wig style with curls, 18th century. (*Tennent*)

CURLED DARLINGS (1) Well dressed, idle young men, 16th century. (*Shakespeare, Othello*, 1604)
(2) Military officers. Mid 19th century.

CURLED GOD, THE Sol, the Roman sun god.
'Those precious locks, that might out-vie
The trim curl'd god, who lights the sky;' (*Somervile*, 1727)

CURLED HAIR (1) 'When a lock of hair turns round and round in itself.' 17th century. (*Holme*)
(2) In postiches and growing hair – hair that has been artificially curled, *cf* curly. Not a natural curl which is referred to as curly hair.

CURLED MARTEAU (1) A Marteau, *qv*, that has been constructed of frisure forcée.

(2) A curled marteau which has been dressed into a curly style.

CURLED TAPER HAIR Tapered hair that has been curled.

CURLER (1) A small circular pipe or toggle of clay, metal, wood, plastic or other suitable material on which hair is wound and treated with chemicals and/or heat for curling the hair.
(2) Any appliance for curling the hair.

CURLER CADDY A woman's small bag for carrying curlers and other toilet necessities, 1965.

CURLER EXHIBITIONIST A woman who exhibits herself in a public place with her hair rolled on jumbo plastic curlers. A common but unlovely sight in many English and American towns.

CURLET A little curl or ringlet.

CURLEY ROY (Curly Roy) A man's 18th century wig style, advertised by one, Pickeaver, wigmaker, Dublin. (*Dublin Gazette*, 1724)

CURL-HAIRED Curly haired. (*Miege*)

CURLICUE (1) A fantastic curl.
(2) A curl worn by men in the centre of their foreheads in the 19th century.

CURLIE Scot. (1) Curled.
(2) One whose hair falls naturally in ringlets. 18th century. (*Burns*)

CURLIE-WURLIE (1) A fantastically curled ornament.
(2) A large diameter flat curl.

CURLINESS The state of being curly.

CURLING (1) Subs. A curl. That which has been curled. 'Chignon Normand adorned with curlings.'
(2) Adj. That which curls.
(3) The process of making curly.   *394*

CURLING A LA PAPILLOTE Curling hair by means of curl papers and pinching irons.

CURLING BODKIN 17th Century curling pin. (*Guillim* p 290)

CURLING CLAMP (1) A square (approx 3″ × 3″) of hard wood ½″ thick with two circular holes ³⁄₁₆ diameter bored ³⁄₈ apart with the grain of the wood running between them. A leather bootlace is threaded through the two holes, and to its ends a strong piece of string or another leather bootlace is tied and the loop left hanging to within 2″ of the floor. Also called a Jigger. (*Sutton*). Used for holding a strand of hair when winding it up preparatory to making frisure forcée.
(2) A metal vice. See figure   *89(13), 462*

CURLING COMB A tail comb with a rounded tail for the rolling of hair to form curls. The same as roller comb, tail comb and curl comb.

CURLING FLUID An oil with which the hair was lightly anointed before iron-curling. It consisted of olive oil, 1 pint; oil of origanum, 1 drachm; oil of rosemary, 1½ drachm. (*Stevens Ms*)

CURLING IRON See Curling irons (2).

CURLING IRON BRACKET A metal gas bracket on which curling irons are heated.

CURLING-IRON HEATER See Curling iron stove.

CURLING IRONS (Curling iron; Curling tongs) (1) An iron instrument with two prongs, one rounded and the other, in which the round prong fits, fluted. The edges on the fluted prong are thinner on curling-irons than on waving irons. Heated, the irons are used by grasping the tips or points of a tress of hair and winding the irons up the hair, or spirally twining the hair around them. 'Twisted locks delicately curled by the iron of those adorning her.' (*St Adhelm*, 8th century reference Planché). Curling yrons, 1592. (*Iyly*). Until the 18th century both prongs of many of the curling irons were solid and rounded. (*Cox*). Until the middle of the 19th century pinching irons were called curling irons and small diameter curling irons were called frizzling irons, *qv*.   *444, 450*

(2) A single iron rod like a gauffering iron was also used to curl hair and the 8th century reference above probably refers to this type of curling iron. 'Are they not in dayly thraldome, and perpetuall bondage to their curling irons.' (*Prynne*, 1628)

CURLING-IRON STOVE A gas, electric, oil or methylated spirit stove on which curling or Marcel waving irons are heated.

CURLING KID Small pieces of chamois leather used to roll the hair to produce a temporary curl.

CURLING NEEDLE A steel needle about $\frac{1}{12}''$ in diameter used to facilitate winding the points of a strand of hair round a hair curler in handwinding for a permanent curling process, using the croquignole method of winding.

CURLING PATTERN The type of curl and their arrangement on the head.

CURLING PEG See Curl stick.

CURLING PINS Folding clips, used cold, for curling the hair.

CURLING ROD See Curler (1).

CURLINGS (Subs.) Curls, especially in a postiche.   *334*

CURLING STICK See Curl stick.

CURLING TONGS See Curling irons. '1758 Oct 19 A pair of Curling Tongs £0. 2. 8 (*Woodforde, J, Diary of a Country Parson 1758–1802*)

CURLLESS Without curl.

CURL MIXTURE (for hair and whiskers) Olive Oil $1\frac{1}{2}$ oz; spirit of Hartshorn (aqueous solution of ammonia) 1 oz; Well mix and dress the hair thoroughly with the mixture every two days, comb and brush well, arrange the hair in ringlets as required and wear a tight cap over it, and it will form into natural curls, or so it was claimed in 1832. (*Toilette*, 1832)

CURL PAPER (1) A small square of paper in which a tress of hair is held in a curled form and heated with a pinching iron.   *87 (16, 17)*

(2) A small piece of paper (usually newspaper) used for twisting hair into and producing a curl after being in the curled position for some hours. See also End paper.

CURL-PAPER IRONS See Pinching irons.

CURL PATE (1) A curly head;

(2) A curly headed person.

CURL PATED Curly headed.

CURL PEG A cigar shaped implement of wood, used for rolling the hair strands into curls. 18th century. (*Stewart*)

CURL RAG A small piece of rag used for twisting hair into and producing a curl after being in the curled position for some hours.

CURL SIZE A method of accurately referring to curl size and avoiding such imprecise expressions as loose, large or tight curl is to use the measurement of the diameter of the curl. One of $\frac{1}{2}''$ diameter being small and tight, whereas a curl of $2''$ diameter would be large and loose.

CURL STICK (1) A long, polished, slightly tapered wooden rod or stick ($10''$ to $18''$ in length and of varying diameter as needed), on which dry curls are dressed. The curl is wound round spirally, commencing at the root end of the curl and the end of the greatest diameter of the curl-stick, which can then be freely withdrawn on account of its taper. 18/19th century. (*Creer*)

CURLY (1) Having curls.

(2) A curly-headed person; slang. (*B and B*)

CURLY BOYS (1) Boys whose hair was dressed to copy the Pear's soap advertisement 'Bubbles'.

(2) A late 19th century gang of London tough boys.

CURLY CHIGNON A chignon dressed in curls.

CURLY HAIR (1) Hair for postiche that has a natural curl.

(2) Growing hair having natural or induced curl *cf* Curled hair.

CURLY LOCKS A curly headed person; slang. (*B and B*)

CURLY MURLY A fantastic curl.

CURLY PATE A curly headed person. Slang. (*B and B*)

CURLY POW A curly head. Cumberland usage.

CURLY WIG A facetious appellation for a person (especially a child) with a head of curly hair.

CURLY WURLY See Curlie Wurlie.

CURT Adj. Short. '. . . in more temperate climes hair is curt,' (*Herbert*)

CURTAIN OF HAIR A length of wefted hair.

CURTAINS Two flat swirls of hair hanging, one on each side of the parting, and covering both sides of the forehead. 19/20th century.

CURTANE A part-fringe at the side of the forehead. American usage.

CURVED SCISSORS Haircutting scissors with curved blades. Usually used for tapering hair.

CURVILINEAR Taking the course of a curved line; bounded or formed in or by curved lines. 'She has the new Curvilinear Coiffure.'

CUR WIG An effeminate white powdered wig worn by fashionable young men *c* 1734, *c* 1775, 'powder'd and appearing like the twigs of a gooseberry bush in a deep snow'; also called adonis wig, *qv*. (*Lon. Mag*, 1734)

CUSHION (1) Pad to dress hair over, 18th century.
'Don't let your curls fall with that natural blend,
But stretch them up tight 'till each hair stands on end;
One, two, nay three cushions, like Cybele's tow'rs;
Then a few ells of gauze, and some baskets of flow'rs.'
(*Venus Attiring the Graces*, 1777)

(2) A soft block on which to dress small pieces of postiche. See Malleable cushion.

(3) A malleable transformation block. Birmingham usage. (*Symonds*)

CUSHION HEADDRESS A 19th century term for a woman's early 15th century hairdress that incorporated a padded roll.

CUSHION ROLLER A large diameter, soft hair roller. Used for setting curls.

CUSHION STROP A hand strop, *qv*. (*Foan*)

CUSPIDOR A spittoon. An ever-present convenience in American barber's shops of the 19th century, and an often-present nuisance in English barbers' shops in the 19th and early 20th century.

CUSTER, GEORGE ARMSTRONG (1839–1876) American general. Prior to Custer's 'last stand' at the Little Big Horn River in Dakota Territory, he had his hair very closely cut. His Indian opponent said it was a sign of Custer's impending death. (*Bergen, T, Little Big Man*, p 342)

CUSTOMARY PLUMES See Court coiffure.

CUSTOM-MADE WIG Made to a client's special requirements. Not mass produced. Made to measure. American usage.

CUT BEARD A beard style in which the hair is trimmed short. (*D'Urfey*)

CUT BLUNT, TO See To club. American usage.

CUT BOB A man's 18th century wig style. (*London Mag*)

CUTICLE The outer horny layer of the hair shaft. It is composed of minute overlapping scales and gives the hair elasticity.

CUT OF THE COUNTRY 16th century hair style for men. (*Stubbes*)

CUT OF THE COURT 16th century hair style for gentlemen. (*Stubbes*)

CUT-THROAT RAZOR A razor with a fully exposed blade.
440

CUTTING The process of severing hair by means of a sharpened implement such as scissors or razor. *302*

CUTTING COMB (1) Small or medium sized comb used during the hair-cutting process.
(2) A comb incorporating a sharp blade which by combing also cuts the hair.

CUTTING DOWN Cutting the hair to style in a finished wig, especially a man's wig.

CUTTINGS Tresses of hair cut from the head.

CUT WIG An 18th century short-hair plain wig with no tail. Same as Scratch wig, *qv*.
'What plaudit would he draw if cut or scratch
Debas'd his temples and his cheek expos'd?'
(*Woty, Shrubs of Parnassus*, p 52 1760)

CYANOTRICHIA Blue or bluish-green coloured hair. (*Wheeler*)

CYBELLE HAIRDRESS See A La Cybèle.

CYBELLE'S TOWER An 18th century hair style for women. See A La Cybèle.

CYDONIUM See Quince seed.

CYMOTRICHOUS Having wavy hair. 1909.

CYMOTRICHY Wavy-hairedness. 1909.

CYMRIC FRINGE Worn by Welshmen in the 19th century and early 20th century. Two main varieties were the vogue:
(1) Part of the front hair was plastered with an oleaginous preparation and dressed downward over the forehead to the eyebrows, the ends of the fringe being finished as a scroll.
(2) The second variety, that was known as the *friseur*, was dressed over the forehead in a frizzed brush. See also Cymric toupée.

CYMRIC TOUPEE A fringe, as worn by Welshmen, that extended from ear to ear as a border of frizziness.

CYPRIAN COIFFURE A prostitute's hairdress. 'A fashion which pursu'd by Cyprian dames.' (*Brome*, 1659)

CYPRIOTE CURL A stand-up ringlet or palm curl built up upon a wire frame and forming part of a front of curls extending over the front part of the head from ear to ear. The style originated in Cyprus and became popular in classical Greece and Rome.

D

DACKED HAIR'D The same as dagged hair'd, *qv*.

DAFFODIL See Narcissus.

DAGE Hairdresser to Madame Pompadour. (*Johnson*)

DAGGED HAIR'D Shock-headed, *qv*, 'Dagged', a south-west dialect word, is derived from 'dag': a clotted lock of wool at a sheep's backside.

DAGGER PIN A single prong tortoiseshell or horn, etc, decorative hair ornament.

DAGLOCKS Dirty, bedraggled locks of hair. 'A doctor whose beard hung in daglocks down to his heels.' (*Quevodo, Y Villegas*, 1697). This word as *dag-loakes*, was originally used in the early 17th century to describe the dirty, clotted wool on the rumps of sheep.

DALMAHOY A bushy type of bob wig worn by tradesmen in the 18th century and very popular with chemists and druggists.

DAMASK POWDER FOR THE HAIR 18/19th century recipe:
16 lb fine starch powder, ½ lb fine damask perfumed powder. Mix and sift. It is the perfumed powder that makes the mixture brown. (*Lillie*)

DAMNRUFF American slang for dandruff. (*B and B*)

DANDER Dandruff, 18th century. (*Earle*)

DANDER COMB A dandruff comb, 18th century. (*Earle*)

DANDIZETTE A woman devoted to fashionable smartness in dress and hair style, *c* 1800.

DANDRIFF See Dandruff. (*Wheeler*)

DANDRIFF COMB (1763) See Dandruff comb. (*Earle*)

DANDRIFFE Dandruff. 'Like hair and dandriffe shed.' (*Alarbas*, 1709)

DANDRUFF See Pityriasis.

DANDRUFF COMB A small, fine-toothed comb for drawing through the hair and removing loose scales of dandruff.

DANDRUFF GARAGE Hair of the head. American slang. (*B and B*)

DANDY A man devoted to fashionable smartness in dress and hair style.

DANE A red-haired man. Devon usage. (*Gregory*)

DANGLER A hanging curl; a loose hanging corkscrew curl. West Country usage.

DAPPLING CAP A rubber or plastic head cap, evenly punctured with small holes through which strands of hair can be pulled by means of a hook in the highlighting process. Before 1965.

DARK-HAIRED MAN Regarded in Scotland and many parts of England as bringing luck to the house if he first-foots it in the New Year. In a very few places the fair-headed are regarded as bringing luck by first-footing the house. First-footing means the first man to cross the threshhold of the house on New Year's day. (*Radford*)

DART A V-shaped section cut from a flat piece of wig net that is being shaped to conform to the curved surface of the wig block. See also Tuck.

DAUBIGNY (A la mode de) A woman's powdered hair style, 18th century. The hair is frizzed, raised in front, then carelessly rolled back over the fingers. Strings of pearls are then disposed between each rouleau. (*Creer*)

DAUPHINE HAIRDRESS See A la Dauphine.

DAY, CHARLES Son of a barber and perfumer in Covent Garden who left his father's barber shop with another assistant, Mr Martin, to set up as Blacking Manufacturers. Their 'Black Diamond' made Day a fortune of about half a million pounds. (*Procter*)

DAY DRESSING A hair style suitable for wear during the daytime. Casual styles for holidays and more formal styles for work are usual.

DAY HEADDRESS See Day dressing.

DAY NET A net for wear on the head during daytime. It is usually an invisible net.

DAY-TIME STYLE See Day dressing.

DEAD HAIR See Cadaver hair.

DECALVATION To make bald by removing the hair, 1650. (*Bulwer*)

DE CASTRO, JOHN He pledged his whiskers at Goa for £10,000. (*Fitzpatrick*)

DECOLOUR To deprive of colour. See Bleaching; not to be confused with discolour which usually means undesired change or spoiling of the colour.

DECOLOURANT A chemical that will remove colour from hair.

DECOLOURIZATION The removal of colour from the hair. See Decolour.

DECOMPOSED LEECHES Used as a black hair dye in classical Greece. (*Forbes*)

DECORATE To adorn with colour or ornament.

DEEP-CLEANSING SHAMPOO See Shampoo, Deep cleaning.

DEEP COMBING Hair combing so that the teeth of the comb penetrate to the surface of the scalp.

DEFLUVIUM The rapid loss of hair.

DEFLUVIUM CAPILLORUM Diffuse hairfall, *qv.*

DEFLUVIUM MYSTAX Shedding of hair from the moustache and thinning of it. (*Wheeler*)

DEGAGER (les cheveux) Fr. To disentangle the hair.

DELACQUER SHAMPOO A shampoo to remove applied lacquer from the hair.

DELAYED HEATING The application of heat to the permanent waving heater before it is applied to the head.

DELILAH A woman of the Philistines who betrayed Samson by cutting off his hair. (See Samson)

DEMARCATION LINE A narrow line or band of colour differing from the colour above and below, produced in retouching by overlapping the hair dye on the previously dyed lengths.

DEMELOIR Fr. Large hair comb; a dressing comb. (*Creer*)

DEMI-ELEGANTE A comparatively fashionable woman.

DEMI-TRANSFORMATION The same as semi-transformation, *qv.* (*Vasco*)

DEMI-TRANSFORMATION TOUPEE The same as semi-transformation *qv.* (*Black and White Budget*, 15 Dec 1900)

DEMI-WAVE Half of the head hair permanently waved.

DEMON BARBER See Sweeney Todd.

DEODORANT A substance which will destroy or mask an offensive odour.

DEPILARISTE A Greek household slave whose special duty was the removal of superfluous hair. (*Forbes*)

DEPILATE To remove hair from.

DEPILATION (1) The action of removing hair.
(2) The condition of being without hair.

DEPILATOR One who removes hair. A shaver.

DEPILATORY (1) A hair remover. An oriental formula used in Turkish harems was:
Fresh quicklime ½ lb; liquor of potash 2 oz; sulphuret of potassium 1 oz; (*EDM*) Other depilatories included parsley water; acacia juice; gum of ivy; milkthistle juice mixed with oil; gum of cherry tree; oil of walnuts; quick-lime in various mixtures of such as: 1 oz quick-lime; 3 drachms orpiment; 2 drachms orris; 1 drachm saltpetre; 1 oz sulphur; ½ pint soap lees. A modern formula is: barium sulphide, zinc oxide, powdered starch, equal parts. Work into a paste with water before using. (*Niemoeller*)
(2) Having the quality of removing hair.

DEPILATORY WAX Numerous waxes have been used for removing unwanted hair in a similar manner to Burgundy pitch, *qv.*

DERIVATIVE Subs . A thing deriving from or originating from another.

DERMA The true skin or corium. The layer of tissue lying beneath the epidermis and forming the general integument of the organs of the body.

DERMATITIS Inflammation of the skin. See also *Dermatitis venenata*.

DERMATITIS VENENATA Inflammation of the skin caused by an external poison such as a 'para' dye.

DERMATOLOGIST A medical practioner who specializes in diseases of the skin.

DESIGN The general conception or plan for the arrangement of a hair style, including proportion and outward form, by the skilful control of shape, line, colour and texture.

DES MAHONNOISES A French hair style for women in which hair towers rose from the coiffure. (See Assisin, L')

DETACHED BUCKLE A man's 18th century wig style. (*Lon Mag*)

DETANGLER A substance, usually an oil, used on very frizzy hair to facilitate combing and disentangling. American usage.

DETERGENT A cleansing agent such as soap, or a soapless shampoo.

DETROIT CUT A flat-top crew cut.

DEVELOPER A substance that will induce the development and effective working of a dye. Hydrogen peroxide is one of the commonest developers.

DEVELOPMENT TIME The time taken for the chemical in a dye, bleach or permanent curling process to produce the desired result. Timing commences at the end of the application.

DEVIL In most early pictorial representations, the devil is depicted as being hairy.

DEVIL IN THE BEARD See *Tinea sycosis*. (*Wheeler*)

DEWEY MOUSTACHE A style similar to that worn by Thomas Edmund Dewey (and named after him) born 1902, Governor of New York, 1942. American usage, *c* 1943.

DE-WIG (1) To remove the wig.
(2) To tear a person's hair out. Slang.

DEWLAP A hanging loop of hair. Probably named after the loose skin hanging from the throats of dogs, or the pendulous fleshy lobe of the turkey.

DIACHYLON An adhesive plaster made by boiling together litharge (lead oxide), olive oil and water. Used on oiled silks to secure scalps to the head. 19th and early 20th century. (*Creer*)

DIADEM A curved postiche or dressing on top of the head. It frequently incorporates jewels. *200*

DIADEM COMB A large curved comb, highly ornamented at the top. 1830–1840.

DIADEM PLAIT A hair plait worn across the top of the head.

DIAMANTE SLIDE (or comb) A hair slide or comb decorated with material scintillating with powdered crystal, etc.

DIAMOND FRONT A wefted front sewn on a diamond-shaped foundation and secured at the back of the head by tying the extended galloons of the foundation.

DIAMOND MESH Also Honeycomb mesh. An arrangement of weft (including a fine wire) in a diamond-shaped pattern suitable for a cluster, a marteau or a cache-peigne.

DIAMOND MESH CLUSTER A cluster of curls worked on diamond mesh, *qv.*

DIAMOND MESH FOUNDATION A foundation for a dressed postiche of diamond mesh, *qv.*

DIAMOND MESH MARTEAU A marteau of hair worked on a diamond mesh, *qv.*

DIAMOND PARTING A knotted-hair parting for a postiche of which the net foundation is woven in a small diamond pattern.

DIAMOND PARTING FOUNDATION The diamond patterned foundation to which hair is attached to make a parting for a postiche.

DIANA (Luna, Isis) In ancient mythology, goddess of the moon and hunting. Depicted by the ancients with long, golden hair. (*Salmon*)

DIANA STYLE A 19th century hair style for women in which the neck hair is combed upwards. (*Mallemont*)

DIANE DE POITIERS, à la. After the style of Diane de

Poitiers, (1499–1566), mistress of Henry II of France. (*Creer*)

DICKER-OF-RAZORS Ten razors. (An act for . . . granting . . . duties. Dublin, 1799)

DICK FRIZZ The barber in the poem *The Stage Struck Barber*. (*The Universal Songster*)

DICK A louse. Yorkshire slang. (*Symonds*)

DIDO (Queen of Carthage) Legendary founder in 853 BC of Carthage. The ancients depicted her with yellow hair, tied up with spangles and knots of gold. (*Salmon*)

DIETZ, JOHANN Surgeon in the army of the great Elector and Barber to the Royal Court.

DIFFUSE HAIRFALL Severe and rapid loss of hair from all areas of the scalp.

DILDO (1) Sausage corkscrew curl of a man's wig. From 17th century. The dildo formed part of the dressing of the Campaign wig, *qv*, and was the origin of the pigtail of the Ramilies wig, *qv*. Originally the dildo (from the Italian diletto: delight) was an artificial substitute for the *membrum virile*, *cf* dildo-glass: a cylindrical glass. (*Grose*)
(2) A slang term for a bigoudi or curling stick.

DIMINISHING CURL (Clockspring curl) A curled tress of hair in which each succeeding circle, working inwards, diminishes in diameter, *cf* also Snail curl.

DIOGENES (412–323 BC) The Greek cynic and philosopher who, meeting a man with a smoothly shaven chin, asked whether he shaved as a reproof to nature for having made him a man and not a woman. The ancients depicted him with a hairy, rough beard. (*Salmon*)

DIP Subs. (1) Hair that hangs looped on the cheek or neck. A loop of hair. (*Moler*)
(2) A forward wave onto the face.
(3) Verb. To dip for a wig. Formerly in Middle Row, Holborn, wigs of different sorts were put into a close-stool box, into which anyone on paying 3d might dip and take out a wig. If dissatisfied with the one drawn, by paying three halfpence and returning the wig he could draw again. (*Grose*, ed 1823)

DIPILOS Bald. (*Hartrampf*)

DIP TRANSFORMATION A transformation, *qv*, in which the front dressing dips forward onto the face (*AH*, 1915)

DIRECTIONAL-KNOTTING Relating to the direction in which the hair lies when knotted to the net foundation of a postiche.

DIRECT-DYE A dye that penetrates the hair and remains there chemically unchanged.

DIRECTOIRE HAIR STYLES Hair styles in the form of those worn at the time of the Directory, the Supreme Executive Council of France, 1795 to 1799.

DIRECT WIG A full wig fully dressed before being laced on the head and worn by ladies who were bald. 18th century. (*Stewart*). Also called French tête.

DISC JOCKEY CONTOUR Man's hair style, 1960.

DISCOLOURATION The changing or spoiling of a colour from a desired to an unwanted colour.

DISENTANGLING COMB See Rake.

DISHEVEL To tousel, disarrange or make untidy (especially hair).

DISINFECTANT A substance that will kill micro-organisms.

DISPENSARY A closet or section in the saloon where hair dyes, shampoos and other materials for the hair are prepared for use.

DISPENSER (1) A container from which the material therein is readily obtained or 'dispensed'.
(2) Person who prepares and dispenses the shampoo, hair dye, etc, in the dispensary.

DISPLAY BLOCK A stand shaped like a human head on which wigs and other postiches can be displayed.

DISPLAY BUST Similar to display head, *qv*, but including the upper part of a woman's bust.

DISPLAY HEAD A waxen, wooden, china or plastic head shape used to display wigs and other forms of postiche.

DISPLAY MANIKIN Artificial head for the display of wigs.

DISPOSABLE TOWELS Towels of a cheap and easily disposable tissue, such as paper, that are used once and destroyed.

DISPOSABLE WIG See Wig hat.

DISSEMBLING-COLOUR The colour of hair that has been dyed.

Rosalind: His very haire
 Is of dissembling colour.
Celia: Something browner than Judasses:
 Marrie his kisses are Judasses owne children.
Rosalind: I'faith his haire is of a good colour.
Celia: An excellent colour:
 Your chessenut was ever the onely colour:
Rosalind: And his kissing is as full of sanctitie,
 As the touch of holy bread. (*Shakespeare, As You Like It*, act 3, scene 4)

DISTAL Terminal. Situated away from the centre of the body. Opposite to proximal.

DISTAL END The end furthest from the point of attachment. Terminal. 'The distal end of a hair' = the point.

DISTICHIASIS A congenital abnormality in which two distinct rows of cilia occur on an eyelid. (*McCarthy*). See also Dystichia.

DISTILLED VINEGAR Dilute acetic acid.

DISTINCTION HAIRDRESS See A la Distinction.

DISTORTION A deviation from the normal in shape or form.

DISTRICT ATTORNEY HAIR STYLE A short hair style for men. American usage.

DISWOUND HAIR Hair that has been unwound from a curler.

DIVERGENT CURLS Curls arranged back to back. Curls turning away from each other.

DIVIDED BANG A bang or fringe having a break or division.

DIVIDED BEARD A divided or forked beard was regarded as the sign of a cunning man. See Forked beard.

DIVIDED FRINGE See divided bang.

DIVIDING See Sectioning.

DIVIDING CLAMP (or **GRIP**) A spring-operated grip opened by pressure on the handles, closed by the pressure of its spring and used to hold hair away from the immediate area of operation. This instrument facilitates the division of hair for dyeing, permanent waving, etc., hence its name.

DIVOT American slang term for a wig. Derived from the golfing term, divot, a piece of turf. (*Berrey*)

DIZZY BLONDE A 'fast' blonde woman, slang. (*B and B*)

D J CONTOUR See Disc Jockey Contour.

DO Subs. Shortened form of Hairdo, *qv*. Slang.

DOCK To cut short. West country and Scottish usage. (*Henderson*)

DOCTOR A ship's cook who also acted as ship's barber. 19th century Slang. (*HC* 1 September 1925)

DOCTORED HAIR Hair that has been dyed, bleached, curled or treated in a manner that changes its nature from its virgin state, *cf* treated hair.

DODYPOLL A blockhead, a silly ass. Poll = head, dody (from dotty) = silly. The verb *dote* = to be foolish or silly. (*The Wisdom of Doctor Dodypill*, A comedy, 1600)

311

DOG BARBER One who trims and strips dogs. 18/19th century.

DOG COMB Slang term for a metal hairdressing comb.

DOG'S EAR The bent-back points of a strand of hair when winding hair on a curler for a permanent wave or shaping a curl.

DOG'S EARS, THE See En-oreilles-d'epagnent.

DOG'S LEG COMB See Boomerang comb.

DOG WIG A wig of nylon or human hair for wear by pet dogs. Called a 'doggie-wiggy', USA, 1967. 'Nylon wigs cost £4, but wigs made from human hair and coming in black, dachshund brown, yorkie blond, silver grey and white are £7'. (*Daily Express*, 22.11.67)

DOLICHOCEPHALIC Long-headed (skull with breadth less than 4/5th of length).

DOLL'S WIG Usually made directly on the doll's head and until the 19th century human hair was usually employed and still is for the best dolls. Mohair is also used for inferior wigs. Legros, the 18th century Parisian wigmaker, exhibited thirty coiffured dolls at the annual fair of Saint-Ovide in 1763. (*Von Boehn*)

DOLLY BOB (American style) Similar to Buster Brown hair cut but a little longer with a slight curl on ends of hair. A girl's style popular in the 1920s. (*Rohrer*)

DOLLY CURL A small curl.

DOLLY LOOK A woman's hair style of waves and curls. 1968, *cf* Little Girl Coiffure.

DOLLY VARDEN HAIRDRESS Dressed to a centre parting with shoulder length loose ringlets. So named after a character in Charles Dickens's *Barnaby Rudge*, 1841, illustrated by Hablot K Browne. Bonnets of the shape worn by this character, also gay coloured gowns with a pointed bodice and skirt are also named after her. Creer illustrated the 'Dolly Varden' headdress as a double plait, the ends tied by a bow of ribbon; but this is not the style illustrated by H. K. Browne, whose drawing must be regarded as authoritative. *419(3)*

DOME FALL A loose fall of false hair, the root ends of which are dressed over a pad to give height at the head.

DOMINO MASK A half mask to cover the eyes.

DONA SOL A woman's hair style of 1865. (*Bysterveld* p 64)

DONDEL Famous French Coiffure, born 1833 at Rennes, died 1903; a creator of world-famous coiffures and friend of hair masters such as Leroy, Leblond, Balade, Amelin, Dufour, Robert, etc. (*J. de la C*, No. 19 1903)

DON SALTERO Barber to Oliver Cromwell.

DONUT (1) A small round chignon with a hole in the centre. (2) A small round chignon. Both named after the doughnut confection.

DONUT BUN See Donut.

DONUT BUN PAD A round pad with a centre hole over which is dressed the Donut, *qv*.

DONUT NET A net of human hair to enclose a donut.

DOODLE (also Noodle) An 18th century man's flowing wig. Described in the 18th century burletta of Tom Thumb. (*Smith, JT*)

DOOR KNOCKER STYLE Woman's hair style 1857. *289*

DOOR MAT American slang term for a wig. (*Berrey*)

DOPE Word used for the liquid used in hot permanent waving systems. Hairdressing craft slang *c* 1925 to *c* 1939.

DORÉ-E Fr. Golden or Gilded.

DORLET A hair net ornamented with jewels. 15/16th century.

DOUBLE ADHESIVE An adhesive patch having adhesive on both its sides. Used for securing toupets and scalpettes to bald heads. See Double-sided adhesive.

DOUBLE BRUSHING With a brush in each hand brushing a head of hair with the two brushes alternately.

DOUBLE COMB Two combs, one clasped into the other. 17th century. (*Holme*)

DOUBLE CROWN A head of hair having two natural crowns.

DOUBLE-DIP POMPADOUR A woman's pompadour hair style in which a wave dips forward over each eye.

DOUBLE EIGHT PLAIT A twist of hair coiled into a double eight formation.

DOUBLE-ENDED-SWITCH A stem of wound hair made by sewing the centre of a length of weft to the centre of the stem cord and winding one half; the cord is then reversed and the remaining unwound half of the weft wound. Both ends have a loop and the points of the hair on each half of the stem point to the centre of the cord, *cf* Double-loop-cluster.

DOUBLE GRECIAN PLAIT See Plait.

DOUBLE HAIR DYE A dye comprising two ingredients that are mixed before use or applied one after the other. A 'two-bottle' dye, eg Para and hydrogen peroxide.

DOUBLE HAIRPIN A hairpin with two prongs constructed from bent wire, as opposed to the single pronged hairpin or bodkin.

DOUBLE KNOT The two knots, *qv*, used to secure a pinch of hair to the wig net. See Knotting.

DOUBLE KNOTTING Forming a double knot; tyeing a wisp of hair to a net foundation by means of two knots at the root end of the wisp. Used on soft net foundations, *cf* Single knotting used on stiff foundation net.

DOUBLE LOOP CLUSTER A small postiche or hair piece made of woven hair on a tail cord with a loop at either end to secure it to the head. It is dressed in a cluster of curls.

DOUBLE-O A very close hair cut. From the number 00 on hair clippers. American usage.

DOUBLE QUEUED WIG An 18th century wig with two tails or queues.

DOUBLE SHAMPOO Two complete shampoos, including two latherings and two rinses. All thorough shampoos are double shampoos.

DOUBLE SHAVE See Close shaving.

DOUBLE-SIDED ADHESIVE Tape, cloth or waterproof material with adhesive on both sides for securing toupets and other hair pieces to the scalp or face.

DOUBLE-TOOTH-COMB A hair-cutting comb with teeth on both sides of the spine. American usage. (*Smith*)

DOUGHNUT See Donut.

DOW Black. Generally applied to hair. Gaelic origin. (*Mac-Neill*)

DOWER BRUSH A hairbrush made from specially selected boar bristles. American usage.

DOWN The fine hair as it first shows itself on the human face.

DOWNDO A hair style dressed hanging over the neck, forehead and ears. 20th century.

DRAB (1) Adj. and subs. A colour or tone which contains no red or yellow. Dull in colour. (2) Verb. To remove red or yellow tones from the hair.

DRABBING A process to tone down bright hair colours such as auburn by means of a rinse.

DRABBING AGENT A suitable chemical used to produce ash-blonde or mouse-coloured hair.

DRAB SERIES Hair dyes that contain no red or yellow. Dull colours.

DRAGON See Serpent.

DRAGONNE See a La Dragonne.

DRAKE See Drake tail curl.

DRAKE TAIL CURL When only the ends of the hair turn up and all the rest hangs smooth. 17th century. (*Holme*)

DRAW Subs. A thin strand of hair left unplaited and running through plaited hair which is used as a runner over which the plait can be pushed to shorten, widen and thicken it.

DRAWING The process of pulling hair from between the brushes with the drawing knife.

DRAWING-A-PARTING Parting the hair with a comb.

DRAWING BLADE See Drawing knife.

DRAWING BRUSH The brushes that are used to hold hair to be drawn off for mixing, matching, knotting or weaving.
172, 462

DRAWING CARD Wire prongs with bent teeth set in leather and used to hold hair that is to be drawn off for mixing, matching, knotting or weaving. *173*

DRAWING GAUZE See Parting gauze.

DRAWING HOOK A very fine hook used for drawing hair through the parting silk to make a drawn-through parting, *qv*.

DRAWING KNIFE A blunt-edged knife or razor used to draw off hair. (*Creer*)

DRAWING MAT See Drawing card.

DRAWING NEEDLE A fine barbed steel needle for drawing hair through silk in making a drawn-through parting.

DRAWING OFF See Drawing.

DRAWING WIRE See Drawing card.

DRAWN PARTING See Drawn-through parting.

DRAWN-THROUGH PARTING The parting of a wig or other postiche having a parting so constructed that the hair after being knotted to the foundation net is drawn through a white or parchment-coloured fine silk that has the appearance of the natural scalp. In England, this type of parting began to replace the knotted hair-lace partings, *c* 1917.

DRAW OFF Verb. To pull hair with the drawing knife from between the brushes.

DREADLOCKS A hair style consisting of hanging locks of hair with metal beads secured at the points. 1977.

DREDGE To sprinkle with flour or powder. See Powder dredge.

DREDGE BOX A box or container with perforated top used to sprinkle powder or flour on hair. (*Pindar, Hair powder*, ed 1795)

DREDGER See Dredge box.

DRESSING Subs. The dressed hair. The hairdress, coiffure or hairdo. 'This is a very lovely dressing.'

DRESSING BLOCK A malleable block, *qv*, on which are dressed postiches.

DRESSING COMB A medium sized hair comb used in dressing hair.

DRESSING HAIR Arranging the locks into a desired hair style. The elements of a coiffure can be secured by the use of (1) pins, (2) grips, (3) slides, (4) combs, (5) back-combing, (6) gums and lacquers, (9) ties such as ribbons, head binds, etc, (8) nets.

DRESSING NEEDLE See Hair needle.

DRESSING-OUT-LOTION A liquid such as (1) Brilliantine, or
(2) Scented spirit, used to spray on the set coiffure preparatory to the first dressing out.

DRESS OUT Verb. To comb and arrange the tresses after setting, drying and the combout or brushout.

DRESS WIG A formal wig worn on social occasions; any formally dressed wig worn as a fashionable article of dress, as opposed to a wig of necessity, *qv*, which is made in imitation of nature.

DRESS-UP HAIRDO A coiffure for formal or evening wear. American usage.

DROOPING MOUSTACHE Any type of moustache that hangs low over the mouth or corners of the mouth, such as a walrus moustache, *qv*.

DROOPY MOUSTACHE See Drooping moustache.

DROP A man's 18th century wig style. 'Drop wigs are in fashion.' (*Lon Mag*, 1753)

DROP CURL A curl or ringlet in spiral or corkscrew form.
325

DROP LOCK (1) a man's 18th century wig style. (*Tennent*)
(2) A tress of hair hanging free in a hairdress.

DROP ORNAMENTATION Hair or hair ornaments worn in a hanging position.

DROP WIG See DROP; also En-point.

DROWNED COLOUR A colour which has been added to, or bleached, dyed or interfered with to such a degree that any further attempt at lightening or darkening would have unpredictable and undesired results.

DR PANGLOSS WIG A wig of the style worn by the pedantic old tutor to the hero in Voltaire's *Candide*, 1759.

DR SYNTAX WIG A wig of the style depicted in Rowlandson's drawings of Dr Syntax in the *Tours of Dr Syntax* (1819–1821) by William Combe.

DRUG STORE BLONDE (1) Bleached hair on the head. American slang. (*B and B*)
(2) A woman with artifical blonde hair. American slang.

DRUIDS' HAIR Long moss. Wilts usage. (*B and H*)

DRYAD HAIRDRESS See A la Driade.

DRY BURN A burn occasioned by dry heat.

DRY EGG SHAMPOO A shampoo for which only the white of an egg is used.

DRYER An apparatus for drying the hair. Basically all hair dryers consist of a system whereby the air is heated and blown onto the head. In most dryers both the heating and blowing are electrically activated, but in the 19th century gas heated dryers with electrically driven fans were commonly used. There are hood dryers which cover the head, spider dryers that have long fingers with holes for the hot air to issue from, and which are placed over the head; and hand dryers which are small hand-held nozzles emitting hot air.

DRY SET A hair set on dry or slightly damp hair by the use of rollers, the fingers and a comb and then heating under a hot dryer for a few minutes.

DRY SHAMPOO (1) A shampoo in powder form which is applied to the head as a powder, massaged in and then brushed out, carrying absorbed grease with it. An early 19th century formula was: 8 oz cassia lignum reduced to a very fine powder, with 1/2 oz white vitriol (zinc sulphate), well mixed and sifted. A modern 20th century formula is: Borax 6.6%, sodium sesquicarbonate 16.5%, Fullers earth 16.5%, talc 60.4%, perfume *qv*. Other formulae include: corn meal, powdered orris root, powdered starch, etc.
(2) A shampoo composed of industrial methylated spirit or isopropyl alcohol and water with the addition of a foaming element such as saponin. This type is also called Liquid dry shampoo and Spirit shampoo. The latter is to be preferred. Both the other terms are long-standing misnomers as this formula is as wet as any normal wet shampoo.

DRY SHAVER An electric or tension spring operated shaving machine.

DRY TETTER See *Psoriasis Capitis*. (*Wheeler*)

DTP Drawn-through parting, *qv*.

DU BARRY COIFFURE The style of hairdress worn by Comtesse Marie Jeanne du Barry (1746–1793), mistress of Louis XV. She was guillotined for conspiring against the French Republic. In 1891 there was a short curled style with forehead curls, dressed away from the neck, called by this name.

DUCHESS A bow of ribbon worn high with the Fontange Headdress. (*Cunnington*)

DUCHESSE DE LONGUEVILLE COIFFURE Long waved and curled hair combed back from forehead and arranged over the neck and ears; a short fringe extending across the forehead. After the style worn by Anne (1619–1679) only daughter of the Prince of Condé. She married, 1639, the Duc de Longueville.

DUCHESSE D'ORLEANS 18th century style as worn by her. *260*

DUCHESS OF DEVONSHIRE COIFFURE A hairdress in the style of that worn by Georgiana, Duchess of Devonshire (1757–1806), wife of the 5th Duke of Devonshire. This coiffure is possibly one of the finest English designed hair styles of all time. *376*

DUCK-BILL-IRONS A hair-former, similar to Marcel waving irons, but having the hollow rod and solid rod ovoid-shaped, rather like a duck's bill, instead of rounded. Overall width of outer (hollow) rod, ½″. (*Symonds*)

DUCK'S ARSE A vulgarism for the Duck's tail hair style for men, *qv*, *c* 1959. American usage.

DUCK'S TAIL A fish-hook, *qv*.

DUCK'S-TAIL COIFFURE A woman's short hair style of *c* 1935 in which the lower ends of the hair were turned up into half curls, like a duck's tail. This became a popular style for several years.

DUCK'S-TAIL HAIR STYLE A man's long hair style in which the neck hair turned up like a duck's tail. Popular from *c* 1958.

DUCKTAIL BEARD An American beard style. 19/20th century. *97k*

DUCK TAIL CUT See Duck's tail coiffure. (*Ingerid*)

DULAPE See Dewlap.

DUMB BLONDE A physically attractive, but mentally dull or stupid, blonde-haired woman.

DUMMY A dummy head on which wigs were displayed. 18/19th century. (*Thornbury*)

DUMONT, JULES Born 1856 in France. Is said to have had a beard 11′ 11½″ long.

DUNDREARY WHISKERS Long, drooping side whiskers and no beard. From the character of Lord Dundreary in Tom Taylor's *Our American Cousins*, 1858. A late 19th century style, also called Piccadilly Weepers and Weepers, *qv*. (*Rogers and Allen*)

DURABLE CURL A long-lasting curl, but not necessarily permanent.

DUST COMB See Dandruff comb.

DUTCH A man's 18th century wig style. (*Colman*)

DUTCH BANG A straight fringe.

DUTCH COIFFURE A hair style for women consisting of long curls, dressed close to and around the head, with a bow or ribbon at the crown, *c* 1730.

DUTCH CUT (1) Similar to a bob cut, *qv*, but used from an early period on children's hair to avoid the tangles that were the invariable result of all long-haired styles for children.
(2) A plain hair style for men, 16th century. (*Stubbes*)
(3) Flat-top crew cut.

DUTCH DOLL Short straight hair style for women. A bob.

DUVILLIER WIG A very high dressed wig named after the famed French wigmaker of late 17th century. Also called a falbala and furbelow periwig. 'Huge falbala periwigs.' (*Steele. The Tatler*, 1709)

DWYER, EDWARD The first recorded Irishman to wear a wig. (*Doran*)

DYE (1) Subs. Colour or hue produced by dyeing. See Hair dye.
(2) Subs. A substance (especially in solution) used for dyeing hair.
(3) Verb. To diffuse a colour or tint through; to colour or stain; to impregnate hair or fix a colour in the substance of hair.

DYE BACK The dyeing of bleached hair back to its natural colour.

DYE BRUSH A small brush like a tooth-brush or a flat paint brush used for applying hair dye.

DYE CAPE A covering of rubber or plastic or thick cotton material worn around the shoulders to protect the client from any spilt dye.

DYEING Subs. The process of impregnating the tissue of the hair with colour.
An Assyrian recipe of 600 BC was: 'Gall of a black ox (V. Gall of a snake), gall of a scorpion, gall of a pig, punpulla . . ., suadu, thou shalt reduce; these five drugs in equal parts thou shalt mix . . . which have been buried (?) take up and together mix, in the oil of a cyprus of the cemetery . . . press on the head, seven days anoint, and the grey hair will turn black.' (*Stubbs and Bligh*) Frequent allusions to hair dyeing occur in works of the 16/17th century. 'If any have haire of her owne natural growing which is not faire enough, then they will die it in divers colours.' (*Stubbes, Anatomie of Abuses*, 1583). Before the introduction of aniline dyes in 1859, most hair dye was of vegetable origin. A hair dye may be permanent or temporary. It may be a coating dye or a penetrating dye; synthetic (aniline derivative), metallic or mineral, vegetable or compound; and act 'instantaneously' or progressively; and in form may be applied as a liquid or a paste. No dye can be semi-permanent; the expression is a contradiction in terms. It can only be permanent or temporary, albeit long-lasting. The term semi-permanent is an Americanism adopted by some hairdressers in Britain and introduced by dye manufacturers' advertising material.

DYE-REMOVER A liquid suitable for the removal of hair dyes. The type of chemical used will depend upon the type of dye to be removed.

DYE STICK A short round or flattened rod of glass, wood (often cane), bone or other suitable material, with cotton wool wound around one end, used for the application of hair dye or bleach.

DYNEL A synthetic fibre used instead of hair in the manufacture of cheap wigs. (*Hanle*)

DYSTICHIA A double row of hairs on the eye-lids. 1707 (*Glosso*)

E

EAR CURL See pincurl.

EAREJEWEL A love lock, *qv*. (*Prynne*, 1628)

EARE LOCKE (Ear lock) Another name for love lock, *qv*, especially a lock hanging over the ear. Described by Prynne, 1628, as 'badges of infamie, effeminacy, vanitie, singularitie, pride, lasciviousnesse and shame, in the eyes of God.'

EAR GUARD (1) Side whiskers, slang.
(2) A small circle or square of a suitable material used to protect the ears during the drying process. (*Mitchell*)

EAR HAIR (1) The hair that grows in or on the ear.
(2) The hair that grows on the head in the vicinity of the ear.

EAR LAPPET A wave or loop of hair dressed over the ear. Early 20th century.

EAR-PEAK The hair adjacent to the top and front part of the ear.

EAR PHONES Coiled plaits over the ears, *c* 1916.

EAR PLUG A small plug to fit in the ear as a protection against the roar of the hair dryer.

EAR POINT See Ear peak.

EAR PROTECTOR See Ear guard.

EAR PUFF See Ear guard (2).

EASY CURL A loose sausage curl. 'The toupee dressed in easy curls.' (*Chapman*, Vol 1 p 387)

EAU (Fr) Water.

EAU D'AFRIQUE A 19/20th century 'secret' preparation for dyeing the hair black, consisting of three liquids that had to be applied in succession: (1) A solution of 3 parts of silver nitrate in 100 of water, (2) An 8% aqueous solution of sodium sulphide, (3) A solution of silver nitrate, as (1) but scented. (*Koller*)

EAU D'AMERIQUE See Plumbiferous hair water.

EAU D'APOLLON See Plumbiferous hair water.

EAU DE BAHAMA See Plumbiferous hair water.

EAU DE CAPILLE See Plumbiferous hair water.

EAU DE CASTILE See Plumbiferous hair water.

EAU DE CHINE An early 19th century hair-dye made of 1 part silver nitrate and 4 parts hydrated lime. (*Debay*)

EAU DE COLOGNE A perfume made at Cologne in Germany, where its manufacture was first established by the Italian, Giovanni Maria Farina (1685–1766), who settled there in 1709. There are numerous formulae each claiming to be the original. The following example will suffice: Oil of Bergamot, oil of lemon, of each 2 fluid drachms; oil of orange 1 fluid drachm, Neroli ¾ fluid drachm, oil of Rosemary ½ fluid drachm, essence of ambergris, essence of musk, of each 3 or 4 drops. Rectified spirit 1 pint. (*Cooley*)

EAU DE FLORIDA See Plumbiferous hair water.

EAU DE JOUVENCE Hydrogen peroxide. 19th century. (*Mallemont*)

EAU DE QUININE A 19th century tonic for the hair: Quinine sulphate 2 parts, tincture of Krameria 4 parts, tincture of cantharides 2 parts, spirit of lavender 10 parts, glycerine 15 parts, alcohol 100 parts. (*Hiscox*)

EAU DES FEES (Fairy water) A proprietary dye for hair and beard marketed by Madame Sarah Felix, Paris, in 1873.

EAU DE ZENOBLE A 19/20th century 'secret' hair dye, consisting of a solution of sodium hyposulphite, sodium sulphate and sodium acetate, with free acetic acid, and a sedimental deposit of lead sulphide. (*Koller*) This could have been injurious.

EAU D'INNS See Plumbiferous hair water.

EAU HAMILTON See Plumbiferous hair water.

EAU MAGIQUE See Plumbiferous hair water.

EAU SUBLIME DE FEUILLES A 'secret' hair dye, 19/20th century. It consisted of a 1½% aqueous solution of lead acetate with glycerin and sulphur. This could have been dangerous. (*Koller*)

EBENE Fr. Ebony. *Des cheveux d'ébène* raven hair.

ECAILLE Fr. Tortoiseshell. *Peigne d'écaille*: tortoiseshell comb.

ECCLESIASTICAL PERUKE Wigs of the 18th and early 19th centuries suitable for wear by the clergy. (*London Mag*, 1764)

ECKERT'S HAIR WASH A 19/20th century 'secret' preparation which consisted of water, alcohol, glycerin, lead acetate, fruity-ether, and a sediment of undissolved lead acetate and precipitated sulphur. This could have been dangerous to health. (*Koller*)

ECOLE Fr. Academy or School.

ECONNOMME See A L'Econnomme.

ECTODERMIS The outside of the skin.

EDWARD OF THE WIG Edward Dwyer, the first recorded Irishman to wear a wig. (*Doran*, p 153)

EEL FAT 18th century remedy to make hair grow. (*Stewart*, p 266)

EFFILAGE (1) Hair tapering.

(2) Tapering haircut. See also Effilate. (*Ray*)

EFFILATE To cut hair by slithering the scissors up and down the hair strand. (*Trusty*)

EFFILATION The act of cutting the hair by slithering the scissors up and down the hair strand. See also Effilate. (*Trusty*)

EFFILE Fr. Tapered.

EFFILEING Slither cutting hair.

EFFLEURAGE A stroking massage movement in which a light, continuous rubbing without pressure is applied to the scalp or skin.

EGAN A London wigmaker and a Roman Catholic in whose house James Boswell lodged in 1760. (*Boswell's Journals of a Tour to the Hebrides*, ed Pottle, FA and Bennett CH, 1936)

EGG CURL See French curl (1).

EGG-HEAD (1) A head shaped like an egg.

(2) An intellectual. American usage.

EGG JULEP A stimulating shampoo for the hair: Rectified spirit 1 pint, Rose water 1 gallon, extract of Rondeletia, *qv*, ½ pint, transparent soap ½ oz, hay saffron ½ drachm. Shave up the soap and boil it and the saffron in a quart of rose water; when dissolved add remainder of rose water; then the spirit finally the rondeletia, which is used to perfume the mixture. Although called egg julep, the egg is absent. (*Piesse*). See also Egg shampoo.

EGG JULEP SHAMPOO See Egg julep.

EGG SHAMPOO Popular in the Victorian and Edwardian periods. Valuable in hard water areas, good for dry, overbleached and damaged hair. For best results the egg white and yolk should be beaten separately and then mixed and applied to the hair. Two to six eggs were usually sufficient for a complete treatment. The use of egg as a shampoo avoided the formation of scum by the action of soap and hard water. It also left the hair with a remarkable lustre.

Of recent years egg shampoos containing less than 10% of emulsified or dispersed egg powder have been marketed. In earlier years there were some who used only the yolk of the egg, and others who used only the white, and for very greasy hair the juice of half a lemon was added. (*Family Economist*, 1859; *Piesse*, 1855)

'To clean the hair, Mr Nesbit recommends the yolks of a couple of eggs, beat till they form a cream, to be rubbed into the hair, and then washed out with tepid water, well brushed and wiped, as bestowing the most silky and beautiful appearance.' (*Walker*, 1837)

EGG YOLK SHAMPOO Egg yolk emulsifies readily with the grease of the hair, facilitating its rapid removal by the water rinse. See Egg shampoo.

EGYPTIAN BOB A woman's hair style in which the hair is cut to a bob with a fringe and worn straight. Style of the 1920s and 1960s. (*Rohrer*) 262

EGYPTIAN HENNA See Henna.

EGYPTIAN HENNA SHAMPOO See Henna shampoo.

EGYPTIAN LIQUID Synonym for Chinese wash, *qv*.

EGYPTIAN LOOK A woman's hair style in the fashion of Ancient Egypt. See Cleopatra look, and Egyptian bob.

EGYPTIAN PRIVET See Henna.

EGYPTIAN WATER A 19th century American hair-dye consisting of: Nitrate of silver 1 oz; nitrate of bismuth 1 oz; subacetate of lead 4 oz dissolved in warm water. One hour after application concentrated sulphuretted water was applied to the hair. A very dangerous process. (*Dussauce*)

EGYPTIAN WIG Wig worn by the ancient Egyptians. A strong taboo concerning the head or hair of a King being seen by his subjects seems to have been the origin of wig-wearing. Later the habit spread to other members of the ruling class. (*Murray*). These wigs were constructed from human hair or vegetable fibre (date palm fibre and grass). (*Lucas*) For details of manufacture see 'The Construction of an Ancient Egyptian Wig (*c* 1400 BC) in the British Museum' by J Stevens Cox, Toucan Press, 1978.

248

ELASTIC A tensile rubber thread used in some types of wig to hold them securely to the head.

ELASTICITY OF THE HAIR The hair's capacity for being stretched.

ELASTIC SPRING Tension Spring, *qv*.

ELDER (*Sambucus Ebulus*) The Romans used the juice of the black elder as a hair dye. (*Fernie*)

ELECTRIC CLIPPER A hair clipper motivated by electricity.

ELECTRIC HAIR BRUSH A hair brush constructed of an ebony type material which generated electricity when brushing the hair. An advertisement in *The World* of June 1882 for Dr Scott's Electric Hair Brush warranted it to cure nervous headache, bilious headache or neuralgia in five minutes. It was also claimed that its use would prevent baldness, cure dandruff, arrest greyness and soothe the weary brain! Supplied to the Prince and Princess of Wales and W E Gladstone. Price 12/6d. post free.

ELECTRIC HAIR CUTTING MACHINE See Electric clipper.

ELECTRIC RAZOR A razor motivated by electricity in which a cutting edge oscillates or rotates rapidly over a stationary edge. See Electric shaver.

ELECTRIC SHAVER Invented by Col Jacob Schick in 1928.

ELECTRIC SHAVING MACHINE First patented by Jacob Schick in 1928. See Electric razor.

ELECTRIC WAVING IRON A waving iron connected by flexible, insulated electricity wire to a supply of electricity by which it was heated.

ELECTROLOGIST One skilled in the removal of superfluous hair by electrolysis, *qv*. American usage.

ELECTROLYSIS The destruction of hair roots by means of an electric needle.

ELEGANCE (THE) A woman's hair style of the period of Louis XVI. (*Bysterveld*, p 56)

ELEGANT (Fr) Elegant, fashionable.

ELEMENTARY BLEACH The same as Simple Bleach, *qv*.

ELEPHANT See A l'Eléphant.

ELEVATED PINCURL A pincurl with a stem standing at right angles to the head.

ELF LOOK A hair style for women of an impish or tricksy appearance; 1960s.

ELF KNOT See Elf lock.

ELF LOCK Tangled hair. 'The clotted, matted locks of wicked elves.' Lodge in his *Wits Miserie*, 1599, describes a devil named Brawling-Contention as 'his haires are curl'd, and full of elves locks and nitty for want of kembing', It was said that one of the favourite amusements of Queen Mab was to tie people's hair in knots. (*Douce*)

ELITE (Fr) Select body of persons.

ELIXIR A sovereign remedy for disease and thus adopted as a name for quack remedies.

ELIZABETH I, QUEEN OF ENGLAND She wore yellowish-red false hair. 'Crinem fulvum sed factitium.' (*Hentzner*, ed p 135, 1612)

ELIZABETHAN HAIR STYLES Hairdresses similar to those worn during the reign of Elizabeth I. See Neo-Elizabethans.

ELLIPTICAL CURL A curl formed in the shape of an ellipse, a regular oval.

ELL WIG A child's wig made of cloth or wool. Long ell was a particular kind of cloth made in Devon. 'The monstrousness of their children's ell wiggs.' (*Englands Vanity*, 1683)

ELSNER'S BEARD DYE A 19/20th century 'secret' preparation consisting of two liquids; one contained pyrogallic acid, the other was an ammoniacal solution of silver nitrate. (*Koller*)

ELVIS PRESLEY STYLE A hair style for men named after the popular singer, 1956.

EMOLLIENT A substance that has the power of softening or relaxing living animal tissues.

EMPIRE COMB A hair comb decorated with small cameos, mock pearls, coral, etc, in the Empire style, *qv*. (*Smith, HC*)

EMPIRE CURLS Loose hanging or drop curls worn at the neck.

EMPIRE-FRINGE A fringe of curled weft with clusters of curls worn over the temples, *c* 1906.

EMPIRE HAIR STYLE A hairdress in the fashion of those worn at the period of the first Napoleonic Empire or of the second Empire after the marriage of Napoleon III with the Empress Eugénie.

EMPIRE KNOT A figure-of-three knot composed of a long twisted, one-spill-tail formed into three circles and worn as a chignon. Edwardian period.

EMPIRE PUFF (1) A large frisette incorporated in a hairdress.
(2) A bunch of pin-curls used in the dressing of the Empire coiffure, *c* 1900. (*Vasco*)

EMPIRE STYLE See Empire hair style.

EMPRESS BANDEAU A style of *c* 1898 in which the hair was drawn back from the face, rolled behind the ears, drawn down beside the neck and united to the chignon. (*Mallemont*) *297*

EMPRESS EUGENIE COIFFURE A hairdress in the style of that worn by Eugénie de Montijo (1826–1920), wife of Napoleon III (m 1853). After the fall of the Empire she retired to England, living at Farnborough. Method of dressing the style: Divide the hair by a cross parting, fasten the back hair on top of the head, divide the front hair to make a plait over each temple. Comb up the hair and with the short hair make a light fringe curl over the middle of the forehead, leaving the temples free. Position a chignon of very long curls mounted on a comb well forward, only a few inches from the front, then pin the curls back from the ears, leaving them to hang down the neck. Lastly adjust the Imperial diadem. (*Mallemont*)

EMULSIFIER See Emulsifying agent.

EMULSIFYING AGENT A substance that, added to a mixture of two liquids, will hold them in permanent emulsion. Examples: Soap, sodium carbonate, lanoline, albumen, casein, egg, gum arabic, size, etc.

EMULSION A mixture of two liquids in which particles of one are in suspension with the other.

EMULSION BLEACH The same as oil bleach, *qv*.

EN BEGUILLE (The crutch) A man's wig style of the 18th century. (*Lon Mag*, 1764)

EN-BOUCLE-DEMI-NATURELLE (The half natural) A man's wig style of the 18th century. (*Lon Mag*, 1764)

EN-BOUCLE-DETACHEE (The loose buckle) A man's wig style of the 18th century (*Lon Mag*, 1764)

EN-CHAINES (The chain buckle) A man's wig style of the 18th century. (*Lon Mag*, 1764)

EN CHEVEUX Fr. Bareheaded (of a woman). Nu-tête (of a man).

EN COQUE Fr. A hair style incorporating a smooth loop or bow of hair dressed erect.

EN-CUE-D'ARTICHAEUX (The artichoke bottom) A man's wig style of the 18th century. (*Lon Mag*, 1764)

END PAPER A small piece of paper used to facilitate the correct winding of the hair points preliminary to a permanent wave.

EN-ECHELLE (The ladder) A man's wig style of the 18th century. (*Lon Mag*, 1764)

EN-ESCALIER (The staircase) A man's wig style of the 18th century. (*Lon Mag*, 1764)

EN-ESCARGOT (The snail buckle) A man's wig style of the 18th century. (*Lon Mag*, 1764)

ENGINE 18th century term for curling irons; also any apparatus used in the preparation or arrangement of the hair.

'What tho' untaught by art thy Ringlets twine.

No engines scorch, or Papillotes confine.' (*The Art of Dressing the Hair*, a poem by *Ellis Pratt*, Bath 1770)

ENGLISH CURL Loose ringlet curl, 17th century. French and Low Countries usage – Boucle Anglaise. (*Villermont*)

ENGLISH CUT (1) A 16th century man's style. 'The English Cut is base, and gentlemen scorne it.' (*Greene, Quip*, 1592)

(2) American name for a man's hair style in which the hair is long at the top, long and full at the sides and back and combed away from the forehead. 1950s.   *102K*

ENGLISH-DRAWN-THROUGH-PARTING   See Drawn-through-parting.

ENGLISH HAIR DYE A 19th century American preparation consisting of green shells of walnuts, 5 oz, litharge 2 oz, slaked lime 2 oz. This produced a soot-like colour. (*Dussauce*)

ENGLISH LOOK Long, straight hair style for teenage girls. From April, 1965. American usage.

ENGLISH PARTING A drawn-through parting made by knotting hair to the foundation net or gauze and then drawing it through the parting silk. (*Botham and Sharrad*). See also French parting.

ENGLISH STITCH See Stitching.

ENGLISH THINNING To thin the hair from underneath, leaving, depending on the style, the outside hair longer. (*Trusty*)

EN GRAIN D'EPINARDS (The spinage seed) A man's wig style of the 18th century (*London Mag*, 1764)

EN LONG (The long bob) A man's wig style of the 18th century. (*London Mag*, 1764)

EN MEDAILLON Fr. Descriptive name of an 18th century hair style in which is incorporated, and worn hanging down between the shoulder blades, a medaillon-like structure composed of ribbon and other suitable material.   *191*

EN NEGLIGEE (The negligée) A man's wig style of the 18th century. (*Lon Mag*, 1764)

ENOBARBUS Branch of the Roman family to which Nero belonged; the name meaning copper-coloured or red beard. (*Gowing*)

ENOOREILLES-D'EPAGNEUL (The dog's ears) A man's wig style of the 18th century. (*Lon Mag*. 1764)

EN PLI Fr. Wet hair that has been set for a style preparatory to drying and dressing out.

EN POINT (The drop wig) A man's wig style of the 18th century. (*Lon Mag*, 1764)

EN QU'ES ACO? A woman's hair style of 1774 incorporating a banging chignon. This style was caricatured for several years after its advent.

EN ROULEAUX Fr. (1) Hair rolled or wound on curlers. (2) Hair dressed in long rolls.

EN SERPENTEUX Fr. Hair dressed in straggling, loosely waved serpents, *qv*.

ENSIGN (ENSEIGNE) A provocative curl dropping on the face and worn to attract men.

EN SOLEIL-LEVANT A woman's late 18th century hair style. (*Villermont*)   *224*

EN TAURO 18th century term for hair curled on the head, resembling that on a bull's forehead. (*Stewart*, p 289)

ENTIQUITEE See A L'Entiquitée.

EN VERGETTE A sort of basket weave or plaiting, 18th century. 'Tis a wig en vergette, that from Paris was brought.' (*Anstey*)

EPI (de cheveux) Fr. Tuft of hair

EPIDERMIS The scarf skin.

EPILATE Verb. To pull out or eradicate hair.

EPILATION The action of pulling out hair.

EPILATION FORCEPS Forcepts used to remove hair.

EPILE HAIR Hair that has been pulled from or fallen from the scalp. Combings.

EPINGLE (à cheveux) Fr. Hairpin.

EPINGLE ONDULINE (Anglicised French expression.) Waving pin.

EPISCOPAL WIG See Bishop's wig.

EPITHELIAL HAIR Hair growing from the epithelium, the non-vascular tissue forming the outer layer of the mucous membrane. Hair growing from inside the nose.

ERASMUS WILSON'S HAIR PROMOTER A 19/20th century 'secret' preparation that consisted of 300 parts of almond oil, 300 parts of ammonia, 500 parts of Rosemary spirit, 60 parts of cantharides tincture and 35 parts of lemon oil. (*Koller*)

ERECT HAIR STYLE A style in which the hair is dressed standing up from the scalp.

ERECTORES PILI The small muscles that cause the hair to stand erect.

ERIOCOMUS Woolly.

ERYSIPELAS ALOPECIA Loss of hair from the head resulting from erysipelas. (*Wheeler*)

ESILLAG'S BEARD-FORCING POMADE A 19/20th century 'secret' preparation of ordinary fat pomade, with traces of bergamot oil, Peruvian balsam and similar additives. (*Koller*)

ESILLAG'S TEA HAIR WASH A 19/20th century 'secret' preparation which consisted of camomile. (*Koller*)

ESPRIT FEATHER See Aigrette.

ESQUIRE-WIG A gentleman's natural full wig. 1968.

ESSENCE (1) A perfume or scent.

(2) A substance obtained, usually by distillation from a plant and containing its characteristic properties in a concentrated form.

(3) Alcoholic solution of an essential oil.

ESSENCED-HAIR Perfumed hair.

'What courtly youth, with essenced hair,

Shall at thy board the giblet bear.' (*Horace*. Tran P Francis, 1742)

ESSENTIAL OIL Volatile oil of vegetable origin, derived by distillation from plants, barks, flowers, leaves, woods, etc. Soluble in alcohol. Examples: Eucalyptus oil, oil of Roses, *qv*.

ESSENTIA-ODORIFERIA A popular early 19th century perfume compunded of grain musk, balsam of Peru, civet, oil of cloves, oil of rhodium, salt of tartar, and spirits of wine. (*The Ladies' Treasury*, 1859)

ESQUISSE Fr. A preliminary sketch for a hair style.

ETAGER Fr. To taper the hair.

ETAMINE (Estamin, estamine, parting gauze, parting net, knotting gauze, etamine gauze.)

(1) A white, ivory or pink coloured gauze used beneath the parting-silk of a wig to secure the knotted hair for a drawn-through parting.

(2) An open woollen fabric used for making sieves and theatrical wigs. 19th century.

ETHYL ALCOHOL See Alcohol anhydrous.

EUCALYPTUS OIL Dinkum oil. A volatile oil from the fresh leaves of *eucalyptus globulus labill*, and of some other species of eucalyptus. Has been used to mask the unpleasant odour of depilatories containing inorganic sulphides. (*Sagarin*)

EUGENE (1) A permanent waving system named after its inventor, Eugene Suter.

(2) Verb. By extension of meaning this word came to be used as a verb meaning 'to permanently wave'. I am going to have my hair eugèned. (1928)

EUPLYSIA A 19th century proprietary hair wash manufactured by Rowland and Sons, London.

EUREKA PUFF A lightly dressed artificial front of hair, *c* 1892. *286*

EURIDICE See A L'Euridice.

EUROPEAN HAIR Hair from the head of an inhabitant of Europe. Usually finer than Asiatic hair and preferred for wigs for everyday wear.

EUTRAPELUS Barber referred to in the works of Martial, the Roman satirical poet, 1st century AD.

EUXINE BOX WOOD See Box wood.

EVENING DRESSING See Evening hairdress.

EVENING HAIRDRESS A hair style suitable for evening wear. These styles are usually more formal than the day dressings.

EVENING STYLE See Evening hairdress.

EVERY OTHER, EVERY OTHER A wigmaking term. Knot every other hole on every other line; in other words knot a hole, miss a hole. Knot a line of every other hole, and miss a line.

Every hole, every other – Knot every hole on alternate lines, etc.

EXCLAMATION MARK HAIR Straight hair that stands away from the head.

EXOTHERMAL PERMANENT WAVING A system of hot permanent waving that used two chemicals which when mixed together liberated the degree of heat required to permanently wave hair. The Va-per-Marcel system of Peter Sartory in the 1920s was the best known exothermal system.

EXOTHERMIC A chemical action in which heat is evolved.

EXOTHERMIC PAD A pad containing chemicals that will produce heat.

EXPRESSED OIL Pressed out or extracted by mechanical pressure. A fixed oil. These oils are called *expressed* because they are not extracted by distillation like the essential oils.

EXTRADOS The outer curve of a curl. (A borrowed architectural term), *cf*, Intrados.

EXTRAVAGANZA (1) A mountainous hair style for women, 1776. *83*

(2) An excessive or immoderate style.

EYEBROW The arched fringe of short hairs adorning the upper orbit of the eye.

'Her eye-brows from a Mouse's hide,
Stuck on with art on either side,
Pulls off with ease, and first displays 'em,
Then in a play-book smoothly lays 'em.' (*Swift, A Beautiful Young Nymph Going to Bed*, 1731)

EYEBROW ARCHING The artificial removal of unwanted

hair from the eyebrow in order to reduce it to the required shape, usually a distinct arch.

EYEBROW COMB A small comb of ivory, boxwood, etc, with teeth at the end of a slender, pointed handle, used for combing eyebrows. (*Connoisseur*, 24 April 1755)

EYEBROW LINER A pencil shaped cosmetic for colouring the eyebrow and, if necessary, extending its length and shape by marking the skin.

EYEBROW PENCIL See Eyebrow liner.

EYEBROW TWEEZERS Metal tweezers used to pull out unwanted hairs from the eyebrows.

EYELASHES The rows of hairs fringing the lids of the eye. See Artificial eyelashes.

EYELASH BLACK Elderberry juice; burnt cork, or cloves burnt at the candle. 18/19th century. (*Toilette*, 1832)

EYELASH CURLER A small finger-operated apparatus that, by pressure, will impart a curved shape to the eyelashes.

EYEPIECE A lock of hair that hangs in the vicinity of the eye.

EYE PROTECTOR A transparent spectacle-like cover for the protection of the eyes during hair cutting.

'Its use effectually protects the eye and outer folds of the eye-lids from sharp, irritating clippings, when the beard or moustache is being trimmed,' 1888.

EYE TABBING The fixing of single artificial eyelashes to the natural eyelashes.

F

FACE CONE A cone of thick paper to hold over the face to protect it during the application of hair powder. 18th century.

FACE FUNGUS Whiskers. 19/20th century slang.

FACE LACE (1) A beard. American slang.

(2) A false beard. American slang. (*B and B*)

FACE MASK (1) Used in the 18th century to protect the face during the application of the hair powder to the coiffure.

(2) A plastic transparent mask with a handle to protect the face and lungs from sprayed lacquer. 1950s.

FACE SHAPE Seven basic face shapes are recognised by hair style designers:

(1) Oval – considered the perfect shape.

(2) Round

(3) Square

(4) Oblong or rectangular

(5) Pear (broader at chin than at temples)

(6) Heart or inverted triangle (the opposite of No 5), having greater width at temples than at chin.

(7) Diamond (narrow at temples and chin, broader at cheek bones). *278–284*

FACE TOWEL A small towel of huckaback material, *qv* used to protect the eyes and make-up during a shampoo.

FAIR CURLS In the classical theatre of Greece and Rome they symbolized a youthful hero. (*Haigh*)

FAIR EDWY (Edwig) King of Wessex, 10th century. In this and the following eleven entries *fair* relates to beauty, not to light coloured hair.

FAIR GERALDINE, THE Lady Elizabeth Fitzgerald, the supposed mistress of Henry Howard, Earl of Surrey, who dedicated poems to her. 16th century.

FAIR-HAIRED (1) Harold I, King of Norway, *c* 850–*c* 933. See also Harold Fairlocks.

(2) Duncan Macintyre (1724–1812); Gaelic poet.

FAIR-HAIRED HELEN Helen of Troy. (*Winter*)

FAIR MAID OF ANJOU, THE Lady Edith Plantagenet, kinswoman of Richard Coeur de Lion and wife of David, Prince Royal of Scotland.

FAIR MAID OF BRITTANY, THE Eleanor, daughter of Geoffrey, second son of Henry II of England. She died in Bristol Castle in 1241.

FAIR MAID OF GALLOWAY, THE Margaret, daughter of Archibald, Fifth Earl of Douglas. Died *c* 1514.

FAIR MAID OF KENT, THE Joan, daughter of Edmond Plantagenet, and wife of Edward, the Black Prince (1328–1385)

FAIR MAID OF NORWAY, THE Margaret, daughter of Eric II of Norway, 1283–1290.

FAIR PERDITA, THE Mary Robinson, English actress, novelist and poet. (1758–1800)

FAIR QUAKERESS, THE Hannah Lightfoot, whom George III, when Prince of Wales (1759) is reputed to have married.

FAIR ROSAMUND Rosamond Clifford, daughter of Walter de Clifford and mistress of Henry II of England.

FAIRIES' HAIR The common Dodder plant (*Cuscuta Epithymum*). Jersey usage (*B and H*), Guernsey folk-usage (*McClintock*).

FAIRY-HEAD (1) A fossil sea-urchin.
(2) A man with an effeminate hair style.

FAIRY FRAME A light-weight frisette.

FAIRY PUFF A bunch of curly hair sewn to a four-pronged hair comb and used on the head to dress in with the natural hair to give bulk or curl where needed. (*Hearth and Home*, 1903). Similar to a frisette on a comb, *qv*.   396

FALBALA WIG See Duvillier wig.

FALCONER, WILLIAM (1732–1769). Poet son of a hair-dresser. Chief poem, *The Shipwreck*, 1762.

FALL (1) American usage. A hair piece usually a weft (sometimes a switch or swathe) used to thicken or lengthen the back hair while using the wearer's natural hair at the front edges. Chiefly employed for down-hanging styles such as the long bob or page boy bob. See also Marteau, Torsade, Diamond mesh cluster, etc.
(2) Hair hanging loose on the shoulders, 17th century. Also in that century called a 'flat'. (*Holme*)

FALSE BEARD An artificial beard of crêpe or natural hair worn affixed by an adhesive or, in the case of full Father Christmas beards, a wire loop to pass over the ears.

FALSE CHIGNON A chignon composed of hair other than the growing hair of the wearer.

FALSE COMB See Under-comb.

FALSE EYELASHES Either single hairs stuck to existing eyelashes or eyelashes implanted on a suitable foundation and stuck to the eyelids.

FALSE HAIR (1) Natural hair worked on a postiche for wear on the head.
'So are those crisped, snaky, golden locks, which make such wanton gambols with the wind, upon supposed fairness, often known, to be the dowry of a second head, the skull that bred them in the sepulchre.' (*Shakespeare, M of V*, III, 2).
'Before the golden tresses of the dead,
The right of sepulchres, were shorn away,
To live a second life on second head;
Ere beauty's dead fleece made another gay.' (*Shakespeare, Sonnet* 68)
(2) Hair manufactured from vegetable substances or synthetic material.

FALSE HAIR-PIECE An artificial addition of hair secured to a suitable foundation, 18th century. (*Stewart*)

FALSE KNOT A coil, plait or other small hair-piece added to the coiffure. See False chignon.

FALSE LOCKS See False hair-piece, 18th century. (*Stewart*)

FALSE NATURAL CROWN A natural looking crown worked on net for incorporation in a wig. 18th century. (*Stewart*)

FALSE TAIL A switch or tail of hair made up from cut hair or combings, 18th century. (*Stewart*)

FALSE TOP A small postiche such as a scalpette. 18th century. (*Stewart*)

FALSTAFF An 18th century wig used for the characterisation of Falstaff in *The Merry Wives of Windsor* and *Henry IV*, as worn by the actors James Quinn (1693–1766), John Henderson (1747–1786) and Robert William Elliston (1774–1831) in the name part. (*Stewart*)

FALWE Yellow, 14th/18th century. 'Her falwe coloured hair.'

FAN BEARD A beard in the shape of a fan, 16th century. 'They were kept in that order by means of a wax preparation which gave the hair an agreeable odour . . . at night . . . it was done up in a sort of purse.' (*Dulaure*)

FANCY COMB Any decorated comb for display in the coiffure.

FANTAIL COMB See Comb brush, also Brush-comb.

FANTAIL WIG A man's wig style in which the queue or tail hangs loose in several curls, unsecured by a tie and not enclosed in a bag. Early 18th century.

FANTAISIE Fr. Fantastical, odd, whimsical.

FANTASTIQUE Fr. Fantastic.

FANTASY A woman's hair style of 1865. See also Fantasy style. (*Bysterveld*, p 70)

FANTASY COIFFURE See Fantasy style.

FANTASY COLOUR A colour not found in natural hair.

FANTASY SHADE Any colour, such as blue, green, etc, applied to the hair, that does not occur naturally.

FANTASY STYLE Any extreme or fantastic style used in competitive hairdressing or for display purposes; being unsuitable for normal daily wear except by such persons as mannequins.

FAN WAVING See Blow waving.

FARD (FARDE) Fr. (1) Subs. Paint (make up) for the face. 16th century.
(2) Verb. To paint the face with fard.

FARMER GILES A beard style, similar to Collier, *qv*.

FASHION (HAIR) The prevailing form, mode, shape or manner of dressing and wearing the hair. From the Latin *factio*, a doing or making, through the French term façon. 'Fashion wears out more apparel than the man.' (*Shakespeare*)

FASHION BALDNESS See *Alopecia compressio*.

FASHION-WAVING Cutting and permanently waving hair for a fashionable hair style. 1965.

FASHION WIG A wig for wear by persons with normal natural hair who wish quickly to change the colour or style of their hairdress without the necessity of having their own hair treated, *cf*, Necessity wig.

FATHER CHRISTMAS BEARD A long white bushy beard made of crêpe hair.

FAUCIOUS Without a beard. (*Josselyn, J New England's Rarities Discovered*, p 99, 1675)

FAUN BOB A woman's hair style *c* 1927.   270

FAVORI Fr. Whisker.

FAVORIE Fr. See *Au Favorie*.

FAVORITES Locks dangling on the temples. 17th century. (*Evelyn*)
'The comely Fav'rites with adorning grace,
Wave on the Breeze, and flow upon her face.' (*Prior*) 360

FAVUS Honeycomb ringworm. A contagious skin disease that can affect the scalp.

FEATHER (1) Verb. To taper, *qv*.

(2) Subs. A popular 19th century design for a hair brooch or pendant.

FEATHER BLOWN Wind blown.

FEATHER CROWN (1) A wig crown dressed in a stand-up frizz, 18th century.

(2) A wig crown made of 'the single feathers in mallards tails', 18th century. (*KP*, May 1739)

FEATHER CURL A flat tapered half curl.

FEATHER CUT The process of cutting hair relatively short and tapered, *qv*.

FEATHER EDGE A tapered edge.

FEATHERED LADY A high dressed hair style for women of 1778, topped by ostrich feathers. *475*

FEATHERED LINE A soft, minutely irregular line.

FEATHERED TOP An 18th century description of the top dressing of a wig.

FEATHERING See Tapering.

FEATHER TOP A man's 18th century wig style. (*Colman*)

'The Tyburn scratch, thick club and temple-tie,

The Parson's feather-top, frizzed broad and high,

The coachman's cauliflower, built tier on tiers,

Differ not more from bags and brigadiers

Than great St George's or St James's styles

From the broad dialect of broad St Giles.' (*Garrick, D Bon Ton*, 1775)

FEDER, LOUIS Austrian-born wigmaker who emigrated to the USA. In 1914 he established the House of Louis Feder Inc. and popularised his Tashay, a form of toupée that he advertised as 'A hurricane-resisting-hairpiece that can be combed and brushed, kept on in high winds and when swimming, and worn for weeks without removal'. When he retired in 1964 he claimed his company had sold over 100,000 hair pieces. He was known in America as the King of the toupée makers. He died of cancer at Miami, Fla. January, 1969, aged 77.

FELICITE Fr. See La Félicite.

FELL (OF HAIR) A head of hair. From 16th century.

'My fell of haire would at a dismall treatise rowze . . .' (*Shakespeare, Macbeth*)

FELTED The condition of badly matted hair.

FELTING The matting or entangling by movement and pressure of hair into a Hair Mouse, *qv*.

FER Fr. An iron.

FER A CHEVAL Fr. A beard style, short and divided like a horseshoe.

FER A FRISSER Fr. Curling irons.

FER A ONDULER Fr. Waving iron.

FER A PAPILLOTE Fr. Pinching iron.

FER A REPASSER Fr. Pressing iron.

FERN CURL A very loose, delicate and highly tapered curl.

FERRET A kind of narrow ribbon used in wigmaking, 19th century.

FER ROND Fr. Curling iron.

FERRONNIERE A band of fine gold or velvet ribbon and sometimes strings of beads on a silken cord worn round the head with a jewel in the centre of the forehead. From about 1820. (*Smith, H C*)

FESTOON A chain of hair arranged in a curve between two points on the head. 'The back of the coiffure had a festoon of curls.'

FETID HAIR See *Bromidrosis capitis*.

FIBRE Any fine thread or thread-like substance. (*Draper's Dictionary*)

FIBRIL A small fibre.

FIELD HAIR Hair that has been bleached by exposure to the sun in the open air. It was either laid on the ground or hung on a line like a clothes line.

FIGARO (1) A barber of extraordinary cunning, dexterity and intrigue in Beaumarchais' *Le Barbier de Seville* (1775), the basis of the opera by Mozart bearing the same title.

(2) A barber.

FIG SOFT SOAP A combination of oils, principally olive oil of the commonest kind, with potash (*Piesse*)

FIGURE OF EIGHT DRESSING A coiffure which incorporates a figure eight knot, *qv*. *298*

FIGURE EIGHT KNOT A double twist of hair in the form of a figure 8.

FIGURE OF EIGHT WEFT Weft on two silks in which the strand of crêpe or hair is intertwined 'under bottom silk, between the silks, over the top silk, between the silks, etc. until the whole strand is woven on the silk, with no loose ends.

FIJI WIG Made from the hair of victims killed in battle and sold as curiosities to the Americans for one dollar each (mid-19th century) (*Rowland*)

FILAMENT CURL A very narrow curl, composed of a few hairs only, like a curled length of fine string. Narrower than a tendril curl.

FILET Fr. Fillet, net.

FILLE DE CHAMBRE Fr. Lady's maid.

FILLER A preparation that is applied to the hair to correct over-porosity by filling or covering the pitted hair surfaces.

FILLET (1) A head band of any suitable material used for keeping the head dress in position, binding the hair, or as an ornament.

(2) In the 18th century, a hair net to cover the head at night. 'Large fillet must be big enough to cover the head.' (*Stewart*)

(3) An artificial front of hair. (*Procter*)

(4) A fringe of hair. 17th century 'Hair lying the whole breadth of the forehead.' (*Holme*)

FILLETTE Fr. Lass, young girl.

FILTRATION The action or process of filtering.

FIMBRIATE Adj. Bordered with hairs. 17th century. From Latin *Fimbria*; a fringe.

FINE NET See Stiff wig net.

FINE SILK NET See Stiff wig net.

FINE-TOOTHED COMB See Dust comb.

FINGER BLEEDER See Needle beard.

FINGER CAP Thimble.

FINGER GUARD See Finger shield.

FINGER-HAIR TEST A method of determining origins amongst Europeans, which concerns the presence or absence of hair on the middle joints of the fingers. (*Somerset and Dorset* Ns and Qs, Vol 28, p. 170)

FINGER SHIELD A metal sheath open at both ends, one end being circular, the other elliptical. Although worn on the index finger of the left hand it is not worn to shield the finger, but to guide and lift the needle point out of the wig foundation during the sewing process.

FINGER STALL See Finger shield.

FINGER WAVE A wave produced by the fingers and a comb. See Finger waving.

FINGER WAVING The process of shaping the hair into waves by the use of the comb and the fingers on wet hair.

FINIAL LOCK A dressed lock of hair standing high above the head. 'Crowned with a finial of curls.'

FINISHING KNOT The tie knot at the end of a piece of weft.

FINN BARR An Irish saint whose name signified grey beard. (*Reynolds*)

FIRE ALARM A red-haired person, slang. (*B and B*)

FIRMAMENT Diamonds or other precious stones heading the pins which are stuck in the Tour and hair, like stars. 17th century. (*Evelyn*)

FIRST DEGREE BURN Superficial burn affecting the outer layer of the skin. See also second and third degree burns.

FIRST HAND The senior or highest qualified assistant in a hairdresser's salon who has the first choice of those clients who don't express their preference for an assistant. Also second hand, third hand, etc.

FIRST PLI See Pli.

FISH HOOK (1) The doubled back point of a badly wound curl. See Wrinkling.

(2) The knotting needle hook; Scottish and Northern English slang. (*E G French*)

FISH SKIN Used in a postiche under the parting to protect the parting gauze from discolouration by perspiration.

FISH TAIL See Fish hook (1).

FIVE ORDERS OF PERIWIGS A caricature by William Hogarth upon the Five Orders of Periwigs as they were worn at the coronation of George III (1761). Hogarth's print is said to have been a satire on Stewart's *Antiquities of Athens* in which, with minute accuracy, are given the measurements of all the members of Greek architecture.

FIXATIVE (1) Any substance that fixes the hair in position, such as lacquer or thick setting lotion.

FIXATURE See Fixative.

FIXED NITRE See Potassium carbonate.

FIXED OIL Non-volatile oil of animal or vegetable origin. Insoluble in alcohol (exception castor oil). Examples: Almond Oil, Olive Oil, etc. *qv.*

FIXER (1) In cold permanent curling, the oxidant used to rebuild in their new position the linkages broken down by the cold-wave chemical reagent. (Usually ammonium-thioglycollate).

(2) A sticky substance such as a gum based setting lotion.

(3) A hairpin or other similar accessory used to fix hair in position.

FIXING SPRAY An atomized liquid that is sprayed on the completed hairdress and when dry holds it in position. Various types of resins, gums, etc are dissolved in suitable solvents to make the liquid.

FIXOLINE A 19/20th century 'secret' balsamic hair restorer, compounded of wax, lard, Peruvian balsam, alcohol and inert aromatic substances. It was without effect. (*Koller*)

FLACKIN COMB A wide-toothed comb. A rake. Northamptonshire usage. (*Sternberg*)

FLACKING COMB A wide-toothed comb, 19th century. Oxfordshire usage. (*Holloway*)

FLACON Fr. A small bottle or flask.

FLAMES A red-haired person. Slang. (*B and B*)

FLAMMABLE Inflammable.

FLANDAN A kind of pinner joining with the bonnet. (*Evelyn*)

FLAPPER HAIR STYLE Single, or short sleek bob commonly worn by teenage girls, from *c* 1925.

FLARE (1) Subs. A spread out hair motif.

(2) Verb. To dress hair in a spread out or displayed position.

FLARE CURL An erect curl that is flared or spread out.

FLARE PINCURL A pincurl that is spread out.

FLASH (1) 18th century slang word for a periwig. (*Carew*) See also Queue flash.

(2) A blonde or coloured streak in a head of hair.

FLAT COLOUR Dull, lacking warmth and richness.

FLAT CURL A clock-spring curl with little thickness dressed flat on the head.

FLAT MARCEL A Marcel wave with shallow troughs and low crests.

FLAT PINCURL A clock-spring wound pincurl, dressed flat.

FLAT SPRING Positional Spring, *qv.*

FLAT TOP A man's hair style cut flat on the top of the head – the hair then standing straight up, and short back and sides. (*Trusty*)   *104E*

FLAT TOP COMB A comb of plastic or light metal, approximately 5″ wide, with teeth 6″ long, a short handle and a small spirit level attached to one side of the comb's spine. Used for cutting flat-top hair styles by pushing the teeth through hair on top of the head, holding the comb flat and cutting the hair protruding through the interstices of the teeth, thus ensuring a 'flat top' to the style. (*Werrington*)

FLAT-TOP CREW CUT Similar to the Flat top, *qv.* American usage, 1962. Also called California cut, Detroit cut and Dutch cut.

FLAT TOPPER See Flat-top comb.

FLAT TOP WITH FENDERS Man's hair style with two rolls or quiffs running from the middle of the forehead to over the ears. American usage.

FLAT WAVING A method of waving hair by interlacing it on a large hairpin in the same manner as figure-of-eight-weft, *qv.*

FLAT WEFT The commonest type of hair weft, woven on three silks. (*Symonds*)

FLAT-WIND Hair wound on a curler, flat without bulges. (*Smith*)

FLAX Hair of the head. 16th century.
'I will take thy fingers and thy flax,
I will throwe them well in virgins wax;' (*Percy*, III 266/93)

FLEA COMB See Dust comb.

FLEAM A Barber-surgeon's knife of steel with two or three moveable lancets for bleeding the patient.

FLEMISH KNOT See Figure-eight-knot.

FLESH-COLOURED HAIR NET Invented in 1805 by Mon Leguet, Hairdresser of Lyons, France. Postiches had hitherto been so coarsely made that this improvement caused a sensation. In 1810 Leguet, who had found that his wigs did not keep the desired firmness (being badly knotted) sold his patent to Mons Tellier, Hairdresser at the Palais Royal, Paris.

FLESH-COLOURED SILK Used for drawn-through partings.

FLESH SILK A flesh-coloured fine silk fabric through which hair is drawn for a drawn-through parting.

FLEUR Fr. Flower, bloom, blossom.

FLICK (1) Point end of a slightly curled wisp of hair.

(2) Flick curl, *qv.*

FLICK CURL A loose curl flicked into position usually on the cheek or forehead. There are: Ear flicks, Forehead flicks, Cheek flicks, etc, *c* 1960.

FLICK UP (1) Hair style in which the side hair is loosely curled and brushed up towards the crown. 1962.

(2) Loose half curl turning outwards from the head.

FLIES OF SPENYIE Cantharides, Scottish usage. (*Scot*)

FLINK-TAIL COMB A lady's long-handled dressing comb. Devon usage. (*Hewett*)

FLIP (1) A casually arranged tress that has been flipped into position.

(2) A strand of rubber with an eye at either end, used to secure a wound curler in the permanent waving process.

FLIP UP See Flick up.

FLIP-UP CURL See Flick curl.

FLIRTATION RIBBON The two hanging ends of a ribbon tied to the hair. 19th century.

FLOATING SOAP A soap that will float. Made by beating air into the soap mixture as it cools.

FLOP LOCKS A term of abuse hurled at long-haired males in the 1960s.

FLORAL HEADDRESS A coiffure which includes some form of floral decoration such as a red rose worn behind the ear.

FLORENCE OIL See Olive oil.

FLORENTINE CUT See Zazzera.

FLOSS (1) Silk in fine filaments.
(2) Denatured, overbleached hair resembling candy floss. Bristol usage. 1920s.

FLOT Verb. To souse with water. 'She flotted the clients dress during the shampoo.' S W England usage. 1920s.

FLOTTANT SOAP A soap with a low specific gravity that floats on water. (*Morfit*)

FLOUNCE (1) The lower hanging edge of a hairdo.
(2) To curl or frizz hair.
'Toss'd her locks, flounc'd t'express a gallant mein,
Tho', to say truth, not over sweet nor clean.' (*Killigrew*, 1695)

FLOUR Cornflour used in 19th century to give grey effect to hair of actors for theatrical purposes.

FLOWING STYLE Any hair style in which the long locks are dressed flowing freely. A coiffure of loose waves and curly ends. 277

FLOW WIG A wig in which the hair (medium or long) is hanging loosely on the shoulders of the wearer.

FLUFF (1) Loosely to puff out hair by backcombing.
(2) The short very fine hair on an old person's head.

FLUID HAIRDO A style in which the locks of the finished hairdress can move like natural hair.

FLUID HAIR STYLE A loose, free moving style without lacquer.

FLUX To wash a wig. 18th century. 'The Doctor's black coat could not possibly undergo another scouring, nor his perriwig another fluxing.' (*The Parasite*, 1765)

FLY-AWAY-COMB Boomerang comb, *qv*.

FLYING BARBER A barber who visited his clients in their homes, 17/18th century. By the early 19th century this character was rarely seen in London, but continued in the country. (*Hone EDB*) See visiting barber.

FLY RINK A bald head. Bristol usage, *c* 1920. Slang.

FLY WEFT (1) Very small strands of hair woven on two silks. From the rear of bottom silk push the hair between the silks, over the top silk, through the silks, under the bottom silk, through the silks, over the top silk, through the silks. Also called Starting weft. used to commence weft for a switch.
(2) The same as once-in-weft, *qv*. (*Creer*)

FOAM BLEACH Similar to a cream bleach, *qv*, but the released oxygen forms bubbles and changes the creamy consistency to a foam.

FOAM BUILDER A chemical that when added to a shampoo, will produce the required quantity and type of foam. Although foamless detergents will cleanse as well as foaming detergents the public generally has more confidence in the cleansing properties of a shampoo that foams.

FOAM-CUSHION CURLER A hair curler constructed of polyurethane foam and having a plastic locking device to secure the curler when the hair is wound on it during the set.

FOAM ROLLER A hair curler composed of foam rubber. See also Foam-cushion curler.

FOETAL HAIR Hair growth on a foetus.

FOIL A thin guard on an electric razor which protects the skin from the cutting edge.

FOLD The turning back of one half of a strand of hair upon the other half. Equivalent to a loop. 19th century. (*Procter*)

FOLDING HAIR BLOCK A block, on which to dress wigs, that collapses and folds up into a 3″ × 6″ package. Invented by Gustave Sattler, an American. (*AH* 1915)

FOLDING MOUSTACHE IRONS Moustache irons whose handles will fold against the prongs.

FOLEZ German barber poet. (*Smiles*, p 26)

FOLIAGE The natural beard; also a false beard. Slang American usage. (*B and B*)

FOLK HAIRDRESSING Hairdressing by untrained persons of humble stock such as peasants who dress their coiffures in traditional styles that have remained unchanged for many years.

FOLLET Fr. Downy (of hair).

FOLLICLE The involuted sac or bag which contains the hair within the skin. The cavity from which the hair grows.

FOLLICULITIS Inflammation of a follicle or follicles.

FOLLOW-ME-LADS Curls hanging over the shoulders. Slang. American usage. (*B and B*)

FOND Fr. foundation or base.

FOND DE CARDE Fr. Waste hair.

FONTANGE A topknot of ribbon so called from its first wearer Marie-Angélique, Duchesse de Fontanges (1661–1681). She was the successor of Mme de Montespan as favourite of Louis XIV.

FONTANGE COIFFURE A hair style for women *c* 1700, in which the front hair was curled and supported by wire in a high dressing and this was topped by the Fontange headdress of rich lace with which this coiffure was adorned and which formed an integral part. See also Fontange.

FORCED CURL See Frisure forcée.

FORCED WAVED HAIR Frisure forcée, *qv*, set in waves.

FORCEPS 18th century term for Curling irons.

FOREHEAD COMB A semi-circular, narrow comb used in the coiffure to secure the front hair. (*Ogee Cat*, 1905)

FOREHEAD CURL A flat curl dressed on the forehead.

FOREHEAD FRINGE A small postiche for wear as a fringe. 'For ladies who do not wish their own hair cut, also as a means of dressing the hair . . . without hairpins'. (*Nash*)

FOREHEAD HAIR The hair that grows immediately above the forehead.

FOREHEAD PIECE Foretop, *qv*. 17/18th century. (*Fairholt*)

FOREHEAD WAVE A wave that overlies any part of the forehead, *cf* Cheek wave.

FORELOCK (1) A lock of hair growing above the forehead at the fore part of the head.
(2) The dressed portion of a wig above the forehead. See also Topping.

FORELOCKS 'The hair of the head before' (at the front part of the head). 17th century. (*Phillips*)

FORELOCK-PIECE A small postiche for wear at the front of the head.

FORENSIC WIG The wig of a judge, barrister or other officer connected with the law. In the mid-19th century a patent was taken out for 'a Forensic wig, the ends whereof are constructed on a principle to supersede the necessity of frizzing, curling or using hard pomatum and for forming curls in a way not to be mauled; and also for the tails of the wig not to require tying in dressing; and further the possibility of any person untying them'. (*Rowland*, p 165)

FORETOP (1) The forepart of the crown of the head, or a wig. (*Holme*)
(2) A tuft or strand of hair turned up from the forehead,

16/18th century. (*Fairholt*) 'Her foretop was long and turned aside very strangely' (John Evelyn's description of Catherine of Braganza on her first visit to England). The style was possibly of Portuguese origin.

(3) A toupet, *qv*.

(4) The name of a wigmaker in Sir John Vanbrugh's play *The Relapse*, or *Virtue in Danger*, 1697.

(5) Tyburn top wig, *qv*.

(6) A strand or bunch of hair hanging on the forehead. 17th century. (*Comenius*)

FORETOPMAN'S LOCK A lock of hair worn on the foreheads of foretopmen showing below the cap. A privilege afforded them as the elite among the seamen of the ship's company. (*R B Kay-Shuttleworth*)

FORFEITS IN A BARBER-SHOP The barber-shop was formerly a place of popular resort for the purpose (in addition to barbering processes) of discussion. To preserve order during noisy sessions, forfeits were inflicted. (*Shakespeare, Measure for Measure*, II, ii; *The Mirror*, 15 July 1826)

FORFEX A pair of scissors. 1712. Pedantic use in 1982. 'The Peer now spreads the glittering forfex wide, To enclose the Lock; now joins it, to divide.' (*Pope*)

FORGOTTEN WAVE In Marcel waving or setting the waves on top of the head that taper into the parting.

FORK COMB A comb with two long prongs. Used to form and secure a Catogan. 19th century.

FORKED BEARD A broad beard style cut to two peaks. 14/18th century. (*Holme*) 'A Marchant was ther with a forked berd.' (*Chaucer*)   99 (1.2.3)

FORK PARTING See Open-Fork Parting.

FORKY HAIR See *Trichosis distrix*.

FORMALDEHYDE LIQUOR A colourless liquid with a characteristic pungent odour. Inhaled it can irritate the air passage. Miscible with water or alcohol in any proportion. Caustic in contact with the skin. An excellent germicide, which has been employed (30%) successfully for ringworm of the scalp. The vapour of formaldehyde is a good disinfectant as no damage is caused to hair. It is best generated by volatilising Paraform tablets (a polymer of formaldehyde) over a flame or heater.

FORMALIN A synonym for Liquor Formaldehyde, *qv*.

FORMALISM Strict conformity to set custom in the hair style.

FORMER A curling stick.

FORSTER, ROBERT The Cambridge flying-barber (d 1799). So famous for his professional dexterity that the gentlemen of the University presented him with a silver barber's bason. To be shaved out of Forster's bason was regarded as a great honour. (*Hone, Year Book*)

FORTUNA BARBATA A goddess whose votaries sought by her propitiation to grow fine beards. (*St Augustine, De Civitate Dei*)

FORWARD BOOGIE The same as Boogie style, *qv*.

FORWARD BRUSH Man's hair style. American usage.

FORWARD CURL A curl which is wound towards the face. 20th century. See also Backward curl.

FORWARD SHAMPOO A hair shampoo given to a client who is leaning forward over the basin. See also Backward shampoo.

FOUL SHAVE A shave from which a client contracted barber's rash.

FOUNDATION The substance upon which the hair is knotted, woven or sewn in the manufacture of a postiche.

FOUNDATIONAL POSTICHE The same as Foundation postiche, *qv*.

FOUNDATION BLOCK American usage for a wig block, *qv*.

FOUNDATION-CURL (WAVE) The preliminary curl or wave which forms the starting point for the formation of a hair style.

FOUNDATION-MAKER A boardworker skilled in the art of cutting and mounting postiche foundations. 19th century.

FOUNDATION NET The net, usually waterproof, which forms the bulk of the foundation of a postiche and upon which the hair is knotted, woven or sewn. See Stiff wig net.
                                                                                         119

FOUNDATION POSTICHE A postiche made on a foundation of net, gauze, coloured silk, etc, in contrast to postiches such as pincurls or switches in which the hair is secured to macramé, cord, silk or wire.

FOURIAU (Pl Fouriaux) Sheaths, often of silk or gold thread, used in pairs for enclosing the two long hanging plaits of hair worn by noblewomen of the 12th century.   344

FOUR-PUFF DRESSING A hair style incorporating four puff curls, c 1954.

FOX EAR An 18th century wig style for a man. the same as Temple tie wig, *qv*.

FOXTAIL OR FOX'S TAIL 18th century theatrical wig style. (*Stewart*)

FOXY A trade term describing an old worn wig whose colour is fading. (*Creer*)

FRAGELLI'S BEARD PRODUCER A 19/20th century 'secret' preparation consisting of a spirituous extract of lavender, benzoin, cinnamon, and sandalwood oil. (*Koller*)

FRAGILITAS CRINIUM See *Trichorrhexis nodosa*.

FRAGILITAS MYSTAX Splitting or brittleness of the moustache. (*Wheeler*)

FRAISEAU or FRESEAU A back-comb of metal (gold, silver, bronze) decorated by knots and held in position by an encircling ribbon.

FRAMED HEADDRESS See Nebuly Headdress.

FRAME ROLLER A metal spring roller covered in plastic netting.

FRANCAIS Fr. French.

FRANCIS JOSEPH Beard style of the 19th century named after that worn by Francis Joseph, 1830–1916, Emperor of Austria.

FRANCIS'S PILOSITOUS COMPOUND A liquid advertised in 1851 in America for the cure of baldness, removal of dandruff, imparting gloss to the hair, and the cure of insect stings, at 25 cents per bottle. (*Belden*)

FRANCOIS CURL See French curl (2).

FRANCOISE See A La Française.

FRANGIPANI (1) An exquisite perfume probably introduced into Europe from Antigua in the 15th century by Mercutio Frangipani, a botanist and traveller and member of a noble family of Rome. *Plumeria alba* is the plant from which the essence was distilled and its flower is still known as the frangipani blossom. (*Piesse*)

(2) The perfume of red jasmine.

FRANZ-JOSEF BEARD See Francis Joseph.

FRANZ'S PURITAS REJUVENATOR A 19/20th century 'secret' preparation for treating grey hair. It consisted of glycerin 40 parts; water 106 parts; soda crystals 3 parts; cadmium sulphide 15 parts and zinc sulphide 1–3 parts. (*Koller*)

FRATER Village barber. (*Creer*)

FRATRES BARBATI (Bearded Brethren) An order of Cistercian monks who wore beards. (*Gowing*)

FREE-MOVING HAIRDO See Mobile hairdo.

FREE STYLE A loose naturalistic hairdress.

FREGATE LA JUNON, LA 18th century hair style for women. (*Uzanne*)

FRELAN Bonnet and pinner together. (*Evelyn*)

FRENCH BEARD See Olympian beard.

FRENCH BRAID A plait or braid formed from relatively short hair by working the plait close to the head and incorporating fresh strands of hair in the developing plait, thus giving the finished plait an appearance of length greater than the length of the hair of which it is composed. 265

FRENCH CLIPPING Backcombing strands of hair to erect the points and cutting the protruding points. (*Korf*)

FRENCH COMBING A method of combing the hair outwards and upwards to create the illusion of abundance when nature has ill-provided the commodity. The term is sometimes used for back-combing, *qv*.

FRENCH CREPE TOUPEE A small front of crêpe hair, *c* 1745. (*Stewart*)

FRENCH CURL (1) A curl shaped like an egg. These curls first appeared after 1745. 'They look like eggs strung in order on a wire and tied round the head.'
(2) A frizzed curl. One that is back-combed and worn loosely disposed.

FRENCH CURVED COMB See Boomerang comb.

FRENCH CUT 16th century hair style for men, with a love lock down to the shoulder. (*Stubbes, Anatomie of Abuses*)

FRENCHED HAIR (1) Hair dressed in the French fashion. 'Mrs Tibbs in a new sacque, ruffles and frenched hair' (*Goldsmith, Citizen of the World*, 1762)
(2) Frizzed hair.
(3) Backcombed hair.

FRENCH FALL A heavy fall constructed with about 7 oz of hair 22″–24″ long.

FRENCH-FIBRE-FOUNDATION A foundation of imitation hair. 19th century. (*Brodie, Price List*, 1890)

FRENCH FLOW The setting of hair in curves as opposed to waves or curls by means of a blow-comb or other methods. 1976.

FRENCH FIXEURE A stick pomade for holding the hair in position. Mid 19th century.

FRENCH FORK BEARD A forked beard, *qv*. American usage. (*Trusty*)

FRENCH FRIZZ Backcombed hair.

FRENCH FRIZZING Backcombing hair.

FRENCH FRONT This front was distinguished by a cluster of curls made with 8″ tapered hair the curls were called frizzed or French curls. The roots as well as the points were woven in together on wire. There were five, six or seven of these curls on each side, *c* 1830. (*Creer*)

FRENCH HAIR Raw hair of good quality collected in France, mostly brown in colour.

FRENCH HAIRCUT A short haircut for men, the top hair standing upright.

FRENCHING (1) Thinning by tapering. American usage. (*Trusty*)
(2) Frizzing.

FRENCH KNOT A coil that has its point end pinned to its root end and the resulting loop twisted one, two or three times and pinned in the desired position. (*Schaefer*)

FRENCH LOCK Love lock. (*Fairholt*)

FRENCH PARTING The system of working a drawn through parting by inserting the gauze hook through the parting silk and the gauze or net, knotting the hair to this material and then drawing it through the parting silk. Only very skilful wigmakers can successfully work a drawn-through parting by this method.

FRENCH PIN See Italian pin.

FRENCH PLAIT See French braid.

FRENCH RAZOR See Solid razor.

FRENCH RINGLET FRONT A front of hair for a woman on a double diamond shaped foundation. *285, 416 (1,2)*

FRENCH ROLL A method of securing the ends of hair by tucking them under and pinning flat. See also French braid.

FRENCH ROLL FOUNDATION A pad of crêpe hair over which a French roll is formed.

FRENCH SCISSORS Scissors with a finger brace.

FRENCH SOAP A plain, unmarbled, dirty-white sort of soap from France. It was almost as soft as the old crown soap made in London. Of little use to the perfumer. 19th century. (*Lillie*)

FRENCH SOLID RAZOR See Solid razor.

FRENCH STROP See Concave strop.

FRENCH SWIRL A lightly backcombed Swirl curl, *qv*.

FRENCH TETE See Direct wig.

FRENCH TWIST (1) The same as French roll, *qv*. (*Creer, Lessons p 48*)
(2) The same as Torsade Dondel, *qv*. *416(6)*

FRENCH WAVING A method of waving hair by first curling with curling irons and breaking the curl into waves.

FRENCH WEAVING STICKS The weaving silk is accommodated on three revolving pegs inserted in the right hand weaving stick.

FRENCH WIG See Full-bottomed wig.

FRENCH WOVEN RINGLET FRONT A wefted front of three to twelve drop curls on both sides, the curls dressed turning towards the face. 19th century. (*Creer*)

FRENCHY Fluffy, frizzy. 'The girl had Frenchy hair.'

FRESEAU Fr. A backcomb, *qv*. See also Fraiseau. *351*

FRET A hair ornament of jewelled network.

FRICTION (1) A massage movement in which the fingers press and rub the scalp surface, imparting their effect in depth.
(2) A Friction lotion, *qv*.

FRICTION LOTION A perfumed alcohol that is gently or vigorously rubbed into the scalp to stimulate the blood.

FRIENDLY MUTTON CHOPS Beard style. *97C*

FRIG BEARD A beard stroker. (*Rabelais, Motteux trans*, 1708)

FRIGHT WIG A wig designed to frighten or strike horror in the onlooker. (*DT*, 17 March, 1978)

FRINGE (1) A portion of the front hair combed forward onto the forehead and cut short (1883). Also Bang, *qv*.
(2) A row of short hair on the neck, called a neck fringe.
(3) A border of hair with loose ends.
(4) A short narrow band of postiche worn at the front of the head and dressed to a fringe, 19th century.
(5) A front of hair with a fringe.

FRINGE COMB Small comb for securing a fringe. (*Ogee* 1905)

FRINGE CURLING IRONS Curling irons which have small diameter prongs for use in curling fringes. Similar to moustache-irons, but of slightly larger diameter.

FRINGE CUT (1) A hair trim confined to the hair ends.
(2) The cutting of a fringe.

FRINGE EMPERATRICE (*sic*) A narrow band postiche of short curls, *c* 1900. (*Vasco*)

FRINGE FOUNDATION (1) An inch or so of the edge of the wig adjacent to the forehead, ears and nape.
(2) The foundation of a fringe, *qv*.

FRINGE HEDGE The beard. Slang. American usage. (*B and B*)

FRINGE NET A net of human hair or, exceptionally, of silk or nylon used to confine a fringe of hair, that is the dressed front hair of a hairdress. See Cap net and Bun net, etc.

FRINGE-PIN A short, very fine hairpin used to secure the dressed hair (especially curls) of a fringe.

FRINGE POMPADOUR A pompadour hair style, *qv*, with a fringe.

FRINGE SCISSORS Scissors with slight serrations on one blade for cutting fringes. The serrations prevent the hair 'running' from the closing scissors.

FRINGE-TONGS See Fringe curling irons.

FRISE Fr. (1) See frizzed hair.
(2) A 1965 style of half curl and slight wave.

FRISEE The client of the friseur. 18th century. 'tax friseurs; it matters not if the burden do fall on the frisée . . . and perfumery of all sorts.' (*Hill*, 1782)

FRISER Fr. To curl hair; to fall into curl.

FRISETTE Also frisett, frizette, frizzett, etc.
(1) A cluster or band of small curls, usually artificial, worn above and on the forehead.
Frizette 1818 Lady Morgan.
Frisette 1858 O W Holmes.
Frisett 1868 *Daily News*.
Frizzett 1877 Creer (*Lessons in Hairdressing*).
(2) A pad of crêped hair sometimes mounted on a comb used as a foundation over which to dress the growing hair. 19/20th century. (*Creer*) See Puff drawing wire.
126, 205, 421 (3, 4, 5)

FRISETTE DRAWING WIRE See Puff drawing wire.

FRISETTE TUBE See Puff tube.

FRISON (1) Famous French hairdresser who in 1763 helped to found the earliest recorded Ladies' Hairdressers' Guild. (*Johnson*)
(2) Small tight curls at the hollow of the temples worn by Lady Mary Wortley Montagu, (1689–1762). Named after Frison (1) who popularized them.
(3) A very small ringlet. Named after the coiffeur Frison in 1762. (*Ménard*)

FRISSED HAIR 'Hair that is full of small crispings and when one will not sort or fall into order with another but stand bunching out.' 17th century. (*Holme*)

FRISSEUR A male hairdresser. (*Art of Hairdress*, 1770)

FRISURE (1) Curling, curliness, curls.
(2) Mode or fashion of curling the hair, 1775.
'The frisure of her head.' (*Smollett, Humphrey Clinker*, 1771)

FRISURE-CROQUIGNOLE (American usage). The same as Frisure-Forcée, *qv*. (*Nazzaro and Nothaft*)

FRISURE FORCEE Fr. A forced or induced curl produced by rolling the hair on pipes or bigoudis, and boiling or baking it.

FRITZ FRIZZLE The dancing barber of the stage. (*Procter*, p 215)

FRIZ A hairdresser.
'Ditisse pines at home in Bedford Square,
Till Friz from Piccadilly sends her hair.' (*Halhed*, 1793)

FRIZETTE See Frisette, also Frisett, Frizzett, etc.

FRIZEUR See Friseur.

FRIZZ (or FRIZ) (1) Subs. The state of being curled or frizzed. A mass of very small crisp curls.
(2) Verb. To curl or crisp hair. 'Is't not enough you read Voltaire whilst sneering valets frizz your hair.' (*The Goat's Beard, a Fable*, 1777)
(3) The horsehair loops on a judge's wig and on the crown of a barrister's wig.

FRIZZED CURL A type of curl made from 7″ tapered hair and worn in a cluster at the front of the head. Fashionable *c* 1837. Also called French curl.

FRIZZER A hairdresser. Slang. Bristol and West Country usage. 19/20th century.

FRIZZETT The anglicised spelling used by E. Creer in his *Lessons in Hairdressing*, 1877. Frisette being the French spelling and the best form for English use. See Frisette.

FRIZZETTE See Frisette.

FRIZZING (1) Subs. Hair which is frizzed.
'Frizzings adorned her brow.'
(2) Adj. Covered with frizz. 'Frizzing hair and great whiskers.'

FRIZZING TONGS See Crimping iron.

FRIZZLE (1) Subs. A short, crisp curl.
(2) Subs. A Frizz wig, *qv*.
(3) Subs. Frizzed hair.
(4) Verb. To curl hair in small, tight curls. 16th century. (*Legros*, 1768) 'A long lock he has got, and the art to frizzle it.' (*Brathwait*, p 283)
(5) Verb. To dry and partly burn hair with a too hot iron, 19/20th century.
(6) Subs. Any small curled or frizzed postiche, such as a pincurl.
'She has had to sell her two frizzles and corneleun (*sic*) ring and lots of other nice things that she had to catch her husband with.' (*Holley*, *c* 1896)
(7) Subs. 18th century slang name for a hairdresser. (*The Evening Brush*, 1807)

FRIZZLING (1) Subs. A bunch of frizzed hair with loops to secure it to the hairdress. Used to give bulk to hair dressed over it. 'A frizzling for wearing underneath coques.' (*Coiffure Européan*, Feb 1866)
(2) Adj. Having the quality of being able to frizzle. 'A frisling or crisping pinne of iron.' (*Coryate*, 1611)

FRIZZLING IRONS Small diameter curling irons used to produce a frizzle in the hair.

FRIZZLY Adj. Full of frizzles or tight curls.

FRIZZURE See Frisure. 'All this curling was to be undone, and another frizzure to take place.' 18th century.

FRIZZ WIG A wig with short, tight crimped curls, 18th century.

FRIZZY Adj. Pertaining to or resembling frizz.

FRIZZY FORSEY Frisure Forcée, *qv*. Slang. Derbyshire usage. (*Symonds*)

FROND CURL A loose curl that forms only part of a circle. A curl of incomplete circination.

FRONT An artificial covering of hair for wearing on the front of the head.
'There is, however, a kind of semi-wig, commonly called a front, which is in great vogue under a bonnet or cap.' (*The Weekly Entertainer*, 9 June 1823)

FRONTAL PIECE A postiche for wear at the front of the head.

FRONT FOUNDATION The foundation of galloon and net in which is implanted hair for a front.

FRONTLET A small front of hair.

FRONT PIECE See Front.

FRONT POSTICHE Worked hair postiches worn on the front of the head.

FRONT WEFT See Twice-In weft.

FROSTING (1) Bleaching small strands of hair throughout the head and blending them with the darker hair, giving a light frosted effect over the whole coiffure.
(2) The bleaching of parts of the surface of a hairdress. See also Streaking and Tipping.

FROTH CURL A loose backcombed curl formed on well tapered hair.

FROTHING AGENT A substance that will promote froth.

FROUFROU HAIRDRESS A medium length, curly hair style for women, 1871. (*Coiffeur Européen*, 1871)

FROUNCE To crisp, curl or frizz the hair.
'Schall frounce them in the foretop'. (*Skelton*)
'They nourish, (yea, frizle, curle, colour, crispe, adorne

and frounce) their Hair.' (*Prynne*, p 35)

FROWZE (1) Subs. A wig of frizzed hair 16/17th century or, by extension, a frizzed hair style on a person's own hair. (*Shadwell*)

(2) Verb. To curl; to frizz. (*Florio*, 1611)

FROWZLETOP Untidy or unkempt hair on the head. Slang.

FROWZYTOP (1) Untidy or unkempt hair on the head. Slang.

(2) A person with untidy or unkempt hair. Slang.

FRUGILITIS Split ends of the hair.

FUDGE Verb. To contrive a result in the manufacture of a hairpiece without the correct materials.

FUGITIVE COLOURING MATERIAL Colouring material or dye that is susceptible to fading due to strong light, atmospheric chemicals, sea water or other commonly met conditions.

FUGITIVE DYE See Fugitive colouring material.

FUKES Locks of hair. Northern usage. (*Holloway*; also *Grose*, Prov. Glos)

FULL, THE A man's 18th century wig style.

FULL BAG Name of an 18th century wig style for men. Dressed fuller than the rose bag, with the back hair secured within a bag topped with a large bow.

FULL BEARD Hair growth on chin, back of cheeks and upper lip. No part of the face is shaved.   98D

FULL BOB A man's 18th century wig style. (*Dublin Gazette*, 1724)

FULL BOTTOM (1) Name of 18th century wig style. See full-bottomed wig. (*Dublin Gazette*, 1724)   194

(2) A judge, 18/19th century slang. (*Grose*, ed 1823)

FULL-BOTTOMED WIG Late 17/18th century wig style with long curls hanging over the shoulders. Worn by professional men and the aristocracy. 'The full-bottom formally combed all before, denotes the lawyer and the politician.' (*The Guardian*, No 149, Sept 1713)

'I must have a physician's habit, for a physician can no more prescribe without a full wig, than without a fee.' (*H Fielding*, *The Mock Doctor*, 1732)

Introduced by Duvillier to hide a natural defect on the shoulders of the Dauphin. (*Lambert*)

According to Lord Chesterfield, first made for Duke of Burgundy to hide his hump back.

Today (1965) the full-bottomed wig is worn as part of the ceremonial dress by –

(1) Judges on the Queen's official birthday and other specially ordered days;

(2) Queen's Counsel when pleading in the House of Lords;

(3) The Lord Chancellor when sitting on the Woolsack;

(4) The Speaker of the House of Commons.

The full-bottomed wig comprises a curled or frizzed crown with long flaps, composed of from twenty or more rows of curls made from the manes of horses. On ordinary occasions judges wear what is known as an undress wig, which is frizzed all over, and has no curls.   194

See also Judge's wig and Barrister's wig.

FULL DRESS Man's wig fashion from 1760. 'Full dress bobs from £1 10s.' (*Ipswich Journal*, January 1761)

FULLER'S EARTH A powdered clay sometimes used to degrease very oily hair before washing it.

FULLER'S EARTH SOAP Curd soap, 10½ lb, marine soap 3½ lb, Fuller's earth (baked) 14 lb, Otto of French Lavender 2 oz, Otto of Origanum 1 oz. (*Piesse*)

FULL FRONT The frizzled and curled front hair of a peruke; the brow hair.

FULL MOON Woman's hair style, *c* 1857. (*HTATH*)

FULL POMPADOUR A pompadour hair style having a wave dip only over each ear.

FULL SET Beard and moustache. See Full beard.

FULL TRANSFORMATION See Transformation.

FUME CABINET See Sterilizing cabinet.

FUNGICIDE A disinfectant.

FUNGISTATIC An antiseptic substance used to prevent the growth of fungi. (*PPB*)

FUNKE'S CRININE A 19/20th century 'secret' preparation for the hair which consisted of an ammoniacal solution of silver nitrate. (*Koller*)

FUN WIG A wig made of synthetic hair and dressed in a flamboyant or 'way out' style and worn assertively as a wig. In the 1960s many women had a dozen or more of this type of wig in different styles and colours.

FURBELOW WIG See Duvillier wig.

FURRING See Tapering.

FURZY-HAIR Coarse, frizzy, prickly hair. West Country usage.

FUZZ (1) Fuzzy or frizzed hair.

(2) Adolescent beard. Slang. American usage. (*B and B*)

(3) Pubic hair.

'For things like fuzz, you should be well paid, Such old commodities do well in trade,' (*Thompson*, *The Courtesan*, 3rd ed 1765)

FUZZ-FACE Face of a youth with adolescent beard. Slang. American usage. (*B and B*)

FUZZ MERCHANT (1) A hairdresser or barber. Ilchester, Somerset usage, 19/early 20th century.

(2) One who over-indulges in promiscuous intercourse.

(3) A pimp.

(4) A man who sexually interferes with girls.

FUZZ WIG The same as Bushy and Buzz wig, *qv*.

FUZZY PUSS A face with an adolescent beard. Slang. (*B and B*)

FUZZY WUZZY (1) The Beja of North East Africa, so named in the Mahdi War by the British because of their fashion of frizzing out their hair into a large mop. (*B M Ethno*) The same hair fashion was also common amongst the Baggara people of N E Africa and those of Fiji, New Caledonia, New Britain and New Guinea.

(2) Current English slang usage to describe the high backcombed hair styles of the 1960s.

G

GALA COIFFURE A hair style suitable for a festive occasion.

GALATEA COMB A comb for wearing in the hair, its top curved and surmounted by an ornamental looped dressing or decoration. In 1882 Galatea was a cotton material striped in blue on a white ground, commonly used for boys' sailor suits. The name was derived from HMS Galatea which was named after Galatea, a sea-nymph in Greek mythology.

GALATHEE Fr. form of Galatea above. A woman's hair style of 1864. (*Bysterveld*)

GALLANT The rosette or bow at the end of a Cadanette, *qv*.

GALLIA BONCELLE A permanent waving system originated by Gaston Boudou and Arnold H Bongers and introduced in England in 1923.

GALLIA COMATA (The Hairy Gauls) Nickname for Gaul in the Roman period because of the long hair of the inhabitants. Gauls considered it distinguished to have long hair. Caesar on subduing this land compelled them to cut short their hair as a token of submission.

GALLIPOLY SOAP A soap made from cheap oil, but free from dirt. 19th century. (*Lillie*)

GALLIPOT An earthen glazed jar of about 1 pint capacity, used to hold the warm water when setting postiche.

GALLOON Narrow, close-woven ribbon or braid of silk thread or other suitable material in different colours, used in the foundation of wigs and other postiches. See also Ferret.

GALWAYS A beard which follows the chin line from ear to ear. American usage. (*B and B*)

GAME WIG A necessary wig for everyday wear. A wig worn to disguise the ravages of time and excess, *cf* Game leg, a lame leg. In Game wig the word game is used in a transferred sense. 18th century. (*Rowlandson, T*) See also Theatrical wig, Legal wig, Clerical wig, etc.

GAMIN HAIR STYLE A woman's hairdress of 1954; short and straight like a street urchin's and combed forward onto the forehead. It was worn by the French theatrical star, Zizi Jeanmarie.

GAMMABENZENE HEXACHLORIDE (Findane) Used as a parasiticide by the hairdresser and the wigmaker. Used to destroy nits (louse eggs) adhering to the hair shaft.

GANGLY Long and hanging loose. 'Her hair be all gangly.' (West Country saying), ie long hair draping onto the shoulders.

GANYMEDE A beautiful youth of Phrygia, son of Tros. He succeeded Hebe as cup-bearer to the gods, and was carried away by an eagle to satisfy the unnatural and shameful desires of Jupiter.

GANYMEDE HAIR STYLE A curly, girlish hair style affected by a man.

GARCETTE (1) A light, short fringe from temple to temple, curled or straight. 17th century.
(2) A woman's hair style of the 17th century with a short fringe. (*Villermont*)

GARCON Fr. Hairdresser's assistant. 19th century. London usage.

GARCON BOB A boyish, short hair style for women; also called Eton crop and boyish bob. 1920s.

GARNISH Hair ornaments, 19/20th century. (*Hairdressers' Chronicle*, 1 June 1926)

GARRICK CUT A small wig with five crisp curls on each side worn by the actor David Garrick (1717–1779). (*Stewart*) An 18th century wig with five curls on each side. Brought into fashionable use by David Garrick, the dramatist and actor. Its cut is precisely engraven by Sherwin in his portrait of the actor for Davies's memoirs. (*Smith, J T*)

GAS BRACKET CURLING IRON HEATER A metal bracket to support the irons with a series of holes in a central gas tube, from which gas is burnt.

GASH BEARD A protruding chin. Scottish usage. (*Ramsay*)

GASOLINE Petrol. Used for the cleaning of wigs and other postiches that are worked on net foundations.

GASOLINE SHAMPOO A dangerous method of cleansing head hair that was popular in the early 20th century. Serious tragedies in the form of burnings have resulted from this type of shampoo and it should never be practised. American usage.

GAUCHE Fr. Clumsy, awkward.

GAUL NET Caul Net, *qv*. American usage. (*A H April*, 1915)

GAUZE A woven fabric of transparent texture used in wig-making, for partings and foundations. Originally made of silk; now (1965) either silk or synthetic material is used.

GAUZE FOUNDATION A postiche foundation made of gauze, *qv*.

GAUZE HOOK A fine barbed hook fixed in a short wooden handle and used to draw hair through the gauze 'skin' for the drawn-through parting of a postiche. See also Knotting needle and Ventilating needle.

GAUZE HOOK HOLDER The wooden or bone holder for the Gauze hook.

GEL SETTING LOTION See Jelly setting lotion.

GENDARME see A La Gendarme.

GENERAL An English moustache style.   *101J*

GENTIAN VIOLET JELLY An antiseptic of first aid use in cases of scalp burns. (*Kibbee*)

GENTILLY See A La Gentilly.

GENTLEMAN'S COMB A dressing comb with relatively short teeth.

GENTLEMEN'S CUT 16th century hair style for men. (*Stubbes*)

GENTLEMEN'S HAIRDRESSER A person skilled in the art and craft of cutting, shaving, shampooing, colouring, curling, waving, styling and dressing a man's head of hair or beard.

GENTLEMEN'S HAIRDRESSING The art and craft of cutting, shaving, shampooing, colouring, curling, waving, styling and dressing a man's hair (head and face). See also Hair styles.

GEOMETRIC-CUT Hair club-cut at differing angles to the head.

GEORGIA HAIR Another name for refined Chinese hair, *qv*. (*Creer*)

GEORGIAN HAIR STYLES Hair styles in the fashions of the Georgian period, 1714–1820.

GEORGIAN WIG Wigs in the fashions worn from 1714–1820.

GERM Microbe or micro-organism, especially one of the disease-causing organisms.

GERMAN CURL A roll-shaped curl. (*Ladies' Companion*, 1851)

GERMAN CURLS A mixture of scollop-shell and French curls in the front of the dressing, curled all over behind; also known as Tête de Mouton, 18th century. (*Stewart*)

GERMAN CUT See Flat top.

GERMAN FLY WEFT Fine weaving on three silks. Through the top space, over the top silk, through the top space, under the bottom silk, through the top space, over the top silk, through the top space, through the bottom space (*Symonds*, p. 76)

GERMAN HAIR Raw natural hair of good quality, collected in Germany and mostly blond in colour.

GERMAN RAZOR A hollow ground razor of German or Sheffield steel and ground by the German method. (*Foan*)

GERMICIDE A substance which will destroy micro-organisms. (*PPB*)

GERMINATIVUM The innermost layer of the epidermis adjoining the stratum mucosum.

GET OUT COMBINGS, TO To disentangle hair combings preparatory to rooting.

GHIRLANDAIO STYLE A hair style after the manner of those depicted by the Florentine artist Ghirlandaio (1449–1494).

GIBSON GIRL COIFFURE A high pompadour with a short looped coil hanging down the back of the neck. 1904.

GIDDY FEATHER TOP. See Feather top.

GIGOLO BOB A woman's bobbed hair style of 1926.

GILD To cover with gold powder.

GILDA BOB A woman's hair style of *c* 1927.   267

GIMMICK A trick, gadget or characteristic in, of, or for mannerism, dress, presentation, voice, etc. to attract publicity or aid identification.

GINGER Slang term for a red-haired person, 19th century.

GINGER HEAD See Ginger.

GINGER MOP A red haired person, Slang (*B and B*)

GINGER HACKLED Red haired. See Ginger pated. 18th century. Slang (*Grose*)

GINGER PATED Red haired. A term derived from the cockpit where red cocks were called Gingers. 18th century. Slang (*Grose*)

GINGER ROGERS-COIL A thick coil of hair named after the film actress. 1940s.

GINGERSNAP A red-haired person, slang. (*B and B*)

GINGER TOP A red-haired person. Slang. (*B and B*)

GIORGIONE STYLE A woman's hair style in the fashion of those depicted by the Italian painter Giorgione (c 1478–1510).

GIRAFFE, THE A woman's hair style of the early 19th century consisting of a pyramid of rolls or bows of hair supported by a tall comb and heightened by flowers. The back was one straight line from the shoulders to the top of the comb. (*Ladies' Companion*, 1851)

GIRAFFE COIFFURE A high-dressed hair style for women that first became fashionable in 1827 as a result of a gift of live giraffes, one each to George IV of England and Charles X of France, from Mehemet Ali, Pasha of Egypt. (*Country Life*, 2 Dec 1965)

GIRAFFE COMB A high ornamental hair-comb for wearing in the coiffure. 1874+ (*Cunnington*)

GIZZ (Scottish) A periwig. 18th century. (*Burns*)

GLABROUS Lacking hair, smooth.

GLASS WIG Lettsom, *qv*, the physician, unusually wore a wig of glass. 'Soon . . . you will have the man who dresses Dr Lettsom's glass wig, to know how he ought to replace a deficient curl, or how much of its possessor's face it should cover, so that his forehead might be seen to the best advantage'. (*Smith, J T*)

GLAUVINA PIN An ornamental pin with a decorated detachable head, used to decorate the head dress. 1820-1840. (*Cunnington*)

GLAZE A semi-transparent or transparent, colourless film, or film of colour, applied to the hair.

GLEEBE (Glib) A long lock of hair. The Irish 'having a long head of hair with curled gleebes, much affected by them, and they take it hainously if one twitch or pull them'. (*Camden, Britannia*, ed 1695)
In 1571 an ordinance was proclaimed at Limerick ordering the inhabitants of cities and corporate towns not to suffer their hair to grow glib. (*McClintock*)   *102H*

GLIB Long lock of hair. See Gleebe.

GLINT Subs. (1) A gleaming or shining appearance.
(2) A momentary appearance of light.

GLOUCESTER, THE English hair style for men.

GLOUCESTER LANE ROLL A Bristol term, Gloucester Lane being a typical habitat for the kind of man who wore this roll in the 19th and early 20th century.

GLOVES See Rubber gloves.

GLUED WIG A quickly-made cheap wig for theatrical use, in which the hair is glued to the foundation.

GLUE HAIR Lacquered hair. Slang, *c* 1958.

GLYCERINE A sweet, syrupy hygroscopic liquid. Used as a solvent, plasticizer, emolient and humectant in the manufacture of cosmetics, liquid soaps, permanent waving lotions, hair-grooming aids, hair lacquers, shaving soaps and creams, and wave setting lotions.

GLYCEROL See Glycerine.

GOATEE A medium length beard with no side whiskers.
        97HJ

GODDESS A woman of superior charm.

GOD-OF-THE-HAIR See Hsüan Wên-hua.

GOD'S EYELASHES The slanting evening rays of the sun,
piercing the clouds and giving a streaked effect downwards. (Inf *Miss E Fowler*)

GOFFERING IRONS The double pronged goffering iron was commonly used by women in the 17th, 18th & 19th century for curling their hair. Unlike the curling irons these have two solid circular prongs.

GOING-AWAY HEADDRESS See Travelling Head-dress.

GOLD DUST Used for powdering hair to give it a sunny appearance. Referred to in 1857 as 'a new fashion'. (*NQ* 28 March 1857)

GOLDEN-GROMMET A woman's pubic hair. Naval slang.

GOLDEN HAIR A symbol of the highest aspirations of the mind. (*Gaskell*)

GOLDEN HAIR FLUID Peroxide of hydrogen, *qv*. (*Thompson*)

GOLDEN HAIR POWDER In modern times first worn by the Empress Eugenie, at the festival of Boeuf Gras, 1860. It consisted of crushed gold leaf. An inferior type was manufactured from powdered bronze. (*Piesse*)

GOLDEN LOCKS Venus. 'No more of Venus and her golden locks'. (*Thompson*, 1765)

GOLDEN WASH A 19th century 'secret' hair liquid for bleaching the hair. It consisted of 10 vol hydrogen peroxide. (*Nash, Stevens Ms*, 1896)

GOLD HAIR A true story of Pornic. A young girl died there in the odour of sanctity and was buried near the high altar of the Church of St Giles. Some years later the paving was removed from her grave and 30 double louis were found, which had been buried in her gold hair at the girl's own request. (*Browning*, Poems, 1864; *Brewer, RH*)

GOLDIE A blonde woman, slang. (*B and B*).

GOLDILOCKS (1) A blonde-haired girl.
(2) The fairy tale heroine.

GONK LOOK Men's hair style, 1964. Very long hair worn over the ears and eyes. 'The eyes peeping through.' (*Daily Telegraph* 11 September 1964.)

GOOSEBERRY CUT A hair style for men in which the hair is cut short to the contour of the head and stands erect. English, 1950s.

GOOSEBERRY WEFT Untidy weft with short hairs standing out like the hairs on a gooseberry.

GOOSEBERRY WIG A large, frizzled wig; perhaps from its supposed likeness to a gooseberry bush. (*Grose*, ed 1823)

GOOSEFLESH The rough, bristling condition of the scalp or skin caused by fright or cold.

GOOSE-GREASE Used as a base for powder dressings. It had the disadvantage of turning rancid.

GORDIAN KNOT (1) An intricate knot of hair consisting of involved convolutions.
(2) A figure eight knot.   *384*

GORGONE An 18th century hair style for women, dressed high and in which the curls were loose and moveable and could writhe or twist with the motions of the head. Named after the gorgones, three female monsters with snakes for hair; Medusa, Stheno, and Euryale. (*Elegant Arts*)

GOSLING GREEN Pale yellowish colour, 18th century. (*Goldsmith*)

GOSSAMER WIG A light-weight wig of hair knotted on net. Mid-19th century (*Hunt's Directory of Dorset*, 1851)

GOTHIC HAIR STYLES Hairdresses of the 13/14th century. The whole consistent logic of Gothic beauty is evident in the deeply religious feeling and purpose of the hair styles – dignified, restrained, severe. Men's hair was worn below the ears, hanging over the neck; that of married women being covered with head dresses of wimples, headbands, toques, calottes, etc. Young girls, before marriage, allowed their hair to hang loose and flowing.

GOUT Fr. Style, manner, fashion, taste.

GOUTY WEFT Unevenly woven weft.

GOWN A loose flowing protective garment of a suitable material, such as nylon, which covers the clothing of a seated client receiving attention.

GOZZAN An old wig, grown yellow with age and wear. Cornish use. 18th century. (*Grose, Prov Glos*)

GRACE, W G England's greatest bearded cricketer.

GRADUATE, THE A hair style of the 1960s for men.

GRADUATE Verb. To cut the hair in a regular series of imperceptible steps or gradations from the short hair of the neck to longer hair near the crown. 'His hair was skillfully graduated from the neck towards the crown without a single step being visible.'

GRADUATED CUT A cut in which the hair lengths are graduated. See Graduate.

GRADUATING Subs. The process of cutting in gradations. See Graduate.

GRAFTED WIG This had a turn on the top of the head in imitation of a man's hairy crown. 17th century. (*Holme*)

GRAIL A comb-maker's file. (*Creer*)
'A comb-makers grail . . . is a long, flat, and broad tool on the back, and the other side wrought into teeth like a saw.' (*Holme*, 1688)

GRAILED Comb teeth filed or cut with a grail, *qv*.

GRAILED COMB A saw-cut comb, *qv* finished with the grail, *qv*.

GRAILING The process of finishing the teeth of a comb with the grail, *qv*.

GRANULAR LAYER The stratum granulosum of the skin.

GRAPE OF CURLS A hanging cluster of curls. Mid-Victorian expression. (*Coiffeur Européen*, 1867)   322(3)

GRAPPE Fr. Bunch (of grapes or currants). The word Grappe was employed for hair as grappe boucles – bunch of curls; grappe de coquet – cluster of bows, etc. See Grape of curls. 19th century. (*Creer*)

GRAPPE BOUCLES Fr. A bunch of curls.

GRASS BLEACHING Exposing hair to air, light and moisture by spreading it on grass in the open air. Slower than chemical bleaching. Hair so bleached is referred to as field hair.

GRASS HAIR A species of long, fine, tough grass was used in 1914–18 war to make imitation hair switches to wear on the head in place of genuine hair. Made and sold by Mrs F Stevens, 45 High Street, Bristol, from 1914 to 1918. See also Vegetable hair.

GRASSHOPPERS Lucian in *Navigio* refers to old men tying up their locks of hair in 'golden grasshoppers'. (*Stukeley, Ms*)

GRATEAU, MARCEL Usually referred to as Mons Marcel, the inventor of the Marcel wave. See Marcel. (*Rambaud*)

GRAVE FULL-BOTTOM WIG See Full-bottom wig.

GRAVE HAIR See Cadaver hair.

GRECIAN BANDEAU A band of ribbon two or three times encircling the head; around the front of the head to the neck, over the top of the head to the neck and then encircling the low loose curls at the back of the head. A triple bandeau.

GRECIAN COIL A kind of spiral roll by which the front hair on either side of a middle parting is brought forward onto the forehead and from the forehead rolled spirally towards the ears.

GRECIAN CURL See Grecque.

GRECIAN FLY A man's 18th century wig style.

GRECIAN KNOT A way of dressing the chignon of a woman's hair in imitation of a style of Ancient Greece.
293, 416(4).

GRECIAN PLAIT Divide the hair into two equal parts; from the outside of the left part turn a strand of about a sixth part, pass it over into the centre and unite it with the right hand portion. Do the same from the right hand portion and pass it over into the centre, uniting it with the left hand portion. Proceed thus: taking the small and even-sized lock alternately from the left and right hand portions until all is plaited. This plait was kept very smooth. (*Ladies' Companion*, 1851 and *Elegant Arts*). See also Plait.

GRECIAN PROFILE A profile with a Grecian nose, ie a straight and continuing forehead line without any dip at the top of the nose.

GRECIAN WATER A 19th century hair dye to colour the hair black, consisting of nitrate of silver dissolved in syrup of buckthorn. (*Francis*)

GRECQUE Fr. Greek. A horseshoe-shaped curl across the front of the head, from ear to ear. See also A La Grecque. (*Ipswich Journal*)

GREEK BEARD A long full oriental type beard.

GREEK FUNERAL CUSTOM It was customary to hang the hair of the dead on their doors, previous to interment and the mourners sometimes tore out or cut off their own hair which they laid upon the corpse. (*Speight*)

GREEK HAIR STYLES These were represented in sculpture and painting with certain peculiar forms of hair styles as follows: Jupiter; magnificent head of hair rising in full upright locks from the forehead and falling thickly upon the shoulders, Apollo; curling hair, sometimes tied in a woman's knot on the crown of the head, Hercules; The hair of a bull, Virgins: Hair worn tied in a knot across the top of the head, Matrons; Hair worn in a knot on back of head or in double knot on the top with the ends turned towards the front and back of the head, Diana; Hair in a double knot with ends pointing to the ears, Amazons; Represented with the Maiden's knot with dishevelled hair. See also Classical hair styles.

GREEK WASH BALLS These took their name from an old man named Lyon, a Greek by birth, who was accustomed to go about to the most celebrated London coffee-houses to sell wash-balls. They were similar to Jerusalem Wash-balls, *qv*, but without added colour. 19th century (*Lillie*)

GREEK WATER An 18/19 century preparation of silver filings dissolved in spirit of nitre. Used as a hair dye to change red or light coloured hair to brown. (*New Family Receipt Book*)

GREEK WAVE A very deep wave in which the crest hangs over the succeeding trough.

GREEN HENNA See Henna.

GREEN SHAMPOO See Green soft soap shampoo.

GREEN SOFT SOAP Made by saponification of potassium and sodium salts of coconut and/or palm oil fatty acids. These soaps are yellowish-white to brownish-yellow, or green in colour, soft in consistency and more readily soluble than hard soaps. (*Merck*)

GREEN SOFT SOAP SHAMPOO A shampoo composed of a solution of green soft soap, perfumed by oil of verbena, or oil of Citronella, *qv*.

GREENWICH BARBERS Retailers of sand in the 18th century from the pits of Greenwich in Kent. Probably so-called on account of their constant 'shaving' of the sandbanks. (*Grose, Lex Bal*)

GREGARINE Minute creatures alleged by a Dr Lindemann to live in false hair and procreate rapidly. Apart from the worthy doctor no-one else saw the insects. This, like the

Chignon fungus, *qv*, was part of a 19th century attack on women's hair fashions which included hair. (*Creer*)

GREGORIAN (1) 'A kind of cap so call'd, as being the device of one Gregory, a barber.' 17th century. (*Phillips*)

(2) A wig style for men, 18th century. See Gregory.

(3) A wig, 18/19th century.

GREGORIAN TREE The gallows, after Gregory Brandon, a hangman, 17/18th century. (*Grose, Lex Bal*)

GREGORY A famous 17th century London wigmaker, buried at St Clement Dane's Church, London. (*Aubrey*)

GRESELDE Grizzled, grey. Medieval usage. (*Fisher*)

GRETCHEN STYLE A hair style usually worn by young girls, in which the hair, 6″ to 10″ long, is worn in tightly plaited stiff plaits hanging over or just behind the ears.

GRETEL Hair style for women. (*Ingerid*)

GREY Adj. A colour intermediate between black and white with little or no positive hue. Of hair: that is turning white with age.

GREY BEARD (1) 18th century name for earthenware jugs used for drawing ale, having on them the figure of a bearded man. See Greybeard jug.

(2) Dutch earthen jugs used on coasts of Essex and Sussex for smuggling gin. (*Grose, Lex Bal*)

(3) An old man.

GREYBEARD JUG (or Bellarmine) A jug incorporating a bearded face and modelled on Cardinal Bellarmine. First made by the Netherlands Protestants to caricature the Cardinal. 16th century. See also Bellarmine beards.

GREY COURT See Court wig.

GREY HAIR POWDER An 18/19th century recipe was: 2 lb black hair-powder; 2 lb fine starch powder; 1 lb fine orris powder; 4 oz calcined salts. Mixed and sifted well. (*Lillie*)

GREYNESS Canities, *qv*.

GRIMWIG A character in Dickens's *Oliver Twist*.

GRIP See Hair grip.

GRISAILLE Fr. Hair partly grey.

GRISON Fr. Grey haired.

GRIT GAUZE A firm wide meshed gauze upon which the hair is knotted preparatory to drawing through silk gauze imitating the human skin. American usage.

GRIZZLE Subs. (1) Grey hair.

(2) A grey wig.

(3) Nickname for grey-haired man.

(4) Verb. trans. to make grey haired.

'I'd wait till white hairs had grizzled my pate o'er.' (*NFH* Vol 2, p. 35)

(5) Verb, intrans. To become grey-haired.

'I am just beginning to grizzle.' (*Lowell, Letters,* 1894)

GRIZZLE BOB A grey bob wig for men. (*The Wig,* 1765)

GRIZZLE CUT BOB A man's 18th century wig style. (*Tennent*)

GRIZZLED (1) Adj. Grey, grizzly. 'Her grizzled locks assume a smirking grace.' (*E. Young, Love of Fame',* 1757)

(2) Having grey hair, 'Send this grizzled head'. (*Shakespeare, Antony and Cleopatra,* 3, XIII, 17)

GRIZZLE TYE WIG A man's grey wig with a tied queue which came into fashion in the early 18th century.

GRIZZLE WIG 18th century, full grey wig style for men, large, long and curled.

'At skittles in a grizzle can I play.'

'All hail, ye curls, that rang'd in reverend row,

With snowy pomp my conscious shoulders hide!

That full beneath in venerable flow

And crown my brows above with feathery pride!'

(*Ode to a grizzle wig by a gentleman who had just left off his bob, O S,*) cf Grisaille.

GROLICK'S ROBORANTIUM A 19/20th century 'secret'

preparation for 'remedying baldness. Was a dilute Eau de Cologne, with a little glycerine. (*Koller*)

GROMMET Bun pad (ring).

GROOM Verb. To make neat and tidy, especially the hair and beard.

GROUND COLOUR The prevailing colour of the hair.

GUARD COMB A comb hinged to a guard to protect the teeth when not in use.

GUARD-DAGGER WHISKERS A small pointed beard popular in France during the second half of the 17th century. (*Dulaure*)

GUARDSMAN An English moustache style. (*Foan*) *101R*

GUICHE Fr. Strand or strap. Part of the segment of the flat curl dressed forward onto the face. See also Side-board and Cheek piece.

GUICHE LOOK A woman's medium length bob style, with a guiche, *qv* on each cheek. 1961. *269*

GUILLOTINE CUT The hair club-cut straight across at the back of the neck. West Country usage.

GUINEVERE HAIRDRESS A woman's hair style of 1963, popularized by the musical play *Camelot*. The hair was worn bouffant on the top, combed to a pompadour and slightly bouffant at the sides combed down over the ears.

GULES Heraldic red.

GUM ACACIA See Gum arabic.

GUM ARABIC (Acacia gum) The dried, gummy exudation from the stems and branches of *Acacia Senegal*, and other species. Used as a mucilage in thin setting lotions and as an emulsifer.

GUM BENJAMIN An aromatic gum used in perfumery. (*Lillie*)

GUM DRAGON See Gum tragacanth, for which it is a synonym. (*Lillie*)

GUM SENEGAL See Gum arabic.

GUM TRAGACANTH The dried, gummy exudation from *Astragalus Gummifer*, an asiatic plant. It is the principal ingredient in many thick setting lotions and men's hair dressings. Also useful as an emulsifying agent.

GUMMED-UP HAIRDO A heavily lacquered coiffure (1955). Slang.

GUT A material used in wigmaking to strengthen the parting.

GUZZLE A filthy drain. Wiltshire usage. (*Akerman*)

GYPSY CURL A spiral curl.

H _____

HACKLE (1) Subs. An instrument set with pointed steel pins for combing tresses of hair in boardwork. See also Card. *174, 175, 462*

(2) Verb. To draw hair through a hackle to disentangle it.

HACKLE BRUSH A square brush for placing on top of the hackle as a safety precaution against anyone accidentally sitting on it, or indeed, catching any part of himself. *175*

HACKLE COVER A wooden cover to envelope the hackle as a protection. See Hackle brush.

HACKLING The same as Carding. The drawing of hair through the hackle to disentangle it.

HADRIAN According to Plutarch the first Roman Emperor to wear a beard. He grew it to hide a face wart and scars.

HAFFIT The side of the head. Scots usage.(*Brown*)

HAGGLE, TO To cut irregularly. Midlands usage. 17/18th century.

HAGS 'A kind of fiery meteor, appearing on men's hair or horses' mains', 17th century. (*Phillips*)

HAIR (1) Subs. A fine filament growing from the skin.

(2) Subs. The aggregate of the hairs growing on the head or body; also, collectively, hairs in the mass.

(3) Adj. Colour name for bright tan, 16th century. (*Cunnington*)

(4) Verb. trans. To depilate of free from hair.

(5) Verb. intrans. To grow hair.

(6) Verb. To cover or edge with hair.

(7) Used as a surname. Fred G Hair (*Thorpe Bay*). (*Daily Telegraph*, 23/9/70)

(8) A musical play in the modern permissive vernacular. First produced in the USA. Presented at the Shaftesbury Theatre, London, November 1968, and described as 'The American Tribal Love-Rock Musical'.

(9) A female. Slang. 19/20th century.

HAIR (Significance of dreams) If in your dreams your hair appears to grow long and hang untied over your shoulders, it is a sign that you will be beloved by a person of quality; but if you dream it is short or falls off, you will lose a dear friend. If your hair is burned in a dream, the person you love will prove false to you. (*Every-Lady's Own Fortune-Teller*)

HAIR, CUT OFF The Greeks and Romans believed that life would not leave the body of a devoted victim until a lock of hair had first been cut from his head and given to Prosperine. When Dido slew herself she could not die until Iris had cut off one of her locks. (*Virgil, Brewer*)

HAIR, LONG The longest hair recorded was 26′ long on the head of Swami Pandarasannadhi, head of the Thiruvadu Thurai Monastery in India. (*McWhirter*)

HAIR, LOOSE AND FLOWING Symbolical of penitence. See *Luke* ch 7, v 37–38. This Biblical story led to the custom of hermits growing their hair long. Virgin Saints are usually portrayed in Christian art with long, flowing hair.

HAIR AERIALIST See Hair Aerist.

HAIR AERIST One who juggles or performs gymnastics while suspended by the head-hair in mid-air. (BBC, 24.12.67)

HAIR ALBUM A blank paper album in which were preserved small bunches of braided and unbraided hair with the names and dates of the persons contributing the specimens. This was a rare form of collecting and analogous to the autograph book. The earliest example dates from the late 18th century and the fashion reached its height in the mid-19th century.

HAIR ARRANGEMENT Useful words denoting different forms of hair arrangement.

Arch, bale, band, bend, bounce, bouquet, braid, bun, bunch, burst, bush, chaplet, coil, convolution, corkscrew, curl, crisp, curlicue, fall, fillet, fold, fringe, gathering, grape, group, halo, hand, hank, head, helix, interlacement, intertwining, knot, lock, loop, mane, mat, mop, parcel, pinch, plait, plication, portion, puff, queue, ravel, ribbon, ringlet, roll, shock, snail shell, snuggle (of curls), spiral, strand, switch, tail, tangle, tendril, tete, tress, tuft, turban, turn, twine, twist, wave, wavelet, weft, whorl, wisp, wreath.

HAIR ARTIST (1) (Also Artist in hair) 19th century name for a designer and manufactuerer of jewellery made from or incorporating hair.

(2) Since *c* 1920 the description is also applied to a hairdresser who is, or claims to be, an artist in the creation and/or execution of hair styles. Sometimes the French spelling 'artiste' is affected.

HAIR ATTACHMENT (1) Any worked hair that can be attached to the head hair, eg pin curls, hair tails, back dressings, etc.

(2) Any device such as a slide that can be secured to or in the coiffure.

HAIR BAG (1) A bag to receive a woman's combings.

(2) A bag to hold the queue of a bag wig, *qv*.

(3) One who talks of past events or ancient scandals. (*W and F*)

HAIR BALL The mass of combings that was accumulated by women and kept in a 'combing container' on the dressing-table. The hair ball was later sometimes used to stuff pin cushions or was sold to the wigmaker as combings. The word is also used for the ball of hair sometimes found in the stomach of cats and some other animals.

HAIR BAND A band or fillet to confine the hair.

HAIR BEARD Luzula Campestris, a wood rush. (*Webster*)

HAIR BIND See Hair binder.

HAIR BINDER A length of any suitable pliable material such as silk, silk or cotton covered lead wire, elastic, etc, that can be used to hold together firmly the hairs in a tress on or off the head.   299

HAIRBIRD The chipping sparrow, an American bird which lines its nest with hair. (*Webster*)

HAIR BONES Cockney nickname for a very thin man. (*Franklyn*)

HAIR BOUTIQUE See Boutique.

HAIR BOW (1) Tresses of hair formed into a bow, a bow of hair.

(2) A bow of ribbon tied on the hair.

HAIR BOYS Young American men of the 1950s, also called hotrodders and greasers, who affected strange attire and rode fast motor bikes. They combed their hair straight back without a parting over a backcombed base of hair that made them look like minature 18th century Macaronis.

HAIR BRACELET A woman's bracelet made of plaited human hair. 18/19th century. (*Martin*)

HAIR BRACKET In ship building, the moulding on a sailing vessel which comes at the back of the figure, and breaks in with the upper part cheek. (*Burney*)

HAIR BRAIDER See Hair threader.

HAIR BRAINED See Harebrained. The form Hairbrained is often found but is quite erroneous.

HAIR BRAMBLE The European dewberry, *rubus caesius*. (*Webster*)

HAIR BREADTH ESCAPE A very narrow escape from danger or evil.

HAIR BROOM A long handled sweeping broom with hair bristles.

HAIRBRUSH (1) A small hand brush for disentangling and smoothing the hair, 1599. The best types have bristles of whalebone, boar and other animal hair. Of recent years nylon and other synthetic materials have been used for bristles. Metal bristles have been used, but these tear the hair.

(2) An explosive bomb with a handle. American military slang, 20th century. See Hairbrush grenade. (*Weseen*)

(3) A head of hair. Slang. (*Davies*)

HAIRBRUSH CACTUS *Pachycereus pecten-aboriginum*. The common tree cactus (15 to 40′ high) of Sonora and Chihuahua, Mexico.

HAIRBRUSH CLEANER A small, stiff bristle brush, a strong comb or a small wire rake for removing hair from between the bristles of hairbrushes.

HAIRBRUSH GRENADE Slang name for a type of hand grenade used in the 1914/1918 War. so called from its hairbrush-like shape, (*F and G*)

HAIR-BRUSHING MACHINE See Rotary hairbrushing machine.

HAIR BUBBLES 'Bubbles' of air in the hair shaft which reflect light and give the hair an appearance of greyness.

HAIR BULB The bulbous indented root-end of a hair; the indentation fitting over the papilla.

HAIR BUTCHER A hairdresser of inferior skill in cutting. slang.

HAIR BUTTONS Buttons made of hair. (*Miege*)

HAIR BUYER (1) One who buys hair. 1721. (*London Gazette*)
(2) A procurer, 18th century slang. (*Ward*)

HAIR BUYER, THE Henry Hamilton, Lieut Governor of Detroit, America, 1775-9. During the American revolutionary war it was said that he paid bounties only for scalps and not for prisoners. Called the Hair Buyer by American patriots because of his tactics in instigating Indian raids and scalpings of frontier settlers. (*Havigurst*)

HAIR CAP (1) A toupet, slang.
(2) A cap composed of hair.
(3) Facetious name for a short bob wig, 18th century. (*L C March*, 1762)

HAIR CARDER A person who cards, *qv*, hair.

HAIR CHARM (1) Hair cut off and cast into the sea to appease a storm. (*Lean*)
(2) a small lock of human hair carried for good luck. Hair from the tail of an elephant is often worn for good luck in the form of a bangle or finger ring.

HAIR CLAMP (Hair vice) See Jigger (3).

HAIR CLASP (1) An ornament for the hair, of steel, silver, etc, often set with jewels, to secure the braided back hair. 18th century. (*Earle*)
(2) A slide that clips on the hair. 18th/20th centuries.

HAIR CLIPPER(S) See Clipper.

HAIRCLOTH Cloth made of hair, used for shirts by ascetics and penitents; also for tents, etc.

HAIR COIL See Coil of hair.

HAIR COLLECTOR An itinerant buyer of human hair for the manufacturers of wigs, tails and other postiches. (*Speight*)

HAIR-COLOURING CRAYON *cf* Water cosmetic.

HAIR-COLOURING PAD (1) A comb with an absorbent pad attached, which when impregnated with a hair-colouring liquid is combed through the hair to dye it. American usage.
(2) A rod of wood, bone or glass covered with an absorbent material and used as (1) above.

HAIR COLOURIST A person who dyes or bleaches the hair.

HAIR COMPASS A compass that can be regulated to the utmost precision.

HAIR CONDITIONER A preparation whose constituents are intended to improve the condition of the hair by bringing it back to or nearer a state of normality. For instance excessively dry hair can be improved by the application of certain fats and oils in correct combinations with other chemicals. Among the ingredients that have been used in hair conditioners are egg and beer, various ranges of oils and fats and more complex mixtures such as lecithin and lanolin.

HAIR CONDITIONING External treatment designed to improve the condition of the hair by means of lotions, creams, massage and the application of steam to the head and hair.

HAIR-CONDITIONING CREAM See Conditioner.

HAIR CONTOUR See Contour.

HAIR COPPER Chalcotrichite, a red, semi-translucent variety of cuprite, characterised by its capillary habit. (*Chambers*)

HAIR CORD A kind of cotton, the warp of which consists of

coloured ribs. (*Franke*)

HAIR CORD MUSLIN Finely woven cotton cloth (38″ wide) the threads running the long way and presenting the appearance of fine cords. Used for infants robes. (*Caulfield SFA* Ad; *Saward, B, Dictionary of Needlework*, 1882)

HAIR COURT Sexual connection, 19th century slang.

HAIRCRAFT Skill in matters pertaining to hair.

HAIR CRAYON A type of water cosmetic in the form of a crayon used for colour-coating the new growth of hair between applications of hair dye.

HAIR CREAM Hair dressings of a creamy consistency.

HAIR CREPE Crêpe made from hair. See Crêpe hair.

HAIR CROOK A tortoiseshell, bone, or metal crook for drawing small locks or strands of hair through dressed hair in the construction of a hair style. 19/20th century, *cf*, Hairdressing needle.

HAIR CURLER (1) A device for curling the hair. There are many and various forms.
(2) A rod of metal, plastic or other material on which hair is rolled preparatory to permanently curling it.

HAIR CUSHION (1) A small cushion or pad over which the hair was dressed on the head; 18th century. 'Silk and hair cushions, black and white hair pins, and every other article necessary for dressing ladies' and gentlemen's hair.' (*Morning Herald*, 13 Dec 1787)

HAIRCUT (1) The act of cutting the hair to shorten, thin or shape it. 'I am going to have a haircut.'
(2) The style cut by the hairdresser. 'That's a fashionable haircut you have.'
(3) Cockney nickname for a man with very long hair. (*Franklyn*)

HAIR CUTICLE The scaly covering of a hair.

HAIR CUTTER A craft description of a person who offers the limited service of hair-cutting to the public. (19th century Trade cards and advertisements)

HAIRCUTTING Subs. The process of cutting, trimming, thinning or shaping the head-hair by the use of scissors or razor.

HAIRCUTTING AND SHAMPOOING ROOMS The usual 19th century appelation for a hairdressing establishment. Adv.

HAIRCUTTING GOWN A cloak or cover of material which allows cut hair to fall off readily; used to protect the clothing of a client receiving a hairdressing service.

HAIRCUTTING ROOMS Rooms, in contradistinction to an open saloon, in a hairdresser's shop, where the process of haircutting took place. 19th century.

HAIR DEALER A person who buys and sells human hair. See also Hair collector.

HAIR DESCRIPTION A full description of a hair requires the following details: (1) Chemical composition, (2) Elasticity, (3) Tensile strength, (4) Porosity, (5) Colour (this can differ along the hair shaft), (6) Length, (7) Texture (this can be uniform or variable along the shaft), (8) Shape of cross-section, (9) Degree of curl, (10) Cell structure, (11) Presence of foreign bodies (dye, chemicals), (12) Scale structure, (13) Condition (dry, greasy, brittle, etc), (14) Refractive index, (15) Description of root, (16) Widths of cuticle, cortex and if present the medulla.

HAIR DESIGN (1) A style for a hairdress.
(2) A design in hair for a hair-bracelet, hair-brooch, etc.

HAIR DEVICE (1) Designs in hair of landscapes, flowers, patterns, etc, usually set in a trinket 'for wearing as a brooch, locket, ring, watch-guard, etc. (See Hair jewellery. (*Elegant Arts*)

HAIRDO (Pl Hairdos) 20th century. The attention to and dressing of the hair. The writer first heard the word used in

178

conversation at Weston-Super-Mare in 1925. By the 1950s it had become synonymous with coiffure and hairdress, *qv*. *Fowler's modern English Usage*, ed 1965, suggests Hairdo is now to be preferred to the hyphenated hair-do. The present writer agrees.

HAIR-DO See Hairdo.

HAIRDOING The same as hairdressing, *qv*. 'The hairline frequently proves the most challenging hairdoing factor.' (*H F*)

HAIRDO PROTECTOR A hairnet of hair, nylon or other suitable material; plain, or decorated with spangles, patterns or colours. 20th century.

HAIR DRAG The pull on the hair when combing or winding the hair on curlers for a permanent wave.

HAIR DRAW The thin strand of straight, unbraided hair around which a plait is formed. On completion of the plait, the point end of the draw is held in the left hand and the plait pushed up towards the root end of the draw, thus widening the plait. Popularly used in styles of the 18th and 19th centuries.

HAIR DRAWER A person who draws-off, *qv* hair.

HAIR DRAWN Drawn out finely as a hair.

HAIRDRESS (Hair-dress) (1) Subs. Coiffure, Hairdo, Style or Mode of wearing the hair. Hairdress is to be preferred to headdress as the latter can also refer to millinery. The word Hairdress with the hyphen was first used by Robert Southey in his *Common-place Book*; 1849–1851, and has been regularly employed since; in Britain and America. 'No more Curls or Buckles be introduced in the Hair-dress, than there are in the patterns.' (*Le Gros, Ladies' Toilet*, 1768)

Sir Ernest Gowers, in the revised edition of H W Fowler's *A Dictionary of Modern English Usage*, 1965, suggests that hairdo should supersede the alien coiffure. This is unlikely to happen, as the now Anglicised French word coiffure is too firmly embedded in the language of the hairdresser ever to fall completely into disuse. It has for 100 years been, until recently, one of the only three words commonly used to describe a dressed head of hair, the others being hairdress and headdress. Headdress has the serious disadvantage of being used for hats and hair. Hairdress does not suffer from this dichotomy, and the present writer suggests that the three words hairdress, coiffure and hairdo, could and should be used at choice instead of headdress with its double meaning.

Hairdo which started as hair-do in the 1920s has captured the American imagination and is their present preference, as it undoubtedly is of the younger set in this country. See also Coiffure and Hairdo.

(2) Verb. To dress hair. 'He had hairdressed the wench.'

HAIRDRESSER One whose business it is to comb and brush, clean, cut, curl, wave, bleach and dye, design hair styles, arrange and dress hair. Written as Hair-dresser with a hyphen, in *A Second Letter to Her Grace the Duchess of Devonshire*, 1777, and in the 18th century hairdresser was a trade description of a person who offered the service of hair dressing, but not necessarily hair cutting. In the Georgian and Victorian periods it was usual to designate the services offered, eg S Hicks of Angel St, Cardiff, 'Perfumer, Ladies' and Gentlemen's Hair-Cutter, Dresser and Ornamental Hair Manufacturer.' (Trade Card, 19th century)   *460*

HAIRDRESSER'S REGISTRATION COUNCIL Founded 15 February, 1922, to secure statutory registration of hairdressers. In 1964 it was successful in its efforts. Parliament set up under statute the Hairdressing Council to register those hairdressers who had by examination demonstrated that they had reached the standard of proficiency demanded by the Hairdressing Council. Since March 1966, the HRC has continued its educational and examination duties under its new title: The Hairdressers' Technical Council.

HAIRDRESSER'S SIGNS At a time when few could read or write, trade signs were commonly displayed outside shops to indicate the goods or services offered. In addition to the commonest hairdressing sign – the barber's pole, others included locks of hair, curled and tied, used by John Aklen, hairdresser, on London Bridge, in the 18th century; Lock of hair and shears; a periwig; blue peruke and star; white peruke; hand and lock of hair; a major wig; a hair-cutter; absalom hanging. (*Garwood*)

HAIRDRESSER'S WEEKLY JOURNAL First published 1882 by William Wise, 4 Crane Court, London, EC, now published under the title *The Hairdresser's Journal*.

HAIR-DRESSING A liquid preparation of a creamy consistency used to anoint the hair of the head to improve its condition, impart a sheen, facilitate its dressing or hold it in position.

HAIRDRESSING The practice of the hairdresser, consisting of cutting, shampooing, dyeing, bleaching, curling, waving, styling and dressing hair.

HAIRDRESSING ACADEMY See Academy. In the 18th century in Paris these academies were described as follows: 'The academy for teaching the art of female hair-dressing, according to the present high *gout* . . . wherein you see a great number of the dirtiest female drabs the streets afford hired to sit, not for their pictures but for their patience, and to have their heads and their hair twisted and turned about in various forms according to the taste of the operator. . . . When the head is finished the whole chamber of artists examines the workmanship, and after each has given his opinion the pyramid is thrown down and re-erected by some other student.' (*Gents Mag*, 1770s)

HAIRDRESSING CLOTH A cloth to cover the client during a hairdressing process. Until the late 19th century it was usually a long, white cloth. Later it had a neck slit and smooth, coloured, patterned cotton fabrics came into use. (*Chambers Journal*, Nov 1866)

HAIRDRESSING COUNCIL See Hairdresser's Registration Council.

HAIRDRESSING GOWN A cloak or cover with or without sleeves, used to cover and protect the client's clothing during hairdressing processes.

HAIRDRESSING NEEDLE See Hair needle.

HAIRDRESSING OUTFIT The complete collection of implements and materials necessary to conduct a hairdressing business. In 1887 R Hovenden advertised a complete outfit for 7 guineas. (*Creer*)

HAIRDRESSING SUNDRIES The items and accessories, supplies and oddments needed by a hairdresser for the practice of his craft. The following are some prices advertised in 1887 (*Creer*): Curling irons 10d to 2/- each; pinching irons 1/3d to 4/9d each; crimping irons 2/- to 9/- each; mounting blocks 4/6d each; weaving silk 2/- per oz; sewing silk 2/3d per oz; drawing brushes from 6/6d to 15/- per pair.

HAIRDRESSING UNDERTAKINGS WAGES COUNCIL (GREAT BRITAIN) Established under Statutory Order No 1879 in the year 1947. This compulsory order replaced the voluntary non-statutory body 'The National Joint Industrial Council for Hairdressing' which had in itself been reconstituted in 1943. The Council consists of 13 employees, 13 employers and 3 independent members. An independent member acts as Chairman.

HAIRDRESSING WAX A preparation of wax (such as

beeswax) or incorporating wax for dressing moustaches and hair.

HAIRDRESS POCKET Some of the natives of the Congo made a secret fob in their woolly hairdress of which, as Labat writes, the worst use they made of it was to carry poison in it. The Matolas, a long-haired race who border upon the Kaffirs, formed their locks into a kind of hollow cylinder in which they carried their little implements. (*Southey, The Doctor*)

HAIRDRYER An apparatus which blows hot or cold air as required, used to dry wet hair. See also Hand dryer, and Hood dryer.

HAIR DYE The Organ Cactus (*Marginatocereus Marginatus*) is commonly used as a hair dye in Mexico. It is prepared by stripping the branches of their thorns, cutting the cactus into small cubes and putting them into water to remain three days. The mixture becomes glutinous and is rubbed into the scalp as an ordinary scalp tonic. It is said this has the effect of causing the new growth of hair to emerge with its original colour and within a few months the whole of the hairs will have reverted to their former hue. (*Mitford*) See Dye and Tint.

HAIRE Cloth made of hair. See Haircloth.

HAIR EATER (1) A small parasite which destroys hair. (*Belcher*)

(2) A compulsive eater of hair.

HAIRED Adj. With hair; covered with hair; having hair.

HAIRE DECEIT False hair or artificial colouring of the hair, 16/17th century. (*Tuke*)

HAIRED STAR Cancer (Astronomy).

HAIREN Adj. Consisting of hair.

HAIRESTER One who works in horsehair.

HAIR FALDERAL Ornament for decorating a woman's hairdress. Somerset usage.

HAIRFALL The slight or excessive loss of hair from the scalp, over a short or long period. See also Diffuse hairfall.

HAIR FANDANGLE A fancy comb, slide or other hair ornament. Somerset usage.

HAIR-FASHION CONSULTANT One who holds himself out as an expert whose taste and knowledge qualifies him to advise an enquirer on payment of a fee which fashionable hair style is the most suitable for him or her. American usage. (*Cordwell*)

HAIR FETISHISM The attraction of a person to hair because of its associations, especially erotic. (*Berg*)

HAIR-FETISHIST One who, because of its associations, is attracted by hair and often, through unconscious elements, with varying forms of erotic pleasures, such as the cutting off of girls' hair plaits. (*Berg*)

HAIR FIDDLER A person who fiddles with the hair, usually by drawing the thumb and fingers down a strand, or twisting a small strand round and round. A common nervous affliction of students and persons whose time is occupied more by thought than action.

HAIR FINGER (1) The second finger of the right hand, which is used with the thumb to feel the texture of hair; the skin of the index finger being less sensitive than the second finger.

(2) A narrow tress of uncurled hair.

HAIR FIXATIVES Preparations to hold the hair in position.

HAIR FLOWER *Calliandra Cenomala*. An evergreen shrub of the *leguminosae* family with hair-like flowers in a hemispherical head.

HAIR FOLD A strand of hair folded back upon itself. A constituent of many 18th century and Victorian coiffures. (*Miscellaneous and Fugative Pieces*, 1773, Vol 2, p 336)

HAIR FOLLICLE The small sac or vesicle in the skin from which hair grows.

HAIR FORK A two-pronged fork with a tapered and pointed handle made of plastic, tortoiseshell, etc, used for picking out curls and arranging tresses in a hairdress. 1920s.

HAIR-FOUNDATION NET A foundation net for postiche made from human hair. This type of net, in the 19th century, was principally made in Normandy and Brittany by peasants working in their own homes.

HAIR FRAME (1) A hair covered, hollow, wire frame used as a pad or foundation for incorporating in a hairdress. 18th/20th century.

(2) Ditto, but covered in a light-weight, loose weave material. 18/20th century.

Both made in many shapes and sizes such as pompadour; three-quarter circle; all-round frame; half sausage; side frame; oval frame; round frame; parting frame, etc.

HAIR GAME A game or play of children in which human hair plays a part. Example: Hair tugging, in which the loser is the first one to cry out.

HAIR GLOSS (or Crème de mauve) A 19th century preparation consisting of glycerine 4 lb, spirit of Jasmine 1 pint, aniline 5 drops. (*Piesse*)

HAIR GLOVE A glove of horse hair used to massage the skin.

HAIR GOODS Articles such as wigs manufactured from human hair; also objects connected with boardwork, such as galloon, wig net, etc.

HAIR GOWN See Hairdressing gown.

HAIR GRASS The botanical species *aira*. (*B and H*)

HAIR GRIP A device of bent metal, used to hold hair in position.

HAIR HARVEST The cutting and collecting of human hair from the peasants at Continental fairs and other places of female congregation by agents or collectors who travelled from village to village at regular intervals for the purpose of obtaining hair of peasant women in exchange for money or trinkets. F Trollope in *Summer in Brittany* gives a lively description of such a scene. 19th century.

HAIR HAT A craft term of contempt for a cheap fashion wig of the 1960s made of synthetic hair or oriental hair.

HAIR HAWKER A prostitute. 18th century slang. (*Ward; Heron*)

HAIR HOLD See Hair tidy.

HAIR HOOK A large hook of tortoiseshell, bone, metal or other suitable material, similar to a crochet hook and used for pulling strands of hair through the intersteces of skeleton wigs, streaking caps, etc. 19/20th century.

HAIRHOOF, SCENTED The plant *asperula odorata*. (*B and H*)

HAIR HYGROMETER An instrument of which the vital constituent is a human hair used for measuring the humidity of the air. The expansion of the hair when exposed to damp is indicated on a dial.

HAIRILY Adv. With hair or hairiness.

HAIR IMPLANTATION The anchoring of human hair by various means to a postiche foundation.

In 1805, Leguet, hairdresser at Lyons, invented the flesh-coloured hair-net. Postiches had hitherto been so coarsely made that this improvement in the manufacture of wigs caused quite a sensation. The fame of the inventor soon reached Paris, and M Tellier, hairdresser at the Palais Royal, tried to buy Leguet's patent. In 1810, Leguet, who had found that his wigs did not keep the desired firmness (the hair being badly knotted), easily agreed to cede his patent to Tellier. An English firm having heard of Leguet's invention, procured one of his wigs, which they imitated and improved. This came to the knowledge of Tellier, who went to London to study the improvements. Meanwhile, Carron, another coiffure at the Palais Royal, bought from a Lyons silk weaver the process for the implantation on silk of a different kind, which, though less suitable for men's wigs than that of Leguet's gave much neater partings for women's work. Tellier on his return to Paris, intending to considerably extend his novel industry, associated himself with a stocking weaver of the Cevennes. Hence arose a law suit between Carron and Tellier. But contrary to the ordinary rule, this law suit, instead of ruining the parties more immediately concerned, helped to make their fortune. All the papers were full of this suit, and every bald-head – feminine or masculine – in the kingdom was eager to see and perchance try to rejuvenate itself by the novel inventions. The poor Lyons weaver who parted with his patent, being unable to witness others amassing fortunes by its means, while he remained in misery, put an end to his days. In the law suit M Tellier, having produced the patent bought of Leguet, got the best of it.

Michalon, a weaver, invented the silk parting, produced with a long piece of silk without head which he put on his shuttle. Dufour invented the knotted hair foundation, knotting the hair by means of a gauze needle. Then a workman established himself in the Faubourg St Denis, who made partings in the way Carron made them. He was the first to make partings in heart shape. The brothers Lavacquerie perfected the work of the latter. Valon, one of Dufour's workmen, further perfected the wig by giving a tighter and better fit.

In 1822, Souchard took out a patent at Bordeaux for implantations made with an embroidery needle, and having in the course of time perfected his invention, he tried to implant hair on a pig's bladder, which, being lined with *gros de Naples*, made an excellent bald-wig for theatrical performances, and produced a very good effect.

In 1823 Souchard went to England to study the manner in which the English made their silk-net wigs. He found the English silk net infinitely superior to the French, and he adopted the former for his wigs. (*Moniteur de la Coiffure*, 1836; *Creer, Boardwork*, 1887)

HAIRINESS The state of being hairy. Hirsuteness.

HAIRING (1) The action of dressing or manipulating hair. Hairdressing. 'A hairing implement.' (*She*, May 1968)

(2) Adj. Tearing, furious. 20th century. Public School slang. 'A hairing great row.' (*Partridge*). Derived from the tearing of hair from a person's own head when in an uncontrollable rage.

HAIRISH Partly hairy.

HAIR JEWELLERY (1) Jewellery constructed from human hair, in the 17th to 19th century, and offered by ladies to their lovers as a mark of their favour.

'Your four mistresses beg you to accept of their bracelet, 'tis the work of all four, compos'd of their own hairs, and wrought with their own hands.' (George Granville, Lord Lansdowne. The She-Gallants, act 1, scene 1, 1969. First acted 1695.) See also Hair ring.

(2) Jewellery for the hair such as ornamental slides incorporating precious or semi-precious stones, gold or silver. *436, 437*

HAIR KNOT A decorative twist or fold of hair in a hairdress.

HAIR LACE (1) A tie or string to bind hair; a fillet. 'A haire-lace. Fascia crinalis vel texta tae.' (*Clerk*, p 256). 16/17th century.

(2) A fine lightweight diamond mesh net made of hair and used for the finest partings and foundations of postiches.

HAIR-LACE FOUNDATION A foundation of hair lace.

HAIR-LACE FRONT A front of hair worked on hair lace.

HAIR-LACE PARTING A nearly invisible hair parting worked on hair lace and revealing the natural scalp through the lace. The hair knots are very fine and this gives the illusion that the hair is growing from the wearer's scalp.

HAIR LACQUER A solution of or similar to the following (1–4) and used to hold the dressed and styled hair in position in a static hairdress or hairdo; (1) Shellac dissolved in alcohol; Shellac 9%, Triethanolamine 2%, Ethyl Alcohol 20%, Distilled water 69%, Water-soluble perfume QS; (2) Polyvinyl acetate resin dissolved in industrial ethyl alcohol; (3) Polyvinyl pyrollidone dissolved in industrial ethyl alcohol; (4) Dimethyl hydantoin formaldehyde resin dissolved in industrial ethyl alcohol. Glycerine or triacetin can be added in small quantities to the above formulae to soften the resin and prevent it flaking. Lacquer spraying can, in certain concentrations, endanger both operator and client. M Bergman and others have reported cases of serious illness and three deaths resulting from its use. See M Bergman and others *The New English Journal*, 12 April 1962. Also *Savill, The Hair and Scalp*, ed 1962.

'A half-filled container of hair lacquer exploded on a dressing table cracking two walls, knocking a door jamb out of true and setting fire to bedding. Mr R Peck of Blandford Road, Chilwell, Notts, said yesterday. No one was in the room. (*Daily Telegraph*, 13 June 1966)

HAIRLESS Adj. Without hair, bald.

HAIRLESS COCONUT A bald head. Slang.

HAIRLET A small hair. (*Davies*)

HAIR LICHEN A fungoid eruption that attacks the root of the hair.

HAIR-LIFT COMB A narrow comb with about six widely spaced teeth. Used for lifting bouffant styles. USA 1970.

HAIRLIKE Adj. Resembling a hair. Fine like a hair.

HAIR LINE (1) The outline of the growing hair on the head. (2) The line or outline of the dressed hair; the outline of the hairdresses silhouette. (3) A line or rope composed of hair. (4) A very thin line.

HAIRLINE LETTER A very thin-faced printing type.

HAIR LOCK (1) A lock of hair on the scalp. (2) A cut lock of hair often given as a gift to a lover or friend; also kept in memory of a person.

HAIR LOCKET A locket set with a small lock of human hair. See Hair ring.

HAIR LOOP See Loop.

HAIR MASTER A supreme craftsman in the art of hairdressing.

HAIR MAT (1) A mat composed of hair. (2) A thick mass of entangled hair; matted wad of hair.

HAIR MATTRESS A mattress stuffed with human or other types of hair.

The ex-King of Bavaria is not the only sovereign who has had the offer made him of a mattress of soldiers' beards. During the war of Liberation in Portugal, and in Oporto at the time of the siege there was a corps in Her Majesty's service styled The Sacred Battalion, composed chiefly of officers, for whom there were no vacancies in the regular regiments. These gentlemen all wore beards of prodigious length as was customary with the whole army and had all sworn never to shorten them until the Queen, Donna Maria, was seated upon her throne, when they were to be cut off, and devoted to the purpose of making a mattress for Her Majesty. (*Dorset County Chronicle*, 9 October 1856)

HAIR MEMENTO A piece of jewellery incorporating a pinch of hair in memory of a loved one.

HAIR MEMORIAL RING (Locket, etc) A ring composed of

human hair or a locket enclosing human hair in memory of someone.

HAIR MERCHANT One who buys and sells human hair. Most of the human hair used in England is imported from Europe. The merchant cleans, sorts, grades and curls much of the raw hair he purchases and then sells it to the wigmaker. (*Ladies' Companion*; 1851; *GSB*)

HAIR MILK Skimmed milk, sometimes used as a setting lotion on fine hair.

HAIR MOLE A mole on the skin having a hair or hairs growing from it.

HAIR MONGER (1) A dealer in hair. 1840. (*T A Trollope, A Summer in Brittany*). See Hair merchant.
(2) A pimp.

HAIR MOULD a mould which appears on bread. Scots usage. (*Brown*)

HAIR MOUSE The same as Hair rat (2), *qv*, but smaller.

HAIR MOVEMENT The directions in which the strands of hair in a coiffure are pointing. The arrangement of the tresses in a coiffure.

HAIR NEADELL An ornamental hairpin. Medievel usage. (*Earle*)

HAIR NEEDLE (1) A large-eyed, flat bodkin of ivory, bone, horn and rarely metal. Used for threading strands of hair in a coiffure. Much used in the 18th century and 19th century for constructing the intricate hairdresses of that period.
(2) A single pointed hairpin. A bodkin (*Norman; Franke*)

HAIR NET (1) A net of hair, silk or other suitable material used to enclose the hair of the head and prevent its disarrangement.
Shangtung was the centre of the human-hair-net industry. The hair nets were made by women in the evenings and kerosene lamps were used to enable them to do their work. When the bobbed hair fashion started in Europe and spread rapidly, hair nets were no longer in great demand. (*Cartwright*)
(2) A net made of hair. See also: Back net, Bun net, Cap net, Caul net, Chignon net, Day net, Donut net, Fringe net, Setting net, Shingle net, Sleeping net, etc.

HAIR-NET WIG A wig made on a foundation of human hair net with all the sewing done with human hair. Hair was knotted onto this foundation which was made to fit the head exactly. There were no springs and everything in the wig was of human hair. My grandfather was making this type of wig in the 1870s when the price was £8–8–0. By 1920 the price had risen to £25 and by 1945, when the last one was made by my family business, the price had risen to £75. The parting could be changed to several positions. There was no shrinking. It was smooth and soft to the scalp and the last wig made, a short-haired one, weighed 1 oz. The foundation had six ¾" circular holes for ventilation. It is doubtful if a wig such as this will ever again be made. Certainly the price today would exceed £1000.

HAIR NOMENCLATURE Physicians distinguished human hair by the following Latine names: Hair of the head *Capillus*; that of women particularly, *Coma*; that of men, *Caesaries*; that of the back of the head, *Juba* and *Crines*; that hanging behind the ears, *Cincinni*. (*Chambers*)

HAIR-OF-THE-EARTH The grass.

HAIR-OF-MACROPROSOPUS A symbol of the divine life emanating from the source of all life and truth, in forms of infinite diversity. Macroprosopus – godhead. (*Gaskell*)

HAIR-OF-MEAL A few grains. Hair a very small quantity.

HAIR-OF-THE-HEAD (1) The average number of hairs on the human scalp is: Red hair 90,000, Black hair 103,000, Blonde hair 140,000, the overall average being 120,000. The average diameter of head hair is ¼₀₀". (*Leftwich*)

(2) A symbol of faith or the highest qualities of the lower mind. (*Gaskell*)

HAIR-OF-VENUS The herb *Adiantum Capillus – Veneris*. Maidenhair made into a lotion was believed to strengthen the hair and make it curl. (*Level*)

HAIR OIL An oil that is used as a dressing for the hair. A popular 19th century recipe: Finest olive oil 3 lb; castor oil ½ lb; essence of lemon 1½ oz. To colour steep 1 oz of alkanet root (bruised and tied in muslin) to every 20 oz. Apply heat by means of water bath and filter. (*Creer*)

HAIR-OIL BAZAAR A large bazaar in Cairo, where nothing but scents, oils and gold lace for the hair was sold.
'On each divan sat one or more moos'lim coiffeurs, whose profession was stamped on their delicately turned moustache and glossy silken beards.' (*Griffith*)

HAIROLOGIST One who purports to read character by growth, quality and substance of the hair. (*Aurand*, 1938. *BBC* March, 1969)

HAIROLOGY The study of the growth, quality and substance of the hair with a view to deducing the character of its grower. (*BBC* March 1969)

HAIROMETER A measuring device for recording the tensile strength of hair. (Invented by JSC)

HAIR ON THE TONGUE Amatus Lusitanus tells of a person who had hair growing upon his tongue. (*Speight*)

HAIR ORNAMENT Any ornamental device to add to a hairdress, such as a slide, comb, pompon, coque, etc.

HAIR PAD (1) A puff or frisette, *qv*.
(2) The same as Hair frame, *qv*.

HAIR PALM The hair or fan palm of Southern Europe.

HAIR PARCEL 56 lb of uncleaned human hair.

HAIR PASTE A mixture of soap lather and flour used by army officers as a dressing for the back hair, 18th century.

HAIR PATCH (1) A small postiche to cover a thin or bald area of the scalp.
(2) Hair cloth.

HAIR PEDLAR An itinerant buyer of human hair for the wig trade. (*Cox*, editor, *Hair Pedlar in Devon*, 1968)

HAIR PEG A device with a single point and often with an ornamental head, used to secure the hair; a hair pin. (*Earle*)

HAIR PENCIL Small brush used by artists made of the fine hairs of the polecat, marten, badger, etc.

HAIR PICTURE A representation on a flat surface of scenery, still-life, portraiture, etc, worked in hair and framed for hanging as a watercolour.

HAIR PIE (1) A pie of paste in which hair, already wound on earthenware rollers was placed to be baked to fix the curl. (*Stewart and Temple Bar*, p 250, 3 September 1861)
(2) The vulva. 20th century American slang. (*W and F*)

HAIR PIECE A wig or other postiche; an artificial addition of real or false hair in the form of a wig, toupee, front, semi-transformation, chignon, switch, pin curl, etc, for wearing on the head. (*Daily Telegraph*, 3 April 1959; the *Lady*, 1963)

HAIRPIN (HAIR-PIN) (1) A kind of pin used in dressing and fastening the hair. In ancient Greek and Roman times and during the medieval period they were single-pointed, like a bodkin, *qv*, but by the 18th century the double pointed hairpin had become popular. In June 1775 both double and single hairpins were being advertised for sale by Harriet Paine of Boston, New England. (*Earle*)
'The hair at the sides was stuck out in stiff curls, or rolls, tier above tier, fastened with long double black pins.' 1782. (*Southey, Letters*)   *134, 167, 171*
The single-pointed hairpins were made of bronze, silver, jet, bone, ivory, wood, etc, and the double-pointed ones of wire, horn, tortoiseshell, etc, with curves and indentations

to catch in the hair and prevent the pin from slipping out. Modern hairpins carry names descriptive of their shapes such as: straight, waved, curvilinear, holdfast, etc. (*Longman*) Essential requirements of a good hairpin are:

(A) Wire strong enough to support the hair,

(B) Adaptable to adjustment by bending,

(C) Smooth finish,

(D) Points that will not scratch the scalp,

(E) Sufficient curvature or irregularity to hold fast the hair without dropping out.

(2) Humerous term for a man. 'That's the sort of hair-pin I am,' American usage, first popularly employed about 1880. (*Walsh*)

(3) a strange or unusual person. A crackpot. 20th century. American slang. (*W and F*)

(4) A woman. 20th century. American slang. (*Weseen*)

(5) Cockney nickname for a very thin man. (*Franklyn*)

HAIRPIN BEND An acute bend in a road or path, like a hairpin in form.

HAIR PINCER Pinching irons, *qv*.

HAIR PLUCKERS (1) The Jains of India.

(2) Eyebrow tweezers, *qv*.

HAIR PLUME A plume of feathers worn as a hair ornament.

HAIR POSTCARD A postcard on which a picture of a human head has hair stuck on it.

HAIR POWDER A scented powder made of finely ground starch, flour, gold dust or other suitable particles, used to powder dressed wigs or hairdresses and secured to the hair by a previously applied pomade. (*Youth's Behaviour*, 1650) First used by the Romans, and in France by 1590 (*Yeats*). Hair powder of fine ground orris root, nutmeg, etc, was used on natural hair in the 16th and 17th century. 'Nutmegs for your hayere 10d.' (*Account Book*, Viscount Scudamore, 1632; *Rimell*, p 208). William Vaughan in *The Golden Grove*; 1600, refers to hair powder and periwigs being worn by women. A recipe of 1670 was: 1 lb rose leaves; 10 lb starch powder; mix well together every 3 hours; The next day sift and add the same number of fresh rose leaves again. Do this for three days. White, yellow, rose pink, and black powder was used for hair powdering in the 18th century. (*The Mirror*, vol 30)

On 20 October 1745, 51 barbers were fined £20 each for having in their possession hair powder not made of starch, and on the 27 October 1745, 49 other barbers were similarly convicted and fined. (*Lambert*, p 27)

'Lewis Hendrie . . . continues to make and sell Hair Powder, manufactured from the finest starch.' (*Morning Herald*, 13 Dec 1787)

Hair Powder was often adulterated with flour, rice powder, plaster of Paris, and slaked lime. (*Francis*)

HAIR-POWDER PERFUME Popular hair-powder scents were: orange flower water, jasmine, orris root, lavender and ambergris. (*Francis*, p 167; *Merle*, p 123)

HAIR-POWDER TAX In 1795 Parliament imposed a tax of one guinea per annum, effective from 5 May 1795, on persons wearing hairpowder. This tax yielded up to £20,000 per annum, but at the time of its repeal, 24 June 1869, the yield had dropped to about £1,000 per annum. The *Hull Advertiser* 11 July 1795 recorded that nearly one thousand hair-powder certificates were issued to persons in that town. (*Edwards, An Act*, 1795)

HAIR PREPARER A boardworker skilled in the art of preparing hair (drawing off, mixing, curling, colouring, etc) for the making of postiches.

HAIR PRESSING A method of temporarily straightening over-curly or kinky hair by means of a heated metal comb which is drawn slowly through the hair and the hair is allowed to cool in the straightened condition. This is called a soft press. Hard pressing is the application of a second treatment with hot Marcel waving irons over the comb dressed treatment. (*Thomas*)

HAIR-PRESSING OIL An oily preparation used in the process of hair pressing. A commonly used formula is: Petrolatum (petroleum or paraffin jelly) 90% per cent; Paraffin 10%; perfume and colour, *qs*.

HAIR-PROCESSING SALON A hairdressing salon. 1960s.

HAIR PUFFER A curling stick with a groove down its length to facilitate the entry of the pin of a safety-pin type of hairpin, *c* 1880.

HAIR PYRITES A native sulphuret of nickel which occurs in capillary filaments, of a yellow-grey colour. (*Franke*)

HAIR RAG Strips of rag used by women to roll or twist their hair into curls. The rolled hair was left in the rags for several hours and produced a temporary curl in otherwise straight hair. (1827. *Illustrated Life of G C* by Jerrold, p 108, Vol 1 My extra illus copy)

HAIR RAISER A subject that causes anger, fear, argument or amazement. (*Weesen*)

HAIR-RAISING Terrifying. An eerie story with a frightening plot is said to be a hair-raiser.

HAIR RAT (1) Hair pad. American usage, 19th to early 20th century. (*Cocroft*)

(2) A crêpe pad or puff.

HAIR RECEIVER See Hair tidy. American usage.

HAIR REGENERATOR (1) An apparatus to heat or steam the hair in combination with suitable chemicals to improve the condition of the hair and/or increase its growth.

(2) A dye to colour the hair.

(3) A hair restorer to renew hair growth. (*A H*, 1915)

HAIR REMOVER A substance which will remove hair. See Depilatory.

HAIR RESTORER A preparation to encourage or restore the growth of hair. See also Colour restorer.

The earliest known hair restorer appears to be that mentioned in the Papyrus Ebers (1552 BC). It was a prescription prepared for Scherch (an Egyptian queen of the third dynasty) and consisted of equal parts of the heel of an Abyssinian greyhound, date blossoms and asses' hoofs, boiled in oil. (*Lawall*)

The Poor Man's Physician published in Edinburgh, 1731, gives: 'To cause hair to grow on bald heads. To wash with dogs piss causeth hair to grow on bald heads'. Presumably the ammonia acted as a stimulant. Most 19th century to early 20th century hair restorers contained an irritant, such as spirits of Rosemary and acetic acid.

'Pigeons dung and honey equal quantities simmered together over a slow fire. Anoint the parts every day.' (18th century Ms receipt book in the writer's collection)

An Assyrian remedy, recorded on a clay tablet (incised cuneiform), from the Great Library of Minevah, collected by Ashur-bani-pal, of *c* 650 BC was: 'Incantation to preserve the hair of a woman's head. Spin a thread . . ., a Pa-stone of its seven colours, taniba-stone, a meteorite, stone(?) of Gutium, copper, bronze, . . . thereon Thou shalt thread: seven and seven knots thou shalt tie: as thou tiest (them) thou shalt recite the charm; bind them on her hair and the falling hair shall be stopped.' (*Stubbs and Bligh*). The number 7 was a sacred number.

HAIR RIBBON A ribbon with which to bind the hair. Popularly worn as a bow in the hair by schoolgirls in the early 20th century.

HAIR RING (1) A hair curl.

'Her glossy hair outvy'd the ravens' wings,

And curl'd about her neck in wanton rings.' (*Rowe, History of Joseph*, 1736)

(2) A ring made of plaited human hair. 18th/19th century, *cf* Hair-bracelet.

(3) A finger ring set with a small lock of human hair. Worn as a memorial ring or as a charm against evil. A Roman finger ring found at Heronval, Normandy, had a small recess for containing hair. (*Edwards*)

HAIR ROLLER A hair curler. There are flexible or rigid curlers, made of metal, plastic, foam rubber and other suitable materials.

HAIR ROOT That part of the hair shaft which lies within the follicle.

HAIR ROPE Rope manufactured from human hair. A miniature in the Manesse MS in the State Library, Zurich, Switzerland, depicts rope being twisted from human hair. (*Zemler*)

HAIR RYME Hoar frost. Scots usage. (*Brown*)

HAIR SAC Hair follicle.

HAIR SALT Alunogen. Native sulphate of magnesia, occuring as a fine capillary incrustation. (*Franke*)

HAIR'S-BREADTH A measure of length, very narrow. Among the Jews the forty-eighth part of an inch. (*NCD*)

HAIR-SEATING Woven horsehair used for covering chairs, sofas, etc.

HAIR-SET (1) The formation of waves or curls, etc. on wet hair preparatory to drying the set. See Set (2).   *324*

(2) *A setting lotion. American usage.*

HAIR-SET-PATTERN The arrangement and alignment of the wound curlers on a head for the composition of a hair style.

HAIR-SET-TAPE (1) A type of sticking tape to hold set curls in position when the hair is being dried.

(2) Narrow white tape used to hold the dressing of a postiche in position when being dried.

HAIR SHAPER A razor combined with a safety guard; used for hair-cutting and tapering.

HAIR SHAVED OFF The Chinese shaved all of the head except the top, where the hair was allowed to grow into a long pigtail. This was a Tartar custom. Buddhist priests shave the whole head. Some Catholic priests shave the crown of the head. The part shaved is called the tonsure. St Peter's tonsure is shaved right round the head to indicate the crown of thorns. St Paul's tonsure denotes the shaving of the whole head. Simon Magus's tonsure is shaved from ear to ear, above the forehead, but not extended to the back of the head. (*Brewer*). St John's tonsure was semicircular. (*Speight*)

HAIR SHAVEN FROM THE CROWN OF THE HEAD A symbol of contrition for the short-comings of the lower nature and a fervent desire to contact the source of power and truth. (*Gaskell*). In the Catholic and Buddhist orders the tonsure 'marks the passage from the worldly to the religious life.' See Tonsure. (*Oldenberg*)

HAIR SHEATH The hair sac or follicle.

HAIR SHEEN (1) Brilliantine.

(2) Lacquer.

HAIR SHINE Brilliantine.

HAIR SHIRT A shirt of hair cloth, worn by ascetics and penitents.

HAIR SIEVE A sieve with a bottom of finely woven hair, usually horsehair, used for straining liquids and powders.

HAIR-SINGEING-MACHINE See Singeing machine.

HAIR SLIDE A hair clasp that slides into place and is then clipped shut.

HAIRS OF KYNOCEPHALUS See Kynocephalus.

HAIR SOFTENING The pre-dye bleach to increase the porosity of the hair and facilitate penetration of the dye into the hair shaft.

HAIR SORTER One who sorts raw hair into its different grades of quality, length, etc.

HAIR SPACE the narrowest space used by printers.

HAIR SPECIALIST A person who claims to be a devoted student of matters pertaining to hair.

HAIR SPLITTER (1) One who argues over trifles or makes cavilling distinctions.

(2) The virile member. 18/19th century slang. (*Grose*)

HAIR SPOOL A small plastic hair curler.

HAIR SPRAY Any liquid or powder sprayed on the hair such as scent, colour, fixative, bloom, etc. Before *c* 1940 the term mainly referred to scented 'setting lotions', but since *c* 1945 it applies mainly to perfumed lacquers and other fixatives for keeping the hair-set in position.

HAIR SPRING The fine hair-like spring of a watch.

HAIR STAIN A colourant that impregnates the hair. A hair dye. A popular formula in the 19/early 20th century was: Sulphate of iron, 2 drachms; Rectified spirit, 2 oz; Rose water, 20 oz. This gradually darkened the hair.

HAIR STANDING ON END A sign of extreme fright. Also caused by a sudden and intense drop in temperature.

HAIR STANE (Scottish use). A hoar stone that marks the boundary of an estate or domain. Also called Hour-Stone, Hare Stane, etc.

HAIR STICK A water cosmetic in the form of a stick used to temporarily cover white or grey hair between dyeing treatments, *c* 1920.

HAIR STOCKINGS 'Stockings made from human hair and worn by Chinese fishermen as the best preventive of wet feet. They are drawn over ordinary cotton stockings, being too rough for putting next the skin.' (Unpublished letter from an English resident in China, 8 June 1891)

HAIR STONE Sagenite.

HAIR STRAIGHTENER (1) a chemical in liquid or paste form used to remove curl or kink in hair.

(2) A type of iron used to straighten hair that has unwanted curl or kink.

HAIR STREAK (1) A lock of hair of different colour from the rest of the head hair.

(2) Hair-streak butterfly of the genus theola.

HAIR STREAM The natural direction in which a group of hairs lie.

HAIR STROKE A very fine line in writing or painting.

HAIR STUFFER A womanizer. Vulgar slang. Bristol and West of England usage.

HAIR STYLE The mode, manner or fashion of dressing the hair. The names of hair styles may be (A) Descriptive of appearance, eg Bouffant, Heart-shaped, etc.

(B) The name of the first wearers or popularisers, eg Beatle, Marie Antoinette.

(C) That of a recognizable period of history, eg Empire.

(D) Descriptive of a human quality, eg Winsome.

(E) That of a recognizable group, eg The Military.

HAIR STYLING The creation and execution of a hair style. It is a semi-plastic form of art and consists in the judicious moulding and arrangement of hair and ornamentation on a globular surface. The hair artist has to have an understanding and feeling for line and contour, colour and tone, pattern and texture.

HAIR STYLING CO-ORDINATOR One who professes an ability to suggest a hair style or styles suitable for a particular dress design or historical period. They are found in the world of the film, stage, and television. American usage. (*Cordwell*)

HAIR STYLIST (1) A person who offers himself as an expert in the designing and dressing of hair styles. This expression was first noticed in the 1920s and by the 1930s had become a common appellation of many hairdressers.

(2) One who can copy and dress different styles of hairdressing.

HAIR SWINGER A dancing girl of Arabia. These dancers swing their long black hair from side to side in a repetitive dance to the chant of the men. The dancers of Abu Dabi were shown on British television, 29 August 1967.

HAIR TAIL The cutlassfish. *Sic*

HAIR TEDDER A witch's ladder. (*Tongue*)

HAIR TEST A test made on a small strand of hair before the main treatment of dyeing, curling, etc, to discover the hair's reaction to the proposed treatment.

HAIR TEXTURE The degree of fineness or coarseness of the hair.

HAIR THIEF During the 18th century when wigs were commonly worn and hair for their manufacture was in steady demand hair thieves flourished. They cut hair from the living head and procured cadaver hair from graveyards.

HAIR THREADER See Hair needle (2).

HAIR TIDY A cloth bag, also a metal or pottery container to receive the combings from a woman's head.

HAIR TONIC Any preparation that has a tonic effect on the hair or scalp. The term in connection with products for the hair is now illegal in America, as being inaccurate and misleading. It has been replaced by the term *Scalp Lotion*. (*Wall*)

HAIRTORIUM Barber's shop. American usage. 20th century. (*Weseen*)

HAIR TRAINER The hair net used on men or women to hold a set in position during the drying process. (*Stecklyn*)

HAIR TRAP A device to trap hair in the pipe mouth of the hairdresser's sink and prevent it blocking the drains.

HAIR TRIGGER (1) The secondary trigger on a firearm which sets free a spring mechanism called the hair and releases the main trigger by very slight pressure.

(2) Hair-trigger flower. An Australian plant of the genus stylidium.

HAIR TUFT BETWEEN BUDDHA'S EYEBROWS An emblem of spiritual truth within the soul. (*Gaskell*)

HAIR TUGGER See Hair fiddler.

HAIR-UM A facetious play on the words Harem and hair-room. American usage for Beauty Parlour, seen by the writer in Omaha and Los Angeles, 1965.

HAIR VICE See Curling Clamp, also Jigger (3).

HAIR VITAMINS For prevention of grey hair: Pantothenic acid, folic acid and paraaminobenzoic acid. (*Gayelord Hauser, Look Younger, Live Longer*, 1951).

HAIR WASH (1) Shampoo or prepared soap for washing the hair.

(2) The process of shampooing hair.

HAIR WASHER One who shampoos or washes the hair.

HAIR WATER (1) An 18th century term for a mixture of silver nitrate diluted in water, used for dyeing hair a dark colour. (*Stewart*, 1782)

(2) A toilet water for the hair. '12 handsfull of Rosemary, 12 do of vine runners, 12 do of fumatory, 1 lb of honey. To be distilled in a cold still with water and no spirit. This to make 2 quarts.'

(Duchess of Marlborough's recipe, 18th century. From Ms receipt book in the collection of the writer.)

HAIR WAVER (1) An implement such as waving irons by the use of which hair can be waved.

(2) Any apparatus such as a permanent waving machine which heats the hair wound on curlers during the permanent waving process.

(3) A person who waves hair.

HAIR WAVING The transformation of straight hair into waved hair, or the setting of curled or curly hair into waves.

HAIR WEAVER A boardworker who weaves hair.

HAIR-WEAVER'S JOINING KNOT This is used to join a broken silk, which usually happens near the weft. Take the long end (right hand) of the broken silk O and make a simple knot R. Do not pull it tight. Put the end N in the loop thus formed and make another loop P, which can be called the second loop, into which place the short end of the broken wefted silk Q. Pull to the right the end N of the longer silk and the two loops which it forms will tighten. When the knot is almost tight and you have the short end well held, quickly draw the end N in the opposite direction, that is, from the right to the left and when you hear a click the knot is firmly tied.

This method of joining silks has been used from at least the mid-18th century. (*Garsault*), and is still employed by the weaver in 1984. *89(11) 439*

HAIRWEED (Hairy-bind) The plant *Cuscuta Europoea*; dodder. A parasitic, slender, twining plant.

HAIR WHITENER Liquid colour for whitening or greying hair for theatrical use.

HAIR WHORL The natural 'lie' of hair around a focal point. The crown of the head or vertex.

HAIR WORK (1) Postiche, *qv*.

(2) Wigmaking, postiche manufacturing, boardwork. Any kind of work on human hair off the head for the production of postiche.

(3) Hair devices inset in brooches, lockets, etc. The most popular Victorian designs were the aster, ear of barley, feather cluster, flowers, heart's-ease, leaf, pearl band, rose spray, star, tomb and willow tree, wheatsheaf, and wreath.

HAIR WORKER (1) A person who works in hair off the head, such as a wigmaker; boardworker, or posticheur.

(2) A person who works in hair for the production of hair devices inset in brooches, lockets, etc.

HAIRWORM A slender, unsegmented roundworm belonging to the phylum *nemathelminthes*.

HAIRY (1) Hirsute; covered with hair.

(2) Consisting of hair; made of hair.

(3) Old and out-of-date, ie so old that it has grown hairs. Frequently used with regard to gossip or jokes. Slang.

(4) A strong, virile man. American slang, 20th century. Expression: 'He's hairy.'

(5) The Hairy: Glasgow slum girls, poor and hatless. Late 19th century. (*Partridge*)

(6) To get angry or excited. Similar meaning to *get shirty*. Slang.

HAIRY AINU The indigenous inhabitants of Japan. (Ainu pronounced eye-new).

HAIRY APE A person of low social position or intellectual capacity. Slang.

HAIRY APE, THE Yank, a character in Eugene O'Neill's play of that name, 1922.

HAIRY ARMS Said to be the sign of riches to come. (*Radford*)

HAIRY ARSED Old. 19th century. Slang.

HAIR BIND See Hairweed.

HAIRY BIT An amorous female. Slang.

HAIRY BOB A bearded man. Scarborough and Yorks. usage. (*Symonds*)

HAIR BREECHES Regner of Denmark (9th century) so called because he wore hairy breeches when he went forth to conquer an enormous serpent. (*Brewer*)

HAIRY CRUPPER A woman's private parts. (*Phillips*, 1678)

HAIR DEVIL A fox-bat or flying fox.

HAIRY-FAIRY An effeminate but masculine looking man. 20th century. Bristol and West of England usage.

HAIRY-FEATHERY Rough, uneven. Devon usage.

HAIRYFORDSHIRE The female pudendum. 19th century. Slang.

HAIRY GAUL, THE The Gauls in the Roman period wore their hair very long, and this custom, wrote Pliny, gave the whole country the name *Hairy Gaul* (*gallia comata*).

HAIRY-GENTLEMAN See Old-Hairy-Gentleman.

HAIRY-HEART See Aristomenes, Hermogenes and Leonides.

HAIRY-HEELED Lacking manners or breeding. Slang.

HAIRY-KING, THE Clovis, King of Salic Franks, 481.

HAIRYMAN, THE Elias the prophet, so called because he wore garments made of hair. (*Powell*)

HAIRY-MANOR A female's genital fissure. 17/18th century. (Miscellaneous Works of His Grace George, late Duke of Buckingham, 1707)

HAIRY-MARY Name of a railway engine camouflaged with closely draped ropes trailing to the ground, used in the Boer War, 1899/1902. (*Treves*, p 94)

HAIRY-MEG A spirit believed to haunt Tullochgorm and give warning of the approaching death of a Grant. (*W G Stewart, Highland Superstitions and Amusements*, 1823)

HAIRY-MOLE See Hair mole.

HAIRY ONE, THE (1) The devil. West Country usage.
(2) The virile member. West Country usage.

HAIRY ORACLE The female pudendum. Low slang.

HAIR-PARMER The common hairy caterpillar. Parmer is the Somerset form of palmer. Somerset usage. (*Elworthy*)

HAIRY-STONE, THE Asbestos.

HAIR-TASSEL The penis. West Country usage.

HAIRY-WHEEL The female pudendum. 19th century Australian slang. (*Partridge*)

HALF-A-CURL See Half curl.

HALF-BOB A woman's head of hair bobbed at the sides, but worn long at the back. 1920s.

HALF-CREPE Hair that has been crêped from the root and half way down its length. (*Redgrove and Foan*, p 26; *Symonds*)

HALF-CREPE WEFT See Half-crêpe.

HALF-CURL Duck's tail, often worn on nape of neck.

HALF-MOON CURL The same as Arc curl, *qv*.

HALF-NATURAL A man's 18th century wig style. (*London Mag*) See En-Boucle-Demi-Naturelle.

HALFPENNY BARBER A term of derision applied to the poorest type of barber; a halfpenny being the charge for the cheapest shave or hair-cut that could be obtained in Britain in the Victorian period. *133*

HALF-TRANSFORMATION See Semi-transformation.

HALF-TWIST-WIND In the permanent curling process a twist-wind with a twist intermediate between a full twist and a quarter twist. (Smith)

HALF-WIG (1) A wig so dressed that half is as nature and the other half as art has dressed it. 18th century. (*Fenton*, p XIV)
(2) A front or back postiche, so constructed that the natural hair can be blended with it.

HALO (1) A three-quarter circle of curls worked on a galloon-covered clock spring and worn across the top or front of the head.
(2) A circlet of dressed postiche such as a halo-plait, halo-tendrils, etc.

HALO PLAIT See Halo.

HALYCONEA An extract from the sea swallow's nest used as a depilatory by the ancient Greeks. (*Forbes*)

HAMMER A boardworker's tool used to insert block-points

to hold the foundation ribbons and bracings in position on the wooden block.

HAMMER CURL A barrel-spring curl; a croquignole curl. 19th century.

HAMMER-CUT BEARD Similar to Roman T. *qv*.

HAND CLIPPER A hair clipper worked by the pressure of the thumb and fingers. See Clipper. *105*

HAND DRYER An electrically operated hair dryer which blows warm air through a nozzle and is held in the hand during the drying process.

HANDEL George Friedrick (1685–1759), the son of a barber. Famous German composer, born at Halle, Saxony and lived and composed in England for many years.

HAND-OF-HAIR A substantial group of hairs; larger than a wisp or tress. That quantity of hair which can be conveniently held in the hand.

HAND KNOTTING Knotting a wig foundation by hand.

HANDLEBAR MOUSTACHE A moustache with protruding ends, like the handlebars of a bicycle. A popular style in the Royal Air Force during the Second World War, 1939–1945. *98H*

HANDLEBAR-MOUSTACHE CLUB A club organised for a charitable purpose, whose members had handlebar moustaches, *qv*.

HANDLED RAKE A lady's large-toothed dressing comb with a handle. (*Ogee*, 1965)

HAND-MADE WIG A wig made entirely by hand, without the use of a machine.

HAND-MASSAGE VIBRATOR A vibrator that is fixed to the back of the masseur's hand and vibrates his fingers as he massages the client's scalp.

HAND MIRROR A small mirror with a handle used to reflect the back of the head in the large mirror in front of which a client usually sits to have his or her hair dressed.

HANDSOME BEARD Baldwin IV, Earl of Flanders. 'The Bearded King', 1160–1186. (*Brewer*)

HAND STROP A rigid strop held firmly by a handle. See also French strop.

HAND-TIED WIG A wig with hair knotted to the foundation as opposed to a weft wig. American usage.

HANGING CHIGNON An elongated chignon that hangs partly below the neck-line. *312*

HANGING CURL 19th century usage. The same as Corkscrew or Drop Curl, *qv*. *325*

HANGING STROP A strop for sharpening razors, consisting of a leather strip, usually horse hide, about 2½″ wide and 20″ long; or of leather one side and canvas the other, with a hook at the end to secure the strop and a handle at the other end to hold it taut.

HANGING TORSADE A torsade worn in a hanging position.

HANK Two or more skeins of thread tied together.

HANMAN'S-HAIR DYE A 19th century hair dye composed of: litharge 21 grains, quicklime 375 grains and hair powder, *qv*, 186 grains. (*Francis*)

HANOVER CUT A woman's hair style introduced from Germany by Princess Anne, daughter of George I. It consisted of an erection of gauze and ribbon. The hair was arranged on pads over the forehead in a semicircle and plastered with pomatum and powder. 'How can you reconcile yourself to this odious Hanover Cut.' 1714 (*Arch Cant* Vol V)

HANOVERIAN HAIR STYLES Hair styles worn by the Whigs or Court party in the early years of the reign of George I. So-called because they were favourable to the Hanoverian section. Their opposers were the Jacobites or favourers of James II who had abdicated.

HARDING, SYLVESTER Miniature painter, born New-castle-under-Lyme, 1745. Taken to London in his youth and apprenticed to a wigmaker. His son George Perfect Harding was also a miniaturist of high ability.

HARD PRESSING See Hair pressing.

HARD WATER Temporary hardness in water is caused by calcium and magnesium bicarbonates. Permanent hardness is caused by calcium and magnesium sulphates. Hard water will not lather readily with soap.

HARD-WATER SOAP Soap made from coconut oil with a little free sodium carbonate present.

HAREBRAINED Inconstant; unsettled; wild as a hare. The word has no connection with hair, but is frequently presumed to be, eg
'. . . our poetry
Unfit for modest ears, small whores, and play'rs,
Were of our hair-brain'd youth the only cares . . .' (Buckingham, 1707)

HARE'S FOOT In the 18th and 19th century a dried haire's foot was used to powder the faces and necks of clients.

HARLENE A hair tonic popular in the early 20th century. An analysis of a sample bottle revealed: borax 0.5 parts, anhydrous sodium carbonate 0.04 parts; 10% solution of ammonia 0.12 parts; glycerine 0.4 parts; alcohol 5.7 parts; colouring matter and perfume traces; water to 100 parts. (Schofield)

HARN-PAU The skull. Scots usage. (Brown)

HAROLD I, KING OF NORWAY See Harold Fairlocks.

HAROLD FAIRLOCKS or FAIRHAIR Harold Haarfagre (c 850–c 933), first King of Norway; so called from the length and beauty of his hair.

HARSH COLOUR An unpleasing, jarring tone, such as brassy blond.

HAT-AND-WIG A Guernsey schooner privateer of 2 tons named by Touzel, a hatter, and Rabey, a barber. Late 18th century. (Uttley, Story of the Channel Islands)

HAT-HAIRDRESSING Dressing hair to suit a woman's hat when it is the central theme of the head-dress; the hair then being complementary to the hat.

HATTAT A composition used in Turkey to blacken the eyebrows of women. (Toilette, 1832)

HAUT(E) Fr. High, tall, lofty.

HAUT DE COIFFURE Fashionable head-dress. From the French, cf Haut Ton – High fashion.

HAUTE COUTURE High fashion. The fashionable world; the very height of fashion in tailoring and dressmaking.

HAY-BAG A term of abuse in reference to a middle aged woman of doubtful or 'free' morals, who heavily bleaches her hair to retain a youthful appearance.

HAYDEE A woman's hair style of oriental inspiration, c 1864. (Bysterveld, p 38)

HAZELNUT OIL One of three ingredients in beef pomatum of the 18th century. the others were beef marrow and essence of lemon. (Legros)

HEAD (1) The cranium
(2) All the hair growing on a human head; the head of hair. 'The hair collector purchased her head.'
(3) A collection of hair from one scalp removed at one cutting. Peasant girls' heads of long hair yielded from ¾ lb to 1½ lb of hair when sold to the hair-collectors of France and Germany. (Yeats)
(4) A wig. Mainly theatrical usage 18/20th century. 'He will wear his comic head in the next act.'
(5) The hair as dressed in a particular manner. 'Pray how do you like this head?' (Goldsmith)
(6) Adj. The scalp end of a growing hair is sometimes known as its head end.

(7) Enough hair to make a wig. The quantity varies from 1½ oz to 5 oz or more of prepared hair, according to the style of wig required. 'That style of wig will need a head of 3 oz. best frisure forcée.'

HEAD BRUSH A hairbrush, qv. (Guillim)

HEAD-CAST The plaster cast of a head for mounting a made-to-measure wig to ensure a perfect fit. 19/20th century

HEAD-CLOATHES (-Clothes) Decorative additions to a coiffure.
'To Day, as at my glass I stood,
To set my head-cloathes, and my hood;
I saw my grizzled locks with dread' (Barber)

HEAD COMB (1) A dressing comb, 16/17th century. 'We have head-combes, beard-combes, I, and cox-combes too.' (Heywood, T)
(2) 'A decorative comb worn in the hair.' (A Visit to the Antipodes)

HEAD COWL Dome-shaped, metallic, or preferably, non-metallic cover to encompass the human head and used as an integral part of a hair dryer or hair steamer, qv.

HEADDRESS (1) A dressing or covering for the head (early 18th century) applied to hats, bonnets, etc., or any material added to the growing hair for decoration. 'A head-dress of flowers.'
(2) A wig or added hair pieces. 'She hangs her head-dress on a mushroom at night.'
(3) The dressed or arranged hair. 'Where the head-dress is to be decorated with any plumes of feathers.' (Legros, 1768). Hairdress, Hairdo or Coiffure are to be preferred to head-dress for describing dressed hair on the head. Head-dress is confusing. The other three words can only mean, dressed hair.

HEAD-DRESSER A hairdresser. (Brown, 1702; also trade card of W Winter, 205 Oxford Street, London, c 1840)

HEAD-OF-A-HAIR Root end of a hair. (Crosby) See Head (6)

HEAD-OF-HAIR The growth of hair on the head. See Head.

HEAD-OF-SKIN A bald head. (BBC, American commentator, 26.5.69)

HEAD LOUSE See Pediculus Capitis.

HEAD MOULD A wax or plaster of Paris mould of the head. See Head-Cast.

HEAD SHELL A faceless, hollow head shape for displaying postiche. Usually made of papier maché and covered with green, blue or red velvet. 19/early 20th century.

HEAD TIRE A coiffure, 17th century.

HEAD TURBAN See Turban.

HEARE Hair, 16th century. (Fry). 'A bracelet of her heare'. (Skelton)

HEART-BREAKER (1) a long lock of hair, similar to the Love-lock, qv, that became fashionable among women and men in Charles II's reign. (Speight)
(2) A curl, 20th century. (B and B)
(3) A pincurl, 20th century.

HEART HAIR The hearts of Aristomenes, the Messenian; Hermogenes, the rhetorician; and Leonides, the Spartan, were reputed to have been hairy. (Speight)

HEART-SHAPED COIFFURE A short hair style for women designed by William George Cox, the writer's father at Bristol in 1926.

HEART-SHAPED HEADDRESS See Horned Headdress.

HEAT BURN A burn caused by heat such as a too hot and badly protected permanent waving heater. See also Pull burn.

HEAT-CUT A drastic thinout of the hair. So called because in hot weather it is a comfort to have thick hair thinned appreciably.

HEATER (1) Curling-iron heater, *qv*.

(2) Permanent waving heater, *qv*.

HEAT-PERMANENT-WAVING A method of permanently curling the hair by means of the application of heat to hair that has been saturated with a suitable chemical and wound round a cylindrical object. Before the introduction of cold permanent waving the usual term was simply Permanent Waving, but since the advent of the cold system from *c* 1939, the new term has come into common use to distinguish the heat system from the cold.

HEAVY CUT (1) A club cut.

(2) The removal of a large quantity of hair.

HEBE Daughter of Jupiter and Juno. Goddess of youth and cup-bearer to all the gods until dismissed by Jupiter because she fell down in an indecent posture as she was pouring nectar to the gods at a grand festival. Ganymede succeeded her as cup-bearer.

HEBRA'S SOAP A shampoo composed of equal parts of soft soap, rectified spirit, and spirit of lavender. (*Savill*)

HECKEL American usage. See Hackle.

HECKLE American usage, See Hackle.

HECTOR The Trojan son of Priam and Hecuba, depicted with fine long hair hanging on his shoulders. (*Stukeley*)

HECTORIAN HAIRCUT Short at the front and long at the back. (*Classical Quarterly*, NS Vol XXIII, No 23, p 196)

HEDGE A false beard. (*B and B*)

HEDGEHOG HAIRDRESS (1) A hairstyle for men in which the hair is short and dressed partly standing up. Natural hair or a wig, *c* 1796.

(2) A hair style for women in which the hair of the wig is dressed in a bouffant frizz. Also called Hérisson, *c* 1780. (*Uzanne*) 330

HEDGEHOG ROLLER A large-diameter roller incorporating numerous bristle spikes to facilitate the winding of the hair. Used to curl the hair in a hair set.

HEEL BRUSH A small bent brush used for postiches, back-brushing, etc, in dressing-out a hair style. Also called boomerang brush.

HEEL OF SCISSORS See Crutch.

HEFTINGS The short hair and dross which are discarded when getting-out combings. Bristol usage, 19th and early 20th century.

HEGEWALD'S ANTIPHILATHRON A 19/20th century 'secret' preparation for preventing the hair falling out. It comprised: filtered extract of gall nuts with a mixture of 50% strong spirit and 30% water, scented with several aromatic oils. (*Koller*

HEIDRICH'S HAIR FLUID A 19/20th century 'secret' hair dye which contained a large quantity of lead acetate. It could have been dangerous to health. (*Koller*)

HELICAL Spiral; screw shaped.

HELICAL WINDING See Spiral winding.

HELICONE CURLING ROD A curling rod on which hair is spirally wound. American usage.

HELIX Subs. Spiral, shaped like a cork-screw; or in one plane, like a watch spring. A spiral curl or a clockspring curl.

HELMET COIFFURE A short cut style for women (1966), shaped to the head and similar to the shingle of the 1920s. Popularized by Twiggy Hornby, the fashion model. (*Evening News*, 9 March 1966)

HELMET DRYER See Hood dryer.

HEM The turned-under edge of the wig net. So done to avoid fraying.

HEMIPHALACROSIS One-sided baldness. (*Wheeler*)

HEMIPHALACROSIS MYSTAX Hairlessness on one side of the lip. (*Wheeler*)

HEMMING Sewing and shaping the hem, *qv*

HEM STITCH See Stitching.

HEN CAUL A kind of netting or hair cap used by women to enclose their hair. Northern usage. (*Holloway*)

HENLE'S LAYER One of the layers of the inner root-sheath of the hair follicle, composed of clear, non-nucleated cells.

HENNA The powdered leaves of *Lawsonia Inermis*, called Egyptian Privat (*Lawsonia Spinosa* or *Lawsonia Alba*). A brown sweet smelling powder which, in the form of paste mixed with water, has for many centuries been used by the Arabs to dye their beards after the example set by Mohammed and his successor Abu-Beker. (*Planché*). Also used in the East to dye the body. Commonly employed as a hair dye in England since the 18th century giving only red shades, the final result depending upon the original body-colour of the hair. Light coloured hair will redden more noticeably than dark hair, which will take on a dark auburn shade after an application of henna. As a dye pure henna is relatively safe and is very unlikely to cause dermatitis, unlike the para-dyes or a compound henna. Mohammedans who have made the pilgrimage to Mecca henna their beards to show they have made the journey.

HENNA (COMPOUND) Egyptian Henna, *qv*, with added metallic salts. These preparations can cause dermatitis in susceptible subjects and need a skin test before use.

HENNA (EGYPTIAN) *Lawsonia Inermis* (Egyptian privet). The common Henna of commerce.

HENNA (GREEN) Henna made from the leaves of *Lawsonia Inermis* before they have ripened. This Henna gives a deeper red than the ordinary Egyptian Henna.

HENNA (JAPANESE) A henna powder which gives strong shades of red. Made from green henna.

HENNA (PERSIAN) Henna powder with added indigo.

HENNA (SPICED) A henna powder made with 1 teaspoonful of mixed cloves added to 1 tablespoonful of Egyptian Henna.

HENNA (TUNISIAN) A compound Henna, *qv*.

HENNA (WHITE) A euphemism for a bleach pack, no henna being present. The so-called white hennas contain magnesium carbonate, kaolin, peroxide of hydrogen and ammonium hydroxide or allied substances in varying proportions.

HENNA CAP (1) Henna application in paste form.

(2) A plastic or other cap to cover the hair and head and retain the natural heat to accelerate the dyeing process.

HENNA PACK A prepared henna paste, *qv*, for application to the hair and left until the hair receives the required colour. The applied paste is usually covered with a turban of paper, waxed paper, or plastic, etc, to prevent dripping and to retain the heat and speed the process.

HENNA PASTE Henna powder and hot water mixed to a thick, creamy consistency.

HENNA POT A double saucepan, like a porridge pot, but made of earthenware, in which the henna paste is prepared.

HENNA-RASTICK See Rastick-henna.

HENNA-RENG A hair dye consisting of a combination of Henna and Indigo in varying proportions according to the colour desired.

HENNA RINSE A hair rinse of very warm water in which has been steeped a small quanty of henna powder.

HENNA SAUCEPAN A double saucepan like a porridge pot, the inner pot usually being earthenware. See Henna pot.

HENNA SHAMPOO A soft soap shampoo incorporating a small quantity of Egyptian henna.

HENRY'S COSMETIC A 19/20th century 'secret' preparation for preventing falling hair and greyness, consisting of

180 parts of spirit, 3 parts of lemon oil, 1 part each of bergamot oil, rosemary oil and lavender oil. (*Koller*)

HERALDIC ARMS OF BARBERS COMPANY 'Quarterly, the first sables, a chevron between three flewmes argent, the second quarter per pale, argent and vert on a spatter of the first, a double rose gules and argent, crowned golde. The third quarter as the seconde, and the fourth as the first, over all; on a crosse, gules, a lyon passant gardant golde; and to their crest upon the heaulme on a torce argent and sable an opinicus, *qv*, golde mantelled gules doubled argent, supported with two lines in their proper colour; about their necks a crowne with a chayne argent pendant thereat, as have plainly appearith depicted in this margent.' (*Lambert*)

HERBAL SHAMPOO A shampoo in which is incorporated a herb or herbs such as rosemary or celandine. (*Sagarin*)

HERCULES The celebrated hero of great physical strength who, after his death was ranked among the gods. He was represented with a thick, bushy head of hair and bushy beard but also with much body hair; hair being commonly regarded as a sign of strength and virility from early ages. (*Lemprière and Stukeley*)

HERISSE (CHEVEUX) Fr. Shaggy, rough hair, from Herisson – hedgehog.

HERISSER Fr. To bristle, to bristle up.

HERISSON COIFFURE See hedgehog hairdress.

HERMES The legendary inventor of the razor, wash-ball and toilet powder.

HERMOGENES, THE RHETORICIAN His heart, according to Coelius Rhodiginus, was hairy. (*Speight*). See also Aristomenes.

HERRINGBONE STITCH See Stitching.

HESSIAN SOAP Made from goats' tallow and ashes of beechwood. So called from being made in Hesse, Germany. This same mixture, Martial the Roman poet informs us, was used in his time to stain wigs to give them a flame colour. (*Toilette*, 1832)

HEXAGONAL NET Stiff foundation net with six sided holes for use in wig-making. For the front and nape of wigs and the whole foundation in transformations and semi-transformations. Also called honeycombe net.

HEYRECLOTH Hair cloth. Cloth of woven hair. Medieval usage. (*Fisher*)

HIDEOUT A false beard. American slang usage. (*B and B*)

HIDING POWER The power of an opaque dye or other colouring material, when applied to hair, to cover or hide its existing colour.

HI-FASHION Americanism for high fashion, *qv*.

HIGH BOB A bobbed hair style, worked and dressed high on the head. Popular in the 1920s. (*Rohrer*)

HIGH DRESSING Any hair style that is dressed high on the top of the head.

HIGH FASHION See Haute couture.

HIGH FREQUENCY An electric current of high voltage and very low amperage, used in scalp treatment. Also called violet ray because of the violet light produced in the glass applicator. (*Flitman*)

HIGH FREQUENCY MACHINE An apparatus that delivers an electric current of high voltage and very low amperage. See High Frequency.

HIGH HAIRDRESS A high-dressed coiffure for women, fashionable from 1771 to 1787.

HIGH-LIGHTS Those parts of the hair's surface that catch and reflect the most light.

HIGH-LIGHT CAP A plastic head cap with holes in it used for drawing a strand or strands of hair through to bleach without bleaching other hair.

HIGHLIGHTING See Highlighting tint.

HIGHLIGHTING TINT The tinting or bleaching of parts of hair to a lighter or a different colour from the overall tint, causing the bleached parts to catch and reflect highlights.

HINDES The firm of Hindes were manufacturers of hair curlers and for some years early in the 19th century this name was used for hair curlers generally, *cf* Inecto.
'Walking about in a striped petticoat and Hindes.' (*The Perfidious Welshman*, 1910.)

HIPPOLYTUS A mythical Greek god to whom the virgins of Troezene consecrated their hair before they entered into marriage bonds. Hippolytus was the son of Theseus and died for his chastity. (*Potter*)

HIRCUS Armpit hair.

HIRSUTE Hairy or shaggy.

HIRSUTE APPENDAGE Hairy attachment.
(1) A weakly facetious term for the beard.
(2) The private parts of a man. Slang.

HIRSUTENESS The state of being hairy, hairiness.

HIRSUTIES (1) Hypertrichosis. An excessive and unnatural growth of hair on parts of the body where it is not usual for it to grow, such as the face of a woman.
(2) Hairy or with superfluous hair. From the latin *Hirsutus*, hairy. (*Wheeler*)

HISTOLOGY The science which deals with organic tissue structure.

HISTORICAL HAIR STYLES (1) Hair styles that were worn by men and women of past ages.
(2) Modern copies of the hair styles of the past.

HITCHHIKE A finger wave. Slang, American usage. (*B and B*)

HOARE-BEARD White beard. (*Percival*).

HOARIE (HOARY) Grey or white.

HOARY HEADED Grey haired.

HOC NET Stiff waterproofed wig net, invented in the 1890s by Philippe Hoc, 43 Richmond Road, Westbourne Grove, London. Hoc was a human hair foundation manufacturer. By 1900 Hoc net had come into general use in England. (*HC*). See Stiff wig net.

HOG GUM Gum tragacanth.

HOLBEIN BEARD A short beard parted in the middle of the chin and then brushed to each side, giving it a broad look. So named after Hans Holbein the younger, who wore this style. (*Mitchell*)

HOLD-ALL A bush beard. Slang. (*Mitchell*)

HOLDING COMB A comb used to secure a constituent part of a coiffure and forming part of the hairdress. See also Fancy comb and Dressing comb.

HOLLOW-GROUND RAZOR A razor whose blade is ground slightly concave or 'hollow'. These razors were introduced to the English barbers in the 1880s and were regarded as being easier to set than the solid type. They needed only honing and stropping to maintain the sweetness of the razor's edge. See also Solid razor.

HOLLYWOODIAN BEARD A short beard and joined moustache but with that part of the chin immediately beneath the lower lip shaven. (*Trusty*)   98a

HOME-HAIRDRESSING (1) Hairdressing by one of the family in the home, *cf* Folk hairdressing.   422, 429
(2) Hairdressing by a qualified hairdresser who visits clients in their own homes.   422, 429

HOME PERM A permanent wave that has been produced by an amateur using a home permanent waving outfit, simplified to make it possible for members of the public to produce an acceptable wave upon the head.

HOMME (COIFFEUR D') Fr. Gentleman's hairdresser.

HONE A whetstone for sharpening the edges of metallic

implements especially razors. There are numerous kinds of hone, but they can conveniently be divided into two main groups. (i) Natural stone and (ii) artificial stone. Examples are: (i) Belgian hone. From natural rock formed by alkaline deposits, a slow cutting wet hone, lubricated by oil, water or lather. German hone, also called water hone. A natural fine-grained slate hone. Very slow cutting wet hone, lubricated by water or lather. (ii) Swaty hone. The modern synthetic swaty hone may be used wet or dry and is a medium fast cutting hone. The old Swaty which was probably the earliest synthetic hone was first manufactured by an Austrian chemist. They were harder and slower cutting than the modern version. Carborundum hone. A synthetic hone incorporating silicon and carbon. May be used wet or dry and are made in varying degrees of coarseness. German hones cut the slowest of any and carborundum the fastest. *86 (9, 10)*

HONEY AND FLOWERS A harmless dressing to discipline the hair. The term is a euphemism. It sounds sweet and nourishing. Were it composed of the substances indicated by its name it is obscure what value perfume, invert sugar and flower petals could have for hair, but like many modern toilet preparations the name-appeal is to vanity or to fear. A common 20th century formula is: ¼ oz perfume essence; 1 pint spirits; 3 pints yellow mineral oil. (*Preemo*)

HONEYCOMB An overall pattern of hexagons similar to that of the bees' comb.

HONEYCOMB COIFFURE A hair style worn by Roman women and popular at the court of the Emperor Domitian (AD 81–96).

HONEYCOMB MESH Se Diamond mesh.

HONEYCOMB NET See Hexagonal net.

HONEYCOMB TOWEL Of cotton material, used by barbers as a face towel when shaving clients.

HONEYPOT HAIRDO A high, rounded hairdress for women, similar in shape to a honeypot.

HONEY SOAP Best yellow soap 1 cwt; Fig soft soap 14 lb; otto of citronella 1½ lb. (*Piesse*)

HONEY-WATER (1) Fashionable hairwash of the 19th century consisting of:

Essence of ambergris	1 dr
Essence of musk	1 dr
Essence of bergamot	2 dr
Oil of cloves	15 dr
Orange flower water	4 oz
Spirits of wine	5 oz
Distilled water	4 oz

(2) Distilled from honey and mixed with spirit of rosemary has been used in England and other countries as a wash for promoting the growth of hair. (*Fernie*)

HONGROIS Fr. Hungarian.

HONGROIS POMADE See Pomade hongrois.

HONING The process of sharpening a razor upon a hone.

HONKIL A hair style worn between the time of circumcision and the growing of the beard by males of the Bega tribe in Africa. It consists of plaited hair and the neck and temples shaved. (*De Rachewiltz*)

HOOD A loose head covering. Women's headdresses were called hoods in Tudor times.

HOOD DRYER A hair dryer in the form of a hood secured to a pedestal. Hot air is blown or rises from internal apertures in the hood onto the head. *454*

HOOK AND EYE FASTENER A fastener consisting of a small hook and eye used in postiche work on transformations and semi-transformations to secure them and hold them on the head.

HOOK CURL A straight lock of hair of which the points are formed into a half circle.

HOOK-HOLDER A knotting hook handle.

HOOK NET See Hoc net.

HOOKS, MAJOR THEODORE A character whose hair was greying and thinning, to remedy which he annointed it with 'an infallible specific' and kept his night-cap on for 24 hours as directed, only to find that all his hair had come away with the night-cap. (*Speight*)

HOOTENANNY HAIRDO A hairstyle incorporating a gadget or gimmick. American usage. (*Hanle*)

HORACE GREELEY American beard style, similar to French Collier. (*Reynolds*)

HORIZONTAL PAD WEFT A method of weaving hair on three silks. The hair is woven through the top space, over the top silk, through the top space, under the bottom silk, through the top space, over the top silk, through the top space. (*Symonds*)

HORN COMB A hair comb made of cow or ox horn. 17th century. (*Holme*)

HORNED HEADDRESS A women's hair style in the form of two horns, like rams' horns. Late 13th to 15th century. 'What shall we say of ladies when they come to festivals? They look at each other's heads, and carry bosses like horned beasts; if any one be without horns, she becomes an object of scandal.' (Trans late 13th century French Ms in Brit Mus printed in *Reliquias Antinquiae*, Vol 1, P. 162) That the horns were often made of or supported by false hair appears evident from an early 14th century French Ms poem (Bibliothèque Royal, Paris, No 7218) partly printed by M Jubinal in *Jongleurs et Trouvères* under the title *Des Cornetes* (of horns). This poem describes how the Bishop of Paris preached a sermon against the extravagent dress of women and he criticised particularly the bareness of their necks and the wearing of horns. 'If we do not get out of the way of the women, we shall be killed; for they carry horns to kill men. They carry masses of other people's hair upon their heads.' (Translation). For an article by *T Wright* on 'The Horn-shaped Ladies' Headdress' see *Archaeological Journal*, No 1, March 1844.

HORNY Of a texture resembling horn.

HORSE COMB See Mane comb. 17th century. (Holme)

HORSEHAIR Hair from the mane or tail of a horse. Used for legal wigs and, very occasionally, as thread in an all-hair foundation for a wig. 'White horsehair wiggs' worn by some household slaves in America, 18th century. (*Earle*). Today the horsehair for legal wigs is imported from Japan.

HORSEHAIR FRAME Circular and semi-circular hair-frames made entirely of horsehair with no wire.

HORSEHAIR PAD Made of créped horsehair they were used in the 18th and 19th century to construct high hair styles or give the desired shape to a coiffure.

HORSEHAIR WORM See Hairworm.

HORSESHOE FRONT A weft of hair on a horsehoe-shaped pad, worn at the front of the head and dressed in pompadour style.

HORSESHOE MARCEL See Aureole Marcel.

HORSESHOE MOUSTACHE A drooping moustache that hangs over each corner of the mouth and reaches below the chin, in the shape of a horseshoe. American usage.

HORSESHOE PAD A long hair-pad of crêpe hair which was worn on the head and shaped like a horseshoe.

HORSESHOE SET OR MARCEL A style with no parting in which the waves run from the face in a semi-circle around the head and return to the other side of the face, *cf* A waved pompadour. (*Rohrer*)

HORTENSIA, THE A women's hair style of 1865. (*Bysterveld*, p 55)

HORUS LOCK The lock of hair that was left uncut to fall over the ear of young men in ancient Egypt. (*Asser*)

HOT COLOUR An exceptionally rich and deep colour.

HOT COMB An electrically heated metal comb used for drying, setting, straightening and setting curly or frizzy hair. American usage.

HOT-OIL SHAMPOO (1) A shampoo incorporating oil and used hot on the hair and head.
(2) An application of hot oil to the hair, followed by a shampoo.

HOT-TOP Auburn haired. American usage. (*B and B*)

HOT-TOWEL APPLICATION The application of hot towels to the face after a shave. This practice was originated in Boston, America by A. S. Shultz of Auburn, Mass. in 1878. (*Foan*)

HOT-WATER URN A metal urn in which is kept hot water ready for use in shaving, etc.

HOUPPE Fr. Tuft, top-knot, powder-puff.

HOUPPER Fr. To comb.

HOURI A nymph of the Mohammedan paradise.

HOWIE MOUSTACHE A thin moustache tapering towards the turned-up ends. (*Trusty*)   101C

HUBSHEE A person with woolly hair. Indian usage. (*Partridge*)

HUCKABACK A linen with raised pattern used for making small towels which are used by the client to protect the face, when having a shampoo, and less usually to dry the hair. See also Huckaback towel.

HUCKABACK TOWEL Made of strong linen fabric with a rough surface. Small huckaback towels are the familiar face towel of the hairdressing saloon and are used by the client to protect the eyes and make-up. In the 19th century before the use of linen, these towels were made of hemp. (*Beck*)

HUFFING-PERRIWIGS Puffed-up, flowing wigs. 17th century. (*England's Vanity*)

HUILE Fr. Oil; hair-oil.

HULIHEE BEARD See Mutton chops (with moustache also). Called after the Hawaiian King. American usage. (*Trusty*)   98G

HUMAN HAIR Hair from the head of a human being.

HUMAN HAIR FOUNDATION A foundation for a postiche composed of human hair upon which hair is knotted.

HUMAN-HAIR-GIRDLE Worn by the otherwise naked Australian Aborigines of Queensland. (B M Ethno)

HUMAN-HAIR-GOODS See Hair goods.

HUMAN-HORNS See *Cornua Humana*.

HUMAN IVY The beard. Slang, American usage. (*B and B*)

HUMECTANT A substance that moistens or wets, 1822. From the 1940s a word commonly used by hairdressers in connection with hair treatments.

HUMIDITY Dampness, moisture.

HUNGARY WATER An obsolete perfume which contained a dozen or 20 ingredients of which rosemary was the most prominent. (*Rouse*) A 19th century substitute was: 1 part oil of rosemary, 49 parts spirit of wine.

HUNTING-BUN A bun of hair attached to the back of a woman's hunting hat, beneath the brim. Worn to prevent the woman having a 'bald' appearance when the short hair styles of the 1920s were fashionable.

HUNTING-PERUKE 18th century man's wig style. (*Encyc Brit*)

HURE Hair. Lancs dialect. (*Gent's Mag*, vol 16)

HURLUBERLU A hair style, originating in Paris in 1671, comprising masses of curls close to the scalp, with a few longer ringlets hanging down the neck. (*Letters of Marquise de Sévigné*)

HUXLEY'S LAYER One of the layers of the inner root sheath of the hair follicle composed of coarsely granular, epithelial cells derived from that portion of the epithelium lying over the papilla. (*McCarthy*)

HSUAN WEN-HUA According to the Yün Chi Ch'i Ch'ien was the mythological Chinese god of the hair. His height was supposed to be one and one tenth of an inch, and his hair black. The same work also gives the name as Shou Ch'ang; the gods of the hair being seven star-spirits. (*Werner*)

HYACINTH CURL A small natural falling crescent curl, not set or prosaically dressed. 'His head was covered with hyacinth curls, light flaxen in colour'. (*L C Powys, The Powys Family*, Yeovil, 1952)

HYACINTHINE (Hyacinth) A poetical epithet pertaining to hair. 'Locks like the hyacinthine flower.' (*Homer*)
'Thy hyacinth hair, thy classic face.' (*Poe, E A*)
Tawny, auburn or curly. See Hyacinthine locks.

HYACINTHINE LOCKS (1) Tawny (brownish-yellow) or auburn coloured hair. (*Ovid*). 'Hyacinthine locks round from his parted forelock manly hung clustring.' (*Milton, Paradise Lost*)
(2) Curly hair.

HYACINTHUS The son of Amyclas and Diomede of Greek mythology, beloved by Apollo and Zephyrus, but killed by Apollo and from his blood sprang the hyacinth. (*Greek Mythology*)

HYDROGEN PEROXIDE H_2O_2. Discovered by Thenard in 1818. First used for hair bleaching at the Paris Exposition of 1867 when E H Thiellay of London and L Hugo of Paris used a 3% solution for this purpose. Its use for hair bleaching quickly spread throughout Europe and America and superceded all other methods. (*SDP*)
Marketed as a solution in water in concentrations from 3 to 90% by weight. Agitation or contact with rough surfaces, metals and many other substances will accelerate decomposition. The presence of mineral acid renders it more stable. H_2O_2 is a colourless, unstable, slightly acid liquid, miscible with water. Protect from light and store in a low temperature. Used in concentrations of 5 to 30% by weight for hair bleaching, 20% is the usual strength. In excess of 30% serious damage to the hair and scalp could result. (*Merck*; *Sagarin*). Also used as an oxidant with certain types of dye especially aniline derivative dyes.

HYDROXOMETER An instrument for measuring the strength of Hydrogen Peroxide.

HYGEIA Goddess of health. Her status represented her veiled and matrons usually consecrated locks of their hair to her. (*Lemprière*)

HYGIENE The principles of good health. Sanitary Science.

HYGROBAPTON A proprietory liquid hair dye. Early 19th century.
'Hygrobapton, or liquid dye, for changing the hair any tint required, in five minutes.' (Adv by J H Harper, *Hairdresser*, Dorchester, 1851; *Hunt's Dorsetshire Directory*)

HYGROMETER An instrument for measuring the humidity of the air.

HYGROSCOPIC The ability to absorb water.

HYOGO A Japanese hair style for women 17/18th century, in which a standing knot of hair at the crown is the particular feature. (*Hashimoto*)

HYPERAPHIA Tenderness of the scalp. (*Wheeler*)

HYPERTRICHOSIS An excessive or abnormal growth of hair, either locally or over the whole body.

HYPERIDROSIS CAPITIS Excessive perspiration of the scalp. (*Wheeler*)

HYPERION The Sun God and incarnation of beauty. (Greek Mythology)

HYPERMACROTRICHIA See Macrotrichia. (*Wheeler*)

HYPOGYNOUS HAIR Pubic hair of the male. A word of botanical origin, loosely applied to human hair.

HYPOTRICHOSIS An abnormal deficiency of hair.

HYSTRIACIS Porcupine hair; thick, rigid and bristly hair. (*Winter*)

I

ICED SHAMPOO LOTION A spirit shampoo containing menthol.

ICE SHAMPOO A spirit shampoo containing menthol.

IDIOSYNCRACY A physical reaction or mental constitution peculiar to an individual person. Persons who react to certain dyes and other chemicals are said to have an allergy to them.

IMAN, PIERRE An internationally famous French manufacturer of wax models for wig display.

IMBRICATE Verb. To overlap like tiles or scales of a fish.

IMBRICATED Overlapping as roof tiling or fish scales.

IMBRICATIONS OF HAIR The overlapping of the hair scales.

IMCO HOME PERM A home permanent waving outfit produced by the writer in 1939, but abandoned owing to the war and other duties.

IMMISCIBLE That propensity of a substance which prevents it mixing with another substance. Unmixable.

IMPASSIANT Fr. See A l'Impassiant.

IMPERIAL (1) The name for a small beard being a tuft of hair growing beneath the under lip. So called because Emperor Napoleon III wore this kind of tuft in 1839.   *97B*
(2) A pointed beard. 19/20th century.

IMPETIGO A very contagious pustular disease of the skin.

IMPLANT (1) To knot hair on to a net or other foundation.
(2) To insert hair into the wax of a wax model head to simulate growing hair.

IMPLANTATION (of hair) The action or process of inserting or fixing hair in a suitable postiche foundation.

IMPLANTED BUST A wax display bust in which the hair is implanted in the surface of the head to simulate hair growing from the follicle.

IMPLANTED PARTING A drawn-through parting, *qv*.

IMPLANTER Fr. To knot.

IMPLEMENT A tool, instrument or apparatus.

IMPROVER A worker in the hairdressing craft who has served an apprenticeship but who has not obtained full qualification. Used from *c* 1860 to 1965. (*Creer and others*)

INCONSTANCE See A l'inconstance.

INCOMPATABILITY TEST (1) Before permanently waving, dyeing or bleaching a head of hair it is sometimes necessary to test a small section first, using the chemicals proposed for the process to be performed, in order to ensure that no untoward chemical action takes place owing to the presence of unsuspected chemicals already on the hair.
(2) Skin test, *qv*.

INDIAN MELISSA OIL See Verbena oil.

INDIFFERENCE See A l'indifference.

INDIGO A dye obtained from the shoots of *Indigofera Tinctoria* from India and Java. The pure substance has the composition $C_{10}H_{10}O_2$. In the 18/19th century it was popularly used for hair dyeing, especially in the preparation of hair for postiches, for which it is still sometimes employed. A recipe was: Henna 1 part, Indigo 2 parts. To obtain a light brown the application was left on for 1 hour and 1½ hours for darker browns.

INDUCED CURL Hair that is made to curl by artifice. Not natural curl.

INDUSTRIAL SPIRIT (Industrial methylated spirit) A mixture of 19 volumes of 95% alcohol and 1 volume of wood naptha. Used in toilet preparations. Highly flammable; can be purchased only on production of a Customs and Excise permit.

INECTO (1) Subs. A proprietary hairdye of an aniline nature. For many years this was the most popular of any dye in its field.
(2) Verb. To dye hair, from *c* 1925. 'She has had her hair inectoed', may mean – She has had her hair dyed with Inecto hair dye, or she has her hair dyed (with any dye). The word was long used as a synonym for dye.

INERT Lacking active chemical properties or power of action.

INFANTA COIFFURE A young girl's hairdress similar to that worn by the infanta Margarita, daughter of Philip IV, King of Spain and depicted by Velasquez in his painting.

INFILL (1) The dressed hair enclosed within a specified area.
(2) Knotting hair within a specified area.

INGROWN HAIR A hair that unnaturally grows beneath the skin.

INNER-BRACING Those bracings of a wig foundation that lie within the contour galloon.

INNU An Egyptian female hairdresser of the 11th dynasty (*c* 2000 BC). (*Forbes*)

IN-PLI Hair that has been set in waves and/or curls. It remains in-pli in its wet state, during and after setting, until dressed-out. It can then be put into second-pli. See Pli.

INSANITARY Not sanitary or healthful, unclean.

INSECTICIDE An insect killer.

INSERTED STEM (1) The second or subsequent stem or stems added to or inserted in a hair switch to make it a two, three, four or five stem switch. (*Creer*)   *419(5)*
(2) Made of half-crêpe hair. The crêped root-end is woven on the silk leaving part of the crêped root and the straight ends free. Completed it presents a full, yet smooth, appearance, the crêped ends being almost covered by the straight ends of the hair. With a top row of carefully créoled long hair it is valuable in providing a long tail mostly from short hair as the stem is long and the woven hair incorporated in it is short, except for the top row length.

INSET HONE A stone hone for setting razors, set in a base of wood, with a wooden handle.

INSOLUBLE That which cannot be dissolved or solved.

INSTANT BEARD The donning of a false beard. A gimmick expression, 1967, *cf*, Instant hairdo – the donning of a dressed wig, instant coffee – needing only to be dissolved in hot water, etc. (*The Glasgow Herald*, 1967)

INSTANTANEOUS Occurring or done in an instant.

INSTANTANEOUS HAIR DYE A quick-acting hair dye that, although not instantaneous, effectively acts within minutes.

INSTANT HAIRDO The donning of a dressed wig. (*Hanle*)

INSTRUMENT CABINET The sterilizing case in which hairdressing implements are stored in a sterile atmosphere.

INSTRUMENT TABLE The table on which the instruments are arranged during a hairdressing process. They should later be cleansed and replaced in the instrument cabinet.

INTEGUMENT The skin or other natural covering such as rind or husk.

INTERCELLULAR Between cells.

INTERLACE Verb. To dress hair tresses in an interwoven pattern.

INTERLACED LOOPS HAIRDRESS A 19th century style for women. The front hair is crêped in the back; from the top of the head to the nape the hair is rolled and twisted so as to look like a mass of interlaced loops. (*The Queen*, 15 April 1876) *292*

INTERSTICE An intervening space.

INTOLERANCE Subs. Not having tolerance. A person can be said to have an intolerance to a para dye, ie it will cause dermatitis.

INTRADOS The interior curve of a curl. (A borrowed architectural term). *Cf*, Extrados.

INVERTED EYEBROW A narrow fringe of beard on the chin. Slang. (*Michell*)

INVERTED MOUSTACHE A style in which the ends of the moustache are brushed and stuck in an upright position, ie towards the eyes.

INVISIBLE COVERING An ill-chosen euphemism for a scalpette. If it were invisible the bald head top would still be apparent; the expression is intended to imply that the covering is indistinguishable from the natural growth. 'Indetectable addition' would convey more accurately the meaning intended.

INVISIBLE CURLS Small pieces of curled postiche indistinguishable from the wearers own hair. 'John Caire, also . . . sells . . . double black hair pins and invisible curles.' (Adv. *Star Newspaper*, Guernsey. 14 October 1818)

INVISIBLE PERUKE A wig of 1849/50, not invisible, but the term meant that it was indistinguishable from the subject's own hair. (*Thackeray*)

INVISIBLE PINS Very fine hairpins which are difficult to see when placed in the hairdress.

INVISIBLE TUFT (Postiche patch, *qv*) Hair worked on a small piece of very fine mesh net and worn on a bald patch.

INVISIBLE VENTILATING HEAD OF HAIR A natural looking knotted wig. Advertised by Ross and Sons, Wigmakers to the Royal Family, 1849/50. See Invisible peruke.

IN-WAVE A wave that recedes from the face.

IO A 19/20th century 'secret' preparation for dyeing hair. It consisted of paraphenylenediamine. This could have been dangerous. (*Koller*). Io was a priestess of Argos whom Jupiter loved and changed into a heifer for fear of Juno.

IODINE SOAP See Medicated soap.

IONIAN COIFFURE A woman's hair style of 1863.

IPHINCE See Megarensian virgins.

IRISH MOSS *Chondrus Crispus*. A seaweed from which is obtained a gelatinous substance used in cosmetics, including hair creams. (*Verrill*)

IRISH RAZOR POINT A straight end forming an acute angle with the cutting edge on an open solid razor.

IRISH SOAP A soap manufactured from clean and fresh tallow. It was better than the English tallow soaps. 19th century. (*Lillie*)

IRISH TONSURE See John (apostle), Tonsure of.

IRON BARREL The solid, cylindrical-shaped prong, rod or shaft that fits into the grooved prong of curling and waving irons.

IRON CLAMP (1) Used to secure the weaving-stick holder to the bench.
(2) A clamp to hold hair securely.

IRON FLUTTER The rapid, but slight, opening and closing of the irons in Marcel waving.

IRON GREY Similar to the grey colour of freshly broken iron. 'Her iron-grey hair looked drab and lifeless.'

IRON HEATER A small stove on which curling and waving irons are heated. Charcoal 16/18th century, gas 19/20th century, electricity 20th century, methylated spirit 19/20th century, and meta tablets, have all provided heat in suitably adapted heaters.

IRON MAIDEN Slang name for the early permanent waving machines. So-called because of the discomfort and, at times, pain which a woman suffered during the heating process with this primitive apparatus.

IRONS See Curling irons, Créoling irons, Crimping irons, Moustache irons, Pinching irons, Pressing iron, Waving irons, Whisker irons.

IRONS HANDER An apprentice who heated, tested and handed the hot Marcel waving irons to the Marcel waver. This ensured continuous waving by the operator. Early 20th century.

IRON-WIG Mr Walpole, describing Wortley's election to the Royal Society, wrote, 'The most curious part of his dress, which he has brought from Paris, is an iron wig; you literally would not know it from hair'.

IRRITANT That which causes irritation, eg acetic acid in hair restorer.

ISABEL HEADDRESS A woman's hair style as worn by and named after Lady Isabel Claire Eugène of Austria. (*Bysterveld* p 65)

ISABELLA A name for the colour Light Buff, *c* 1600. From French Isabelle.

ISIS'S HAIR A seaweed found off the 'island' of Portland, Dorset.

ITALIAN, THE A woman's hair style of 1866. (*Bysterveld* p 87)

ITALIAN BROWN An 18th century man's theatrical wig style. (*Stewart*)

ITALIAN CURL See Scollop-shell curl.

ITALIAN CUT (1) A woman's hair style popularised by Italian film actresses. It was sculptured, shaggy, waved deep on the crown, with flat curls at the forehead and cheeks, and a studied disarray at the neck. 1953.
(2) A 16th century hair style for men, cut short and round. (*Stubbes: Repton*)

ITALIAN HAIR A deceptive name applied in the 19th century to hair prepared from combings. Good quality black and brown cut hair, collected from peasants was imported into Britain from Italy for the wigmakers use and this name made the combings-hair sound of better quality than it actually was. (*Creer*)

ITALIAN PIN A hairpin with both points bent back upon the shafts. Wefted hair is sewn onto the pin to make a pin curl.

ITALIAN-TYPE BANG A wispy fringe. 20th century.

ITALIENNE See A l'Italienne.

ITINERANT BARBER, HAIRDRESSER OR BEAUTICIAN A barber, hairdresser or beautician who travels to his client and performs his services on their premises.

IVORY COMB A comb made from an elephant's tooth (or tusk? *JSC*). 17th century (*Holme*)

IVORY POWDER Used for cleansing the hair and scalp. See also Bran. 18/19th century. (*Toilette*)

IVY LEAGUE CUT Short back and sides, fairly short top. American usage. (*Trusty*)

IVY LEAGUE HAIRCUT See Ivy League cut. (*Trusty*)

J

JABORANDI (*Pilocarpus*) Tinture of Jaborandi leaves is used in hair tonics to cleanse the scalp, remove dandruff and give a gloss to the hair.

JACOBEAN HAIR STYLES Hairdresses worn by men and women during the reign of James I (1603–1625).

JACOBITE, MODE DU A style of black wig popular in France in the pre-revolutionary period. (*Truefitt*)

JALOUSIE See A la Jalousie.

JAMAICA MIGNONETTE The henna plant, *Lawsonia Inermis*, See Henna.

JANSENIST BOB A man's 18th century wig style. (*Lon Mag*, 1756)

JAPANESE HAIR Dark, coarse hair imported from Japan for the manufacture of cheap postiches and theatrical wigs. (*Creer*)

JAPANESE HENNA See Henna.

JARDINEE Fr. That single pinner next to the Bourgoigne. (*Evelyn*)

JASCHKE The barber of Kings whose back shop in Regent Street, London, was called the House of Lords, so noble were his clients. King Edward VII regarded him as the perfect barber – hearing everything and saying nothing. (*Mitchell*)

JASEY (1) A bob wig. (*Grose*, 1823)
(2) A wig made of worsted. Humourous and colloquial term 15/19th century. (*Forby*)
(3) Slang name for a judge, because of his big wig, 19th century.
(4) Contemptuous term for a mop of hair. 19th century.

JASMIN, JACQUES Pseudonym of the provincial poet Jacques Boé, who, born at Agen, 6 March 1798, earned his living as a barber, but wrote poetry in his native Languedoc dialect. His first volume Papillotes (curl papers) appeared in 1835.

JASMINE HAIR POWDER Used in 19th century. It was usually scented with orange-flower water. See Hair powder. (*Francis*)

JASMINE POMATUM A 19th century recipe: Lard 1 lb, suet 4 oz, Jasmine water 1 pint, essence of Jasmine 1 oz. (*Francis*)

JAUNE Fr. Yellow.

JAVOL A 19th/20th century 'secret' wash for the hair compounded by W Anhalt of Colberg, and composed of Beef tallow 1 gram; lemon oil 5 grams, tincture of quinine 15–20 grams; potassium carbonate 0.2 gram, water to 100 grams. (*Koller*)

JAZEY See Jasey.

JEHU'S JEMMY An 18th century wig worn by coachmen. A white wig covered with small, close curls, like a fine fleece on a lamb's back.

JELLY BLEACH A hair bleach in the form of a jelly.

JELLY SETTING LOTION A setting lotion having the consistency of a loose jelly.

JERRY JARVIS'S WIG A short story in the Rev R H Barham's *Ingoldsby Legends*.

JERSEY, COUNTESS OF See Countess of Jersey.

JERUSALEM ARTICHOKE (*Helianthus Tuberosus*). The juice pressed out before the plant blossoms was used for restoring the hair when bald. (*Fernie*)

JERUSALEM WASH-BALLS 10 lb white oil-soap; 10 lb Joppa soap; 1½ oz vermillion; 1 pint rosewater; 1 pint thin starch. 19th century.

JERVAS Samuel Pepys' barber.

JESSAMY A Macaroni, *qv*.

JEWISH BEARD Anciently beards were the rule among Jews and in accordance with *Leviticus* XIX, 27, their beards were not to be trimmed. The custom is today followed by only a few orthodox Jews.

JEWISH STYLE OF VEIL A veil covering the whole of the head and face. (*Mallemont* p 64)   307

JEWISH WIG See Wig, Jewish.

JIGGER (1) A weft winding or twisting machine, *qv*. West Country usage.   95A
(2) A jockey, *qv* for keeping weft in position on the silks during the process of weaving. Midlands and Northern usage.
(3) A clamp or vice for holding hair firmly when winding croquignole. See also Curling clamp, Midlands usage. The hair-vice consists of a piece of hard wood 7" or 8" long, 3" wide and ½" thick, with three holes in the form of a triangle, towards the upper end, through which ordinary screws are passed to fix it securely to the work bench. About 3" of this jigger is allowed to project and through the projecting part two small holes are made about ½" apart. A piece of leather bootlace is passed through the two holes, extended to within a couple of inches of the floor and tied in a knot. The jigger is used in the piping or curling of hairs off the head. The pipes for curly hair are about 3½" long and from ¼" to 1" in diameter at the centre of the pipe, but rather wider at the extremeities. A small strand of hair is inserted beneath the leather lace on top of the board and the foot presses down the end of the loop holding the hair firmly while it is wound on the pipe. (*Creer*)

JOBBERNOLE The head. 18th century usage. (*Grose Lex Bal*)

JOCKEY A clip fashioned like a miniature wooden clothes peg and used on the silks in weaving to prevent the end knot loosening. In the 18th and early 19th century, fabricated from wood, leather or cardboard, but since the mid-19th century made of bent watch spring, shaped as in the illustration annexed. The spring ends are tied with twine and covered with sealing wax. The implement 'rides' astride the silks, hence the name Jockey. Mentioned by Creer in his *Board-Work*, 1887.

JOCKEY RIDERS A woman's hair style of 1865, suitable for outdoor wear. (*Bysterveld* p 57)

JOHN (Apostle), **TONSURE OF** The front of the head shaved to a line drawn from ear to ear, this was the method in the ancient Celtic Church, and is hence called the Scottish, or Irish tonsure. See Tonsure.

JOHN THE BEARDED The German artist, John Mayo (temp. Charles V), whose beard was so long that it was tied at his girdle to prevent him walking on it. (*Mitchell*)

JOKE MOUSTACHE Any moustache, usually of an outrageous colour and shape, that is worn for fun at a convivial gathering, or other suitable occasion. Usually made of crêpe hair.

JONKE'S COLOUR RESTORATIVE A 19/20th century 'secret' preparation of an ammoniacal solution of silver nitrate, with alcohol and glycerine. (*Koller*)

JONNICK HEADDRESS A well dressed normal hairstyle, with nothing fancy added. A plain hairdress. West Country usage, from c 1920.

JOPPA SOAP A yellow, mellow soap from Turkey. Excellent for producing a clean (not ropy) shaving lather. 18/19th century. (*Lillie*)

JOURNEYMAN Originally one who worked by the day, but since late 17th century applied to those workers who covenanted to work with another in his trade or occupation by the year. (*Phillips*)

JOWL The jaw or jawbone; also the hanging part of a double chin.

JUBA The hair at the back of the head. See Hair nomenclature.

JUDAS-COLOURED HAIR (1) In the early Mystery plays the hair and beard of Judas were fiery red. 'Let their beards be Judas's own colour.' (*Kyd, The Spanish Tragedy*, 1597) (2) Yellow hair.

JUDGE'S WIG (1) The undress wig is frizzled all over, with one curl at the back and a baby on each of the two tails. The dress wig is the full-bottomed wig, *qv*. Previous to the wearing of wigs English Common Law Judges wore velvet caps, coifs and three-cornered caps. Sir Matthew Hale (1676) refused to decorate himself with false hair. Chancery Judges took to wearing wigs later than the Common Law Judges. (*Speight*) 254
(2) A formation of white curled clouds in the sky is known as Judges' Wigs. (*Cobbett*)

JUGLON The active colouring element in walnut hair stain. (*Wall*)

JULEP A medicated, stimulating shampoo for the hair. See Egg julep.

JULIAN A woman's short hair style *c* 1803. Inspired by and named after the hairdress of Julianus, son of Julius Constantius. (*Lafoy*)

JULIUS DE LA ROVERE He ascended the Papal Throne in 1503, under the title of Julius II, and was the first Pope to allow his beard to grow. (*Chambers, Book of Days*, 1881)

JUMBO DRYER See Trunk dryer.

JUMBO HEAT CURLING IRON A curling iron with shafts of large diameter, 2" to 3". Used in theatrical hairdressing.

JUMBO JUNIOR A man's long full beard style worn without a moustache. American usage. (*Trusty*) 98i

JUMBO ROLLER A large diameter hair roller on which hair is wound croquignole fashion, to produce a large diameter curl.

JUNIOR Euphemism for apprentice.

JUNIOR HAND An apprentice or first year improver.

JUNIPER TAR SOAP Made from the wood of *Juniperus Communis*, almond or olive oil, fine tallow and a weak soda ley. (*Piesse*)

JUNO In Roman mythology, the wife of Jupiter and Queen of heaven. Depicted by the ancients with black hair. (*Salmon*)

JUNON See La Frégate la Junon. (*Uzanne*)

JUPITER The supreme deity of Roman mythology. Depicted by the ancients with long, curled, black hair. (*Salmon*)

K

KAIM (1) A comb. Usage of Roxburghshire and elsewhere in Scotland.
(2) To comb. 'A'll kaim eer haid for ee!' A threat. (*Watson*)

KAISER MOUSTACHE A moustache of which the ends are turned up in the manner of William II, Emperor of Germany, the Kaiser. From 1914.

KALI PRAEPARATUM See Potassium carbonate.

KAME A comb. Scottish usage. (*Ramsay*)

KANEKALON-WIG A wig made with synthetic hair of modacrylic fibre.

KANGLE To entangle. (*Sternberg*)

KANGLIN COMB A wide-toothed comb. A rake for disentangling hair. (*Sternberg*)

KAOLIN Powdered china clay; a hydrated aluminium silicate, insoluble in water, cold acids or alkali hydroxides. Used as an inert carrier in bleaching processes.

KARAYA GUM Indian tragacanth. The dried exudate of *sterculia urens*. A finely ground white powder used instead of the more expensive gum tragacanth. (*Merck*)

KARIG'S CRINOCHROME A 19/20th century 'secret' preparation for the hair, consisting of 10 parts pyrogallic acid in a mixture of rectified wood vinegar and spirit of wine, 500 parts of each; and a solution of silver nitrate 30 parts, in 900 parts of distilled water, with sufficient ammonia to redissolve the precipitate first formed. (*Koller*)

KATE GREENAWAY STYLE Hairdresses for young children inspired by the hair fashions depicted in the coloured illustrations by Kate Greenaway, published between 1879–1895.

KAY, JOHN (1742–1826) Caricaturist and miniature painter. Barber at Dalkeith and Edinburgh until 1785. Etched nearly 900 plates including the chief contemporary Scotsmen.

KEEKIN-GLASS A looking glass. Roxburghshire usage. (*Watson*)

KEEM (Kemb) A comb. Form now obsolete. Verb. To comb. 'Keemed it and weared it.' (*Powell*, 1661.)

KEKSY Dry, brittle. Derived from Keeks, the dried stalks of hemlock. Southern and northern usage. (*Akerman*). 'Hair all keksy.'

KELL (also Kull) (1) A hair net.
(2) A vaul, *qv*.
(3) The hinderpart of a woman's cap. Scots usage. (*Brown*)

KEME (1) A comb.
(2) To comb. Scottish usage. (*Jamieson*)

KEMBE (1) A comb, 14/17th century.
(2) To comb, 14/17th century.
'Such a kemming, such a trimming.' (*Withals*)

KEMP HAIR Coarse hair. (*Levens*, 1570)

KEMPT Combed. From at least 14th century.
'A man have a kempt hed.' (*Wyclif*)
'Shook his wet wings, and kempt his hair'. (*Fitzpatrick*, 1828) cf, Unkempt.

KENWIG'S FAMILY A family of young ladies in Dickens's *Pickwick Papers*, 1837, who wore long plaits at the back of their heads. The style had come from the Tyrol. Dickens's ludicrous verbal portrait of the Kenwig girls hastened a change of fashion from plaits.

KERATIN A nitrogenous substance which forms the basis of hair, nails, horns, hoofs, claws, feathers, quills, etc.

KERATOSIS Inflammation of the hair follicle. (*Wilson*)

KERSHAW, JOHN Started life as a barber. He was one of the first barber's to close on Sundays. Became a publisher. 19th century.

KEWIE A red-haired woman. Slang. (*B and B*)

KID A hair curler made of rolled kid skin. Popular from before 1850 until *c* 1925. 'She always uses kids to curl her hair.'

KIDDING Rolling hair in kids, *qv*, to curl it.

KID-SKIN WIG Worn by the Romans as a cheap substitute for the better class wig but an improvement on the Roman practice of painting hair on bald heads. (*Martial*)

KID TIPPING The process of sticking rectangular pieces of kid leather on the ends of the cut and rubbed down positional springs of wigs to reduce wear by friction on the enclosing galloon.

KIKE-USH-BASHUI See Moustache lifter.

KILLINGWORTH, GEORGE A person at the court of

Ivan the Terrible of Russia. He had a long, thick, broad beard of yellowish hair, five feet two inches long. (*Hakluyt*)

KING-OF-BEARDS The beard of Domenico d'Ancona. (*Southey, The Doctor*)

KINK (1) Subs. A short twist in a hair at which point the hair is bent upon itself.
(2) Verb. To put kinks into the hair; to curl or twist tightly so as to produce frizz.

KINKOUT A preparation for the removal of hair frizz. 20th century. American usage.

KINKS A curly-headed person. American slang. (*B and B*)

KINKY (1) A curly-headed person. American slang. (*B and B*)
(2) Excessively curly.

KINKY HAIR Hair that is excessively curly or frizzy.

KINKY PATE A head of hair with small tight curls. 20th century slang.

KINKY TOP Untidy curled or frizzled hair on the head. Slang.

KIRBIGRIP A proprietary spring hair clip.

KISS-CURL A small, flat curl worn forward onto the face, *cf* Kiss-me-quick.

KISSING THE BEARD Among the Jews it was the custom for friends to salute each other by kissing the beard. To the Turks it was a great affront to take any man by his beard, unless to kiss it.

KISS-ME-QUICK A small, spiral curl worn onto the face, *cf*, Kiss-curl.

KNEIFEL'S HAIR-FORCING TINCTURE A 19/20th century 'secret' preparation which consisted of ethereal oils combined with extracted substances from onions and cinchona bark. (*Koller*)

KNIFE See Drawing knife.

KNIGHT OF THE BASIN A Barber, 18th century. (*The Barber's Wedding*, 1791)

KNOCKER A pendant to a wig. 1818.

KNOT (1) Subs. The point of intertwining and tying of hairs to a net or gauze foundation. See Single knot, Double knot.
(2) Verb. The intertwining and tying of a small strand of hair to a net or gauze foundation in the wigmaking process. 'I shall knot the front quickly.'
(3) A group of intertwined or folded hairs secured in various forms such as a coil or figure of eight. (*Nicol*)
'And her faire lockes, which formerly were bound up in one knott, she lowe adowne did loose,' (*Spenser, Faerie Queene.* ed 1617)   *401*

KNOTTED HAIR (1) Hair that has been knotted to a net foundation.
(2) Trichonodosis, *qv*.
(3) Hair in a matted condition.

KNOTTED PARTING That part of a postiche on which hair is knotted to the foundation to simulate a natural parting. See also Drawn-through parting.

KNOTTED WIG (1) 18th century wig dressed with two hanging knots of hair at the back, and a short queue between. (*Carsault*)   *91(5.6)*
(2) A wig that has the hair knotted onto the net foundation, unlike a weft wig, on which woven hair is stitched.

KNOTTER A board worker skilled in the craft of knotting hair to net.

KNOTTING The process of tying very fine strands of hair onto a net foundation by means of a knotting needle. See Single knot, Double knot, etc.

KNOTTING GAUZE Fine gauze on which hair is knotted in the manufacture of a postiche. See Etamine.

KNOTTING HAND A knotter. A boardworker skilled in knotting hair to net.

KNOTTING HOOK See Knotting needle.

KNOTTING HOOK HOLDER See Knotting needle holder.

KNOTTING NEEDLE A very fine bent needle of spring steel with a fine barbed point, similar to a crochet hook. Manufactured in a series of sizes. The smaller the barb, the fewer hairs will it gather at one engagement. When not in use the needles are inserted into a wooden, metal or bone pencil-like holder.

KNOTTING NEEDLE HOLDER A wooden handle $^3/_{16}$th inch in diameter, 4″–5″ long, with a brass screw collar to secure the needle.

KNOUTSCHEFFSCHLERWITZ, IVAN PETER ALEXIS A Siberian hairdresser working in London in the 18th century who, offering his services in the art of hairdressing, engaged to execute it in a manner peculiar to himself, rejecting the use of 'black pins, hair cushions and the like cumbersome materials so dangerous in their effects. . . .' Instead he filled the 'hollows of the hair with soft aromatic herbs which prevent the disagreeable effect of that perspiration now so generally complained of'. He dressed hair in every mode, and engaged to make a lady's head appear like the head of a lion, a wolf or any exotic beast which she chose to resemble. He also offered to give any colour to the hair which a lady might desire, such as chestnut, blue, crimson or green. (*Speight*)

KOGLER'S HAIR-RENEWING POMADE A 19/20th century 'secret' preparation which consisted of coconut fat, containing, in addition to scent, a little of a sulphur oil, presumably oil of mustard. (*Koller*)

KOHL Powder, usually finely powdered antimony, used in the East to darken a woman's eyelids, etc.

KOHOL A 19/20th century 'secret' preparation that was advertised as a hair dye. It contained Indian ink suspended in a solution of gum arabic, but washed off the hair and was, therefore, useless for the purpose for which it was sold. (*Koller*)

KOJAK BRUSH A pledget of cotton wool. Facetious. After the bald-headed film actor Telly Savalas who played the part of Kojak, popular in the 1970s.

KOJAK CUT A shaved head. Called after the principal character in the television series *Kojak* played by Telly Savalas, 1974. Also Yul Brynner cut.   *104F*

KOKO A popular lotion for the hair in the early 19th century. An analysis of a sample bottle revealed: Borax 1.4 parts; glycerine 1.7 parts; 10% solution of formaldehyde 0.1 parts; alcohol 3 parts; perfume, a trace; water to 100 parts by measure. (*Schofield*)

KORSES The first man who shaved himself in classical Athens acquired by this act the name of Korses – the shaven. (*Doran* p. 166)

KORYMBOS HEAD-DRESS An ancient Greek headdress for a woman. (*Rimmel*)   *341*

KRELLER'S MILANESE HAIR BALSAM A 19/20th century 'secret' preparation consisting of beef marrow 40 parts; cinchona extract 5 parts; 1 part each of Peruvian balsam, styrax and bergamot oil, and ½ part of lemon oil. (*Koller*)

KREDEMNON HEADDRESS An ancient Greek headdress for a woman. (*Rimmel*)   *341*

KRELL'S BEARD TINCTURE A 19/20th century 'secret' preparation consisting of linseed oil, castor oil, charcoal, saltpetre, a little sulphur and pounded bread crust, coloured either light or dark brown. (*Koller*)

KRUGER'S WHISKERS A kind of liquorice sweet. Early 20th century. (*Reynolds*)

KTESIBOS OF ALEXANDRIA Son of a barber who

became famous as an inventor in the 3rd century BC (De Zemler).

KULL See Kell.

KYNOCEPHALUS, HAIRS OF Dill seed. (*Papyrus Ebers*, 1552 BC; *La Wall*)

L

L'APOLLON A woman's hair style of 1865. Named after Apollo, son of Jupiter and Latona of Greek mythology. (*Bysterveld*, p 50)

LA CANDEUR A woman's hair style of 1864. (*Bysterveld*, p 45)

LA COQUILLE A woman's hair style of 1823. (*Bysterveld*, p 32)

LA COUPE A L'ECUELLE Basin cut. A head of hair club cut around the bottom as if a basin had been put on the head and the hair hanging beneath the basin's edge cut.

LA DEESSE Fr – the Goddess, a hair style of 1864. (*Bysterveld*, p 26)

LA FAVORITE A woman's hair style of 1864 (*Bysterveld*, p 40)

LA FONTANGE See Fontange and Fontange coiffure.

LA FORNARINA A woman's hair style of 1865. (*Bysterveld*, p 54)

LA FRISONNE Fr – Friesian (f). A 19th century woman's hair style of North Holland. (*Bysterveld*, p 28)

LA GUERRIERE Fr – Female warrior. A woman's hair style of 1864. (*Bysterveld*, p 33)

L'HIRONDELLE Fr – Swallow or martin. A woman's hair style of 1864. (*Bysterveld*, p 27)

L'INCROYABLE Fr – The unbelievable.
(1) A woman's hair style of 1782. (*Bysterveld*, p 31)
(2) Foppish hair styles for men *c* 1810.
(3) An incredible hair style.

LA JUIVE Fr – Jewess. A woman's hair style of 1865, based on an ancient Greek style. (*Bysterveld*, p 51)

LA MARQUISE A woman's hair style of Louis XVI period. (*Bysterveld*, p 52)

LA MOSKOWA A woman's hair style of 1864, presumably with a Russian appearance. (*Bysterveld*, p 47)

LA NOUVELLE DIANE A woman's hair style of 1864. (*Bysterveld*, p 35)

LA PARABERE Woman's hair style of 1730. (*Bysterveld*, p 30)

LA PARTERRE GALANT Fr – The lover's garden. A high-dressed hair style for women topped by a miniature elegant flower garden; 1774.

LA PENSEE Fr – The thought, or (bot.) pansy. A woman's hair style of 1864. (*Bysterveld*, p 46)

LA POUDRE Fr –. Powder for hair or face.

LA PRINCESS DE LAMBALLE COIFFURE Marie-Therese-Louise de Savois-Carignan, widow of Louis Alexandre Joseph Stanislas de Bourbon-Penthievre, Prince de Lamballe, born at Turin 8 Sept 1749, killed 3 Sept 1792. Two coiffures as worn by her are recorded (see *Sutton, Album*, pp 56, 60 for description)

LA SIRENE Fr – The Siren; a woman's hair style of 1864. (*Bysterveld*, p 43)

LA SOUVERAINE Fr – The Sovereign. A woman's hair style of 1864 (*Bysterveld*, p 53).

LA SULTANE Fr – The Sultana. A woman's hair style of 1823 (*Bysterveld*, p 29).

LA SYLPHIDES Fr – The Wood Nymph. A woman's hair style of 1865 (*Bysterveld*, p 53).

LACE CURTAINS The Beard. Slang American usage (*B and B*)

LACE EDGING A fine flesh-coloured mesh of silk used at the edge of a postiche to give a natural hairline. Make-up is used to blend the front of the lace edging into the natural skin of the wearer. Mainly theatrical use.

LACE NET Hair Lace; wig net made of human hair (see Hair lace 2).

LACE-NET PARTING A parting made of hair lace.

LACE WIG A wig which has a foundation of hair-lace (a fine net made entirely of hair).

LACQUER See Hair lacquer.

LACQUER REMOVING SHAMPOO A shampoo containing chemicals that will remove hair lacquer from the hair. Most of the modern lacquers will shampoo out satisfactorily with a soap or soapless shampoo.

LAC-SULPHURIS See Precipitated sulphur.

LACTINE POMADE See Cocoa butter.

LADDER, the see En-chelle.

LADDER (1) A man's 18th century wig style (*London Mag*, 1753).
(2) An obsolete form of Lather, qv.

LADIES HAIRDRESSER A hairdresser, male or female, who is skilled in the art and craft of cutting, shampooing, curling, waving, dyeing, bleaching, styling, setting, arranging, and dressing a woman's head of hair. The expression 'ladies hairdresser' is always used, *never* 'woman's hairdresser', the assumption being, presumably that every woman is a lady.

LADIES' MOUSTACHES Long ringlets pinned to the side of the head and falling to the shoulders. 16th century.

LADIES' WATER An infusion in white wine of red roses, rosemary flowers, lavender, spikenard, thyme, chamomile flowers, sage of virtue, pennyroyal and marjoram, after which is added, cloves, gum benjamin and storax. Used as a toilet water.

LADY KILLER see Dundreary whiskers.

LADY'S BODKIN A bodkin for securing the hair, a hairpin (*Holmes 2*: p 13).

LADY'S COMB (1) A comb with wide, strong teeth at one end and a stout handle at the other. 18/19th century.
(2) A comb with a handle.

LADY'S HAIR (1) *Briza Media*, 'Maidenhaire grasse.'
(2) *Adiantum Capillus-veneris*, maidenhair fern. (*B and H*)

LADY'S TRESSES (1) Plants of the genus *Spiranthes*.
(2) Grasses of the genus *Briza* (*B and H*)

LAIVER BEARDS Meatless soups; Roxburghshire usage (*Watson*)

LAMBALLE See La Princess de Lamballe Coiffure.

LAMBREQUIN WHISKERS American usage. The same as Dundreary Whiskers, *qv*

LAMP CUT The combined processes of cutting the hair when wet, finger waving it and drying the set under an infra-red lamp. A popularly offered service in 1964. American usage. (*Ingerid*)

LANETTE WAX A fatty acid derivative used in cosmetics and hair preparation as an emulsifying agent.

LANK Hair is said to be lank when it is straight and limp.

LANOLIN Fat from sheep's wool. Emulsified, is used in hair reconditioning creams and shampoos. Sometimes added to permanent waving lotions to counteract the drying propensities.

LANTHORN JAWED Thin visaged, the cheeks being almost transparent. A troublesome type for the barber to shave. 18th century (*Grose, Lex Bal*).

LANUGO Fine soft hair or down on the surface of most of

the smooth skin of the body. The lanugo hairs have no medulla and the Arrector pili muscle is usually absent. The sebaceous glands are often comparatively large. (*Savill*)

LAPPET A hair-finger, or tress of hair hanging loosely on the face or neck.
See Hair-finger (2)
(2) A loop of hair hanging from the coiffure.
(3) A hanging lock of hair.

LAPPET CURL A hanging lock of curled hair, a corkscrew curl 18th century (*Stewart*) *The Bristol Journal* 15 August 1767.
'Monday was committed to the same gaol (Newgate, Bristol) as Daniel Light, for stealing one pair of Lappet Curls, and six ounces of human hair, the property of Jonothan Whitchurch, barber and peruke-maker, of this city.'
(*The Bristol Journal*, 18 October 1766).

LARGE SIDE That side of the parting that has the greatest area of scalp.

LARSEUR Hairdresser to Marie Antoinette. He was followed by Leonard.

LASH To comb the hair. Yorks dialect.

LASH COMB A wide toothed hair comb, *cf* Rake.

LASHING Subs. A combing, the hair being made smooth and straight.
Craven dialect. (*Holloway*).

LATERAL PARTING A parting extending across the head from the left side to the right side (*Elegant Arts*).

LATHER (1) Subs. The froth produced by mixing soap and water.
(2) Verb. To cover with lather
(3) Nickname for a barber 18th/19th century. (*Elliot*)

LATHER BOWL A metal or earthenware bowl in which the barber prepared his lather for softening beards preparatory to shaving.

LATHER BOY The barber's young attendant whose task it was to lather the faces of clients ready for the barber to shave them. He also had other menial tasks to perform, such as sweeping the floor, washing the basins, etc. Few, if any of the breed exist in England today (1965).

LATHER BRUSH A brush for applying lather to the beard to soften the hair preparatory to shaving.

LATHERER One who applies the lather to the face preparatory to shaving. See also Lather Boy.

LATHERIZER A manually or electrically operated machine for producing lather. 20th century. (*Thorpe*)

LATHER-MIXER An apparatus which produces 'instant' lather for the barber. 20th century. (*MH*)

LATTEN (LATEN, LATIN) A yellow-coloured mixed metal like brass. Used for manufacturing barber's basins, 16/19th century.

LAUTENSCHLAEGER'S SCURF ESSENCE A 19/20th century 'secret' preparation which consisted of scented ammonia soap, dissolved in alcohol and glycerine. (*Koller*)

LAVANT See Levant.

LAVATORY BASIN A basin for washing the head, hair, hands or face.
From Latin: *lavatorium*, wash.

LAVENDER OIL Rubbed on the scalp (in Somerset) to promote hair growth. 19th century.

LAVER A container for the barber's shaving water, suspended over the bason. (*Comemius, Orbis Pictus*, 1659)

LAWN MOWER TREATMENT A short, quick, drastic haircut. Slang.

LAWSONE (2-hydroxy-1, 4 napthoquinone). The active colouring agent in Henna. For permanent dyeing the pH

must be about 5.5 and this may be achieved by the addition of citric, boric or adipic acid. Relatively non-toxic, but can cause some irritation to very sensitive skins. (*Merck*)

LAWYER'S TIE WIG See Tie wig. (*Graves*)

LAYER Verb. To cut hair in layers. See Graduating.

LAYER CUT (1) Subs. Hair cut in layers so that they overlap like roof shingles or fish scales. (*Trusty*)
(2) Verb. To cut in layers. See Graduating.

LAYER CUTTING (1) Thinning and tapering hair by dividing it into layers parallel with the parting.
(2) Graduating, *qv*

LAYERED CUT Hair cut in layers. See Layer cutting.

LAYERING See Layer cut.

LE BANDEAU D'AMOUR Fr. A woman's hair style of 1780 dressed with frizz and question-mark curls.

LE BRUN Famous female hairdresser, wife of a wigmaker. Temp. Louis XIV. (*Johnson*)

LE CAPRICE Fr. A woman's hair style of 1864. (*Bysterveld*, p 44)

LE CHIEN COUCHANT Fr – the crouching dog. 18th century hair style for women. (*Uzanne*)

LE COUNTE (*sic*) A beard style. 20th century.

LE COUP DE VENT Fr – The gust of wind. A woman's hair style of 1864. (*Bysterveld*, p 34)

LE MARKIS (*sic*) A beard style (Gent's Acad.) The name appears to be a corruption of Le Marquis.

LE POUF A LA PUCE Fr – The flea pad. 18th century hair style for women. (*Uzanne*)

LE POUF SENTIMENTAL A woman's 18th century hair style.

LE PREMIER PAS Fr – The first step. A woman's hair style of 1864. (*Bysterveld* p 39)

LEAD COMB A comb made of lead and used to colour the hair by the simple but dangerous process of combing it, which often caused lead poisoning. 17/18th century. (*Holme*)
'The specious lead-comb, colour-giving box,
The crisping iron, and the mimic locks.' (*Woman in Miniature*, 18 century)
'When Mercury her tresses mows,
To think of black-lead combs is vain;' (*Swift, Miscellanies in Verse*, 1727) The first line refers to the effect of mercury treatment for venereal disease. This causes the hair to fall off.

LEAD HAIR DYE A popular but dangerous type of hair dye much used in the 19th century. According to Dr Benjamin Godfrey in his treatise *Diseases of Hair*, 1872, the following, which contained acetate of lead, sulphur and glycerine, were the most noted: Rossetter's Hair Restorer, Simeon's American Hair Restorer, Hall's Vegetable Sicilian Hair Renewer, Aqua Amarella, Helmsley's Celebrated Hair Restorer, Melmoth's Oxford Hair Restorer, but Alex Ross's Hair Restorer contained oxide of lead, carbonate of lead and potash.

LEATHER CURLER A small, tightly rolled hair curler made of soft leather so as not to cause damage to the hair. 19/20th century.

LEATHER-ROLL (Roller) An implement formed of rolled leather used to form curls. 18/early 20th century. (*Thornburg; Pyne*)

LEECHES, DECOMPOSED See Decomposed leeches.

LEFT-GOING WAVE A wave, the trough of which is inclined towards the left of the person waving the hair.

LEFT-HAND STICK See Weaving stick.

LEG (of a wig) The queue or tail. 18th century. (*London Mag*, 1764)

LEGERE See A la legère. Fr – light (of weight).

LEGHORN PLAIT A plait made of wheat straw from Leghorn, Tuscany.

LEGROS First recorded hairdresser to dress the hair of manikins (small dolls) and use them to advertise his hair fashion creations beyond his district. They were known as Legros's dolls.

LEGROS'S DOLLS See Legros.

LEIOTRICHY The condition of having straight hair. (*Webster*)

LEMON ACID See Citric acid.

LEMON GRASS, OIL OF See Verbena oil.

LEMON JUICE Used in the 19th century to remove dandruff from the scalp. (*Fernie*)

LEMON RINSE A hair rinse containing a small quanity of lemon juice or citric acid, used after a shampoo to remove any soap or soap-curd residue from the hair, in order to brighten it, to harden bleached hair and facilitate combing, and to give a lustrous appearance. See also Acid hair rinse.

LENTICULAR Shaped like a double convex lens.

LEOMINSTER This town is famous throughout Britain for its 'wigs'. These are cakes, not the wig worn on the head.

LEONARD French coiffeur and hairdresser to Marie Antoinette.

LEONIDES, THE SPARTAN His heart, according to Plutarch, was hairy. (*Speight*)

LEPRA OF THE SCALP Psoriasis capitis. (*Wheeler*)

LEPTOTRICHIA Excessively fine hair. (*Wheeler*)

LESBIAN SPOT A small, circular depilated area on the inside of the left leg. A means of recognition employed by the Caucasian lesbians of Peru.

LES CHEVEUX EN BROSSE Fr – Hair cut short. Standing up like the bristles of a brush.

LETTSOM, JOHN COAKLEY (1744–1815). Physician born in the West Indies and brought to England in 1750. Author of medical and other books. Famous for having worn a glass wig.

LEUCOTRICHIA White hair.

LEUCOTRICHIA ANNULARIS See Ringed hair.

LEUCOTRICHIA TOPICA White hair in patches. (*Wheeler*)

LEVANT Name for an 18th century wig style.

LEXONIC WIG An 18th century wig style for men.   *125*

LEYTENS, TINCTURE DE See Tincture de Leytens.

LIART also Lyart. Adj. Having grey hairs intermixed, grey haired, piebald. Scottish usage. (*Brown*)

LICHTENFELD, J A Famous 19th century wigmaker, hairdresser and writer on hairdressing. He followed his craft at 39 Great Castle Street, Oxford Circus, London, W.

LIEUTENANT COLONEL WIG Also called Brigadier wig and Major wig, qv. (*London Mag*, 1764)

LIFT (1) Verb. To remove colour from the hair. 'To obtain maximum lift apply the bleach cream thickly.'
(2) Verb. To dress a hair style in such a manner that some of the hair stands loosely away from the head.

LIGATURE A band or cord to tie the hair. (*Creer*)

LIGHT CUT (1) Removal of a small quantity of hair.
(2) A taper-cut that leaves the hair tresses tapered at the points.

LIGHTENER A preparation to lighten a hair colour, qv. The word has been used of recent years as a euphemism for bleach. It is thought by some hairdressers to connote a gentler treatment of the hair than the word bleach, which by reason of much overbleaching by incompetent hairdressers in the past and doubtless in the present too, has to some minds associations with harshness, destruction and hair breaking.

LIGHTENER RINSE A hair rinse that slightly bleaches the hair.

LIGHTENING The process of removing colour from the hair. Bleaching.

LIGHT MOUNT A light-weight postiche mount in which all the materials are of the lightest possible weight, and a minimum of galloon is used.

LIGUE BEARD (League beard) A 16th century beard style. (*Dulaure*, p 27)

LILACS The natural beard; also a false beard. Slang American usage. (*B and B*)

LILLIE, CHARLES A celebrated early 18th century perfumer, of Beaufort Buildings, in the Strand, London, friend of Steel, Swift, Pope, Addison and Arbuthnot. Both Addison and Steel frequently called public attention to his Perfumed Compositions, for which see: *Tatler* Nos 92, 94, 96, 101 and 103, 1709; *Spectator* Nos 358, 1712; *Guardian* No 64, 1713.

LIME Used by the ancient Greeks and Romans to lighten hair.

LIME BLONDE A woman with blonde hair of a greenish hue.

LIME FILM The deposited scum, in shampooing, produced by the reaction of magnesium or calcium salts in the water on the soap.

LIME SOAP See Lime film.

L'IMPERIALE A woman's hair style of 1865 based on an ancient Greek hair-dress. (*Bysterveld*, p 49)

LINCOLNIC BEARD A beard resembling that worn by Abraham Lincoln. American usage. (*Trusty*)   *98E*

LINDANE See Gammabenzene hexachloride.

LINE OF DEMARCATION See Demarcation line.

LINEN Cloth of Lint or flax.

LINEN BIN A metal or plastic container in which dirty linen from the saloon is deposited and kept until laundered.

LINEN SKULL A foundation of linen on which hair or imitation hair is secured. Used for theatrical work when a bald crown or front is required.

LINE WAVING Waving a head of hair with the waves parallel to the parting.

LINING NET See Lining silk.

LINING SILK A fine, white silk fabric thicker than parting silk, used to protect the head side of a drawn-through parting.

LINNAEUS WIG A wig style for men of *c* 1720 in which one half of the hair was tied on the left side into a club. The style was adopted by Charles Linnaeus (1707–1778), the Swedish botanist. (*Fenton*)   *252*

LINSEED, (FLAXSEED, LINUM) The dried, ripe seeds of *Linum Usitatissimum*, source of linseed oil.

LINSEED OIL Obtained by the expression of linseed and used as a raw material in the maufacture of soft soap and shampoos.

LINTWHITE Flaxen, fair. (*Macneill*)

LINT WHITE BLONDE A woman with pure white hair. (*Daily Telegraph*, 22 Dec 1965)

LION WIG A name for a physical wig, qv, from its resemblance to the mane of a lion. Late 18th century. (*Gent's Mag*, 1761)

LIP SPINACH A moustache. Slang American usage. (*B and B*)

LIP TICKLER A moustache. Slang American usage. (*B and B*)

LIP-HAIR BLEACH A bleach suitable for bleaching the hair on the upper lip.

LIPPUFF A moustache. Slang American usage. (*B and B*)

LIQUID BLEACH A hair bleach in liquid form.

LIQUID DRY SHAMPOO Flammable liquid dry shampoos

should never, under any circumstances, be used for shampooing hair on the human head. See Dry shampoo (2).

LIQUID SHAMPOO (1) A soap shampoo or a soapless shampoo, in liquid form.

(2) Liquid dry shampoo. See Dry shampoo.

LIQUID SOAP SHAMPOO The base is usually green soft soap and sometimes in addition either coconut oil, olive oil or eucalyptus oil. In the absence of the oils the shampoo is perfumed with oil of citronella or oil of verbena, etc.

LISSE Fr. Smooth, glossy.

LISSOTRICHY See Leiotrichy.

LIT. To dye or tinge. Scottish usage. (*Henderson*)

LITT Verb. To colour or dye, whence the name Litster or Lister. Northern and Midlands usage. 17/18th century. (*Derham*)

LITTLE CAP CUT A short, bobbed hair style for girls with the ends turned up into a loose curl and having a divided fringe. (*Trusty*)

LITTLE-GIRL COIFFURE A coiffure for women of any period, so styled that it imitates the fashion worn by young girls of the same period.

LIXIVIATE Verb. To separate a substance into its soluble and insoluble constituents by percolation of water through it.

LIXIVIOUS WATER An alkaline liquid, formerly used to bleach hair 'by spreading the hair to bleach on the grass, like linen, after first washing it out in a lixivious water; this lye, with the force of the sun and air, brings the hair to so perfect a whiteness that the most experienced person may be deceived.' (*Stewart*)

LOCK (1) A gathering or group of propinquent hair. A tress. See also Bunch, Filament, Strand, Tress, Wisp.

(2) 'The hair lying flat on each side of the cheek.' 17th century. (*Holme*)

(3) A small quantity of hay; also lock of wool and lock of hair.

Wiltshire usage. (*Akerman*)

LOCKER (Lockar) Verb. To curl. See Lockered.

LOCKERED Adj. Curled, c 1400–c 1700.

'The daughter's lockard hair.' (*H More*, 1687)

LOCKS The hair of the head.

LOGWOOD *Haematoxylon Campechianum.* Used in the 19th century for dyeing hair.

LOHSE'S CHROMACOME HAIR DYE A 19/20th century 'secret' preparation, consisting of two liquids, one a tincture of gall nuts, the other a solution of iron acetate, with a little silver nitrate. (*Koller*)

LONG BOB A man's wig style, early 18th century, also called Minister's Bob and Clergyman's Bob. The long bob wig covered the back of the neck, whereas the short bob wig ended at the base of the head, leaving the neck uncovered. (*London Mag*, 1753) See En-long.   *210, 257*

LONG BOB WITH FEATHERED FORETOP A man's 18th century wig style. See Long bob. (*Tennent*)

LONG CURL The row of seven top curls of a barrister's wig.

LONG HAIR Anciently long hair was a sign of high social rank. The Parthians and ancient Persians of high rank wore long, flowing hair. Homer wrote of 'Long-haired Greeks' by way of honourable distinction. Later the Athenian Cavalry wore long hair, as did all Lacedaemonian soldiers. The Goths regarded long hair as a mark of honour and short hair as the mark of thraldom. Long hair was the distinctive mark of kings and nobles in France for many centuries. It was regarded as a notable honour by the Gauls and for this reason Julius Caesar compelled conquered Gauls to have their hair cut off as a token of submission. Both the ancient Germans and Franks considered long hair a mark of noble

birth.

LONGHAIR (1) A young male of the 1960s who wears his hair long over the neck and ears. 'Here comes another longhair.'

(2) A highbrow or intellectual, American usage. 'The fair added more features which might be considered longhair.' (*Newark Evening News*, 22 April 1965). American slang.

LONG HAIRED, THE Clodion, the Frank, was called this and his successors were spoken of as Les Rois Chevelures.

LONG-HAIRED-MOTHER, THE Chicomecoatl, the Aztec goddess of maize.

LONGICILIUM Long, straggling eyebrows. (*Wheeler*)

LONG QUEUE Name of 18th century wig for men, having the front, sides and back dressed rather flat, with a long queue or tail at the back.

LONG-STEMMED PIN CURL A ringlet with a long stem; the stem being the straight between the curl and the scalp.

LONG TAIL An 18th century wig style. American usage. See Long queue. (*Earle*)

LONG-TERM-RINSE A colour, applied to the hair in the form of a rinse, which lasts for several months.

LOOK Subs. The style, fashion or appearance of a hairdress. See New Look, Urchin look, etc.

LOOM Weaving sticks and silks.   *88(21AA)*

LOOP A curved tress of hair that crosses itself. 1830 (*Mallemont*)

LOOP OF HAIR See Loop.

LOOP MARTEAU A small Marteau, *qv*, not more than 2″ across the mount and secured by hairpins through two small loops. (*Symonds*)

LOOSE BUCKLE, THE See En-boucle détachée.

LOOSENING Disentangling by gentle pulling, with the thumbs and first fingers, small strands of hair from the hair-rat or combings ball.

LOTION A liquid preparation for external use on the head or body.

LOTIO-STAPHISAGRIAE, *BPC*. A parasiticidic hair lotion for use in the Nursery. (*PPB*)

LO-TSU TA-HSIEN Chinese mythological god of barbers, beggars and corn-cutters. In private houses represented with bare feet, rolled sleeves and a red face, and in Temples, holding a treatise on haircutting called T'i-fa shu. (*Werner*)

LOUIS Man's 18th century wig style. Name probably derived from St Louis, the patron saint of wigmakers.

LOUIS VII This French monarch submitted to the exhortations of his clergy and had both beard and hair cut short. His shorn and dismal appearance so shocked his Queen (Eleanor) that she obtained a divorce. (*Speight*)

LOUIS XV PUFF An undulating puff. A waved strand of hair, heavily backcombed beneath to produce a light, puffed effect when positioned. 19th century usage. Illustrated pp 4574–4577, *Every-woman's Encyclopedia.* (*Nicol*)

LOUIS, SAINT Patron Saint of barbers, hairdressers and perfumers.

Louis IX, King of France, b at Poissy, 25 April 1215, d of the plague at Tunis, 25 August 1270. Pope Boniface VIII canonised him in 1297. (*Wallon* 4th ed 1893, and *Berger* 1893)

LOUIS STYLE In the mode of the French Kings, Louis XIII to Louis XVI.

(Louis XIII (1610–43), Louis XIV (1643–1713), Louis XV (1713–1774), Louis XVI (1774–1793)).

LOUSE A parasitic insect that infects human hair and skin. It is one of the genus *pediculas*.

LOUSE BAG A black bag worn with a Bag wig, *qv*, and into which the tail was tucked. (*Grose, Lex Bal*)

LOUSE LINE A hair parting. Slang. Somerset and Gloucestershire usage. 19/20th century.

LOUSE TRAPA small toothed comb, 18th century. See also Flea comb. (*Grose, Lex Bal*) Slang name for a dust comb, Somerset usage. (*Elworthy*)

LOUSEWALK A hair parting. Slang American usage. (*B and B*)

LOUSIAD, THE An heroic-comic poem (canto 1, 1785) by Peter Pindar (*John Wolcot*) describing the discovery of a louse by King George III. An edict was, in consequence, passed for shaving the cooks and scullions, to destroy the louse.

LOVE CURL See Love lock. (*W de la Mare, Peacock Pie*)

LOVE LOCK (1) A tress of long, curled or waved hair, combed forward from the neck to hang casually over the front of the shoulder. Its end was often decorated by a ribbon tied in a bow. Greene, in his *Quip for an Upstart Courtier*, 1592, refers to the love lock. It was popularised by James I who allowed a single lock on the left side to grow considerably longer than the rest of his hair. 'Some by wearing a longe locke that hangs dangling by his eare, do think by that lousie commodity to be esteemed.' (*Rich*, 1613). 'I bought him a new periwig with a love lock at it.' (*Beaumont, F, Cupids Revenge*, 1615). 'Some men have long lockes at their ears as if they had four ears, or were prick-eared. Some have a little long lock before only, hanging down to their noses, like the taile of a Wesall, every man being made a foole at the barber's pleasure.' (*Hall, Loathesomnesse of Long Haire*, 1654). Later the meaning was extended to refer to a single tress of long hair hanging from the side of the head. *362*

(2) A lock of hair from the head of his lady, worn into battle (and in peace) by a Man of Arms. It was usually worn in the headgear.

LOVE RIBBAND (RIBBON) A narrow gauze ribbon with satin stripes used to secure and decorate the hair. 18th century.

LOVER'S KNOT A narrow ribbon worn as a bow in the hair or on the trousseau.

LOW TONE Subdued tone or colour.

LUBRICANT A substance which makes the hair or skin slippery or smooth.

LUCCA OIL A fine quality Italian olive oil, obtained from the ripe fruit of *Olea Europea* L, *Oleaceae*. Lucca is the name of a city and province of northern Italy.

LUCIDUM A layer of the skin beneath the corneum, which it resembles, but is less horny.

LUCINA Roman goddess to whom the vestal virgins consecrated their cut hair, hanging it for a monument on a sacred lote-tree. (*Pliny, Nat Hist*)

LUCKEN BROW'D Overhanging, knit brows. Yorkshire usage.

LUCRECIA A woman's hair style of 1866. (*Bysterveld*, p 73)

LUCREZIA BORGIA'S HAIR In a glass case in the Ambrosian Library, Milan, a lock of hair, almost certainly from Lucrezia Borgia's golden tresses, still exists today. The love affair between Lucrezia (1480–1519), daughter of Pope Alexander VI, and Pietro Bembo (1470–1547), who became a Cardinal, is notorious. Almost certainly, too, Lucrezia gave Bembo this lock of hair, and he kept it with her love letters to him, among his papers. Lucrezia's tresses were famous, and their natural beauty enhanced by oil and sun treatment; they appear to have been the subject of several love poems of Bembo. Certainly the youthful Lord Byron was so affected by the lock of hair, now in Milan, that he stole a strand or two from it. There is a colour plate of the lock of hair in Milan, in Bellonci, facing p 480.

Bibliography: For the love affair: M. Bellonci, *L. Borgia* (Milan, rev ed, 1960), of which there is an abridged trans. *The life and times of L Borgia* (London 1953). For the hair and letters: B Gatti, ed, *Letters di L Borgia a P Bembo* (Milan, 1859), P Rajna, 'I versi spagnuoli di mano di P Bembo e L Borgia . . .' *Homenaje a Menéndez Pidal* (Madrid, 1924) II, pp 301 no 1, 309. For the poems: P Bembo, *Prose e Rime*, ed C Dionisotti (Turin, 1960) pp 510–11, 513–14; for Bembo's papers. C. H. Clough, 'The Library of P Bembo . . . ', *The British Museum Quarterly*, XXX (1965) pp 3–17. For treatment of blond hair see Anon, as 'Deux Vénitiens', F S Feuillet de Conches and A Baschet, *Les femmes blondes . . .* (Paris, 1865). For Byron see Gatti. (*C H Clough*)

LUFTLUCKEN Air bubbles in the medulla of the hair.

LUG (1) Verb. To pull by the hair or ears. Midlands usage. (*Derham*)
(2) Subs. A pole. 'A barber's lug', Wilts usage. (*Akerman*)
(3) An ear. North country usage.

LUGGY Adj. Tangled hair. Midlands usage.

LUGS Groups of tangled head hair. Midlands usage.

LUNAR-CAUSTIC Silver nitrate commonly used as a hair dye in the 19th century.

LUNATIQUE See A la lunatique.

LUSTRE Gloss, splendour.

LUSTRELESS Without lustre, sheen gloss or refulgence.

LUTIN Verb. To twist hair into elf locks.

LYART Grey haired. Scottish usage. See also Liart. (*Ramsay*)

LYART HAFFETS Having grey hairs by the side of the cheeks. Scottish usage. (*Brown*)

LYE or **LEY** Any strong alkaline solution, especially one used for the purpose of washing, such as soda lye and soap lye.

LYRATE Shaped like a lyre.

M

MACARONI (Maccaroni) A dandy, a fop, or ultra-fashionable male of 1772–3. The name was derived from the Macaroni Club, formed by wealthy young men of fashion who had travelled in Italy and adopted excessive and eccentric fashions. They affected long curls and spying-glasses and came into prominence about 1760. By 1772 they had assumed an immense knot of artificial hair behind, a very small cocked hat, an extremely close-cut jacket, waistcoat and breeches, and carried an enormous walking-stick. In 1773 a very lofty hairdress was adopted, together with an immense nosegay. (*Forster; Wright*) *247 476*

MACARONI HEAD-DRESS In 1772 the Macaronis, *qv*, were distinguished especially by an immense knot of artificial hair worn at the back, but with the peruke flat on top. By 1773 the wigs worn by the macaronis were dressed very high on top and elaborate. (*Oxford Magazine*, Nov 1772, p 177, ditto Jan 1773, p 17 for illus.) A child's book of the 18th century has the following explanation beneath a figure of a Macaroni – 'M. A Macaroni with loads of false hair.' (*Wright*, pp 259–60; *Holloway*) *247 476*

MACARONI TOUPEE See Macaroni headdress.

MACASSAR OIL (Kusum oil, Paka oil). Derived from the nut kernels of the Ceylon oak. A yellowish-white oil of pleasant odour used as an unguent for the hair since the early 19th century. In England the firm of Rowland and

Son extensively advertised their product as 'Rowland's Macassar Oil', but many such products contained no macassar oil. A 19th century formula was: Expressed oil of almonds 4 lb, alkanet root 7 oz, oil of clove 75 grains, oil of mace 75 grains, oil of rose 75 grains, oil of cinnamon ½ oz, tincture of musk 75 grains. (*Askinson*). See Antimacassar.

431

MACHINELESS WAVING (1) Hot permanent waving in which the required heat is either generated chemically in a pad applied to the hair, or by means of a pre-heated metal clamp.

(2) Cold permanent waving, *qv*.

MACHINE-MADE KNOTTED WIG Made of synthetic curled fibre woven into a light-weight stretch fabric. The finished material can be cut and shaped into a wig with elastic at the nape. The fitting is similar to a woollen cap. 20th cent.

MACHINE-MADE WIG Made from hair weft in which the weft is mechanically sewn in a spiral pattern, pivoting from the crown and spaced ½" to 1" apart. These wigs can be adjusted for size by means of elastic in the nape. 20th century.

MACHINE PARTING A hair parting for a postiche manufactured by machinery and not by hand. In 1912 my father invented a machine for making drawn-through partings but the results were not of a sufficiently high quality to replace the hand-made drawn-through partings.

MACHINE WINDING The spiral winding of hair on a curler by means of a small hand-operated winding machine, preparatory to a permanent wave.

MACINTYRE, DUNCAN See The Fair-haired.

MACRAME Also Macrami. This word is used by wigmakers for macramé linen thread, *qv*.

MACRAME LINEN THREAD Used by wigmakers as the foundation of the stems of switches. All shades from white to darkest brown, including greys and yellows are used, according to the colour of the hair being worked.

MACROCEPHALIC Adj. Large headed.

MACROCEPHALOUS Having a large head.

MACROGENYTRICHIA An exceptionally long growth of beard hair. A Mr Edwin Smith's beard was recorded by Dr Leonard as being 7' 6½" in length. A carpenter at the court of Eidan had a beard 9' long. (*Wheeler*)

MACROPHRYAS See Longicilium.

MACROTRICHIA Extra long hair (24" to 36"). Hair exceeding 36" in length is rare among Europeans, but occurs among Chinese and Indians and some other races. (*Wheeler*)

MACULE A blemish on the hair or skin.

MADAM HAIR STYLE Any formal hair style for a woman. 1960s.

MADAME POMPADOUR'S WASH-BALL Take Brandy 4 pints, add Italian soap cut small 1 lb, quicklime ¼ lb. Let ferment 24 hours, spread and dry, then beat in a marble mortar with ½ oz St Lucia wood, 1½ oz yellow sanders, ½ oz orris root and as much calimus aromaticus, all finely powdered. Knead the whole into a paste with whites of eggs and ¼ lb gum tragacanth.

MADAME ROYALE A woman's hair style of 1790. (*Bysterveld*, p 37)

MADAROSIS Loss of eyelashes or eyebrows.

MADEMOISELLE DE MONTPENSIER COIFFURE The 17th century hairdress worn by Mlle de Montpensier. (*Villermont*, 416)

MADESIS Hair loss due to old age.

MADE-UP HAIR-WORK Postiche, *qv*.

MADONNA FRONT A postiche for women in which the hair is dressed to a centre parting and worn straight, or nearly straight.

MADONNA HAIRDRESS A hair style for women in which the hair is parted in the centre and worn straight, or nearly straight.

MADONNA PARTING A centre parting with straight hair on either side, *c* 1914.

MAEROSE CLUSTER A chignon with puff-curls and three small hanging curls. Popular during the First World War, 1914–1918. (*A H* August 1915)

MAGASIN Fr – Warehouse, storehouse, shop.

MAGDALEN CURL A long hanging spiral curl. Mary Magdalen is represented as having such long hair that she was able to wipe off her tears from the feet of Jesus. Hence a Magdalen curl would mean the long hair of a Magdalen made into a spiral curl.

MAGICIAN, THE A woman's hair style of 1866. (*Bysterveld*, p 95)

MAGNESIA ALBA See Magnesium carbonate.

MAGNESIUM CARBONATE $(MgCO_3)_4$. $Mg(OH)_2$ $5H_2O$. A light, friable, white, bulky powder, used in white henna preparations, *qv*.

MAGNESIUM PEROXIDE MgO_2. A white, tasteless, odourless powder, gradually decomposed by water to liberate oxygen; soluble in dilute acids to form hydrogen peroxide. Used in some white henna preparations.

MAGNETIC ROLLER A roller of large diameter with a smooth plastic surface to which wet hair will adhere as if magnetized by the roller, which it is not, the word magnetic being used tralatitiously.

MAIDEN BARBER The shrub *Berberis Vulgaris*; Burberry.

MAIDEN HAIR Hair which has never been subjected to any process of curling, waving, bleaching or dyeing.

MAIDENHAIR (Maiden hair) (1) The common name for the plant *adiantum capillus-veneris*, maidenhair fern. Recorded by Pliny as having been used to strengthen and embellish the hair. (*Fernie*)

(2) *Nartheciüm Ossifragum* – In Lancashire this plant was 'used by women to die their hair of a yellowish colour', 16/17th century. (*B and B*)

MAIDEN'S HAIR The hair of a maiden.

MAIDEN'S KNOT Hair dressed in a double bow knot across the top of the head. (See Greek hair styles).

MAID'S HAIR The plant *galium verum*. (*B and H*)

MAINTENON A woman's hair style of 1866 based on the style worn by the Marquise de Maintenon. (*Bysterveld*, p 88)

MAISON Fr – The House of, also Maison . . . et Cie, the House of . . . and Company. A mode of address used by many fashionable hairdressers of the Victorian and Edwardian periods. It fell out of favour after the First World War, 1914–1918. The intention was to convey to the public that the firm had a knowledge of French hair styles, methods of hairdressing and postiche manufacture. An example was *Maison Stephens* et Cie, Queen's Road, Clifton.

MAITRE D'HOTEL See A la maitre d'hotel.

MAJOR An English moustache style. (*Foan*)   *101Q*

MAJOR, THE An English hair style for men. From the 1920s. (*Foan*)

MAJOR BOB See Bob major.

MAJOR WIG An 18th century man's wig style with two tails. See Brigadier wig. (*Doran*, p 157)

MAKE-UP (1) Subs. The powder and paint, cream and artificial additions used by women to improve their facial appearance, or so they believe.

(2) Verb. The process of adding the substances in (1) to the face.

MAKSOOS (Pl Makasees) The long lock of hair that hangs down on each side of the face of an Egyptian woman. (*Lane*)

MALE PATTERN ALOPECIA Recession of the hair line at the front region and crown of the head. (*Flitman*)

MALLEABLE BLOCK See Malleable wig block.

MALLEABLE CUSHION A round, velvet-covered cushion, flattened at the top and bottom, and stuffed with hair or other soft material, on which are dressed postiches such as puff curls, pincurls, marteaux, etc.

MALLEABLE TRANSFORMATION BLOCK Similar to a malleable wig block but having a substantial proturberance at the back on which the hair lengths of the transformation can be dressed. A wig block would not afford sufficient surface area for this dressing.   187

MALLEABLE WIG BLOCK An artificial head composed of canvas stuffed with granulated cork or sawdust. The coarctation of the cork holds the canvas in shape. Used for dressing wigs on and for holding a reversed wig for underknotting. These blocks are manufactured in different sizes to suit the varying measurements of wigs, and pins are inserted in the outline galloon and block to secure the wig.

MALLIAC BALL A soap from Mallium in Germany, made from goat fat and ashes and popular with Roman women, *c* AD 100. Used by the ancients to lighten hair. (*Speight*)

MALPIGHIAN LAYER The deeper part of the epidermis.

MALTESE FILAGREE (FILIGREE) HAIRPIN A hairpin of a delicate and decorative kind, finely ornamented. (*Elegant Arts*, p 130)

MAMBRINO'S HELMET (1) A barber's basin.
'T'was Saturday night, six went the clock,
Spruce was the barber's shop;
Wigs decorated ev'ry block,
From scratch to Tyburn-top;
Mambrino's helmet, scoured so bright,
Smiled to receive the suds:
And Labourers flocked to shave o'er night,
To grace their Sunday's duds.' (1867) (*Brighte*, p 114)
(2) The sign of a barber's shop in Mexico and in parts of Europe, 17/19th century. (*Bullock*). Derived from the solid gold helmet of Mambrino, a legendary pagan king introduced by Ariosto into his poem *Orlando Furioso*. In the *Don Quixote* of Cervantes the hero insisted that the barber's basin was the actual gold helmet of the King, Mambrino, and, taking possession of it, he wore it as such. (*Brewer, R H*)

MANCHESTER, THE English hair style for men. (*Foan*)

MANDREL A Curling stick, *qv*.

MANE A profuse growth of long hair on the head. 'Maggie . . . tossing back her mane.' (*Eliot, Mill on the Floss*, 1860)

MANE COMB A strong wooden comb with a thick back. Used for horses' manes and women's long hair, 17th century. (*Holme*)

MANE HAIR Hair from horses' manes. Used, when crêped, in hair pads. Referred to in a diary of Anna Winslow, 1771.

MANICURE The treatment and care of the finger nails and hands.

MANICURIST A person who undertakes the care of the nails and hands.

MANIKIN (1) An accurately proportioned anatomical jointed figure of the human body, used by artists from at least the 16th century.
(2) An artificial head for the display of wigs.

MANNEQUIN (variant of Manikin) (1) A live model used to display a hair style or gown.
(2) An artificial head used to display a hair style, or on which to create a hair style, or work hair for a postiche. See also Manikin (2) and Model.

MANNER The hair artist's way of expressing himself in the principal arts of hairdressing, which are design and colour.

MAN-OF-SUDS A barber, 18/20th century. (*G of L M*)

MANTLE The fold of skin from which the nail grows.

MANUFACTURED HAIR (1) Human hair, which has been worked into postiches, such as wigs, switches, etc.
(2) Artificial hair that has been made from a natural substance (other than hair), or a synthetic substance.

MAN WITH A WIG, THE Dr Samuel Parr (1747–1825), the scholar, is so referred to in *Noctes Ambrosianae*.

MARBLEU, MONS. A French refugee barber, a character in W T Moncrieff's 19th century farce. (*Monsieur Tonson*)

MARBLE WIGS In the Roman period these were used to cover heads of marble statues and keep their hairdress fashionable.

MARCEL (1) Subs. A Marcel wave, *qv*. 'I want a marcel.'
(2) Verb. To Marcel wave hair: 'She had her hair marcelled by Pierre.'
(3) Common English hairdressing trade name, from Marcel Grateau, *qv*, inventor of the Marcel wave. See also Marcelle.

MARCEL CURL A curl produced by the use of Marcel waving irons.

MARCEL FLAT WIND A method of winding hair spirally on a curler by winding the first two circinations flat and the third flat and overlapping the second, but slanted in the opposite direction, and then repeating the sequence until the hair strand is wound. (*Smith, H J*)

MARCEL GRATEAU Inventor of the Marcel wave, which revolutionised the art of ladies hairdressing. He was born 18 October, 1852, at Chauvigny, department of Vienne, France. He was apprenticed to a barber at his birthplace and at 18 years of age moved to Paris, where he practised his craft. At the age of 20 he started his own business in Montmartre. In 1872 he took notice of natural symmetrical waves on the top of his mother's head and practised to continue these waves with curling irons over the rest of the head. Grateau developed his newly acquired technique on suitable heads, without making any charge for the wave, and business prospered and he moved to rue de Dunkerque. In 1875 a client with stiff, sleek and straight hair asked him to wave it. Marcel told her 'Your hair is not sufficiently good for this'. 'Never mind, try all the same' insisted the client, 'I will pay you the price that you desire'. Marcel accepted the offer of money, the first he had received for this special work, his Marcel wave. Five or six weeks passed and the client presented herself to him with her hair still in wave and congratulated him for all the many compliments she had received concerning this novelty. From that moment the Master charged for his wave and as he raised his prices the clients increased. In 1882 he moved to a central address in Paris: 2 rue de L'Echelle. By 1887 the vogue for Marcel waving had commenced and Marcel was overwhelmed with work. Actresses and wealthy women paid up to Fr 500 (£20) to be waved without waiting and for nearly 10 years Marcel earned £4,000 per year. In July 1897, with a million francs saved, he closed his shop and retired, after having published in four languages *La Coiffure Francaise*, illustrating his method of waving hair. He died in June, 1936. (*H W J*, 1 Aug 1908: Biography by E Long)

MARCELLE A common trade name used by ladies' hairdressers from *c* 1914 to *c* 1939, now rarely employed. The feminine form of Marcel, *qv*.

MARCELLER One who Marcel waves hair. Craft word since *c* 1914.

MARCEL-WAVE An artificial hair wave formed in the

manner of that invented by Marcel Grateau using heat«
Marcel waving irons.   3‹

MARCEL-WAVER (1) A person who Marcel waves.
(2) A patented device consisting of two corrugated aluminium rollers which move in opposite directions when the
handles are closed and when closed upon a strand of hair
produce a passable imitation of a wave. (*A H* 1915)

MARCEL WAVING FLUID (1) A liquid used on the hair to
facilitate the process of Marcel waving and to help retain the
wave.
(2) Brilliantine.

MARCEL WAVING IRONS See Waving Irons.

MARCHIONESS WIG A woman's 18th century (*Louis XV*)
wig style.   337(2)

MARECHAL HAIR POWDER A 19th century formula:
oak moss in powder 2 lb; starch powdered 1 lb; cloves 1 oz;
calamus aromaticus 1 oz; Cyperus in powder 2 oz; rotten
wood in powder 1 oz; mixed well together.
Another recipe: Powdered cloves 1 oz, starch powder 2½
lb. (*Francis*)

MARGOT, FIRST WIFE OF HENRY IV Kept yellow-
haired pages as a source of hair for her wigs.

MARGUERITE COIFFURE A head-hugging woman's hair
style dressed in small waves and curls. 19th century.
(Florian Sobocinski Advert)

MARGUERITE D'ANGOULEME COIFFURE Marguerite d'Angouleme or d'Alencon, or de Navarre (1492–1549)
was ancestress of the line of Bourbon Kings and gave her
name to this style of hairdress.   211

MARGUERITE KNOT A knot or coil of hair constructed
from a three spill tail or plait of hair. (*Creer*)

MARGUERITE PLAIT A long, thick plait with a bow to
secure the ends, so named after the character Marguerite
who wore such plaits in the opera Faust, first produced in
Paris in 1859. The plaits were in 4, 5, 6, or 7 strands as
required. (*S D P : O C M and Creer*)   417

MARIE ANTOINETTE BOW (wife of Louis XVI of
France) Divide the hair into the necessary strands, each is
then rolled around all the fingers of the left hand, half a turn
is given and the hair is fastened tightly at the root of the
bow. (*Mallemont*)

MARIE ANTOINETTE CHIGNON A full globular low
dressed chignon.

MARIE ANTOINETTE COIFFURE Hair styles similar to
those worn by Marie Antoinette.   363, 365

MARIE ANTOINETTE PUFF A lightly dressed artificial
front of hair c 1892.

MARIE CHRISTINE COIFFURE Coiffure after the style
of that worn by Marie Christine of Austria. 18th century.
(*Villermont*)   367

MARIE DE MEDICI COIFFURE A coiffure of the style
worn by Marie de Medici (1573–1642).

MARIE LOUISE PUFF A lightly dressed artificial front of
hair as worn by Marie Louise, (1791–1847), wife of
Napoleon.

MARIE STUART COIFFURE (1) A coiffure similar to that
worn by Mary, Queen of Scots. See Mary Stuart.
(2) A woman's hair style of c 1865 based on that worn by
Mary Queen of Scots (1542–1587).
The front hair was divided into two parts on each side so as
to be distinct from the rest of the hair. The top section of
each part was brushed over a narrow roll of brown silk,
stuffed with wool, so as to form *La Marie Stuart*, and the
bottom parts of the two tresses were brought over the ears
so as to conceal them. The back hair was formed into three
and dressed with a crown. (*Elegant Arts*)

MARIE STUART PAD A narrow, hollow, curved pad

constructed of wire and crêpe hair or mohair. 19th
century

MARIENBAD LOOK A woman's bobbed hair style, worn
straight. 1962.   272

MARIE-THERESE COIFFURE The style of hairdress
worn by Marie-Thérèse, wife of Louis XIV. 17th century.
(*Villermont*)   359

MARINE SOAP Soap made from coconut or palm nut oil
containing free caustic soda and salt brine. (*Wall*)

MARION BANDELETTE A waved front of hair.   314

MARMOTTE Woman's head-dress formed of a handker-
chief tied round the head. (*Creer*)

MARQUIS OTTO A corruption of the French word *Marquisotte*, which became Marquisette, *qv*, in English usage. A
close-cut beard style, 16/18th century. (*Mitchell*)

MARQUISE COIFFURE Woman's hair style, time of Louis
XV.   124

MARQUISETTE (MARQUISOTTE: MARQUISETTO,
etc) A close-cut beard style of 16/18th century. From the
French word *Marquisotte*. (*Mitchell*)

MARQUISOTTE See Marquisette.

MARROW POMADE Hair pomade in which is incorporated
bone marrow. A popular 19th century recipe was: Prepared
beef-marrow ½ lb, prepared beef suet ¼ lb; Palm oil ¼ oz;
scent as desired.
Much of the so-called beef marrow of the pomades was
obtained from the knackers.

MARS Roman god of war. Depicted by the ancients with face
all hairy and long curled locks of black hair on his head,
depending even to his shoulders. (*Salmon*)

MARSEILLES SOAP A soap made at Marseilles, France,
similar to but lighter in colour, and superior to Castile
Soap, *qv*, 19th century. (*Lillie*)

MARTEAU (Pl MARTEAUX) A postiche made with flat
sewn weft having two loops at each end, by which it can be
secured, using hairpins or hairgrips; or flat weft mounted
on a hairslide, haircomb or postiche clip. Symonds describes them as flat-topped 'tails' of hair.   398

MARTEAU BOUCLE Fr – A hammer curl, *qv*.

MARTEAU BOW A marteau dressed as a bow of hair.
(*Mallemont*)

MARTEAU CURL A hammer curl, *qv*.

MARTEAU TORSADE See Torsade.

MARUMAGE The rounded chignon of a married Japanese
woman. (*Inouye*)

MARY PICKFORD CURL CLUSTER A hairpiece of drop
curls imitative of the style worn by the famous American
film star, Mary Pickford. The cluster became popular in
March 1914. (*A H* May 1915)

MARY QUEEN OF SCOTS Wore auburn fronts and wigs.
(*Saunders*)

MARY QUEEN OF SCOTS CAP See Paris cap.

MARY STUART A woman's hair style of the 16th century
incorporating raised bandeaux, *qv*. Worn by and named
after Queen Mary Stuart, beheaded 1587. (*Bysterveld* p 69)

MASCARA A cosmetic for application to eyelashes to give
the appearance of greater length and to enhance the
appearance of the eye. One of the oldest cosmetics, having
been used in biblical times. Early mascaras were made of
soap and pigments, or wax and pigments. Carbon black was
a common colouring agent.

MASK (FACE MASK) Used in the 18th century to protect
the face during the application of powder to the coiffure.
                                                           87(42, 43)

MASONIC BEARD A fan-shaped beard.

MASQUERADE WIG A wig that is worn for disguise.

MASSAGE Manipulation of the body's surface tissues and

underlying structures by rubbing, kneading, squeezing, tapping, etc. with the fingers and hands, or electrical or mechanical apparatus.

MASSAGE OIL An oil which is applied to the scalp to aid the process of massage and increase its beneficial effect.

MASSAGIST A person, male or female, who practices massage.

MASSEUR A male massagist.

MASSEUSE A female massagist.

MASTER BARBER (HAIRDRESSER) A self-employed, fully qualified barber (hairdresser) who entered the craft as an apprentice.

MASTER-LATHER A barber. 18/19th century.

MAT Verb. To entangle or entwine hair into a thick mass. Matted hair is in tighter confusion than tangled hair.

MATCHED WAVES (1) Waves that fit perfectly with one another. American usage.

(2) Waves that correspond in size and relative position to each other; eg two identical cheek waves, one on each cheek.

MATCHING (1) In dyeing, producing a hair colour the same shade as the pattern.

(2) In boardwork, mixing hair of different shades to obtain the same shade as the pattern.

MATHEWS, STANLEY A world-famous footballer, the son of a barber.

MATILDA A small bunch of flowers worn in the hair. Mid-19th century. (*Cunnington*)

MATRIX The hair papilla.

MATT An unreflecting surface.

MATTRESS A heavy beard. Slang American usage. (*B and B*)

MATTY Matted, entangled. Somerset, Dorset and Bristol usage.

MAUSOLUS, KING OF CARIA Needing money, he ordered a universal shave among his subjects and had a large number of wigs manufactured which he compelled them to purchase at his price and thus replenished his treasury. (*Speight*)

MAW WORM A long, straight-haired wig with fringe, named after a male character in Bickerstaffe's play *The Hypocrite*, 1768.

MAXIE HAIRDRESS The Maxies wore their hair long on the right side of the head and shaved it on the left side. (*Bulwer*; *Busonii*)   102F

MAYFAIR EXPERIENCE Also 'Late of Mayfair'. Terms used in various forms of advertising by some hairdressers in the provinces (usually Ladies' hairdressers) to convince a gullible public that their skill is as great or greater than actually it is. The claim is sometimes true but not always. Derived from the Mayfair district of London, which is exclusive, fashionable and expensive, the hairdressers of Mayfair offering a very high standard of skill in an extravagant environment of luxurious decor.

MAYO, JOHANN A German painter who had a beard which touched the ground when he stood up.

MAYPOLE CURL A spiral curl.

MAZZARD Head; also head of hair. 16th century S W England usage. 'I'll mall his old mazzard with this hammer –.' (*Woodstock*, ed A P Rossiter. ed 1946)

MEANDER (1) Subs. Ornament, linear or curvilinear, which winds in and out.

(2) Verb. To wind in and out.

MEANE FASHION A 16th century hair style for men. (*Stubbes*)

MEASUREMENTS The needful head measurements for a postiche are – for a wig: circumference; ear to ear over

forehead; ear to ear over top; temple to temple round the back of the head; forehead to nape; width of nape. For a transformation: circumference; ear to ear over forehead.

MEASURING The act of measuring the head for a postiche.

MEAT AXE A beard style, straight and wide at the bottom, 17th century. (*Mitchell*)

MECHANICAL HAIRBRUSH A type of rotary brush driven by a belt suspended from a wheel or a shaft over each client's chair and rotated by a lather boy turning a wheel at the end of the saloon.

MECHANICAL WIGMAKER A wigmaker who manufactures wigs by machinery, 19th century. 'John Stevens, theatrical, mechanical and private wigmaker. 67 Wine Street, Bristol.' See also Private Wigmaker and Theatrical Wigmaker.

MECHE DE CHEVEUX Fr – Lock of hair.

MECKLENBURGH CURL A drop curl, *qv*. (*The Bristol Journal*, 15 August 1767)

MEDICAMENTOSUS Dermatitis, *qv*.

MEDICATED SHAMPOO Any shampoo which contains tar, alcohol, sulphur or any other ingredient that possesses or is thought to possess some medicinal property.

MEDICATED SOAP In the 19th century this was prepared by adding a medicament such a sulphur, iodine, bromine, creosote or castor oil, and many others, to curd soap. (*Piesse*)

MEDIEVAL HAIR STYLES Styles as worn between *c* 476 and 1453. Unmarried girls usually wore their hair hanging free and partly exposed. Married women had their heads covered.

MEDIUM The material in which the hairdresser works, ie human hair and in the 20th century sometimes synthetic hair. Hair is known as the hairdresser's medium.

MEDULLA The pith or central axis of the hair shaft, composed of soft, round cells. Air bubbles, forming among the cells of this layer turn the hair white by reflection of light. This layer is not present in the short, fine body hairs.

MEDULLARY Pertaining to the medulla of the hair.

MEDULLATED HAIR Hair with a medulla.

MEDUSA One of the Gorgons whose head was covered with entwined snakes. Head of Snakes. See also Medusa wig.

MEDUSA-TETE An 18th century over-ornamented wig, locks of its hair twisted and standing out, snake-like, from the head. (*Miscellanies*, *Johnson*, 1773)

MEDUSA-WIG A wig dressed in 'a mass of snake-like curls'. 1800–2. (*Cunnington*, *Procter* 169). See also Medusa.

MEGAERA One of the furies in classical mythology, depicted with snaky locks. (*Settle*, E, *Pastor Fido . . . a pastoral*, 1677)

MEGARENSIAN VIRGINS Offered their hair with libations at the monument of Iphince, daughter of Alcathous, who died a virgin. (*Potter*)

MELACOMIA A 19th century proprietary hair and whisker dye manufactured by Rowland & Sons, London.

MELANIN The dark colouring matter which gives colour to the hair and skin.

MELCHISEDEK AND LOT The traditional play of the Barbers Company at Whitsuntide. (*The Graphical Historical Illustrated*, 1832)

MELROSE'S NEW HAIR WASH See Plumbiferous hair wash.

MENNONITE HAIR STYLES The Mennonites, a religious sect founded by Menno Simon in 1536, have a strong following in Pennsylvania, USA.

Men: Long hair parted in the middle and combed down smoothly, ending in curls over the ears neatly. Front hair sometimes cut to a fringe. Bearded, but upper lip shaven.

Women: Long hair parted in the middle and combed smoothly toward the temple, where two plaits are started, carried around and gathered into a knot just under the edge of the white mule cap above the nape of the neck.

MEPHISTOPHELES BEARD A medium long, sharp-pointed beard. Mephistopheles was the sneering, tempting devil in Goethe's *Faust*.

MEPHISTOPHELES MOUSTACHE A long waxed moustache protruding beyond the corners of the mouth and inclined upwards towards the top of the ears.

MERCURY BICHLORIDE A powerful germicide. Poisonous and corrosive.

MERK See Merkin (2).

MERKIN (1) Counterfeit hair for a woman's privy parts, 17th century. (*Phillips*) A pubic wig. From the French, Mére, a mother, and kin, a diminutive. (*Bailey*). This 17th century device enjoyed a renewed popularity in the 20th century. During and for a period after World War II Neapolitan ladies of pleasure not only bleached their pubic hair, but also wore merkins to provide the blondness demanded by some soldier clients. (*Malaparte*). A 16th century reference to this device occurs in *Tom Longe*, a ballad preserved in Bishop Percy's folio manuscript (ed *F J Furnivall* 1868).

It is
'A health to all ladies that never used merkin,
Yet their stuffe ruffles like Buff lether Jerkin!'
(2) Until after 1910 the expression 'stupid merk' was used euphemistically in some Bristol barbers' saloons as a term of reproach. (*Ivor Westlake*). (3) A small moustache. Officers' banter, 1914–1918 war, referring to a diminutive moustache. 'I don't like your merkin'. (*E Partridge*)

MERKIN COMB A small comb for the merkin. 17th century. (*Holme*)

MERKIN THATCHER A whoremonger. Slang. Somerset, 19/20th century.

MEROVINGIAN HAIRCUT Hair long and tapered and combed over the forehead with no parting. (*Envoy* May 1968)

MERRY WIDOW HAIRDRESS A loosely dressed coiffure of waves and loose fluffy curl. So named after the light opera *The Merry Widow* by Franz Lehar, the Hungarian composer, produced 1905.

MESH One of the open spaces or interstices of a wig net.

MESSALINA Wife of the Roman Emperor Claudius. A woman with a reputation for profligacy who disguised herself in different wigs for her nightly expeditions of debauchery.

METALLIC Made of or relating to metal.

METALLIC BOWL A bowl made of metal. Care should be taken not to mix dyes, bleaches or permanent waving preparations in metallic bowls.

METALLIC DYE A dye in which is incorporated a metallic salt. See Mineral dye.

METIER The particular branch of hairdressing in which the hairdresser specialises; ie Dyeing, Hair styling, Cutting, etc.

MEURTRIERES Fr-Murderers. A certain knot in the hair which ties and unites the curls. (*Evelyn*)

MEXICAN HAIR RENEWER A colour restorer popular in the 19th century. Precipitated Sulphur 1.4%; Lead Acetate 0.13%; and Glycerine 19.0%; Rosewater 79.47%. (*Stevens Ms*)

MEXICAN HAIR STYLE The prevailing hair fashion of Aztec women at the time of the conquest by the Spaniards in 1519 was dressed in two raised loops above the forehead, rather like small horns. (See *Codex Azcatitlan*. Plates V, XI, etc)

MEXICAN MOUSTACHE A thin, drooping moustache dressed along, but not covering, the upper lip and the ends turned down at either side of the mouth.

MICHEL KAZAN See Kazan, Michel.

MICROBE A minute, one-celled, vegetable bacterium.

MICROCEPHALIC Adj. Subs. Abnormally small headed.

MICROCEPHALOUS Having an imperfectly developed, or small head.

MIDDLEDITCH The last operative barber surgeon in London, d 1821. See Barber surgeon.

MIDGET CURLER Very small curler or roller used in hair setting and permanent waving on which the short hair of the neck is wound.

MIGAREE'S MOUSTACHE BALSAM A 19th/20th century 'secret' preparation compounded of fat and resin. (*Killer*)

MILITARY (1) An English moustache style 20th century. (*Foan*)
(2) An English hair style for men 20th century. (*Foan*)

MILITARY COMB A medium length, short toothed comb with fine teeth one end and coarse teeth the other slightly tapering towards the claw tooth of the fine end. Used during cutting processes, especially when cutting over the comb.

MILITARY HAIR BRUSH A hair brush with no handle used by men.

MILITARY MOUSTACHE (1) A moustache as worn by soldiers. The original reason for the soldier wearing a moustache was to give him a fierce appearance. The Gauls, in the Roman period, wore large dangling moustaches. In modern times they were first worn by the Hungarian Hussars in the 18th century and the fashion was soon followed by the French Hussars when it was obligatory for every soldier to adopt the fashion of a bristly, ragged type. Hussars unable to grow a satisfactory walrus had to paint one on the face. The French General, Macard, is recorded by Marbot as saying, apropos wearing a shaggy moustache, 'Look here! I'm going to dress like a beast,' and he stripped to a minimum, exposing a shaggy head, face and body. The British soldiers at the time of the Peninsular War (1808–1814) shaved the upper lip, but it was immediately after this that moustaches began to appear in the British army, probably as a result of contact with continental soldiery during the occupation. By 1828 the practice of wearing moustaches had become common. No regiment of cavalry was without the moustache and it had extended to the infantry, but in 1830 an order was issued which forbade the growing of a moustache except by Household Cavalry and Hussars.

By an order dated 21 July 1854, the wearing of the moustache again became optional with all ranks and has so continued to 1983. See also Poilu.
(2) A moustache style worn by civilians but based on the military fashion of the period. In the 19th century this was bushy, but in the 20th century the various styles were generally close cut.   *101Y*

MILITARY WIG A powdered wig worn by officers in the British Army, and first noticed by Pepys in November 1663. They were discontinued in 1808. See Queue (2).
161, 402

MILK, SKIMMED See Skimmed milk.

MILK-CHOPPED Beardless.

MINERAL Any inorganic natural substance found in the earth's crust.

MINERAL DYE (Metallic dye) Mineral dyes form a metallic

coating over the hair and dye progressively. Continual application will result in brittle hair of unnatural shades. Dyes containing lead turn black, those containing copper turn red, and those containing silver turn green. Permanent curling could not be successfully achieved on hair dyed with these mineral dyes as it either broke or assumed an unnatural colour.

MINERAL OIL Liquid hydrocarbons obtained from petroleum. Insoluble in water and largely insoluble in alcohol. (*De Navarre*)

MINER'S BEARD A long beard cut straight across at the ends. French style *c* 1912.   *102G*

MINGLE A short hair style for women, based on the shingle with 'mingling' waves and curls *c* 1930.

MINIPERM The permanent waving of only a part of a head of hair, *c* 1930.

MINISTER'S BOB A man's 18th century wig style. See Long bob. (*Dublin Gazette*, 1724)

MINNIKEN, JOHN B Maryport, Cumberland, in 1681; d 1793 aged 112. He was remarkable for the fast growth and profusion of his hair which he sold in several croppings to a wigmaker of the town for a penny a day. More than seventy wigs were made from his hair. (*Timbs* 1872)

MINOR BOB An 18th century wig style for men.

MINSTREL WIG A black, short curly haired wig worn by minstrels in the minstrel shows of the 19th/early 20th century.

MIRLITON Short hair in fluted curls dressed around the head, *c* 1760.

MIRON The Greek sculptor who at 70 years of age fell in love with Lois. After she had rejected him he returned the next day with his locks dyed black and renewed his suit. 'How can I,' said Lois, 'grant thee to-day what I refused to thy father yesterday.' (*Speight*)

MIRROR A polished glass surface that reflects images of objects. Anciently made of polished bronze. A looking glass.

MIRROR, ADJUSTABLE A mirror which is supported on adjustable arms and thus can be moved into any position.

MIRROR, HAND A small mirror with a handle, used to reflect the back of the hairdress in the wall mirror or adjustable mirror.

MIRROR, SHAVING A magnifying mirror.

MIRROR, WALL A large mirror of any convenient shape, fixed in front of the client in a hairdressing saloon.

MISCIBLE Capable of being mixed with some other substance or liquid

MIS-CURLING Bad curling.

MISE-EN-PLI 'Putting into set.' Setting. French phrase from *mettre* = to put, and *plier* = to bend. See also Pli.

MISOPOGON A hater of beards. Julian, the apostate *c* 362 ad, was one such.

MISPLACED EYEBROW A narrow moustache. Slang American usage. (*B and B*)

MISTLETOE MOUSTACHE A moustache consisting of two narrow crescentic inverted wings. (*Trusty*)   *101N*

MITE A minute insect or arachnid.

MITRA HEAD-DRESS A woman's hair style of the Graeco-Romano period. (*Rimmel*)   *341*

MITRED HEAD-DRESS See Horned head dress.

MIXED WINDING Spiral (root to point) and Croquignole (point to root) winding on the same head.

MIXING (1) The mixing or intermingling of hairs of different shades, colour, qualities or lenghts to produce a required uniform blend for use in boardwork.
(2) The mixing and preparation of hair dye, bleach or permanent waving lotion, etc.

MIXTURE A blend of two or more ingredients.

MIZZLED Adj. Having hair of different colours. Scottish usage. 'A mizzled head of hair.' (*Henderson*)

MOANA BOB A woman's hair style of 1926, comprising a short cut exposing the ears, with a finger of hair resting on the cheek immediately in front of each ear; a curved fringe, the bulk of hair combed to a pomadour, with a shadow wave.   *414*

MOBILE HAIRDO Any hair style, with long or short hair, that permits the free movement of the hair. See Static hairdo. (*Vito*)

MODE The manner of dressing the hair. The way the hair is styled; the prevailing fashion in hairdress or costume.

MODEL (1) Any object that a hairdresser works by or copies, either after nature or otherwise, in his design for a hair style.
(2) The person or artificial head on which the hairdresser or wigmaker models or displays his hair creation.

MODIGLIANI LOOK A very high hair style for women, 1962. 'Like a long-stemmed flower.'

MOD-LINE A modern hair style. An up-to-date hairdo.

MOHAIR The fine, silky hair of the Angora goat, *qv*. Used for fantasy, theatrical wigs and added postiches for head ornamentation. Takes dye readily.   *425*

MOHAIR CREPE Crêped mohair.

MOHAIR WIG Worn by coachmen in the 18th/19th century. (*Simmonds*)

MOHICAN CUT A man's hair style in which the head is shaven each side leaving a narrow band of short hair standing erect from the forehead to the nape, called the pawnee ridge. Inspired by American Western films and affected by virile groups of aggressively dressed youths, *c* 1960–1980.

MOISTENER A substance such as glycerine that is blended with a permanent waving solution to reduce the risk of dryness or frizz.

MOISTURIZER PERMANENT WAVE A permanent wave in which the solution contains ingredients which reduce risk of dryness and frizz. (*Johnson*)

MONGOLIAN HAIR Dark coloured, straight hair.

MONILETHRIX A disease of the hair, usually hereditary, in which the hair shaft is alternately swollen and constricted. Also called beaded hair, because of its peculair beaded appearance. (*McCarthy*)

MONKS' tonsure See Tonsure.

MONOCHROME Colouring executed in different tones of one colour.

MONSIEUR POWDER-WIG A foppish character in a poem of 1640. See how his perfumed head is powder'd o'er.

MONTAGUE (American) A pin curl mounted on a hairpin. (*Moler* p 86)

MONTAGUE CURLS The front hair dressed in a crescent-shaped fringe of curls stuck to the forehead. 1877+ (*Cunnington*)

MONTESPAN A woman's hair style of the time of Louis XIV, named after Madame de Montespan, mistress of Louis XIV. (*Bysterveld* p 71)

MONT-LA-HAUT Fr. The same as Commode, *qv*. (*Ladies Dicy*, 1694)

MOORISH-GREY HAIR Grey hair consisting of 75% black and 25% white. (*Symonds*)

MOP Untidy hair on head. Slang.

MOPHEAD (1) Untidy hair on head; slang.
(2) A person with untidy or unkempt hair. Slang.

MOP OF HAIR A thick, untidy growth of hair.

MOP-TOP Long, untidy hair of the beatnik.

MORDANT A chemical which, when combined with a dye, forms a fixed colour.

MORE, REV JOHN An Elizabethan clergyman of Norwich who was reputed to have had the longest and largest beard in England at that time. (*Gowing*)

MORE, SIR THOMAS On laying his head on the block, preparatory to being beheaded, carefully moved aside his long beard, asking that it be spared as it, at least, had not offended the King. (*Speight*)

MORNING HEAD-DRESS A hairdress suitable for wear in the morning; 18th/19th century. Females of the fashionable Leisured Class often changed their hair styles three times a day in the Victorian and Edwardian periods. *85A*

MORPHEW A scurfy eruption. (43Ben Jonson, *Timber* 1641)

MORPHOEA ALOPECIATA Patchy baldness. (*Wheeler*)

MOSS (1) Head hair. Slang.
(2) Pubic hair. Vulgarism.

MOSS HEAD A person with thick, short, very curly hair. Slang. Southern England.

MOSS ON THE BOSOM Hair on the chest. American slang. (*B and B*)

MOSSY HAIR Fine, down-like hair on the chin of an adolescent. 16th/17th century. (*Percival*)

MOSY Downy, hairy. (*Levens* 1570)

MOTIF The dominant or distinctive element in a hairdress.

MOTTO A barber character in Lyly's *Midas*, 1591.

MOUCHE Fr. Fly. Patch (on the face); beauty spot. See Charley (1)

MOULD (1) Verb. To form into a shape.
(2) Subs. The head shape moulded in plaster of Paris; essential before making a scalpette for an abnormally shaped head and desirable to obtain the best results before making a scalpette for a normally shaped head.
(3) Top of the head. Dorset usage. (*Barnes*)

MOULDED COMB A comb formed in a mould, *cf* Saw-cut comb.

MOUNT The foundation of a postiche. It includes the net, gauze and galloon on which the hair is anchored by knotting, or sewing in the case of a weft postiche.

MOUNTER A person who puts the mount of a postiche into position on a wooden block by means of braces and block points.

MOUNTER'S PLIERS Small pliers used in boardwork, especially to remove blockpoints from a wooden block.

MOUNTING BLOCK A head-shaped, wooden block used to mount the foundations of wigs and other types of postiche in the process of wigmaking.

MOUNTING CORD A fine cord or thread used as the foundation of switches and around which the weft is wound, forming the stem. Macramé linen thread was commonly used as mounting cord.

MOUNTING HAMMER A small hammer with a thick handle about 5″ long, the head having two round faces, one being ¼″, the other ½″ in diameter. Used for hammering block points when mounting a wig foundation on a wooden wig block. 19th century.

MOUNTING MACHINE See Winding machine.

MOUNTING WIRE Thin wire for mounting postiches. (*Brodie, Price List*, 1890) See Weaving wire.

MOUNTJOY A wigmaker in Silver Street, Cripplegate, London. In 1605 William Shakespeare is reputed to have lodged with him. (*Standen*)

MOURNING COIFFURE A hair style suitable for the period of mourning after a bereavement. The style varies in different countries and is chiefly influenced by religion.

MOUSE-EATEN BEARD A beard that grows whispily with but here and there a tuft. 'growth scatteringly . . . here a tuft and there a tuft.' 16th–17th century. (*Holme*)

MOUSE TAIL A pencil-line thin moustache. Slang, American usage. (*B and B*)

MOUSE TRAP For catching mice that nibbled perukes for the starch and wheat flour. 18th century.

MOUSQUETAIRE Fr-Musketeer. (1) A light fixing liquid for the training of the moustache. Manufactured by E H Thiellay, London, *c* 1875.
(2) See à la Mousquetaire.
(3) See Musketeer beard.

MOUSSE Fr-Froth, foam, lather.

MOUSTACHE (MUSTACHE) (1) The hair growing on the upper lip. The form 'moustache' is now generally used, but 'mustache' was used until late 19th century and was more in accordance with the root, namely the Greek *mustax-the upper lip*, also the hair growing on it. Moustache is the French form of the same word.
The Worcestershire Militia in 1798 are reputed to have been the first English Regiment to wear moustaches. (*Reynolds*) *101, 469*
(2) The long curled lock of head hair hanging down the side of the cheek. 17th century. (*Villermont*)
(3) The hair growing on either side of the upper lip. See Pair-of-Moustaches.
'He twirled first one moustache and then the other' (*Mason, The Four Feathers*, 1902)
(4) The longest moustache of a man recorded was that of Masuriya Din (b 1916) of Uttar Pradesh, India. From 1949 to 1962 it grew to an extended span of 8′ 6″.

MOUSTACHE-BALSAM A 19th/20th century 'secret' preparation for promoting the growth of the beard, consisting of fat, wax and scent. It was utterly useless for its avowed purpose. (*Koller*)

MOUSTACHE-BAND A shaped band of cloth or other suitable material secured around the head by tying or elastic and used to set the moustache in position. German officers in the army of the Kaiser commonly used this apparatus. *101W*

MOUSTACHE CLIP A small clip which grips the central wall of the nose and holds a joke or theatrical moustache in position.

MOUSTACHE COMB A type of small comb for dressing and placing the moustache.

MOUSTACHE CUP A cup with a partial cover to protect the moustache when drinking. 19th/20th century. *245*

MOUSTACHED Having a moustache. 'His moustached lip looked fearsome.'

MOUSTACHE FIXATIVE A preparation for keeping the moustache in position; usually manufactured from pomades with added beeswax or ceresine, perfumed and coloured to taste.

MOUSTACHE FIXER See Moustache fixative; also Moustache clip.

MOUSTACHE IRONS A small pair of irons used to curl the moustache. 18th/20th century.

MOUSTACHE IRRITATION See *Pruritus Mystax*.

MOUSTACHELESS Without a moustache.

MOUSTACHE-LIFTER An implement shaped like a paper knife and used by the male hairy ainu of Japan when drinking, to lift his moustache away from the liquid.

MOUSTACHE PLANT Caryopteris. A shrubby perennial plant.

MOUSTACHE STYLES See Captain, Consort, General, Guardsman, Major, Military, Regent, Ronald Coleman, Shadow, etc.

MOUSTACHE TRAINER See Moustache band.

MOUSTACHE-WAX Various mixtures of white beeswax and pomades were used in the 19th century to fix the hairs of the moustache in position.

MOUSTACHIAL Resembling a moustache.

MOVEMENT OF HAIR Hair movement is understood by the craft to mean the direction in which the groups of hairs in a hairdress are lying, 'backward movement of loose wave'. The term does not imply that the hair is moving.

MOWCHATOWES Moustaches, 16th century. (*Stubbes*)

MR SNIPS A barber.

MR TONSOR A barber, 18th century. (*The Barber's Wedding*)

MRS FRIZZLE (1) A wig. 18th century slang. (*Goldsmith*) (2) A barberess.

MUCILAGE A viscous substance derived from certain gummy secretions of plants or from the roots and seeds of plants by maceration in water. Gum. Many hair setting lotions are mucilaginous.

MUCKASEES The two hair locks that hang down each side of an Egyptian woman's face. They are often curled in ringlets and sometimes plaited. (*Lane*)

MUCOSUM (or MALPHIGHIAN) Layer of the epidermis; contains the colouring matter or pigment.

MUFF (1) A large diameter, thick walled, heavy, side curl, *cf* Bunch.
(2) A false beard, also the natural beard. Slang American usage. (*B and B*)
(3) A film extra with a natural beard. American slang. (*B and B*)
(4) A woman's private parts. Bristol slang. 20th century.
(5) The pubic hairs. (*The Muse in Good Humour*, 1746)

MUFF OF HAIR A puffy postiche hair addition. A kind of chignon. (*Hairdo*, Jan 1965)

MUG A pottery, porcelain, glass or metal vessel, with or without a handle, used for holding shaving soap and hot water.

MUHAMMAD'S HAIR A hair of Muhammad is preserved as a holy relic in the Hazratbal Mosque on the shore of Dal Lake, Kashmir.

MULDER'S HAIR BALSAM A 19th/20th century 'secret' preparation consisting of an aqueous solution of rose leaves, with about 5% of carbolic acid. (**Koller**)

MULIEBRAL WIG A woman's wig.

MULLEIN (*Verbascum Thaupsus*) A plant with large mucilaginous leaves and long flower spike bearing plain yellow flowers. An infusion of the flowers was used by the Romans to tinge their hair a golden yellow. In the 19th century used in Germany as a hair restorer. (*Fernie*)

MULTI-COLOURED HAIR Hair of many colours. See also variegated hair.

MULTIFOIL A many-loved grouping of hair.

MULTI-SPILL SWITCH A switch made of two or more spills. Two spills for coiling, three or more spills for plaiting.

MULTI-STEM SWITCH A hair switch composed of four or more spills or stems.

MURDERER See Meurtrière.

MUSCLE CURL See Poker curl.

MUSH BRUSH A bushy moustache. Slang, American usage. (*B and B*)

MUSHROOM (1) A wig-stand in the shape of a mushroom. 19th/20th century.
(2) A teenage hair style, 1962.

MUSHROOM HAIR STYLE See Toadstool.

MUSK (1) An aromatic secretion from a gland of the musk deer. It is a valuable fixative for stabilising other odours in the manufacture of perfumes.
(2) Hair powder. Scottish usage. (*Henderson*)

MUSK HAIR POWDER A starch hair powder, scented with musk. (*Lillie*)

MUSK SOAP Soap scented with musk. (*Pears*)

MUSKBALL A ball of musk-scented soap, or a receptacle in which musk can be carried about the person. 16th/19th century.

MUSKETEER BEARD A medium length pointed beard. 17th century.

MUST Hair powder. Scottish usage. (*Henderson*)

MUSTACHE Modern American usage; also a 19th century English spelling of moustache, *qv*. (*Webster*)

MUSTACHIO Archaic usage for moustache, *qv*. 16th/17th century.

MUSTACHIO BEARD A moustache.

MUSTACHIOED *qv*.

MUSTACHO(E) Moustache. 16th/17th century.

MUSTACHO HAIRES The hairs of the moustache. 16th/17th century.

MUSTARD The bland oil expressed from the hulls of the seeds of black mustard (*Sinapis nigra*), after the flower has been sifted away. Believed to promote the growth of hair. (*Fernie*)

MUTCH Headdress for a woman. Scottish usage. (*Henderson*)

MUTTON CHOP WHISKERS Side whiskers, rounded at the ends, resembling mutton chops.   97F, 192

MUZZLER The beard. 18th century slang. (*Grose*)

MYSTAX The hair on the upper lip. (*Good*)

MYTHOLOGIC HEADDRESS A hairdress in the styles attributed to the ancient gods and goddesses of Greece and Rome.

N

NAEVIUS, C Latin poet, 3rd century BC who, to convince the Romans of his power as an augur, cut a flint with a razor. Tarquin erected a statue in his honour and the razor and flint were buried near it under an altar. It was usual among the Romans to make witnesses in civil causes swear near the monument. This miraculous event of cutting a flint with a razor was treated as fabulous and improbable by Cicero.

NAGA Tribes, formerly head hunters, inhabiting the hill country on the border of Assam and Burma. The females have shaven heads until marriage.

NAIAD, THE A woman's hair style of 1865. Named after the Naiads of mythology, the water nymphs. (*Bysterveld*, p 60)

NAIL A horny protective covering of modified epidermis formed upon the top surface of the terminal phalanges of the fingers, thumbs and toes of man.

NAIL BED That part of the skin beneath the visible nail, and on which it is bedded.

NAIL BITER A compulsive self-biter of finger nails.

NAIL ENAMEL See Nail lacquer.

NAIL GROOVE The furrowed grooves adjacent to the nail-wall at both sides of the nail edges.

NAIL LACQUER Nitrocellulose dissolved in butyl acetate and allied substances forming, when dry, a hard, tough, resistant film on the surface of the nail. (*Sagarin*)

NAIL MATRIX The part of the nail-bed from which the nail grows at the nail root.

NAIL ROOT The point from which the nail grows at its base beneath the skin.

NAIL VARNISH See Nail lacquer.

NAIL WALL The folding skin overlapping each side of the nail.

NAME BARRETTE A decorative hair clip or bar slide with the wearer's name on the upper prong.

NAME BOBBY PIN See Name Barrette.

NAMED HAIR STYLE A distinctive hair style that has been named, or for which, over the years, a name has evolved. See Hair Style Names.

NANNOTRICHIA Deformed hair; stunted growth of hair. (*Wheeler*)

NAPE (1) The back part of the neck.
(2) The lower back part of the head immediately adjacent to and including the neck.

NAPLES SOAP A soft soap imported from Naples in the 19th century. (*Lillie*)

NAPLES SOFT SOAP A fish oil, mixed with lucca oil and potash, coloured brown for the London shavers. (*Piesse*)

NAPOLEON A hair style of the 1960s for men. Combed onto the forehead and imitative of the style worn by Napoleon the Great of France.

NAPOLEON III BEARD See Imperial.

NAPPER The head. 18th century slang. (*Grose*)

NAPPY Slang name for a barber in India; early 1900.

NARCISSUS A beautiful mythical youth, son of Cephisus and Liriope. He fell in love with his own reflection in a fountain, thinking it to be the nymph of the place. His fruitless attempts to embrace the image so provoked him that he committed suicide and his blood was transformed into a flower, which still bears his name.

NARCISSUS OIL A yellow volatile oil of disagreeable odour, and a brown colouring matter from the flowers of the narcissus (*N Bertolonii*) has been used by the Arabs for curing baldness and for stimulating the sexual organs. (*Fernie*)

NARTHECIUM OSSIFRAGUM Used as a hairdye. See Maidenhair. (*B and B*)

NATAL A beard style, 20th century. (*Gent's Acad.*)

NATIONAL HEALTH WIG A wig or other similar postiche of necessity supplied by a wigmaker for a client whose health is said to be affected by lack of hair, to the order of the Ministry of Health.

NATRON A native carbonate of soda.

NATTE Fr-Plait of hair.

NATURAL A man's 18th century wig style. (*Dublin Gazette*, 1724)

NATURAL BEND Natural curl. 18th century.
'Don't let your curls fall with that natural bend,
But stretch them tight till each hair stands on end.' (*Venus Attiring the Graces*, 1777)

NATURAL BUSH A natural beard, uncut, untrimmed. (*Taylor*)

NATURAL DISPOSITION OF HEAD HAIR In a natural state the hair of the head hangs in tresses from the crown of the head, falling over the face like a veil, and over the shoulders and back like a mantle.   *354*

NATURAL FLY An 18th century wig style worn by country gentlemen. (*Stewart*)

NATURAL HAIR Hair that is grown by nature as opposed to synthetic hair, made by the art of man.

NATURAL HENNA Henna powder from the crushed leaves of *Lawsonia Inermis*, without any additions.

NATURALISTIC A faithful representation of nature in art.

NATURAL PARTING (1) The line at which the hair parts when it is combed straight back and allowed to fall of its own accord on either side of this line.
(2) A natural looking drawn-through parting of a postiche.

NATURAL SKIN PARTING A wig parting drawn through a fabric that has the appearance of natural skin. Used from before 1884 by John Stevens (my grandfather), wigmaker, Bristol, who advertised 'New style of complete wig, with natural skin parting. Price £8 8s 0d. and £10 10s 0d' at that date.

NATURAL WAVE CUT See Wave cut.

NATURAL WIG 18th century man's wig style. (*Garsault*)
91 (10.11)

NAVAL BEARD The regulation requiring naval officers and men to be clean shaven or 'discontinue the use of the razor entirely' was made, by admiralty letter, in 1869.

NAVAL QUEUE The wig tail or queue, *qv*, as worn by naval officers in the 18th century.

NAZARENE FORETOP The foretop of a wig made in imitation of Christ's head of hair as represented by painters and sculptors. 18th century slang. (*Grose*)

NAZARITES Jews of antiquity who were forbidden to touch their heads with a razor or drink wine. They are depicted with long curls. (*Speight*)

NEAT CURD SOAP A good lathering tallow soap. 19th century. An ingredient was neat's foot oil. (*Lillie*)

NEBULY HEADDRESS A woman's headdress of the reign of Edward II (1327–1377), consisting of a close-fitting cap with a broad crimped border hanging down either side of the face to below the chin, completely concealing all head hair. (*Gardiner*)

NECESSITY PIECE Postiche worn because of baldness or other real need, in contrast with that worn for fashionable purposes. (*N and N*)

NECESSITY WIG A wig to cover baldness or other natural deficiency of hair, *cf* Fashion wig.

NECK BRUSH Small, soft bristle brush to remove hair cuttings from the neck.

NECK COIFFURE A hair style of the 1890s in which the hair is combed up from the neck and back from the forehead (pompadour) to be gathered in curls on top of the head, exposing fully the neck. (*Mallemont*)

NECK COMB (1) A small comb worn at the neck to prevent short ends hanging on the neck.
(2) A fine-toothed comb for use when cutting and graduating hair on the neck. American usage. (*Smith*)

NECK HAIR The hair which grows in the region of the neck.

NECKLINE Subs. (1) That part of the neck where the hair growth begins. See Hair Line.
(2) The outline at the neck of a cut head of hair.

NECK LOCK (1) An 18th century wig style in which a hanging lock at the neck formed a distinctive feature.
(2) The vertical curl at the neck of a barrister's wig.

NECKPIECE (1) A chignon. American usage.
(2) See Neck strip.

NECK ROLL (1) The ends of the natural hair worn in a roll at the nape.
(2) A postiche worn at the nape. Also called neck piece.

NECK SPRING A flattened, metallic, coiled spring incorporated in the bind of wigs and transformations to secure them firmly in position on the head.

NECK STRIP A strip of cotton wool or crêpe-type paper wrapped around the neck to prevent cut hair slipping beneath the client's clothing.

NECK WOOL A strip of cotton wool placed around the neck to prevent cut hairs slipping beneath the client's clothes and causing irritation. See also Neck strip.

NECK-WOOL URN A container in which is kept a long strip of neck-wool, from which can be detached a sufficient quantity for encircling a client's neck as needed.

NEEDLE An iron curling rod. 'haire . . . with a hot needle you shall learne it to crispe.' 16th century. (*Wager*)

NEEDLE-BEARD (1) A long, finely pointed beard, 16th century. (*Repton*)

(2) Also Pin beard and Finger bleeder; a very tough beard that often caused the fingers of the lather boys to bleed; the barber continually exhorting them to 'rub in the lather well'.

NEEDLE COMB A tail comb with a thin metal spike for a tail.

NEEDLE GUIDE Finger shield, *qv*.

NEEDLE ROOTER A rooting machine in which a row of contiguous needles formed the stops for the root ends of the hair during the process of rooting.

NEGATIVE CHEEK WAVE A wave that recedes from the cheek.

NEGATIVE SKIN TEST When no skin reaction is apparent after the application of hair dye on a small patch of skin, the test is said to be negative.

NEGLECTED LOCK A loose, free and easy lock of curly hair. A lock of hair deliberately dressed in an untidy fashion. 19th century.

NEGLIGEE, THE See En-negligée.

NEGLIGENT A man's 18th century wig style. (*London Mag*, 1753)

NEGRO HAIR Hair that is frizzy and black.

NEO-ELIZABETHAN A person or article of Britain of the period of Elizabeth II, Queen of England.

NEPTUNE OR NEPTUNUS Roman god of water, son of Saturn and Ops and brother to Jupiter, Pluto and Juno. He was famous for his blue tinted hair, emblematic of his power over the ocean. (*Stukeley*)

Depicted by the ancients with marvellous long hair hanging down over his shoulders, of a very sad and darkish colour. (*Salmon*)

NEPTUNIAN-BEARD A tripartite, fork-shaped beard.

NESTLE SYSTEM The first permanent waving system, invented by Charles Nessler, London hairdresser of Swiss birth, and first publicly offered in 1906. It consisted of borax pads and a gas heater. The hair was wound spirally. In an advertisement in the London Coliseum Sarah Bernhardt souvenir programme of 16 September 1912. C Nestlé and Co, 48 South Molton Street, London, W announced that in 1906 they had waved, with their permanent hair-waving method, 74 heads; in 1908, 108; in 1911, 2,713; and in 1912 to September of that year, more than 5,400.

NET That which is knotted and has interstices between the intersections. Used to make wig and other postiche foundations, the hair being either knotted on the net or, as weft, sewn onto it. See Hair net, Wig net, etc.

NET CURLER A circular, net-covered, wire curler consisting of two hinged circles 1¾″ in diameter to hold a set finger-formed curl in position until dry. 20th century.

NET FOUNDATION A postiche foundation of net which may be of silk, cotton or nylon.

NETTER'S BEARD TINCTURE A 19th/20th century 'secret' preparation which consisted of linseed oil, castor oil, charcoal, saltpetre, with a little sulphur and powdered bread crust. (*Koller*)

NEUROTIC ALOPECIA Baldness due to emotional distress.

NEUTRAL COLOUR A colour such as grey, that has no positive hue.

NEUTRALIZATION The interaction of an acid and a base to form a salt and water. But this word is often used loosely in hairdressing circles to indicate the completion of a development by the addition of another chemical, or the stabilizing of a chemical in a permanent waving process, or the ending of a chemical action by the addition of another substance. When an acid hair rinse is used to neutralize any residual alkali on the hair after a shampoo neutralization would be the correct description; but hydrogen peroxide used in the cold-waving process as an oxidation reagent is not a neutralizer although it is often incorrectly referred to as such.

NEUTRALIZER That which neutralizes, *qv*.

NEUTRAL OIL BLEACH A bleach incorporating oil that has neither an acid nor an alkaline reaction.

NEVADA WHISKERS Long, ragged whiskers, 19th century. American usage. 'How one would enjoy seeing a man – a real one with Nevada whiskers.' (*Leacock, S B; Further Foolishness*)

NEVUS LIPOMARODES A disease of the sebaceous gland in the form of a wen.

NEVUS PILOSUS A mole with a growth of downy hair.

NEW BALSAMIC HAIR DYE See Plumbiferous hair water.

NEWE CUT 16th century hair style for men. (*Stubbes*)

NEWGATE FRINGE A beard growing below the shaven chin.

NEWGATE KNOCKER A beard style. (*Mitchell*)

NEWGATE KNOCKERS The diminished side locks of hair hanging down the cheeks in front of the ears. In the late 18th century, early 19th century worn by men. 'The so-called 'Newgate-Knockers', affected by the vulgar classes of London.' (*King, E, Old Times Revisited*, 1879)

NEW LONDON HAIR RESTORER See Plumbiferous hair wash.

NIDDICK The nape or back part of the neck, also applied to the back of the head and even the head itself. 'A gurt hump 'pon the niddick o'un so big's duck-egg.' West Somerset usage. (*Elworthy*)

NIESKE'S PATENT BIRCH-OIL BALSAM See Plumbiferous hair water.

NIGGER WOOL Negro hair. Slang, American usage. (*B and B*)

NIGHTCAP (1) A covering for the head to keep it warm, or protect the hairdress. See Sleeping net.

(2) A cloche of silver wire to enclose the large wigs of the 18th century and protect them from mice during the night. ('No mouse or even a rat can gnaw through them'.) (*Salisbury Journal*, 1777)

NIGHT-CAP PERIWIG A wig mode adopted by 18th century lawyers in the Court of Common Pleas. (*Connoisseur*, 24 April 1755)

NIGHT-NET See Sleeping net.

NIMBO HEADDRESS An ancient Greek headdress for women. (*Rimmel*)   *341*

NIMBUS An early Roman hair style for women. (*Rimmel*)   *341*

NINON DE LENCLOS A woman's hair style worn by and named after Ninon de Lenclos, of the Court of Louis XIII. (*Bysterveld*, p 72)   *361*

NISUS'S HAIR Nisus was a mythological figure, King of Megara, son of Mars. His fate depended on a single lock, which as long as it grew upon his head, according to an oracle, promised him life and success. His daughter removed it and Nisus was changed into a hawk at the moment of death. (*Lemprière*), *cf* Sampson.

NIT The egg of the louse.

NIT NEST A mass of dirty, tangled hair on the head or on a wig. Slang, Bristol usage.

NIT SQUEEGER See Nit squeezer.

NIT SQUEEZER A hairdresser. 18th century slang. (*Grose, Lex. Bal.*)

NITTER A nitting machine, *qv*.

NITTING The process of removing nits, *qv*, from combings or cut hair by means of a nitting machine, *qv*. (*Creer*)

NITTING-HACKLE (Nitting Machine) An implement with a small tooth comb composed of closely set steel teeth set in a brass base and through which nitted hair can be drawn to remove the adhering nits.   462

NITTING MACHINE See Nitting hackle.

NIVERNOIS-HAT A wig hat. A waterproof hat worn over wigs in the 18th century. (*Lon Mag*, 1764)

NIXIOUS HAIR Hair which is white as snow.

NOB The head. 18/20th century. (*Gross*)

NOB THATCHER A peruke maker. 18th century. (*Grose, Lex Bal*)

NODOSITAS CRINIUM See *Trichorrhexis Nodosa*.

NODULI LAQUEATI See *Trichonodosis*.

NOEUD Fr–Knot, tie, band.

NOIR Fr–Black.

NOKOMIS BEARD A long, full beard, named after Nokonis, a character in *Hiawatha's Wedding Feast*, by Longfellow.

NOLE The crown of the head.

NOLL See Nole.

NONAQUEOUS SHAMPOO A hair cleansing preparation which contains an organic solvent and no water, such as carbon tetrachloride, benzine, ethylene dichloride, petroleum ether, isopropyl alcohol, etc, all of which act as solvents. None of these chemicals can be safely used on hair on the head owing to their toxicity or flammability.

NON-POROUS Not porous; not having minute interstices through which liquids or air can pass.

NONSENSE Melted butter for a wig. Presumably as a dressing instead of pomade. (*Grose, Lex Bal*)

NOODLE AND A DOODLE WIG Slang term for a flowing wig. Derived from 'Noodle and Doodle' in the burletta 'Tom Thumb'. They were bewigged courtiers zealous for the party that was uppermost. At the sale of Mr Rawle, one of the King's accoutrement-makers, one of the lots was a large black wig, with flowing curls, which was stated to have been worn by Charles II. This was bought by Suett, the actor, who wore it for many years in 'Tom Thumb', and other pieces until it was burned when the Birmingham Theatre was destroyed by fire. (*Life of Nollekens*)

NORMANDIN NET A hair-lace foundation for postiches. (*AH*, 1915)

NORRIS SKIPPER BEARD A thick chin tuft. (*Trusty*) 98L

NORTHERN BEAR Bear's grease used for dressing hair and moustaches.

NORWEGIAN PLAIT A long, thick, fair coloured plait.

NOSE CLIP MOUSTACHE An artificial moustache which is held in position against the upper lip by means of a clip that is fixed to the central wall of the nostrils.

NOSEBAG A funnel-shaped paper mask to protect the face from powder.

NOSE PAPER The square of paper used by the old school barbers to hold the client's nose when shaving the upper lip. 'When she got to his upper lip, and took his nose between her fingers with a piece of brown paper, he could stand it no longer,' (*Memoir of Joseph Grimaldi*, 1838)

NOT Short haired. (Obs)
'Not heads and broad hats.'! (*Ben Jonson*, 1620)

NOTCH To cut hair unevenly. 'To notch or pole his head.' (*Clerk*, 1602). The earliest date the *OED*, gives for this use of the word notch is 1747.

NOT-HEADED See Notte.

NOT-PATED See Notte.

NOTTE Cropped short. *Not pated* and *not headed* signified the hair cut close to the head. (*Trone*) 'A notte head had he with a brown visage'! (*Chaucer*)

NOUCHE An ornament for a woman's dress or hair. 16th century. (*Fry*)

NOUVEAU Fr–New, something new or fresh.

NOUVEAUTE Fr–Novelty, innovation.

NOUVELLE Fr–See à la nouvelle.

NOVACULITE A hard argillaceous slate used for the manufacture of razor hones.

NOWLE The top of the head. (*Trone*)

NOZZLE APPLICATOR A container for cream dyes or cream bleaches, having a ribbon-shaped opening from which the cream can be ejected for direct application to the hair, instead of using a brush or cotton-wool-covered stick.

NUMA POMPILIUS Roman philosopher (d 672 bc). The ancients depicted him with white hair crowned with a silver diadem. (*Salmon*)

NUMBER SIXES Curls dressed onto the forehead. Slang, American usage. (*B and B*)

NUN'S WATER See Eau de Cologne.

NURSERY HAIR LOTION *Lotio Staphisagriae*, BPC. (*PPB*)

NYLON HAIR Imitation hair made from nylon thread.

NYLON-SARAN-DYNEL A synthetic substance that approximates to real human hair. It can be woven or knotted and is used in fashion wigs. 20th century.

NYMPH (1) A handsome, young woman.
(2) A fashionable woman under the Directory in France.
(3) A girl's straight and straggly hair style. 20th century.

NYMPHET A young or little nymph.

NYMPHETTE A very young and attractive girl.

NYMPHET HAIR STYLE See Nymph.

O

OAK FERN (*Dryoptoris*) Its bruised root applied to the skin whilst the person is sweating will cause the hair to come away. (*Fernie*)

OAK-MOSS RESIN Obtained from tree lichens, especially oak; used in perfumery. (*Verrill*)

OBSOLETE Out-of-date; a discarded fashion; that which is no longer used or practised.

OCCIPITAL Pertaining to the back of the head.

OCCIPITO FRONTALIS The head muscle that can move the entire scalp.

OCCIPUT The lower back part of the head.

OCCUPATIONAL DISEASE A disease peculiar to and arising from one's occupation, trade or craft, eg determatitis is an occupational disease of hairdressers, skin dressers, dyers, etc.

OCCUPATIONAL SHAVING MUG A shaving mug decorated with the name of its owner and an illustration or design indicative of his occupation. Such mugs were kept in American Barber shops so that clients could be lathered preparatory to shaving from their own individual mugs. (*Ware*)

O'CEDAR MOP Bobbed hair. Slang, American usage. (*B and B*)

OCKAM'S RAZOR A name for the axiom *Entia non sunt multiplicanda* – entities are not to be multiplied; the excision of unnecessary facts in a subject under analysis. William of Ockham (d 1347) scholastic philosopher, dissected every fact as with a razor. (*Allbutt, T C, Science and Medieval Thought*, 1901, p 57)

OCTAVIA HEAD-DRESS A woman's hair style of 1866

inspired by headdresses of Roman antiquity. (*Bysterveld* p 84)

ODORAMENTUM Perfume. (*Bailey*)

ODORATOR A scent diffuser.

ODOUR A pleasant or unpleasant smell.

OFF-COLOUR Not of the required colour or tint.

OFF-SHADE Not of the correct shade, but either paler or darker than the shade required.

OGEE NECK LINE The hair outline at the nape, consisting of two concave curves at each side of the neck running into and joining at a convex point in the middle of the neck.

OIL A viscid, smooth substance having an unctuous feel. Lighter than water and insoluble in it. Many different kinds of oil such as olive, castor, mineral, etc, are used in the hairdressing craft. See Essential oil, fixed oil, mineral oil.

OIL BLEACH Oil bleaches are usually preparations containing Hydrogen Peroxide and ammonium oleate, sulphonated olive or castor oil, prepared at the time of use. (*Sagarin*)

OILCLOTH Waterpoof fabric used to cover work benches to facilitate cleaning them and to provide a perfectly smooth surface which avoids snarling the hair during work.

OILED SILK A waterpoof material sewn in position when needed on the underside of the foundation of a scalpette, patch, etc, and to which adhesive is added to hold the postiche firmly on the scalp.

OIL HONE A razor hone which is lubricated with oil.

OIL SHAMPOO (1) A shampoo that is preceded by the application to the hair and scalp of a suitable oil, such as olive oil or lanolized oil, then followed by a liquid shampoo. (2) A shampoo incorporating in its substance a suitable oil. A modern formula is: Coconut oil 18%, Castor oil 4%, potassium hydroxide (85%) 5.3%, glycerine 4%, borax 0.5%, water 67.8%, perfume to taste.

OIL SOAP An uncoloured combination of olive oil and soda. It is hard, close-grained, and contains but little water. (*Piesse*)

OIL SYSTEM A heat system of permanent waving for which an alkaline solution was used, incorporating glycerine and which felt oily, although oil was not a constituent. The name was a euphemism to give confidence to the client that the hair would not be dried and made brittle by the permanent wave.

OINTMENT An unctuous substance applied to the skin to beautify or heal; an unguent.

OLD BILL See Walrus.

OLD CUT 16th century hair style for men. (*Stubbes*)

OLD DOCTOR A powder made from burnt alabaster and plaster of Paris, used to adulterate hair powder. 18/19th century. (*Lillie*)

OLD DUTCH BEARD A short, square-cut beard with the upper lip and the chin immediately beneath the lower lip clean shaven. (*Trusty*) 97G

OLD HAIRY GENTLEMAN A Roman Catholic who was long imprisoned by his fellow religious and upon his release his face and other parts were overgrown with hair. 1679. (*An Account of the Old Hairy Gentleman*, 1679)

OLD KINGDOM WIG A wig of the Egyptian Old Kingdom period, 2780–2280 bc.

OLD LADY'S CURLS Long drop curls, natural or as a postiche; worn by old women in the 19th century.

OLD MAN'S BEARD A common lichen found on trees and resembling grey hair, hence the name. Used as an adulterant of oak-moss resin, *qv*. (*Verrill*)

Also a vernacular name for the wild clematis in seed.

OLD-MOUSTACHE An old soldier.

OLEUM AMYGDALAE See Almond oil.

OLIGOGENYTRICHIA An absence or deficiency of beard. (*Wheeler*)

OLIVE OIL A yellowish liquid, fatty oil derived from olives. Used in skin and hair preparations and for some shampoos, soft soap, etc. Used in many hairdressing services such as the protection of already curled hair in a permanent curling process, oil treatments for brittle hair, and drunk by Italians to prevent the hair turning grey. Governor John H Volpe of Massachusetts drank olive oil daily to keep his hair from turning grey. (*The American*, 14 April 1967). Unsuitable for use as a hair dressing on account of its propensity to go rancid.

OLIVER CUT A woman's hair style, 1962/3, popularised by the musical play *Oliver*. Described as 'roundly-shaped hair, nibbled at the edges, tumbled on to a face of melting piquancy'.

OLIVIER LE MAUVAIS (Olivier Le Dain) Barber minister of Louis XI, (1423–1453).

OLYMPIAN BEARD A very long, full beard; also called a French Beard. 102i, 103H

OMAHA INDIAN HAIR STYLE The Omaha of the plains cut their children's hair in several styles peculiar to the family group. For instance, one group would remove all the hair from the child's head except a ridge which stood erect and ran from the nape of the neck to the forehead. This symbolized the back hair of a plains buffalo as it stood against the sky. Another group shaved the head except for four square tufts, one at the nape, one at the forehead and one at each side of the head above the ears. This cut referred to the eagle with which the group considered itself connected. These crests were peculiar to the young children only; adults wore their hair long in the usual Indian styles. (*Fletcher, A C and La Flesche, F The Omaha Tribe*. Rep. Bur. Amer. Ethnology, vol.27, 1911)

ONCE-IN-WEAVING Weaving to the pattern of Once-in-Weft, *qv*.

ONCE-IN-WEFT (Flat-weft) Weaving on three silks. From the back of the silk through the bottom silks, over the top silk, under the bottom silk, through the top silks, through the bottom silks. The pattern of the woven hair on the silks is like the letter M.

ONCE-OVER SHAVE The customary shave that removes the heard without causing unnecessary irritation to the skin. See Close shaving.

ONE-STEM SWITCH A switch of hair with only one spill, core or stem. See two-spill tail; Three-spill tail.

ONDE Fr-Undulated.

ONDOYANT Fr-Undulating, waving, flowing.

ONDULATION The action or practice of waving. From the French *Onduler*: to wave.

ONDULER Fr-To undulate, to wave.

ONDULEUR French word, partially Anglicised by the late 19th century. Hair waver.

ONION SOLUTION FOR THE BEARD A 19th/20th century preparation which was claimed to be made from the juice of onions and to raise a strong, full beard on the chins of youths in their fifteenth year.

On analysis the solution was found to consist of dilute scented spirit, coloured with gentian tincture. (*Koller*) In 1928 a dock worker at Avonmouth, Bristol, rubbed slices of onion on his bald scalp. When he was asked if the treatment was succeeding he replied: 'Yes I have gained a few hairs, but lost many friends.' (*I Westlake*)

ON-THE-BOARD Working at the board; boardworking, *cf* At-the-Chair. 'She worked on the board for several years.'

ONUPHRIUS, ST St Onuphrius *c* ad 400. He was an

Egyptian who lived as a hermit for 70 years in the desert in Upper Egypt; a popular saint in the middle ages both in the West and the East. He is the patron saint of weavers and wigmakers probably because he was dressed only in his own abundant hair and a loin-cloth of leaves. He was also Patron of the Milanese Guild of Wigmakers, 17th/18th century.

ONYCHATROPHIA Atrophy of the nails.

ONYCHAUXIS Enlargement of the nails.

ONYCHOPHAGY The habit of biting and/or eating the nails.

ONYCHOPTOSIS The falling off of the nails.

ONYCHORRHEXIS Abnormal brittleness of the nails.

ONYCHOSIS Any disease of the nails.

OPACIFYING AGENT A chemical which will make a preparation opaque.

OPAQUE Not transmitting light.

OPEN-CROWN SKELETON WIG A transformation made in one circular band.

OPEN CURL (1) A round, wide, sausage-type curl which is hollow within. 17th century. (*Holme*)
(2) A curl that is open in the middle when dressed.
(3) A spiral curl.

OPEN-FORK PARTING A postiche parting in which the actual parting is made in the wearer's own hair, which is drawn through the U-shaped aperture and mingled with the postiche hair. The foundation is similar in shape to a hairpin and the net foundation extends 1½" + or − around the outer shape of the U.

OPEN PARTING A small postiche similar in shape to a button stick. The natural hair is pulled through the aperture or open parting and mingled with the knotted hair of the postiche strip. This is only suitable when the client has enough of her own hair in the position of the parting.

OPEN PLAIT A plait with one, two or three 'draws', that is a strand or strands of hair passing down the middle or sides of the plait and incorporated in such a manner that they run in a straight line from the root end to the points. Upon completion of the plait the draw is held firm and the plaited hair slid upwards upon it.

OPEN RAZOR The same as a cut-throat razor. A razor with a free blade that folds into its handle when not being used; similar to a pocket knife but without the spring to keep the blade edge within the safety of the handle.

OPEN SALOON A beauty parlour (parlor) or hairdressing saloon in which clients receive attention in full view of each other, *cf* cubicle. This saloon has become increasingly popular in England since *c* 1945.

OPEN-TAIL-COMB A tail comb with a split tail to facilitate rolling a curl on the tail by engaging the hair points between the split. 1950s.

OPEN HAIR Bareheaded; uncovered hair.

OPEN-MESH FOUNDATION See Open-mesh net.

OPEN-MESH NET Wig net with large apertures between the threads.

OPEN-MESH PARTING A net parting-foundation of open-mesh net. This differs from an Open parting, *qv*.

OPERATA ALOPECIA Loss of hair resulting from a surgical operation. (*Wheeler*)

OPERATOR A person who performs a hairdressing service. See Wages Council Regulations.

OPHIASIS Hair loss in bands.

OPINICUS An heraldic beast with body and forelegs like a lion, the head and neck of an eagle and having a short tail like a camel. Wings are affixed to the body like a griffin. (*Lambert*)

OPISTHOPHALACROSIS Baldness at the back of the head. (*Wheeler*)

OPOBALSAMUM Synonym for Balm of Mecca, *qv*.

OPOPANAX (OPOPONAX) A gum-resin, obtained from the plant *Balsamodendron Kataf*, used in perfumery.

OPOPANAX SOAP Soap perfumed with opopanax.

OPTIC CURL 18th century. See Open curl.

OPTICAL MIXING The mixing and matching by eye of prepared hair (off the head) for use in postiches.

OR (heraldic) Gold.

ORANGE (*Citrus Aurantium*) Common oranges cut through the middle while green, and dried in the air, being afterwards steeped for forty days in oil, were used by the Arabs for preparing an essence famous among their old women because it would darken grey hair. (*Fernie*)

ORANGE-BUTTER Used as a pomade for dressing the hair in the 17th and 18th century. A 17th/18th century Dutch method of making orange-butter was: 'Take new cream two gallons, beat it up to a thickness, then add half a pint of orange-flower water, and as much red wine, and so being become the thickness of butter, it retains both the colour and scent of an orange.' (*Closet of Rarities*, 1706)
'Now make his comely tresses shine,
With orange-butter, Jessamine;' (*Somervile* 1727)

ORANGE-FLOWER HAIR POWDER A starch hair powder scented with orange flower perfume. 18/19th century. (*Lillie*)

ORANGE STICK A small stick made from orange wood, which does not readily splinter, used for manicure. Pointed at one end and blunt at the other.

ORBIS A Roman woman's hair style of the 1st century ad.

ORCHER, JOSEPH Barber of the Faubourg St Antoine, Paris; who murdered and robbed the Marquis de Courzi when shaving him.

ORCHID BOB An almost straight-hair shingle cut, with a loose swirl onto the cheek, terminating in a crescentric curl. Fashionable in 1926/7.   *413*

ORDINAIRE Fr. See l'ordinaire.

ORDINARY, THE A hair style for men, 20th century.

OREILLES DE CHIEN Fr – Dog's ears. A woman's wig style of 1789, frizzed and dressed full at the front, an unbraided queue of hair hanging at the back and held by a bow of ribbon, and two loosely waved tresses like a Spaniel's ears hanging one on each shoulder.

ORFILA'S BALMA A proprietary preparation for restoring, curling and preventing hair from turning grey; manufactured by Leathart & Co, London; advertised as being patronised by the Royal Family and Her Majesty Queen Victoria, mid 19th century.

ORFILA'S HAIR DYE A 19th century preparation consisting of plumbite of lime, made by boiling for 1¼ hours 4 parts sulphate of lead, 5 parts slaked lime with 30 parts of water. The liquid was filtered and the powder collected. This, in a warm solution, would dye the hair a fine black in 1 hour. (*Francis*)

ORIENTAL DEPILATORY A 19/20th century 'secret' preparation which consisted of a mixture of liver of sulphur, calcium sulphide, calcium carbonate and charcoal. There were, at the time, many better, cheaper and more reliable means of effecting the same end. (*Koller*)

ORIENTALE 18th century hair style for women (*Uzanne*)

ORIENTAL HAIR See Chinese hair.

ORIENTAL HAIRDRESS A hairdress of particular magnificence. 20th century.

ORIGO A 19/20th century 'secret' hair dye consisting of an ammoniacal solution of bismuth, containing a large amount of sulphur in suspension, a little glycerine, and strongly perfumed with rose oil. It was not uninjurious.

ORNAMENTAL COMB (1) A hair comb ornamented with jewels or precious metals.

(2) A hair comb that is worn to ornament a coiffure.

ORNAMENTAL HAIR Postiche, such as wigs, fronts, chignons, etc. 18th and 19th century usage.

ORNAMENTAL HAIRWORK (1) Hair-jewellery, ie watch guards, bracelets, etc, manufactured from human hair; or cameos, etc, incorporating designs in human hair.
(2) Postiches and embellishments of hair, incorporated in the hairdress.

ORNE Fr – Adorned or ornamented.

ORPIMENT Native trisulphide of arsenium arsenicum flavum. (*Rouse*)

ORRIS ROOT The fragrant root of three species of iris used in perfumery and, in the 18th and 19th century, commonly used for perfuming hair powder, and in 19/20th century in dry powder shampoos. (*Lillie*)

ORRIS ROOT SHAMPOO Powdered orris root brushed through the hair as a dry powder shampoo, without the use of water.

OSMOSE Subs. Diffusion through a porous membrane.

OSTEOLOGY The science of anatomy, dealing with bones.

OSTRICH-GREASE Unctuous concoctions sold by barbers in the 18th and early 19th century were so-called. (*Chambers Journal*, p 709, 1866)

OTHO, MARCUS SALVIUS (ad 32–69) This Roman Emperor's wig is clearly shown on the obverse of his coins.

OTOTRICHIA See *Pilus Auris*. (*Wheeler*)

OTTELE, JOHN At 115 years old he had a grey beard 1¼ Brabant ells long. (*Derham, W Physico-Theology*, 4th ed, 1716)

OTTO OF ROSES The natural oil of the damask rose used in perfumery.

OUR LADIES HAIR See Lady's hair. (*B and H*)

OUTER-BRACING The wig foundation bracings that lie outside the contour galloon.

OUTER-GALLOON See Contour-galloon.

OUTLINE See Contour.

OUTLINE GALLOON The outer or edge galloon of a postiche.

OUTSIDE TRANSFORMATION A full transformation, ie a foundation with hair that passes right round the hair-line of the head but does not extend over the top of the head, the hair only being dressed to cover that. American usage. (*AH* 1915)

OUT-WAVE A wave directed forward onto the cheek. Also called Cheek wave.

OVEN See Wig oven.

OVERALL An outer garment worn by hairdressers as a protection to their clothing and for hygienic reasons.

OVER-BLEACH (1) To bleach more than the strength of the hair can accept without deterioration.
(2) To bleach over already bleached hair.
(3) To bleach the hair lighter than required.

OVERCASTING See Stitching.

OVER-CURLING (1) Curling too tightly.
(2) Curling over already curled hair.

OVERLAP (1) Subs. That part of the hair shaft on which a dye, colour or bleach in a retouch has overrun the previously dyed, coloured or bleached part of the hair.
(2) Verb. To apply dye or bleach in a retouch to the previously dyed or bleached hair.
(3) In spiral winding in the permanent waving process, the overlapping of one circination *qv*, of the hair strand by the next.

OVER-PROCESS (1) In 'hot' permanent waving, to heat longer than is necessary or than is good for the hair.
(2) In bleaching or dyeing to leave the active substances in contact with the hair longer than is needful for the result

required.

OVERSEWING See Stitching.

OVI ALBUMEN White of egg.

OVI VITELLUS Yolk of egg.

OVID BEARD A beard characteristic of the Latin poet Publius Ovidus Naso (43 bc–17 ad). A slight, graceful beard.

OVIFORM Egg shaped.

OVOID Egg shaped.

OWNDED Having waves or curls. Probably derived from the French *onduler*: to wave or curl.
'Her owndede heer, that sunnish was of hewe.' (*Chaucer, Troilus and Criseyde* 14th century) = Her curly, golden hair.

OXIDATION The action of oxidising; combination with oxygen. The process in which the oxygen of peroxide of hydrogen oxidizes a chemical dye in contact with the hair to produce the required colour.

OXIDATION DYE Any dye that needs oxidation by peroxide of hydrogen to develop colour; sometimes called peroxide dye. See also Aniline Dye.

OYSEAU ROYAL See A la Oyseau Royal.

P

PVP Polyvinylpyrrolidone, *qv*.

PW Permanent wave, *qv*.

PACK The hair covered with henna or paste bleach and formed into a compact mass, within a covering of paper, plastic or other suitable material. See also Henna pack, Bleach pack, etc.

PACKWOOD, GEORGE A celebrated 18th century maker of razor strops, of Gracechurch Street, London. (*Packwood*)

PAD See Sachet, also Hair pad.

PADDED BLOCK Wooden wig block padded with layers of coarse paper stuck on to make the block the size and shape necessary for the postiche to be made on it. 19th century.

PADDOCK HAIR The down on unfledged birds. Scottish usage. (*Brown*)

PAD-WEFT Weft made with crêpe hair and used for the manufacture of pads. When completed the hair sticks out in a frizz from the central stem of thread. Used in the making of do-nut bun pads, as a pad foundation for French rolls, as a pad across the front of the head forming a foundation for a pompadour dressing, obviating back-combing. See Pad.

PAGE BOY A woman's hair style popular from 1936 to 1945. The hair was worn in a long bob, straight or nearly straight, with the ends turned under and hanging on the shoulders.

PAINTED HAIR Among the Romans those who were bald and would not wear a wig had hair painted on their bare skulls. Martial, in one of his *Epigrams* addressed Phoebus: 'Your counterfeit hair is a falsehood of the perfume which imitates it; and your skull disgracefully bald is covered with painted locks; and you have no occasion for a barber for your head, Phoebus; you may shave yourself much better with a sponge'.

PAINTER'S BRUSH MOUSTACHE A narrow moustache neatly cut, extending right across the upper lip. (*Trusty*)
101L

PAIR-OF-MOUSTACHES The hair growing on both sides of the upper lip. 'His moustaches I should say, because he'd a pair.' (*Barham, Ingolsby Legends*, 1842)

PALATE LOCK A small lock of hair on top of the head, at

one time, believed by some Southern negroes of the Unite
States of America to support the palate. (*Puckett*)

PALISADE A wire sustaining the hair next to the Duches
or first knot. 1690. (*Evelyn*)   3:

PALM CUTTING An inferior method of hair thinning b
which a strand of hair is placed on the palm of the left han
and with the point of the scissors hairs are clean cut
intervals. This method, slow, difficult and unsatisfactor
is liable to leave stubble and is not recommended.

PALM CURL A curl with a straight stem, the ends shape
into a half or three-quarter curl. Also called Hook curl.

PALMETTE Radiating curls stemming from a contiguo
gathering of hairs.

PALM OIL See Hair oil.

PALM SOAP A soda soap of palm oil. (*Piesse*)

PAN The Greek god of pastures, forests, flocks and herd
Depicted bearded by the ancients. (*Salmon*)

PANACHE Fr. Upright plumes worn on a hairdress.

PANEL WAVING See Line waving.

PANGLOSS, DR Dr Pangloss was a pompous litera
character in George Coleman's comedy *The Heir at Lav*
1797. He was dressed in a bob wig and hence the name –
Dr Pangloss wig, later shortened in the theatrical world to a
'Dr Pangloss'. (Illus p 47; *Harrison, Theatricals and Tableaux Vivants*)

PANNIKELL Crown of the head. 'Smote him so rudely on
the pannikell.' (*Spenser, Fairy Queen*)

PAPER CAP See Paper hood.

PAPER CURL, TO To put hair in papillotes, *qv*, for
pinching between hot pinching irons to produce curl.
'. . . while my maid papered my curls yester-morning,'
(*Mrs Thrale, Letters*)

PAPER CURLING Pinching hair shaped to the form of a
curl and enclosed within a small piece of folded paper. See
Papillote (1).

PAPER HOOD A cap of paper used to cover the hair and
head to retain the natural heat of the head and accelerate a
dyeing, bleaching or waving process.

PAPERING 18th century term for placing the paper papillotes around the wound hair preparatory to pinching it with
the hot pinching irons. (*Fenton*)

PAPER TOWEL See Towel.

PAPIER POUDRE Decorated booklets, 2″ × 2½″, of
powder-coated tissue papers used for annointing the face,
especially the nose and forehead, to remove face shine. A
common toilet aid from 18th century to early 20th century,
and still used.

PAPILLA A small, nipple-shaped protuberance at the base of
the hair follicle. It is at this point that the hair is formed.

PAPILLARY LAYER The outer layer of the dermis.

PAPILLOTAGE Subs. The action of putting hair in curl
papers.

PAPILLOTE (1) Curl paper. A small triangle of paper to fold
around a flat curl and hold it in position while it is pinched
with hot pinching irons. (*Creer*)
(2) A ringlet curl.

PAPILLOTE COMB A decorated tortoiseshell comb 3″ to 4″
wide.

PAPILLOTE TONGS Pinching irons, *qv*. (*Bailet*).

PARA Paraphenylenediamine.

PARA DYE See Paraphenylenediamine.

PARAFFIN WAX (Hard paraffin) A mixture of hydrocarbons with the general formula $C_nH_2+_2$ obtained from
petroleum. Used in cosmetics.

PARAPHENYLENEDIAMINE (Paradiamino-benzine)
$C_6-H_8N_2$. The most widely used and effective of the
aniline derivative dyes, producing colours ranging from

lightest brown to jet black. Its every action depends on
oxidation, usually effected by hydrogen peroxide and this
reaction results in the formation of an intermediate product
known as Bandrowsky's Base. This type of dye has serious
attendant dangers and can cause disease in persons who
have an allergy to it. Vertigo, anaemia, gastritis, exfoliative
dermatitis and, in hypersensitive persons, even death have
resulted from its application to persons allergic to it. It
should never be used if there is an abrasion, eruption or any
scalp condition other than normality. (*Merck*)

It should never be used on eyebrows or eye-lashes,
nor permitted to enter the eyes or mouth, and before
every application a skin test, *qv*, should be made. If any
doubt at all arises as to the desirability of applying a para-
dye, the treatment should not be given and another type of
dye, such as henna, with its restricted range of colour,
should be used. This type of dye is variously known as an
amino dye, aniline derivative dye, instantaneous dye, oxidation dye, peroxide dye, synthetic organic dye, two
bottle dye.

PARASITE An organism living in, or on another organism,
drawing its nourishment directly from its host.

PARASITICIDE A substance that will destroy parasites.

PARCEL OF HAIR (1) a Collection of heads of virgin hair,
(the hair from each head tied and kept separate) as sent to
the hair merchant from the hair-collector. 18th/20th century.
(2) A collection of treated or virgin hair as sent to the
wigmaker from the hair merchant.

PARE, AMBROSE Famous Barber Surgeon, (1509–1590).
At 19 he was attached to the army and appointed surgeon to
King Henry II of France.

PARESSEUSE Fr. Lazy. See A la Paresseuse.

PARFUM Fr. Perfume, odour, scent.

PARFUMERIE Fr. Perfumery.

PARFUMEUR Fr. Perfumer.

PARFUMOUR Fr. Perfuming dish.

PARIETAL BONES A pair of bones forming part of the
sides and top of the skull.

PARIS BEARD The fashionable beard of the moment in the
17th/18th century. So called because Paris was the centre
and origin of fashion.
'With cloak d'Espagne and Paris beard;
With dangling peruke to his rump.
Invented to disguise his hump;' (*Durfey, The Athenian Jilt*,
1721)

PARIS CAP A woman's head-dress of the mid-sixteenth
century. It fitted the head closely with a jewelled band
running over the top of the head and ending in a point on
the cheeks. (*Gardner*)

PARISIAN CURL An Edwardian name for a pincurl.
London price for a pair in 1906, 7/6d.

PARISIENNE Fr. See A la Parisienne. (*AH*)

PARKING BASE A malleable block shaped like the top of a
head and used to rest toupees on overnight in order that
they shall keep their shape. Toupees are also dressed on it.
American usage. 20th century. (*MH*)

PARSNIP Slang word for the sheathed queue of an 18th
century Macaroni's wig. (*Caricature Print*, 1772)

PARSONIC WIG See Bishop's wig.

PART The parting of the hair. 20th century American usage.

PARTED BEARD A beard dressed parted in the centre and
combed out towards each side. This style broadens the face.
(*Moler p 53*)

PARTERRE GALANT See Au parterre galant.

PARTING (1) The dividing line of combed hair.
(2) A small postiche consisting of a parting only – the hair of

the artificial parting being combed into the natural hair. (*Creer*)

PARTING FRINGE A small fringe worn at the front of the parting of a postiche to disguise the postiche edge.

PARTING GAUZE See Etamine.

PARTING HOOK (1) A fine hooked needle for knotting partings.

(2) A very fine-hooked, straight-shanked needle for drawing hair through the parting silk when working a drawn-through-parting.

PARTING MACHINE 'It consists of a yoke, which, placed over the crown of the head, holds a slotted guide, by means of which the comb is, in making the parting, forced to follow the medial line between the ears of the fair ones, whose ears are supposed to be in an exact horizontal line when their heads are level.' (*Creer*)

PARTING NET (1) Etamine, *qv*.

(2) Fine net used for knotting the partings of theatrical wigs.

(3) Fine-mesh net made of human hair and used for the finest knotted partings. *123*

PARTING SIDE That side of the head where the parting is formed.

PARTING SILK (Flesh silk) A finely woven, white, ivory or flesh coloured silk fabric used for drawn-through partings in wigs, etc. The hair that is drawn-through is anchored to the etamine beneath the parting silk, thus simulating hair growing from the scalp.

PARTING SKIN Fish skin incorporated in a postiche beneath the parting to prevent discolouration of the parting silk by perspiration.

PARTING WEFT A type of weft on three or four silks composed of very fine hair strands woven in the middle of the strand, one strand being woven down, the next up, et seq. Used for the partings of doll's wigs and theatrical wigs.

PARTRIDGE A famous fictional barber, who became the faithful, shrewd and loquacious attendant of Tom Jones in Henry Fielding's novel, *The History of Tom Jones*, 1749.

PARURE Fr. Dress, ornament.

PASSAGERE Fr. A curled lock next the temples. 1690. (*Evelyn* *360*

PASTE BLEACH Bleach prepared in the form of a paste. See also Liquid bleach and Powder bleach.

PASTEL SHADE Soft tints; half-faded tones; pale tones.

PATCH See Postiche patch.

PATCH BOX A small, decorative, flat box to contain the adhesive beauty patches usually black, worn by fashionable women on the face in the 17th/19th century and occasionally by a certain type of man. The patches were of paper, velvet, etc.

PATCHOULI A penetrating and lingering perfume prepared from an odiferous plant *Pogostemon Patchouli*.

PATCH TEST See Skin test.

PATE (1) The head, 18th century. (*Grose, Lex Bal*)

(2) A wig.

PATENT CLIP A small metal hair clip based on a principle similar to that which is employed in a spring door-latch.

PATENT-LEATHER HAIR A heavily greased, smooth, shining head of hair. American usage. (*B and B*)

PATRIARCHAL BEARD See Olympian beard.

PATTERN (1) A foundation pattern for a wig or other postiche.

(2) A strand of hair used as a colour guide.

(3) That which is to be copied in the dressing of a hair style.

PATTERN BALDNESS See Alopecia prematura and Alopecia senilis. (*Lubowe*)

PATTES DE LAPIN Fr. Rabbit's Feet. A wig style in which the side whiskers slightly indent in front of the ears. Popular 18th century American style.

PAUL (APOSTLE), TONSURE OF The Tonsure of St Paul consists in shaving the whole of the head; the usual practice in the Eastern Church.

PAWNEE RIDGE See Mohican cut. The Pawnees were a North American tribe of Indians who affected a similar hair style to the Mohicans.

PEAK The point of a beard (1592). See also Widow's peak.

PEARLASH See Potassium carbonate.

PECTEN A comb-like formation in animals. The scallop shell is known as a pecten or comb from its resemblance to the tortoise-shell combs worn in their hair by Spanish women. (*Cox, I*)

PEDESTAL BLOCK HOLDER A hair block holder on a stand. 19th century.

PEDESTAL DRYER A hair-dryer mounted on a pedestal.

PEDESTAL SHAMPOO BOARD A shampoo board, *qv*, supported on a pedestal.

PEDICULOSIS A louse infested condition.

PEDICULUS CAPITIS Head louse.

PEDICURE Treatment of the feet; chiropody.

PEDIMENT A triangular-shaped dressing crowning the front of a hairdress.

PEDIMENTAL HEADDRESS A woman's head-dress of the first quarter of the 16th century. It lasted until replaced by the Paris cap, *qv*, in the middle of that century. (*Gardner*)

PEEKABOO LOCKS Hanging hair that partly conceals the face and eyes.

PEELS GARLICK See Pill garlick.

PEG See Weaving stick.

PEIGNE Fr. Comb.

PEIGNOR Fr. Dressing gown originally used by women when dressing their hair.

PELADE Spotted baldness.

PELAGE The whole hairy system of the body.

PELE'S HAIR A brittle volcanic glass in the shape of filaments as fine as human hair, found on the volcano Kirauea in Hawaii.

PELOT The side-whiskers worn by Orthodox Jews. (*Jewish Encyc*)

PELT (1) Humorous or dialectal name for the human skin. 20th century.

(2) A wig or hat made of natural animal skin and hair.

PENANNULAR A broken annulet form of curl.

PENCIL BEARD A narrow strip of beard from the lower lip to the chin.

PENCIL LINE MOUSTACHE (1) A moustache consisting of a very thin line of hairs.

(2) A thin line moustache drawn on the upper lip with a coloured cosmetic. (*Trusty*) *101(a)*

PENCILLING Thin streaks of colour differing from the ground colour of a head of hair.

PENDANT BOB A man's bob wig with dildo, or hanging curls. (*Smith*)

PENDANT COIFFURE A hair style in which a substantial part of the hair is dressed hanging as opposed to being dressed high on the head. Cf Pile-up coiffure.

PENDANT CURL See Hanging curl.

PENDANT PLAIT A hanging plait.

PENDETTE Small, loose-hanging ornament for decorating a hairdress. 1977.

PENETRATING DYE A para dye. See Penetrative dye.

PENETRATIVE DYE An oxidation or aniline-derivative dye that penetrates the hair cuticle and cortex.

PENKNIFE SPRING A small, flat, metal attachment for securing toupees to the subject's own existing hair. From mid-19th century. (*Creer*) They opened, as the name indicates, and when closed a small portion of the growing hair was clasped and secured the toupee to the wearer's head. See also Patent clip.

PEPPER AND SALT A head of hair that is a mixture of white and brown hairs.

PEPPERCORN HAIR Frizzy hair growing in small tufts with spaces between the tufts. The Bushmen of South Africa have this type of hair. (*Winick*)

PERAWICKE See Peruke (*Holme*)

PERCUSSION A form of massage which consists of taps or blows with the fingers. See Tapotement.

PEREWYKE 1568. See Peruke.

PERFUME An odoriferous substance derived from animal or vegetable sources, also formed synthetically from chemical substances.

Word derived from the Latin *per* – from, and *fumus* – smoke. The earliest perfumes were wood or aromatic gums which, in burning gave off agreeable odours.

PERFUMED PERUKE A scented wig. 'Your perfumed perrukes or periwigs'. (*Peacham*, 1638)

PERFUMER One who manufactures and sells perfume and scented toilet powders. Hairdressers and Perfumers have been common since the early 19th century but originally in England perfume was vended by the apothecary as well as drugs. 'Give me an ounce of civet, good apothecary, to sweeten my imagination.' (*Shakespeare, King Lear*, Act II, Scene 6)

PERFUMERY The business of a perfumer; preparing and selling perfumes.

PERIMETER GALLOON The outer contour or edge galloon of a postiche.

PERIWICK (Perwicke, Perwigge) False or counterfeit hair, 1617. (*Minsheu*). See Wig and Peruke.

PERIWIG (1) A wig, *qv*, 17th century.

(2) John Josselyn in his *New England's Rarities Discovered*, 2nd ed, 1675, refers to a New England fish called a 'periwig'.

PERIWIG ENGINEER Facetious name for a wigmaker. (*Home*, 1838)

PERIWIGGIAN A periwig wearer. 17th century. (*Hayman, R Quodlibets*, 1628)

PERIWIG MAKER A wigmaker. 17th/18th century usage. (*The Jesting Astrologer*, No 17, 1701 by *Silvester Partridge*)

PERIWIG PATED Wearing a wig. (*Hamlet*, 3 ii 10)

PERIWINCKE (Also periwinkle, etc) – Periwig, *qv*, 'His bonnet val'd, ere ever he could thinke, Th' unruly winde blows off his periwincke.' *Hall, Satires* IV 5)

PERIWIX False hair. (*Youths Behaviour*, 1663)

PERM Subs. Shortened form of Permanent wave.

PERMABLE Capable of being permanently waved.

PERMANENT Subs. A permanent wave, *qv*, 'A permanent helps to give body to any kind of hair.' (Advert, 1940)

PERMANENT CURL (1) A natural curl.

(2) Hair that has been permanently waved, *qv*, and will remain curled as long as the hair itself lasts.

PERMANENT DYE A dye in which the susceptibility to lose colour under conditions has been reduced to a minimum. The term is relative, however, as no hair dye will indefinitely resist the effects of strong sunlight.

PERMANENT TINT A euphemism for permanent dye, *qv*.

PERMANENT WAVE This term is so widespread and long established that it will persist, but strictly it is a permanent curl that is put into the hair, not a permanent wave. It is the hairdresser who sets the permanent curl into waves which, of course, need resetting every time the hair is shampooed.

276

PERMANENT WAVE SHOCK (1) An electric shock sustained in the process of permanent waving.

(2) Hair that has been broken by over-heating or too strong a solution is euphemistically said to have suffered a permanent wave shock.

PERMANENT WAVING SACHET A chemically impregnated pad or sachet to cover the hair, wound on a curler, in a permanent waving process.

PERMEABLE (1) Capable of being passed or permeated.

(2) Capable of penetrating or permeating.

PEROXIDE (1) Peroxide of hydrogen, *qv*.

(2) An artificial blonde, slang. (*B and B*) 'That was a cute peroxide I saw you with.'

(3) Verb. To bleach. 'She has been peroxided.'

PEROXIDE BLONDE A woman with bleached hair. This is a disparaging term employed to indicate and emphasize that the blonde colour of a woman's hair was an artificial production and not a natural colour growth.

PEROXIDE DYE See Oxidation dye.

PEROXIDE OF HYDROGEN See Hydrogen peroxide.

PEROXIDE RINSE A liquid preparation containing hydrogen peroxide and ammonia, which is poured evenly over and through the hair to bleach it slightly. A rinse differs from an application by means of a brush or spatula by virtue of its method of application by rinsing it through the hair.

PEROXIDE SHAMPOO A soft soap shampoo incorporating a small quantity of 20 vol peroxide of hydrogen and two or three drops of .880 ammonium hydroxide.

PEROXIDIZE Verb. To bleach hair. 20th century.

PEROXOMETER An apparatus which can measure the strength of hydrogen peroxide.

PERRIWIG 1592 (*Lyly*). See Periwig and Wig.

PERRIWIG MAKER A wig maker. Wigmaking was referred to by Howell, writing in 1659, as a new trade. 'I am a perriwig maker, and it has cost me a great deal of pains . . .' (*Gent's Mag*, April 1733, p 170)

PERRIWIG THIMBLE 18th century. See Finger shield.

PERRIWINCLE An 18th century slang term for a wig. (*Carew*)

PERRIWINCKE (Periwincle, Perriwinke, etc) An 18th century slang name for a wig. (*Carew; Grose*)

PERRUQUE French word for wig, *qv*. The English periwig, *qv*, was derived from perruque, but the French word was sometimes employed as a kind of affectation in much the same way as the French word *salon* is commonly used for the correct English word Saloon. See also Periwig.

PERRUQUE A BONNET Fr. See Bonnet wig.

PERRUQUE A BOURSE See Bag wig.

PERRUQUE A DEUX QUEUES See Double queued wig.

PERRUQUE A LA BRIGADIERE See Brigadier wig.

PERRUQUE A NOEUDS See Knotted wig.

PERRUQUE A PAPILLONS See Butterfly wig.

PERRUQUE A TONSURE See Abbés wig.

PERRUQUE DE L'ABBE See Abbés wig.

PERRUQUE NAISSANTE See A l'Enfant.

PERRUQUE OF EARWIGS Perruque used as a collective noun, cf gaggle of geese; a 20th century suggestion of L Dawson Campbell. See *C E Hare, The Language of Field Sports*, ed 1949, p 234.

PERRUQUE POINTUE See Pointed wig.

PERRUQUE RONDE See Round wig.

PERRUQUIANA Collection of writings, anecdotes and literary gossip relating to wigs.

PERRUQUIER Fr. A male wig maker.

PERRUQUIERE Fr. A female wig maker.

PERRYWIG See Periwig. (*Porter*, 1678)

PERRYWINKLE, LORD A character in C Anstey's poem *An Election Ball*, 1775. See also Perriwincle.

PERSIAN HENNA See Henna.

PERSONAL TOOL Those hairdressing tools and implements which are owned by the hairdresser's assistant, in contrast to the provided tools. Personal tools may be scissors, hairdressing combs, neck brushes, setting nets, curling sticks, etc. The provided tools include permanent waving machines, sterilizer, hairpins, etc, but the division is sometimes rather arbitrary.

PERSONALITY BOB A short hair style for women similar to the Wind-blown bob, *qv*. (*Wilson, K*)

PERUKE (Perruck; Perrucke; Perrucke; Perrucq; Perruque; Perug; Perucke; Perugo; Peruque)

(1) A natural head of hair, 16th century. 'The heare of a manne's head . . . a peruke.' (*Elyot*, 1548)

(2) A skull cap covered with human hair to represent natural hair growing on the head. 'A false perruke.' 1565 (*Cooper*); a wig.

(3) An heraldic representation of a wig. (*Guillim*)

(4) Verb. To furnish with a peruke. By popular usage Peruke became perewig, perwig, and by elision, wig, *qv*. Many variations of spelling are met with. Some examples and dates when used are: Perawick, 1688 (*Holme*); Perewake, 1661 (*Fuller, Worthies*); Perewig, 1596 (*Griffin, Fidessa*); Perewig, 1641 (*Milton, Anamadversions*); Periwigg, 1667 (*Pepys, Diary*); Perewige, 1656 (*Wood, Life*); Perewincle, 1580 (*Hollyband, French Tongue*); Perriwig, 1592 (*Lyly*); Periwigge (*Fairholt*); Periwincke, 1597 (*Hall*); Periwinke, 1598 (*Hall, Satires*); Periwinkle; Perriwigge, 1596 (*Fairholt*); Perrucke, 1606 (*Holland, Suetonius*); Perruke, 1565 (*Cooper*); Perruque, 1672 (*Wycherley, Love in a Wood*); Perug, 1581 (*Mulcaster*); Peruke, 1659 (*Cotton, Poems*, 1689); Peruque, 1613 (*Hayward, Norman Kings*); Perwick, 1648 (*Hexham*); Perwig, 1614 (*Raleigh, Hist. of World*); Perwyke, 1529 (*Privy Purse Expenses, Henry VIII*); Pery-wig, 1602 (*Shakespeare, Hamlet*); Perywigge, 1579 (*Lyly, Euphues*); Perewyke, 1588 (*Sir F Knollys, Letter to Cecil*, pub in *Antiquarian Repository*. 1808).

PERUKE COMB A comb for dressing wigs. It had 'round, open and strong teeth'. 17th century (*Holme*). A comb with teeth on both sides of the spine, those on one side being wider than those on the other.

PERUKE NAISSANTE See A l'Enfant.

PERUKE 'RIOT' The peruke having declined in fashion to the detriment of the peruke-makers, on 11th February, 1765, a petition to the King, desiring that gentlefolk should be forced to wear wigs, was carried in procession to St James's Palace for presentation to the King. As the distressed peruke makers marched through the streets it was seen that most of them were without wigs themselves. This enraged the London mob as something unfair and inconsistent and so they seized the petitioners and forceably cut off their hair. (*Andrews*)

PERUKE MAKER (Peruq Maker) A wig maker. 'Gregorie, famous peruq maker.' 17th century. (*Aubrey*)

PERUKE MAKER'S SIGN Locks of hair; or black, blue and white perukes, as symbols of their craft. 17th/18th century.

PERUKE MONGER A wig seller.

PERUKER Wig maker. 'See the peruker's shop – the splendid show.' (*Beck*, 1807)

PERUKE WITH LONG TWIST A man's hair style *c* 1679. (*The Country Club*, A poem, 1679. Wing 6525)

PERUKIER A wig maker.

PERUKIERSHIP The art of wigmaking. 'A skillful piece of perukiership.' 1822.

PERUQUE or PERAWICK See Peruke. (*Holme*)

PERUQUEAN ART Wigmaking. (*The Comic Almanac*, 1847)

PERUQUE MAKER 17th century. A wig maker. (*Quevodo*, 1667)

PERUQUIER (Perukier) Wig maker. 17th/18th century.

PERWICK A wig; a cap of false hair, 1694.

PERWYKE See Peruke.

PETAL CURL A flat half curl, the tress of hair curved only and not forming a circle. Similar to Hyacinth curl, *qv*.

PETARD A hair style that has been designed to attract attention by its oddity or extravagence. From the Latin word *Pet* – to break wind, a 'bombshell'.

PETER (APOSTLE) Tonsure of St Peter. May be:

(1) A cross-shaped bald patch on the scalp, two to three inches wide.

(2) A bald circular patch on the crown of the head (worn by secular priests).

(3) The whole upper part of the head shaved, leaving only a fringe of hair, as in some monastic orders. (*Brewer*)

PETERPOL A hair style of the 1960s for men.

PETITE PERUKE A part wig or demi-wig, the hair of which blends with the wearer's own hair. Similar to a Wiglet, *qv*, (*Hanle*)

PETIT MAITRE Fr. See au Petit maître.

PETIT POSTICHE A small piece of postiche. Not a wig. (*Anderson*)

PETRIFIED WIG Lord Erskine, when staying at Knaresborough, by way of a joke, threw his wig into the celebrated dripping well, where it became petrified. It was later added to the collection of the famous manufacturer of forensic wigs, Mr Ravenscroft of Lincoln's Inn. (*Pall Mall*)

PETRISSAGE A kneading massage movement, in which the skin or scalp is grasped between the thumb and fingers, lifted and gently squeezed or rolled with firm pressure.

PETROLEUM JELLY (Petrolatum, Vaseline, Paraffin Jelly.) A purified mixture of semi-solid hydrocarbons, chiefly of the methane series, of the general formula $C_nH_2N+_2$. Insoluble in alcohol, soluble in benzene, ether, carbon disulphide, chloroform and oils. Used in cosmetics, and until circa 1925 commonly as a dressing for men's hair, but has now largely been replaced by emulsion dressings.

PETROL SHAMPOO See Gasoline shampoo.

PEYA (Peyos; Peyot, plural) Hanging curl worn in front of the ear (one on each side) by orthodox Jews. Also called *payus* and *pyus*.

PH A scale of the alkali or acid strength of a substance. The PH rating is indicated on a scale of 1 to 14; 1 being very acid and 14 being very alkali, 7 is neutral. The PH rating of hair averages 5, being slightly acid.

PHALACROSIS (1) Baldness at the crown. (*Wheeler*)
(2) Hair loss that begins at the forehead.

PHARIAN FISH Crocodile dung. Used in Roman times as a beauty aid. (*Ovid*)

PHIALIGE A Greek houshold slave who painted or coloured hair. (*Forbes*)

PHILOSOPHER'S BEARD A thick, long and bushy beard. (*Lambert*)

PHOENIX HAIR DYE A 19/20th century 'secret' hair dye which contained paraphenylenediamine. This could have been dangerous, a case of poisoning following the use of this dye being recorded. (*Koller*)

PHONEY BEARD A false beard. (*B and B*)

PHONEY MOP American slang term for a wig. (*Berrey*)

PHOSGENE GAS A deadly gas emitted if the wig cleaner,

qv, carbon tetrachloride, *qv*, is allowed to drop on a very hot surface.

PHRYAS Eyebrows. (*Wheeler*)

PHTHIRUS-PUBIS See Pubis louse.

PHYSICAL TIE A man's 18th century wig style with a foretop and three hair knots hanging, two at the front on the shoulders, and one at the back. (*L C March*, 1762). This wig was probably so named because it was popular with the physicians who prescribed physic. 257

PHYSICAL WIG A kind of long-bob dressed from the forehead, backwards to beyond the crown, and from that point to the base of the neck, puffed out. Worn by professional men, this style replaced the full-bottomed wig. Also called Lion wig and Pompey, *qv*, Late 18th century.

PHYSICIAN'S DRESSED BOB A man's 18th century bob wig style. See Bob wig. 'Physicians should have their head shaved and wear a round wig.' (*Graves*)

PHYSICS The science that deals with the properties of matter and energy, such as heat, light, sound, electricity, mechanics, dynamics, etc, but excluding chemistry and biology.

PHYSIOGNOMICAL HAIR CUTTING Cutting hair to suit the face of the wearer.

PHYSIOGNOMICAL HAIRDRESSING An expression first used and described by Joseph Lichtenfeld in his work, *Principles of Physiognomical Hairdressing*, circa 1880. 'To make the arrangement of the hair subservient to the natural proportions of the head, with due regard to outline, and to bring the coiffure into harmony with the lines formed by the features.'

PHYSIOLOGY The science of the normal functions of the cells, tissues, organs and systems of the living body.

PHYSIOTHERAPY The use of natural agents such as air, light, heat, water, exercise and massage in the treatment of disease.

PICCADILLY, THE See Regent.

PICCADILLY FRINGE A roll of hair at the front of the head, worn by men. Fashionable in the first half of the 19th century then abandoned by the man of fashion, but worn by costermongers until the early 20th century. Cf Gloucester Lane roll.

PICCADILLY WEEPERS A fashionable style of whisker (*c* 1855–60). Long side whiskers extending down the side of the face and untidily hanging some 6" or so below the chin, which was clean shaven. Also called Dundreary Whiskers, *qv*, (*Rogers and Allen*)

PICK See Roller pick.

PICK-A-DEVANT A 16/17th century style in which the beard was worn cut to a sharp point. Worn by Charles I. (*Holme*) In heraldic language a full face with a sharp-pointed beard was described as 'a man's face with a pick-à-devant beard'. (*Mitchell*)

PICKED BEARD Pointed beard. *qv*17th century. (*Evelyn*)

PICKING See Picking combings.

PICKING COMBINGS The disentangling of hair combings by means of the fingers, preparatory to carding. 19/20th century.

PICTRICE A Greek household slave who brushed hair. (*Forbes*)

PIEBALD Of two colours, especially black and white, irregularly arranged.

PIECE A hair piece or postiche. (*DT*, 24 June 1965)

PIEL'D Shaven, bald. (*Toone*) 'Piel'd priest, dost thou command me to be shut out.' (*Shakespeare, Henry VI*, Pt 1)

PIERRE DE LA BROSSE A French barber of the 13th century who rose to become Prime Minister. He was hanged at Montfaucon in 1278 for plotting against the King.

PIGEON'S WING PERIWIG A man's wig dressed with two horizontal rolls above the ear. The top, sides and back being dressed smooth and plain. This style was worn with different styles of queue. 1750–1760+.

PIGGY A little pigtail. Bristol usage, early 20th century.

PIGMENT (1) Organic colouring matter used as a dye or paint.
(2) The natural colouring matter of tissues, including those of the hair.

PIGTAIL A plait or queue of hair hanging from the back of the head or back of a wig. The name was derived from the resemblance to a pig's tail. 1688.
The military pigtail, about twelve inches long, was dressed as follows: A lock of hair at the back of the head was allowed to grow longer than the rest and upon this was placed a piece of whalebone about ten inches long, of the size of a small quill; a narrow black ribbon was then wound round the lock of hair and the whalebone and continued until near the end of it. Then a separate lock of hair, kept for the purposes, was placed on the end of the whalebone, projecting two inches beyond it and the ribbon wound to the end of the whalebone where it was fastened. The finished dressing resembled a continuous tail of hair, terminating with a curl. (*N and Q*, 1860) The military pigtail was shortened to 7" in 1804, and cut off in 1808.

PIGTAIL PONY TAIL Hair brushed back from the forehead, up from the sides, up from the nape, and fastened securely near the scalp. This loose 'pony tail' is then divided in two and coiled into a hanging two-strand tail, secured at its end by an elastic band, thread or ribbon. 20th century.

PIGTAIL WIG A man's wig style with a long queue, spirally dressed by binding or interweaving with ribbon and tying the queue at both ends with a ribbon bow. 18th century.
'Sir, do not look so fierce, and big,
It is a modish Pigtail wig.' (*The Metamorphoses of the Town* by *Elizabeth Thomas*, 3rd ed 1731)

PILARY Of or pertaining to hair.

PILD See Pilled.

PILE The nap on cloth, fort hair, down. 'This carpet's pile is very fine.' From Latin *Pilus*, a hair.

PILEOUS Consisting of hair; hairy.

PILE-UP COIFFURE A hair style in which the hair is dressed full and high on the head. 1962.

PILI ANNULATI See Ringed hair.

PILI AURICULARES The hair in the external auditory passage. (*Good*)

PILICIOUS Beautifully haired.

PILIFEROUS Having hair.

PILIFORM Hair-like; having the shape of a hair.

PILIGEROUS Covered with hair; bearing hair.

PILI MONILEFORMES See Monilethrix.

PILINE Hairy; having the nature of hair.

PILIOSIS Greyness of the hair; canities. (*Robinson*)

PILL OR PEELE GARLICK One whose hair had fallen off due to disease, chiefly venereal. 17/18th century. (*Grose, Lex Bal*)

PILLED Deprived of hair. 14th/19th century.
'As piled as an ape was his skulle.' (*Chaucer*)

PILLOW A soft, round cushion for dressing postiche on.

PILLOW CURLER A large, soft hair curler.

PILOMANIA An excessive love or mania for hair.

PILOPHOBE A person affected with pilophobia.

PILOPHOBIA An intense fear or dislike of hair.

PILOPHOBIC Adj. Pertaining to pilophobia.

PILOSE OR PILOUS Covered with hair.

PILOSITOUS COMPOUND See Francis's pilositous compound.

PILOSITY Hairiness.

PILOUS Consisting of or abounding in hair.

PILUS AURIS Excessive growth of hair in or on the ears. (*Wheeler*)

PIN A short, thin, metallic peg, pointed at one end and blunt or with a small head at the other. Used to secure postiches to malleable blocks or cushions.

PINAUD'S BRILLIANTINE A 19/20th century proprietary scented liquid which separated into two layers and consisted of about ¾ of olive oil and ¼ of alcohol. (*Koller*)

PINAUD'S EAU DE QUININE A 19/20th century 'secret' preparation for the hair compounded of crameria tincture 2 parts, cantharides tincture 1 part, alcohol 50 parts, lavender spirit 5 parts, glycerine 7½ parts and quinine sulphate 1 part. (*Koller*)

PIN BEARD See Needle beard.

PINCER An 18th century term for curling irons. (*Peter Pindar*, 1795)

PINCHER An instrument for grasping or pinching. Used in boardwork.

PINCHING (1) Compressing the knotted part of wefted hair with a pinching iron.
(2) Compressing papillotes *qv*, with a pinching iron.

PINCHING IRONS Irons with circular, flat-faced ends, which heated are pressed together by means of the handles worked scissor fashion to pinch weft or papillotes.
87 (33,34), 445, 447

PINCH OF HAIR A small strand of hair.

PIN COMB A tail comb with a tail similar to a thin knitting needle.

PINCURL A small postiche of wefted curls secured to a hairpin for easy attachment to a head of hair. Two methods were employed in the 19th and early 20th century. In the earliest method the curls were secured to the looped end of the hairpin. In the later method the curls were secured to the hairpin points and another hairpin was used to secure the pincurl to the head hair. See also Pin curl (3)*329, 415*

PIN CURL (1) A flat curl held in position during the setting process, by a hairpin.
(2) A small flat curl, the dressed-out result of (1).
(3) A small postiche of curls woven and secured to a hairpin for easy attachment to the head hair. Pincurl *qv*, is the best form for No 3. *415*
(4) Verb. To curl hair between the fingers and then to secure the curled hair with pins. 'She had to pin curl her temple hair.'

PINCURL CAGE CLIP Two hinged wire circles covered in net and used to hold the hair of a pincurl in position during the drying process.

PIN CURLING The act of forming curls with the fingers and securing them against the head with hair pins.

PIN CURL MARTEAU A marteau constructed of short hair suitable for dressing as a pin curl, *qv*

PIN CURL WIRE Wire similar to that used for hairpins, which is incorporated in a pin curl as a narrow loop to secure it to the hair-dress.

PINE-TAR SHAMPOO Solution of soft soap and oil of cade (Juniper Tar), coloured with burnt sugar.

PIN FRINGE A postiche of waved or curled hair worn as a fringe and secured on a hairpin for ease of attachment to the head hair.

PIN HOLDER (1) A pincushion for holding hairpins worn on the wrist of the operator.
(2) A magnet worn strapped to the operator's wrist to hold hairpins.

PINKAS'S INVIGORATING HAIR OIL A 19/20th century 'secret' preparation which consisted of a solution of Peruvian balsam and extract of walnut shells with a little cinnamon tincture, in strong spirit. (*Koller*)

PINKY CURL A very small curl, Word derived from the pinky finger, the smallest finger of the hand.

PIN MARTEAU A small marteau mounted on a hairpin. See Pin wave and Pin curl.

PINNE (PIN) A cylindrical metal rod used for curling hair. A curling pin. 'A pinne to crispe the hayre with.' (*Clerk*, 1602)

PINNER A coif with two long flaps, one on each side, pinned on and hanging down. 1652. (*Evelyn*)

PIN PERM See Pin up perm.

PIN TAIL BRUSH A hairbrush with a tail (instead of a handle), similar to a thin knitting needle. Cf Pin comb.

PIN UP (1) Subs. The hair rolled or twisted on curlers or pins to set it into curls in preparation for the dress-out, eg 'It is bad taste to display a pin-up in public.'
(2) Verb. The act of securing the hair on rollers or curlers in position. Eg 'She pins up her hair each evening before retiring.'
(3) Subs. A large photograph of a man or woman with a stylish hairdress for display in the saloon.

PIN-UP PERM A type of cold permanent wave in which the hair is pinned-up in plastic curlers and plastic clips.

PIN WAVE (1) A crinkly type of wave produced by interlacing strands of hair, in figure of eight fashion, over the prongs of a stout hairpin. Popular in the 19th and early 20th century.
(2) A small waved postiche woven and secured to a hair pin for easy attachment to the head hair. Similar to a pincurl but waved. *329*

PINWHEEL Subs. An arrangement of the hair in which it is coiled around a central point to make a pinwheel bang, pinwheel puff, etc. Cf Whorl.

PINWHEEL PONY TAIL A braided pony tail worn coiled into a clock-spring shape and secured to the head by pins or grips. 1940s.

PIPE A cylindrical object of either box wood or baked clay, hollowed a little in the middle length. Used for curling hair in the 17/20th century. Clay tobacco-pipe stems (hence the name), pieces of cane, willow with the bark stripped were also used. (*Creer*) 'The hair was put in pipes and then boiled to impart curl.' 19th century.

PIPED HAIR Hair that has been croquignole or ringlet (spirally) curled on pipes in readiness for the wigmaker.

PIPING (1) The winding of straight hair on clay pipe stems, baked clay or wooden bigoudis, preparatory to boiling for the production of frisure forcée. See also Piped hair.
(2) Curling the ends of the hair with the fingers or around cylindrical objects such as wooden curlers, and fastening them to the malleable dressing-block with pins.

PIPING STICK Pipe, *qv*.

PIQUE DEVANT Fr. See Pick à devant.

PISA BEARD The same as a Stiletto beard, *qv*, 'Play with your Pisa beard; why, where's your brush, pupil?' (*Beaumont and Fletcher, Queen of Corinth*, Act ii Scene 4)

PISS BURNED Discoloured. Commonly applied in the 18th century to a discoloured grey wig. (*Grose, Lex Bal*)

PITYRIASIS A skin disease characterised by the formation of bran-like scales. The (diseased) formation of scurf or dandruff.

PITYRODES The rapid loss of hair brought on by a fine bran-like deposit on the scalp.

PIVOT The point on the head or wig from which the hair falls. The crown *qv*, is the natural pivot of growing hair on the head. American usage.

PIXIE BANG A fringe composed of tapered wisps. (*WO*)

PIXIE LOOK A short hair style for teenage girls, in which wispy locks are a feature. 1950s.

PIXIE WISP A well-tapered wisp of hair coming to a point. (*Trusty*, p 130)

PLAIN HAIRDRESSING The arranging of the hair in a simple, easily managed style.

PLAIN PERUKE See Plain wig.

PLAIN WIG A wig which imitates a natural head of hair, as worn in the 17th century. See Short bob. (*Lambert*)

PLAIT (1) Subs. A contexture of three or more interlaced strands of hair, 1530. Abraided tress of hair.
(2) Verb. To intertwine or braid hair. To interlace three or more strands of hair to form a plait.

Closed plaits incorporate tightly interlaced strands of hair.

Plait of Five Divide the hair into five strands, place three on your right hand and two on the left. Commence with the outside one on the right, and pass it over one and under one. You have now three strands on your left hand. Take up the outside one and pass it over one and under one also. Proceed in this manner unto the end.

Plait of Six Three strands on the right hand and three on the left. Commence with the right hand in all plaits unless told to proceed differently. Pass the outside strand over two. On the left hand pass the outside one under two and over one. This makes a very pretty plait if done carefully, and with a sufficient quantity of hair.

Plait of Seven Over two and under one right; over two and under one, left. Another: Over one, under one, over one, right; over one, under one, over one, left. This pattern makes it a little wider than the preceding.

Plait of Nine Over one, under one, over one, under one, right; over one, under one, over one, under the left. Another: Over two, under one, over one right; over two, under one, over one, left.

Another (Double Grecian) Over two, under two, right; over two, under two, left. This is a pretty plait.

Another (Grecian Centre) Over one, under one, over two, right; over one, under one, over two left.

Plait of Nine (Grecian) Separate the hair into nine strands, and place four upon the left hand, and five upon the right. Commence with the outside one upon the right, and bring it into the middle, passing it over the outer four. Do the same with the hair upon the left hand, and so on alternately. This plait, which looks very pretty when nicely done, is only suitable for thick heads of hair.

Plait of Eleven (Circassian) Six strands on the right, five on the left. Commence over three, under two, right; over three, under two, left. Another: Over two, under one, over two, right; over two, under one, over two, left. Plait of Thirteen Swiss: Over two, under one, over one, under one, over one, right; over two, under one, over one, under one, over one, left.

Another (Double Grecian) Over two, under two, over two, right; over two, under two, over two, left. This is a very pretty plait, and is very suitable for heads of hair of medium thickness. As a general rule, the thinner the hair is the greater number of strands must be employed.

Another (Grecian) Seven strands on the right hand; six on the left. Commence with the outside one upon the right hand, and bring it into the centre, passing it over the other six. Do the same with the hair upon the left hand, and so on to the end. One thing must be particularly observed in all plaits, and that is, that each strand should be of equal thickness, otherwise the work, when completed, will look what is technically called 'gouty'.

Another (Circassian) Over three, under three, right; over three, under three, left. This should be done only when the hair is tolerably long and thick.

Another (Victoria) Under two, under one, over one, under two, right; over two, under one, over one, under two, left. Suitable for a medium head of hair.

Plait of Fifteen (Swiss) Eight strands on the right hand, seven on the left. Over two, under one, over one, under one, over one, under one, right. Over two, under one, over one, under one, over one, under one, left. Another (Double Grecian) Over two, under two, right; over two, under two left. This is a pretty plait and is generally liked. Another (Grecian Centre): Over one, under one, over two, left.

Another (Russian) Eight strands on the right hand, seven on the left. Over two, under two, over three, right. Over two, under two, over three, left.

Another (Grecian) Eight strands on the right hand, seven on the left. Commence with the outside one upon the right and pass it over seven. Repeat the same upon the left hand, and so on alternately to the end.

Another (Victoria) Eight strands on the right, seven on the left. Over three, under two, over two, right. Over three, under two, over two, left. Plait of Seventeen (Double Grecian) Nine strands on the right hand, eight on the left. Over two, under two, over two, under two, right. Over two, under two, over two, under two, left.

Another (Circassian) Nine strands on the right hand, eight on the left. Over four, under four, right. Over four, under four, left.

Another (Tyrolean) Nine strands on the right hand, eight on the left. Over three, under two, over three, right. Over three, under two, over three, left.

Another (Victoria) Over two, under one, over one, under one, over one, under two, right. Over two, under one, over one, over one, under one, under one, left.

OPEN PLAITS, *qv*. To make a nice open plait, a thin strand of hair should be used, as free from short hairs as possible, and it must be rather long. In plaiting, apply a little oil, pomade, or water, in order that the strands may be kept as smooth and compact as possible. It is important for this to be attended to, because, when the hair is afterwards 'pushed upwards' to form the open-worked design, should it be rough, the beautiful appearance will be marred altogether. These plaits are generally made with one, two or three 'draws', that is, one, two or three strands of hair passing down the middle or sides of the plait and incorporated in such a manner as to run in a straight line downwards from the beginning to the end. Upon completing the plaiting of the hair, the 'draw' is to be held firmly between the thumb and fingers of the left hand, while the ends of the remaining strands, must be held equally firm, but distinct, with the right. This being duly attended to, the right hand is to be employed in sliding the hair upwards while the left remains stationary. How far the hair is to be pushed back must be left to the judgment of the executant, for much depends on the length of the hair, the purpose to which the plait is to be applied, and so forth. The strands must be equal in thickness and the work done evenly. It is advisable to separate the strand which is intended for the 'draw' into two portions and twist them firmly together, so as to avoid pushing upwards some of the shorter hairs which it may contain.

Plait of Four (Gimp pattern) Two on the right hand, two on the left. The inner one on the left hand to be twisted so as to form the 'draw'. Over one, under one, right. Under one, over one, left; keeping the twisted strand straight down the centre. When plaited to the end, push up and fasten off securely.

Plait of Four (Gimp pattern) This is worked precisely as the last but when the hair is pushed up, each strand is to be drawn on to the right side by means of the tail comb. They must be put in position singly, the plait arranged in crescent shape, and is to lie flat upon the forehead, cheek, coiffure, or wherever it is intended to be placed.

Plait of Six (Basket plait) Three on the right hand, three on the left. The third strand upon the left hand to be twisted tightly for the 'draw'. Commence over two under one (ie the 'draw'), right. Under two, over one, left. The 'draw' must run down the centre. Plait loosely, push up, and fasten off.

Plait of Eight (Open Swiss pattern) Four on the right hand. Four on the left. The fourth strand upon the left hand to be twisted. Commence over two, under one, over one (the 'draw') right. Under two, over one, under one, left. Plait rather loosely to the end, push up, and fasten off in a secure manner.

Plait of Ten (Open Double Grecian) Five on the right hand; five on the left. The fifth strand on the left hand to be twisted. Over two, under two, over one (the 'draw') right. Under two, over two, under one, left. Push up and fasten off securely. This is a very pretty plait and is sure to give pleasure and satisfaction to the wearer.

Plait of Twelve (Victoria) Six strands upon the right hand, and six on the left. The sixth strand upon the left hand to be tightly twisted. Commence over two, under two, over one, under one (the 'draw'), right. Under two, over two, under one, over one, left. Plait rather loosely, push up and fasten off.

Plait of Fourteen (Open Double Grecian) Seven strands upon the right hand, and seven on the left. The seventh strand upon the left hand to be tightly twisted. Commence over two, under two, over two, under one (the 'draw'), right. Under two, over two, under two, over one, left. Plait loosely, push up and fasten securely. This forms a very pretty plait.

Plait of Sixteen (Tyrolean) Eight strands upon the right hand and eight on the left. The eighth strand upon the left hand to be twisted. Commence over two, under three, over two, under one (the 'draw'), right. Under two, over three, under two, over one, left. Plait carefully, push up and fasten.

Plait of Eighteen (Open Double Grecian) Nine strands upon each side. The ninth one, on the left hand to be twisted rather tight. Commence over two, under two, over two, under two, over one (the 'draw'), right. Under two, over two, under two, over two, under one, left. Plait very carefully, push up and fasten off. This is very rich and handsome, but it requires hair from 24″ to 36″ in length. The following plaits are somewhat different to the preceding ones, inasmuch as the 'draw' is worked in at the side. The effect of this is to produce a light and open plait of a crescent-like form, which is highly useful in elaborate hairdressing. They are intended to be introduced as an embellishment to some heavy styles of coiffure, and also for dressing thin heads of hair when no artificial help is permitted.

Plait of Six (Basket pattern) Four strands on the right hand, and two on the left. The inside one upon the left hand to be twisted, to serve for the 'draw'. Commence over two, under one, over one (the 'draw'), right. Over one, under one (the 'draw') left. Push up, inclining the whole of the plaiting to the right hand, and arrange the strands, if necessary with the end of a tail comb.

Plait of Eight (Open Swiss pattern) Five strands upon the right hand, and three on the left. The third strand upon the left hand to be twisted. Commence over two, under one,

over one, under one (the 'draw'), right. Over one, under one, over one (the 'draw'), left. Push up, arrange as described above, and fasten off securely.

Plait of Ten (Victoria) Six strands on the right hand, and four on the left. The fourth strand on the left hand to be twisted. Commence over two, under two, over one, under one (the 'draw'), right. Over two, under one, over one (the 'draw'), left. Plait moderately firm, push up and fasten off.

Plait of Ten (Double Grecian) Six strands upon the right hand, and four on the left. The fourth strand on the left hand to be twisted. Commence over two, under two, over two (one of these is the 'draw'), right. Over two, under two (one of these is the 'draw'), left. Plait loosely, and be very particular to keep the 'draw' in the right place. The next four plaits are worked with two 'draws', one on each side of the plait. They look very attractive when well done.

Plait of Seven (Fancy Basket pattern) Four strands on the right hand, three on the left. Twist the second strand on each side, counting from the outer ones. Commence on the right hand by passing the third strand over, into the place of the second one, and then plait – over one, under one (the 'draw'), over one, right. There are now four strands upon the left hand. Proceed in a similar way by passing the third strand over the second one (the 'draw'), and plait – over one, under one (the 'draw') over one, left; and so on to the end. Plait loosely, gather all the ends together in the left hand, hold the two 'draws' firmly between the thumb and finger of the right hand, and push up as may be required.

Plait of Nine (Open Swiss pattern) Five on the right hand, four on the left. Twist the second strand on each side. Commence on the right hand, as before described, by passing the third strand over into the place of the second one, and plait – over one, under one, over one, under one, right. Proceed in a like manner with the left hand, and so on alternately unto the end. Finish off as before directed.

Plait of Eleven (Victoria) Six strands on the fourth strands (counting from the outsides) for the two 'draws'. Commence the right side, five on the left. Twist by passing the fifth strand under the fourth one (the 'draw'), and plait – over two, under one, over one (the 'draw') under one, right. Pass the fifth strand under the fourth (the 'draw') on the left hand, and plait in the same manner. Push up as before instructed.

Plait of Thirteen (Handsome Double Grecian) Seven strands on the right hand, six on the left. Twist the fourth strands (counting from the outsides) for the two 'draws'. Commence by passing the fifth strand under the fourth, and plait – over two, under one, over one (the 'draw'), under two, right. Proceed in the same way, with the hair on the left side, and plait each side alternately until the end. Push up and finish off carefully.

The following are examples of open plaits with three 'draws', and they will be found to have a very pretty effect. The designs can be multiplied, *ad infinitum*. But these are sufficiently illustrative of the different styles usually practised.

Plait of Eight (Zephyr) Four strands on the right hand, three on the left, and one down the centre. Twist the second one on each side, counting from the outsides, and twist the centre strand also. Commence on the right hand by passing the third strand over, into the place of the second one, and then plait – over one, under one (the 'draw'), over one, under one (centre 'draw'). Upon the left hand commence by passing the third strand under the second one into its place. Work under one, over one, (the 'draw'), over one, under one (centre 'draw'). Push up and finish off in the usual way.

Plait of Ten (Fantasie) Five strands on the right hand, four on the left, and one in the centre. Twist the three strands, and commence on the right hand side, as described above. Plait over one, under one (the 'draw'), over one, under one, over one (centre 'draw'). On the left hand, work under one, over one, (the 'draw') under one, over one, under one (centre). Finish off in a careful manner.

Plait of Twelve (Unique) Six strands on the right hand, five on the left, and one down the centre. Twist the fourth strand upon each side (counting from the outer one). Commence on the right by passing the fifth strand under the fourth (the 'draw'), and plait – over two, under one, over one (the 'draw'), under one, and over the centre. On the left begin by passing the fifth strand over the fourth strand (the 'draw'). Plait under two, over one, under one (the 'draw'), over one and under one (centre).

Plait of Fourteen (La Sylphide) Seven strands on the right hand, six on the left, and one down the centre. Twist the fourth strand (counting from the outsides), and the centre one. Commence on the right hand by passing the fifth strand under the fourth (the 'draw'). Plait – over two, under one, over one (the 'draw'), under two, and over one (centre). On the left hand pass the fifth strand over the fourth and work – under two, over one, under one (the 'draw'), over two, and under the centre. Do not work it too tight, and use long, fine hair to make these plaits. (*Creer*)

PLAITED CHIGNON A chignon dressed from plaited hair.

PLAITED KNOT A hair twist in which the hair has first been plaited.

PLAITING The action of intertwining or interlacing three or more strands of hair. Pleityng, 1406. (*Little Red Book of Bristol*)

PLAITLETTE A very small hair plait. See also plait and corner plait.

PLAIT ON SPRING A plait mounted on a galloon-covered flat spring shaped to the head and worn as a halo. Also Twist on Spring.

PLASTER CAST A mould of the head in plaster of Paris, *qv*, used to ensure a perfect fit when making a wig for an unusually shaped head.

PLASTER OF PARIS A fine white powder of gypsum made anhydrous by calcination. It sets rapidly when mixed with water and is used for making head moulds. So-called because it was originally made from the gypsum of Montmarte, Paris.

PLASTIC APPLICATOR A pliable plastic container with a suitable nozzle for ejecting a dye of creamy consistency directly on to the hair, eliminating the need of a brush, dish or sponge.

PLASTIC ART Modelling or moulding in clay or other soft material in the making of a head or bust belongs to plastic art.

Some aspects of hairdressing can rightly be regarded as coming within this category; eg the shaping and modelling of wet, curled hair in what is usually referred to as setting the hair to style.

PLASTIC BOWL A small plastic container in the form of a bowl used for mixing hair preparations for holding a preparation during its application. Preferable in many cases to a metallic container as being less likely to have any effect on the chemicals.

PLASTIC CAP See Cap (1).

PLASTIC CURL A curl that has been treated with lacquer; also called a Lacquered Curl.

PLASTIC FOAM WIG BLOCK Light-weight block on which a styled wig can be stored to preserve its shape and dressing. (*N and N*)

PLASTICIZER A substance that softens and makes plastic, synthetic resins used in hair lacquers. Glycerine or triacetin are used as plasticizers to prevent the resin flaking.

PLASTIC LACE Used for the foundations of toupees. The hair line can be extended to the edge of the lace. (*Corson* p 292)

PLASTIFYING LOTION (Plasticizing lotion) A liquid which, applied to dressed hair, coats the cuticle and, when dried, the unevaporated residue holds the hair in position.

PLAT American spelling of the English plait.

PLATINUM BLONDE (1) Adj. A very fair, silvery hued colour popularized by Jean Harlow, the late curvaceous American film star. This colour is produced by bleaching as light as possible and then rinsing with diluted methyl violet or methylene blue to remove residual yellow.
(2) Subs. A fair-haired female.

PLAUTILLA (ad 3rd century) Daughter of Plautianus, favourite Minister of Severus. In the Louvre, Paris, is a stone bust of Plautilla with a moveable stone wig. This enabled the wig to be replaced as fashion changed.

PLEATING The process of making pleats in wig net to ensure a good fit.

PLEUROCOCCUS BEIGELLII See Gregarine.

PLI Subs. Plait, bend, wrinkle. (*Creer*, 1877). The head of water-set hair from drying and combing out. It is in wet pli until dry, after which, until combed through, the hair is in dry pli. Literally in bend, but used by posticheurs as meaning in position – the hair water-set and ready for drying. After drying, the hair, either on postiche or the head, is combed out again, put into position, dampened and once more dried. That is the second pli. It is possible to put a head into third pli or even fourth pli by going through similar continuing processes. See also Mis-en-Pli.

PLICA NEUROPATHICA Matted strands of hair. (*Levin and Behrman*)

PLICA POLONICA Polish ringworm. (*Wheeler*, also *Beigel* p 127)

PLICATE Verb. To fold a strand of hair.

PLICATURA A straight-hair marteau on a double or triple frizette, secured to a comb. (*Creer*)
'15/- a pair. Short hair plicaturas on German shell combs.' (*Waller*). Plicatura is the Latin word for 'a folding', the English derivative, plicature, meaning folding or a fold, has been used since the 16th century.

PLICATURA FRIZETTE See Plicatura Hair Frizette.

PLICATURA HAIR FRIZETTE A Frizette of hair forming part of a Plicatura, *qv*, '1 1s 0d per pair. Made in the best shell comb. For dressing the hair this exquisite style.' (*Waller*)

PLI CLOTH A small rectangle of smooth cloth used in dressing transformations and other postiches. It is pinned over an already waved section to protect it and serves as a base on which to wave another overlapping strand of hair.

PLIERS Small pincers with long jaws having parallel roughened surfaces. Used in boardwork.

PLOCOCOSMIST A hairdresser. (Ms entry in pocket book of *John Savell, Jonathan Royal, Bucks*, 1767)

PLUCK To tug; pull or tear out a hair, etc, with sudden force.

PLUMA A curled bush of frizzled hair by which gallants imitated a feather that was worn in the hat. 17th century.

PLUMAGE HEADDRESS An extravagantly ornamented high-dressed coiffure for women incorporating plumes. Fashionable 1775 to 1783.

PLUMASSIER A worker or dealer in ornamental feathers, especially hair ornaments.

PLUMBIFEROUS HAIR WATERS 19th/20th century.

These were preparations for hair dyeing containing lead in various quantities and combinations. All were, or could be, dangerous. The following were some of the commonest proprietary concoctions: Allen's Hair Restorer, Ayro's Hair Invigorator, Eau de Castile, Eau d'Inns, Eau de Florida, Eau Magique, Eau Hamilton, Eau d'Amerique, Melrose's New Hair Wash, New London Hair Restorer, Rosette's Hair Restorer, Royal Windsor Hair Restorer, New Balsamic Hair Dye, Sterling's Ambrosia, Baume Circassienne, Spring of Life, Eau d'Appolon, Eau de Bahama, Eau de Capille, Nieske's Patent Birch-oil Balsam, Allen's World's Hair Restorer, Milk of Roses Extract (a Viennese preparation). (*Koller*)

PLUMET Fr. Feathers worn as a hair decoration. (*Creer*)

PLUS TUT FAIRE Fr. See A la Plus tôt faire.

PLUTARCH (*King of Sparta*) See Aristomenes.

PLUTO In Roman mythology, the ruler of the infernal regions. By the ancients depicted with long, curled, black hair. (*Salmon*)

PLUTONIAN BEARD A fork-shaped beard having two prongs. See also Neptunian beard. (*Why Shave?*)

PNEUMATIC ROLL An Edwardian postiche consisting of a light-weight, flexible tube or pad with waved hair attached and worn at the front of the head. (30 Dec 1905, *Lady's Pictorial*)

POGONATUS The Bearded Epithet applied to Constantine IV (AD 648–685), Emperor of Rome. (*Baeur*)

POGONIASIS An excessive growth of hair on the male, and growth of beard on the female.

POGONIASTIC An excessively hairy person. Used facetiously in hairdressing circles.

POGONIATE Bearded.

POGONIC Pertaining to the beard.

POGONOLOGIA The science of the beard.

POGONOLOGIST A writer on the subject of beards.

POGONOLOGY The study of beards.

POGONOTOMIST A trimmer of beards or shaver.

POGONOTOMY Beard-cutting or shaving.

POGONOTROPHIST A beard grower.

POGONOTROPHY Cultivating or growing the beard.

POILU The French nickname for a soldier, which means hairy, shaggy, so called from their habit of wearing shaggy moustaches.

POINT A plait of hair: obsolete. 'Her hayre bound into foure severall points.' (*King James's Workes*, 1616)

POINT, TO To fix galloon in position on the wooden wig block with block points. 'Edge the outline of the postiche by pointing ¾" galloon in position with block points.'

POINT CURLING (1) Curling hair by winding it from the points towards the roots.

(2) Curling only the points of the hair.

POINT CUTTING (1) Cutting short lengths only from the ends of the hair.

(2) Cutting hair only with the points of the scissors.

POINTED WIG A shingle wig, made, cut and dressed to a v-shaped point at the neck. Popular in the late 1920s.

POINT FOLDING The bending back of the points of a strand of hair in the winding process for a permanent wave or curling with irons. Also called fish hooking.

POINTING (1) Thinning hair by cutting with the points of the scissors. See Palm cutting.

(2) Trimming, by tapering, short lengths from the points of the hair. 'We must point it, that is take a tress between thumb and fore-finger of the left hand, and, holding the scissors a little inclined in the right hand, cut it obliquely, as it were, hair by hair, By this means the end of each curl becomes smaller, whereas if we were to cut the hair square, the end would be thick and heavy, and prevent the curls keeping in.' (*Walker*, 1837)

(3) In boardwork, securing the galloon and foundation net by hammering block points through them into the wooden wig block.

POINTING HAMMER A small hammer used for driving blockpoints into the wooden wig block to secure the galloon and bracings. *241*

POINTING PLIERS Flat-nosed and pointed nosed pliers used for removing block points from the wooden wig blocks.

POINT KNOTTING Knotting the point end of the hair to the foundation net, instead of the root end, as is usual. After completion of the knotting the shorter points are back-combed and the root ends cut. Mostly used on those areas of a postiche, where the hair is required to be very short.

POINT PROTRUSION That part of the points of a hair wisp that hangs free in weaving.

POINT TO ROOT COMBING Backcombing.

POINT TRESSE A kind of hair work in which human hair is twisted round fine silver threads or plain linen thread, then knitted and worked. True point-tresse resembles extremely fine knitting. Up to the 16th century a lace was made from human hair for ornament. The art was probably practised in much earlier ages when the conquerors returned from war and formed fringes from the hair and heads of the vanquished to adorn their mantles. Point-tresse was made upon the pillow with pins and bobbins. In addition to ornament it was also used to form the foundation or pad over which a lady's hair was dressed. Lace made with grey and white hair was valuable, not only for its variety, but on account of its silvery gloss. A remnant of this type of hair lace making survived until the 1920s when hair lace partings and hair lace for the foundations of wigs were still being made in England and France and probably other European countries. Several portraits of Charles I were worked in point-tresse by ladies loyal to the Royalist cause. They obtained hair from the King for this purpose. (*Caulfield*)

POINTS The ends of the hair furthest from the roots.

POINT WINDING Winding hair on curlers from the hair points towards the root-ends of the hairs.

POINT VICE To be trimmed point-vice – to be trimmed in keeping with the cut of one's clothes. 16/17th century. (*Brathwait, R, The English Gentleman and the English Gentlewoman*, Ed 1641, p 440)

POKER CURL The same as Corkscrew curl; also called in American usage Muscle curl and Tendril curl.

POKER PIN (1) A thin gauffering iron.

(2) A long, coarse hairpin.

POKER STRAIGHT Without a vestige of curl.

POLAND STARCH Starch imported from Hambourg. Of a very fine and clear quality. 18th century. (*Lillie*)

POLE, TO In the 16th and 17th century to cut the head hair. At that time the word trim was confined to cutting the beard.

POLE LOCK (Poll lock) (1) A Dildo. A lock of hair hanging from the head. 17th/18th century. (*Fairholt*)

(2) A corkscrew-shaped lock of hair hanging at the back of the head down the middle of the nape.(*Randle Holme*)

POLIOSIS Premature hair greyness; canities, *qv*.

POLISH PLAIT A dirty, matted condition of the hair, at one time a common condition of many of the inhabitants of Poland, Lithuania and Tartary. (*Enc Brit*)

POLISH RINGWORM Plica Polonica. (*Wheeler*)

POLL (1) The head, 18th century. (Grose, *Lex Bal*)

(2) A wig. 18th century.

(3) Verb. To cut short or crop hair. 'To notch or pole his head.' (*Clerk*, 1602) To be polled – To have a haircut. West Country usage, 18th/20th century. (*Cox* p 246)

(4) The nape of the neck. 17th/19th century. 'Front to poll', one of the essential head measurements for the manufacture of a made-to-measure wig.

POLL COMB A large shell, horn or silver, decorative comb for the dressed hair. 18th/20th century. (*Earle*)

POLLER (POLER) A barber, shaver or hair-cutter. 17th century. (*Home*)

POLT'S RESEDA CURLING POMADE A 19th/20th century 'secret' preparation which consisted of a simple pomade of yellow wax, coconut oil, and olive oil, with an agreeable scent of mignonette and orange flowers. (*Koller*)

POLY BLOCK A wig block composed of a synthetic resin.

POLYPHYMNIA One of the nine muses depicted by the ancients as having orient yellow hair hanging loose about her shoulders. (*Salmon*)

POLYVINYLPYRROLIDONE A water-soluble synthetic chemical used in 'plastic' setting lotions and water-soluble lacquers.

POLYVYNOL BUTEROL Used for scalps with hair implanted.

POMADE A scented ointment for use on the skin or as a dressing for the hair. 'To make a sweete suet called in French and Italian pommade, in Latin pomatum.' 16th century. (*Alexis*) Two groups of pomades were distinguished, one with a soft base, such as lard and beef marrow, the other with a hard base, such as beef or mutton tallow with the addition of paraffin wax or spermacetti to make it firmer. (*Askinson*)

POMADE HONGROISE A perfumed wax for controlling the moustache, until *c* 1918, popular with Army Sergeants and the Police. A 19th century formula was: White wax 1 lb, oil soap ½ lb, gum arabic ½ lb, Rose water 1 pint, otto of bergamot 1 oz, otto of thyme ½ drachm. (*Piesse*) In advertisements of the mid-19th century the firm Unwin and Albert of Piccadilly, London, claimed to be the inventors and sole maufacturers of the genuine Pomade Hongroise. (*Model Men* by Horace Mayhew)

POMADE TOULOUSE See Diachylon.

POMANDER A perfumed ball. From French *pomme d'ambre*, literally an apple of amber.

POMATUM Pomade, *qv* Word derived from Latin *pomum*: an apple, because it was originally made by macerating over-ripe apples in grease. A 1697 recipe comprised: fresh hog's suet 1 lb, sheep's suet 1 lb, wash both in white wine; 16 pom-water apples cleansed and boiled in rose-water; add to these rosewood, sasaffras, roots of orrice, Florentine, of each six drams, of benzoin, storax, calamita, half an ounce of each, and so make it into an ointment. (*NBK*)

An 18th century recipe is as follows: Kid's grease, an orange sliced, pippins, a glass of rose-water, and half a glass of white wine, boiled and strained, and at last sprinkled with oil of sweet almonds. (*Piesse*) A 19th century recipe for common pomatum: 7 lb white mutton suet; 3 lb white hogshead; 1 oz essence of lemon, 40 drops oil of cloves. Melted, refined and mixed well. (*Lillie*)'He pomatumed the hair.'

POMATUMY Covered with pomatum. 18th century. (*Stewart*)

POMP A pompadour front. Vernacular usage. 'Have you finished dressing Mrs Brown's pomp?'

POMPADOODLE A curly pompadour hairdress. Derived from poodle and pompadour. From 1952, when the poodle cut was fashionable. (*Symonds*)

POMPADOUR A style of dressing the hair without a parting, the hair being combed back from the forehead and worn high at the front. So called from a hair style of circa 1745 worn by the Marquise de Pompadour (1721–64). Mistress of Louis XV. (*Bysterveld* p 25)   *400, 405*

POMPADOUR DIP The wave or bend of hair that depends onto the forehead in a pompadour dressing. (*Nicol*)

POMPADOUR KNOTTING Knotting hair on foundation net so that one row is knotted with the knot on the lower left side of the hexagonal mesh, and the next row is knotted with the knot on the lower right side of the hexagonal mesh. This aids the final dressing of the finished postiche and gives height and lift to the coiffure.

POMPADOUR PAD A large pad to give height, over which a Pompadour style may be dressed. 18th/20th century. *408*

POMPADOUR ROLL The same as pompadour pad. Often with loop at both ends.

POMPEIAN HAIR DYE A 19th century proprietary powder hair dye prepared with litharge (Oxide of lead) and quicklime.

POMPEY WIG A name for a physical wig, *qv*. Late 18th century. (*Gent's Mag*, 1761). Probably derived from Pompey, a clown, in Shakespeare's *Measure for Measure*, 1603.

POMPON (Pompom) An ornament attached to a long pin; a tuft or bunch of velvet, flowers, ribbon, etc, worn in the hair, 18th century.

PONY TAIL A hair style for teenage girls, *c* 1950. Identical with hair styles of the Belgic chiefs, 50BC. The hair is worn straight, combed towards the crown and gathered into a single, loose tail of hair secured by a bind near the scalp.

PONY TAIL COMB A circular, hinged comb, used to secure the hair of a pony tail hairdo. See also Round comb.

POODLE CUT Tousled short hair style for women, fashionable in 1952.

POOR MAN'S PERUKE A wig of sheepskin or calves skin with their wool and hair left on. (*Dictionnaire Francois – Celtique*, 1732)

PORCUPINE HAIR See Hystriacis.

PORCUPINE HAIRDRESS A short hair style for women on the growing hair in which the hair on the top and front of the head stands up, *c* 1798.

POROSITY Subs. The state of being porous.

POROUS Having minute interstices through which light, liquids or air may percolate.

PORRIGO A generic name for several diseases of the scalp which are characterized by scaly eruptions.

PORRIWIGGLES Tadpoles, Norfolk usage. Corruption of periwig which, with a queue, resembled a tadpole. (*Holloway*)

PORTLAND A man's hair style popularized in the 1920s by Paul Glaus of The London Gentlemen's Hairdressing Academy.

PORT MAHON See A la Port Mahon.

POSITIONAL SPRING A flat spring used in wig and other postiche foundations to hold the wig's edge firmly in position against the scalp. Also called: contact spring, flat spring, watch spring.

POSITIVE CHEEK WAVE A forward inclined wave.

POSITIVE SKIN TEST When the skin reacts visibly to the test application of hair dye, and becomes inflamed.

POST-CHAISE A hair ornament in the form of a carriage, 18th century. (*Connoisseur*, No 112, 1756)

'Nelly! Where is the creature fled?
Put my post-chaise upon my head.' (*The Mirror*, v 30)

POSTICHE Fr. (Italian: *posticcio*) Counterfeit.

(1) False hair.

(2) An artificial addition of hair, real or false, to the head. (1886, *Pascoe, C E, London To-day*)

Any added hairpiece such as a wig, chignon, pincurl, etc. This word is used by Japanese hairdressers as Posticche. (See *Beauty Book*, 1956/64. Pub Japan).

POSTICHE BRUSH A small brush with a long, pointed handle, for use on postiches.

POSTICHE CLEANING The cleansing of wigs and other postiches by the use of Carbon tetrachloride, *qv*, naptha, benzine, or petrol.

POSTICHE CLIP A small, flat spring clip to which are attached small postiches; used to secure them to the growing hair of a head.

POSTICHE MEASUREMENTS See Measurements.

POSTICHE OVEN A gas or electrically heated oven in which postiches are dried. Also called a Wig oven.

POSTICHE PATCH Any small foundation, of regular or irregular outline, on which is worked hair. Used as a supplement to any part of the head which needs hair or more hair.

POSTICHE PIN (1) A long, round, steel rod, similar to a thin knitting needle and used to give a final arrangement and position to the hair of a dressed postiche.
(2) A hairpin for use in a postiche.
(3) Nickel-plated brass pins. Similar to a dressmaker's pin, but usually with larger heads. Used to hold the hair of a set postiche in position on the malleable block.
(4) A T-pin, *qv*.

POSTICHE RIBBON Galloon, *qv*

POSTICHE STRIP A narrow band of postiche to remedy a local hair deficiency. *203*

POSTICHEUR One who manufactures postiches or artificial additions of hair for the human head. A dresser of postiches, *qv*. French word commonly used in Britain since *c* 1873. See article by Mons Bouchard in *The Hairdresser's Chronicle*, 1873, where he uses this as an anglicized French word.

POTASH SOAP See Soft soap.

POTASSIUM CARBONATE (K_2CO_3) A constituent of some heat permanent waving reagents.

POTASSIUM HYDROXIDE (KOH) Caustic potash. An alkali used in the manufacture of soft soap.

POTASSIUM PERMANGANATE ($KMnO_4$) A chemical which will overdye substances. Used in the 19th century in bleaching processes for the production of fair hair for postiches. The hair was overdyed with a solution of potassium permanganate and then reduced by immersion in sulphurous acid. Hydrogen peroxide has today replaced this method.

POUDRE Fr. Powder, dust.

POUDRE D'OR See Golden hair powder.

POUDRER Fr. To powder the hair.

POUDRE SUBTIL A proprietary preparation for the removal of superfluous hair. Advertised in 1826 by J Delcroix, 158 New Bond Street, London. (*Griffith*)

POUF The same as Puff, *qv*.

POUF A LA PUCE Woman's 18th century coiffure *379*

POUF A L'ASIATIQUE A woman's 18th century coiffure. (*Uzanne*) *466*

POUPEE Fr. Doll. A figure of wax or some suitable material stuffed to the shape of a head and used to display wigs upon or costumes. See Poupée.

POUT To poke or stick out. 'How his hair do pout.' E Dorset usage. (*Barnes*)

POW (1) The head. Northern usage. (*Grose, Prov Glos*)
(2) A haircut. Lancs usage.

POWDER (1) A mass of minute dry particles or granules. See Hair powder.
(2) Verb. To apply powder to the hair by sprinkling or puffing. 'She shall no oftener powder her hair.' (*Ford, Loves Sacrifice*, 1633)

POWDER BAG A small bag with strings, used by hairdressers to carry hair powder when visiting clients to dress their hair. 18th century.

POWDER BELLOWS Small bellows to puff the powder onto the dressed hair, 18th century. Also called Powder puff. *87 (38)*

POWDER BLEACH A bleach prepared from chemicals in powder form. See also Paste bleach and Liquid bleach.

POWDER BLOWER A hollow rubber bulb of convenient size to fit the hand and having several small holes in its vulcanite top through which powder is ejected by squeezing the bulb.

POWDER BRUSH A small brush with soft bristles for the application of powder to the face or hair.

POWDER COLOUR Colour rinses in powder form.

POWDER CONE See Face cone.

POWDER CLOSET (Powdering closet) A small recess, large enough for a person to stand in, the front draped with two hanging curtains. Used in connection with powdering heads in the 18th century. The person stood in the closet and thrust his head between the curtains which protected the clothing.

POWDER DREDGE A small, round, conically-headed tin cannister for storing and sprinkling hair powder onto the hair.

POWDERED HAIR Powder for the hair was abolished for officers by order in 1814 (the common soldier had long ceased to wear it) after the Peninsular Campaigns. The Sovereigns for Russian and Prussia visited England in 1814 after the signing of peace. They appeared with their natural hair and this influenced the Prince Regent to order the abolition of powdering. (*N and Q*, 1860)

POWDERED PUMICE Used for preparing the surface of wax models preparatory to the application of the make-up. Also used for correcting the surface of a razor-setting hone.

POWDERED WIG A wig which needs powdering to complete the dressing.

POWDERER A sort of wicker half-cupola which was fixed to the work bench, partly enclosing the wig block and preventing the powder that was applied to the coiffure from spreading in the room. (*Cox Wigmakers' Art* plate 6)

POWDER GUARD See Powderer and Face cone.

POWDERING APRON (GOWN, DRESS, JACKET or CLOTH) A garment for covering and protecting the clothes when the hair was being powdered. 17th/19th century.

POWDERING ROOM (Powder Room) A small room in which hair was powdered. 17th/19th century. See also Powder closet. Also from the 19th century the small room in a public building where ladies can attend to most aspects of their toilet.

POWDER PUFF (1) Powder bellows. In the 18th century this referred to the puff of hair powder ejected from the puffer on to the hair. (*Gillray*, p 12) *319*
(2) A bunch of swansdown or other suitable material used to apply powder to the hair or face. 19th century. Used in barber shops until about 1914, when they were discarded as unhygienic and replaced by the rubber puffer for after-shave applications of powder.
(3) A contemptuous reference to a man who powdered his hair. 18th/19th century.

POWDER SPRAY A rubber bulb with a neck at the top, having a hole or holes for the emission of the powder. This was half filled with face-powder and by pressing the bulb powder was emitted from the holes. Used by barbers on the faces of clients after shaving and on the necks of clients preparatory to neck clipping. The powder facilitated the passage of the clippers over the skin. See also Powder blower.

POWDER WIG See Powdered wig.

POWTHER Powder. 18th century. Scottish usage. (*Burns*)

PRACTICAL WIG MAKER One who can and does actually make the wig himself, as opposed to a so-called 'Wig maker' who takes the order and then sends the work to a practical wig maker for manufacture.

PRACTICE BLOCK A malleable block knotted with straight hair. Used by apprentices for practice in hair handling, combing, curling, Marcel waving, dressing, etc.

PRACTICE WEFT A piece of strong hair weft upon which a learner can practice curling, waving or winding hair.

PRACTICE WIG A strong wig upon which a learner can practice the various processes of the hairdresser.

PRE-BLEACH Antecedent to a bleaching process; that which is done before the bleach. Often used for the bleach that precedes a hair dye, but that should be called the pre-dye bleach. 'A pre-bleach shampoo is not always necessary before the bleaching of the hair.'

PREDISPOSITION The condition or state of body that renders a person liable to disease.

PREDISPOSITION TEST See Skin test.

PRE-DYE Subs. That which is done before the dye.

PRE-DYE BLEACH Hair bleach, to soften the hair, before the application of a hair dye.

PREEN A pin. 18th century Scottish usage. (*Burns*)

PRENTICE MINOR BOB (Hair cap) A facetious name for short bob wig, 18th century. (*L C March*, 1762) 'Worn short at back to show the stone-stock buckle and nicely stroked from the face to discover seven-eighths of the ears.'

PREPARED HAIR Human hair that has been disinfected, cleansed, rooted, drawn-off, mixed, curled or otherwise prepared, ready for use by the wig maker.

PRE-SATURATION The wetting of the hair with reagent before winding the hair for a permanent wave.

PRESBYTERIAN CUT A man's hair style in which the hair is worn straight and short bobbed.

PRESCRIPTION WAVE A permanent wave that is adapted to the needs of the individual head being treated.

PRE-SOFTENER A substance, usually hydrogen peroxide and ammonium hydroxide, used to sften the cuticle of hair and make it more absorbent preparatory to dyeing it. (But see Pre-bleach for discussion)

PRE-SOFTENER A substance, usually hydrogen peroxide and ammonium hydroxide, used to soften the cuticle of hair and make it more absorbent preparatory to dyeing it. (But see Pre-bleach for discussion)

PRESSER A pressing iron, *qv*.

PRESSING (1) The action of pressing with a pressing-iron seams and knots of hair to flatten them.
(2) The action of combing with a hot metal comb, oiled frizzy hair to straighten it. American usage. (*Wall*)
(3) Sometimes used, but incorrectly, for weft pinching, which is done with pinching irons, *qv*.

PRESSING IRON (1) An iron implement which is heated and used by wig makers to press seams, hair knots and the like. 88 (24, 25), 445A
(2) A metal comb used, when heated, to straighten frizzy hair. American usage. (*Wall*)

PRESSURE BALDNESS See Alopecia compressio.

PRE-TEENAGER STYLE A style suitable for a child under the age of thirteen years. See Sub-teen style.

PRICK EARED One whose ears are longer than his hair. 17th/18th century. (*Grose, Lex Bal*)

PRIMARY COLOURS Red, yellow and blue. From these colours, with the addition of white, the full spectrum range can be prepared.

PRIMP Smart, neat.

PRIMPING Sprucing; touching-up hair or face with the aid of a mirror.

PRINCE ALBERT See Consort.

PRINCE CHARLES FASHION A boy's hair style after that worn by Prince Charles, the eldest son and heir of Queen Elizabeth II of England. (*Miami Herald*, 1965)

PRINCESS COMB A decorative hair comb for a woman's hairdress. 19th century. (*Lich*)

PRINCESS DE LAMBALLE COIFFURE Two 18th century styles of hairdress worn by Princesse de Lamballe (1749–1792); one a high-dressed coiffure, the other full but lower, with a large pendant marteau curl hanging on each shoulder. *368*

PRINCESS EVENING HEADDRESS A woman's hair style for evening wear, *c* 1875. (*Lich*)

PRINK Verb. To dress or adorn ostentatiously, to arrange with nicety, especially the hair. 'Janine is still prinking her hair.'

PRINKED Well-dressed, neat, Exmoor usage. (*Grose, Prov Glos*) 'Her hair all prinked.'

PRISON CROP Very short hair similar to the Convict Crop, *qv*. Prisoners in English gaols had their hair cropped short all over. 'To be cropped as if you were a prison bird.' (*Mrs Henry Wood, Johnny Ludlow*, 1890)

PRIVATE WIG A wig of necessity in contradistinction to a theatrical wig.

PRIVATE WIG MAKER A wig maker who makes wigs for private citizens. See also Mechanical wigmaker and Theatrical wig maker.

PROBLEM HAIR Any head of hair that presents a difficulty not normally met with in relation to the particular treatment involved.

PROCESSED HAIR Hair that has been artificially curled, dyed or bleached.

PROCESSING A series of actions in a hair dyeing, bleaching, curling or waving process.

PROFESSOR OF HAIRDRESSING A skilled hairdresser who offered to teach the art of hairdressing and professed to be competent to do so. 18th/20th century.

PROGRESSIVE DYE A dye which restores or adds colour to the hair gradually over a period of time.

PRONG One of the rods, shafts or tines of a curling or Marcel waving iron. See Marcel waving iron.

PRONGED CRIMPING IRON See Crimping iron.

PROTECTIVE CREAM A Barrier cream, *qv*.

PROTECTOR A collar of rubber or other non-heat conducting material interposed between the scalp and the wound hair as a protection to the scalp in a heat permanent waving process, 20th century.

PROTEIN PERMANENT WAVE A permanent wave in which the solution contains ingredients to prevent brittleness and breaking of the hair. (*Johnson*)

PROVIDED TOOL OR MACHINE Those tools or machines, such as hand-dryers, permanent waving machines and hairpins which are provided by the employer for the use of the employee in the performance of his salon duties. 20th century.

PRUDENCE See à la Prudence.

PRUNE To cut. 16th/18th century.
'And prune the curled tresses of his locks, Which the arts-man neatly had dishevell'd.' (*Sampson*, 1636)

PRUNYIE To trim. Scottish usage. (*Henderson*)

PRURITIS CAPITIS Itching of the scalp. (*Wheeler*)

PRURITUS MYSTAX Itching of the upper lip, 'moustache' irritation. (*Wheeler*)

PRUSSIAN LOCK A man's short hair style. 1965.

PSEUDO Seemingly or professedly, but not actually.

PSEUDOKNOTTED HAIR See Trichonodosis.

PSEUDOPELADE See Alopecia cicatrisata.

PSILOPHRYAS Absence of eyebrows. (*Wheeler*)

PSORIASIS A skin disease that is characterised by red scaly patches.

PSYCHE KNOT A loose twist of hair brought from the neck to near the crown, where it is fastened with hairpins; the remainder of the twist is loosely coiled around the first part of the Psyche knot. (*GOP* 1911)   *382*

PUBES Pubic hair.

PUBIC FUZZ See Pubic hair.

PUBIC HAIR Hair of the pubes or pubis. Caroline Lamb sent a lock of her pubic hair to Lord Byron. (*John S Mayfield*)

PUBIC LOUSE (Phthirus pubis) A variety of louse that infests the pubic region and more rarely the axillary hairs and eyelashes. (*Jarrett, R R*)

PUBIGEROUS Bearing downy hairs.

PUDDING BASIN CUT A common country haircut performed on boys and girls from at least the 17th century (and probably much earlier) to 20th century. It consisted of the simple expedient of placing a pudding basin over the head and cutting off all hair below the rim of the inverted basin.

PUERPERAL ALOPECIA See Alopecia puerpera.

PUFF (1) An 18th/19th century term for a hairdresser or barber.

(2) A hair powder blower. 'To eject powder in your hyre, Here is a pretty puff.' (*Smith, J*)

(3) A rounded, soft, protuberant mass of hair formed by back combing.

(4) Fronts of hair so made and dressed.

(5) A frisette made of crêpe hair, also a crêpe pad.

(6) A loose dressing of puff curls, usually on a diamond-mesh foundation and worn as a chignon. 19th/early 20th century.

PUFF COIFFURE A hairdress incorporating Puffs, *qv.303*

PUFF CURL A soft, loose curl dressed by backcombing.

PUFF CUSHION A circular, velvet-covered, hair-filled cushion about 12″ in diameter, flattened slightly at the top and bottom. Used for dressing puff curls and other forms of small postiches.

PUFF DRAWING WIRE A piece of strong wire with a hook at the end to catch the loop of a frisette or puff, and draw it into the Puff tube, *qv.*

PUFF TUBE (PAD TUBE) A metal tube of 1″ to 1½″ bore and 12″ to 15″ in length which is heated and into which a puff, frisette, or pad is drawn by means of a drawing wire. The hot tube gives shape and regularity to the puff.   *166*

PUFF WIG A man's wig dressed in a full puffy style, *c* 1700. 'Here's ten guineas, get thyself a drugget coat and a puff wig.' (*Farquhar, Inconstant,* 1703)

PUFFER See Powder bellows.

PUFFING The action of puffing hair by back-combing.

PULL-BACK A woman's hair style dressed back from the face. (*Greene*)

PULL BURN (1) A scalp burn resulting from the pulling of a part of the scalp through or clear of a protector during a permanent waving process, and exposing it to a degree of heat which causes burning. Any burn to the scalp while the scalp skin is under tension.

(2) The term is sometimes, but incorrectly, used to denote a soreness or inflammation caused by excessive pulling or a too tightly adjusted protector or curler in the permanent waving process. See Heat burn.

PULL-UP A kind of hair style for women in which the hair is dressed pulled-up and not hanging directly from the roots. (*Greene*)

PULVIL (1) Subs. Perfumed powder for the hair or body. 'Saluted by the fragrancy of powder de orange, jesmine, pulvil.' (*Ames*) A hair powder perfume made from the moss of apple trees, ambergris, musk and civet. 17th/18th century. (*Lillie*)

(2) Verb. To perfume or powder.

PULVIL CASE Powder case; also, cosmetic case. 18th century.

PULVILLO See Pulvil.

PUMICE A light porous lava. Used for removing dye stains on skin. In its powdered form it is used for preparing the surface of wax models to receive the make-up, also for correcting the surface of a razor setting hone.

PUMPKIN HEAD A stupid person. From the 18th/19th century American custom of placing a pumpkin shell over the head and trimming around the rim of the shell. See also next entry. (*Peters*)

PUMPKIN HEAD Hair style for men, 18th century Connecticut, USA (*De Zemler p 259*)

PUNK ROCK STYLE Grotesque hair styles of many colours and shapes, (including mauve, red, yellow, green and blue) worn by members of the punk rock groups and their followers, exemplified by the Sex Pistols and other pop band groups.

PUNTO BEARD A small pointed beard. (*Repton p 11*)

PURCHASED HAIR False hair; a wig.
'If winckles, rotting teeth and purchased hair,
If paint and patches make a woman fair, ... '
(*Killigrew,* 1695)

PURITANS Short locks. From the short hair styles worn by 17th century Puritans.

PURSE WIG See Bagwig.

PUSH WAVE A method of setting wave in curly hair. Comb the hair straight on the head and then by using the comb in the right hand and the left hand resting on the hair strand above the comb push the hair upwards and allow it to break into its natural wave. 19th/20th century.

PUSSY MOSS A woman's pubic hair. Bristol and West of England usage, *c* 1928; also Michegan, USA. usage, 20th century. (inf *Warren Boes*)

PYE-BALD See Piebald.

PYRAMIDAL A 19th century woman's hair style. (*HTATH*)   *290*

PYRAMIDAL MOUSTACHE A moustache in a modified pyramid shape. (*Trusty*)   *101P*

PYROGALLIC HAIR DYE Pyrogallic acid ¼ oz, hot distilled water 1½ oz, dissolve then add when cool ½ fluid oz, rectified spirit. (*Cooley*)

PYR-POINTED HAIRPIN (Ball-pointed hairpin) A hairpin with knobs on the ends. They improve the holdfast and prevent scratching the scalp. (*OG*)   *167*

PYRUS CYDONIA See Quince.

QU See Queue.

QUACK HAIRDRESSER An ignorant pretender to knowledge and skill in the art and craft of hairdressing.

QUADRATE BEARD A 16th/17th century square-shaped beard style. (*Taylor*)

QUADRILATERAL CHINESE RAZOR SHARPENER See Cowvan's canton strop.

QUADRILLED MOUNTING Weft sewn to a squared pattern on a wire foundation for curl clusters and other forms of postiche. 19th/20th century.

QUAKER STYLE A plain, unaffected hair style.

QUARTER TWIST WIND In permanent curling and hair setting, a twist wind, with only slight twisting of the hair. (*Smith*)

QUASSIA The wood, root or bark of the *quassia amara*, a South American tree and of some other trees such as the bitter ash (*Picraena exelsa*) used, with camomile, to brighten hair, and to repel lice.

QUATREFOIL A four-lobed grouping of hair.

QUAYSIDE SHAVER A person who shaved on the quayside at Newcastle-on-Tyne, 18th/19th century. (*Denham*)

QUEBRACHO See Aspidosperma.

QUEEN CUT An effeminate hair style worn by a male person.

QUEER FLASH A miserable weather-beaten Caxon. Slang, 18th centry.

QUERCITRON The inner bark of the *quercus tinctoria* or dyer's oak of N America, used in a yellow hair dye in the preparation of hair for postiches.

QU'ES ACO See A la Qu'es aco.

QUESTION MARK CURL A stand-up curl with a very long stem, like a quaver in music.

QUEUE (1) Subs. Tail of a wig and by extension in word use, the wig itself.
(2) A long plait of hair hanging down behind; a pigtail. The ordinary soldier pipe-clayed his own hair and formed a queue from that. The officers wore queue wigs. (See Queue flash) Regimental queues were ordered to be nine inches long; among the Guards they were fourteen inches. Discontinued 1808. (*James*)
(3) A wig, see (1) above.
(4) Verb. To put up the hair in a queue. 'Their hair was queued', 18th century.
(5) An 18th century nickname for General Pattison. (*Fenton*)

QUEUE CONE A long cone-shaped object used to form the queue. (*Jones*)

QUEUE DE RENARD 18th century wig style. *125*

QUEUE FLASH In 1808 the troublesome queue was abolished to the great delight of the soldiery. The same order directed the hair to be cut short in the neck, and a small sponge added to the soldier's necessaries for the purpose of frequently washing his head. The 23rd Foot (now The Royal Welch Fusiliers) were serving in the West Indies in 1808 and did not receive the order. They were still wearing queues on their return to the UK about 1811. The flash had been worn by all units, attached to the coatee collar to prevent grease and flour staining the coatee when queues were worn, and the 23rd Foot asked, as a special tradition, to continue to wear the flash as the last UK regiment to have worn this embellishment. (*Carter, Austin*)

QUEUE TOUPEE A wig with a tail. (*Ladies' Companion*, July 1851)

QUEUE WIG OR QUEUE PERUKE A wig with a queue or tail, 18th century.

QUICK BLEACH A bleaching mixture of magnesium carbonate, sodium perborate, surface-active agents and hydrogen peroxide mixed at the time of use. Also called White henna, *qv*. (*Wall*)

QUICKSET A setting lotion incorporating alcohol. This evaporates quickly and lessens the drying time for a hairset.

QUICK SWITCH Subs. See Band slip-on.

QUICK SWITCH COIFFURE A dressed wig. American usage. See Instant hairdo.

QUIFF A flat curl or half curl of hair, on the forehead, set in position with water, but more usually human saliva, and allowed to lie flat on the forehead, then oiled with the rest of the hair. A popular early 20th century affectation of soldiers and male manual workers, which persisted in some areas, including Bristol, until as late as *c* 1940. The present writer has not met with it since then, but doubtless there are still a few old stalwarts addicted to this mode.

QUILLAIA The inner bark (soap bark) of a South American tree belonging to the rose family. It contains soponin, which lathers with water. Used in some soapless shampoos. (*Verrill*)

QUILL STYLING COMB A plastic hybrid brush/comb of three, four or five rows of equidistantly spaced teeth.

QUILL TOP COMB A dressing comb with a narrow, rounded spine. 20th century.

QUIM WIG (1) A merkin, *qv*.
(2) A female's pubic hair. Also quim bush, quim whiskers, quim pie, quim scroff, etc. All are of Bristol usage. (Vulgar slang.)

QUINCE SEED Seeds from *pyrus cydonia*. Soaked in water a slimy mucilage is formed which was a common type of setting lotion in the late 19th century, early 20th century and is still used.

QUININE $C_{20}H_{24}N_2O_2$. An alkaloid from cinchona bark. Quinine sulphate and quinine hydrochloride are used in hair tonics. Cinchona (synonyms-Peruvian Bark and Jesuits' Bark) from which is derived quinine, was originally introduced into Europe in the 17th century by the Jesuits from its native habitat, Peru where it had been used by the natives for febrile conditions. In 1638 the wife of Count Cinchon, Viceroy of Peru, suffered an attack of fever and was treated with the powdered bark. Upon her recovery she widely praised its virtues, hence the name cinchona. (*Dorset Folk Remedies*, ed *J Stevens Cox*, 1962)

QUO VADIS A very short hair style for men, cut by clippers and razor. Mid-20th century. (*Trusty*)

QUOIF OR COIF A plain, close-fitting headdress of any material, worn by either sex. A sort of skull cap.

QU PERUKE An 18th century man's wig with a queue, *qv*.

R

RACKET HEAD DRESS A woman's hair style in the general form of a tennis racket, worn high and puffed out at the sides and encircled by jewelled ornamentations, 16th century.

RADIAL BRUSH A hair brush in which the bristles are set around the head of the brush.

RADIATE COIFFURE A hairdress arranged radially, branching out like spokes.

RADICAL VINEGAR Glacial acetic acid.

RADIX PILI Hair root.

RAG CURLS Curls formed by rolling or twisting the hair in short strips of rag and leaving the hair so rolled for several hours. Some women even sleep in this unattractive condition. Expression: 'She's still got her hair in rags', ie the hair not yet having been combed out into curl or, as is more usual with this method, frizz.

RAGGEDY ANN BOB A short hair style for women similar to the wind-blown bob, *qv*, 1940s. (*Wilson, K*)

RAISED BANDEAU A crimped roll of hair at the front of the head, dressed over a frisette. (*Mallemont*) 387, 395

RAISED WAVED COIFFURE A hair dressing in which the waved hair at the front of the head is either back-combed or dressed over a pad and dressed high. (*Mallemont*)

RAISING A WORKROOM ORDER Obtaining an order for a postiche with the necessary details such as type, colour, measurements, style, etc. London usage.

RAKE A strong comb with large even-sized teeth. Used for removing tangles in long hair.

RALEIGH BEARD A pointed beard close cut on the cheek. Named after Sir Walter Raleigh (1552–1618). Similar to the Vandyck.

RAMILLIES TAIL OR QUEUE See Ramillies wig.

RAMILLIES WIG (Ramallie, Ramellie, Ramilie, etc.) A wig with a long, gradually diminishing, plaited queue (called the Ramillies tail), secured at the top with a large bow of black ribbon and by a smaller bow at the tip of the queue. Named after the battle of Ramillies, 1706. By 1731 the pigtail wig had reached its greatest height of absurdity and popularity. By *c* 1780 the plait was often turned up and secured at the nape of the neck. Worn by military officers and others affecting military fashions in the 18th century. (*Smith, Creer*). Lord Bolingbroke (Henry Saint-John, First Viscount Bolingbroke) 1676–1751, is credited with introducing this wig style to the *Elegant World*.

RAM HEAD A cuckold. (*Taylor, J. Cornu-copia*, 1642)

RAMSAY, ALLAN (1686–1758). An Edinburgh wig maker and poet, *c* 1717, abandoned wig making for bookselling. His publications included *Collected Poems*, 1721; *Tea-table Miscellany*, 1724–7; *The Gentle Shepherd*, 1725.

RAM'S HORN CURL A large-diameter partial curl.

RAPHAEL STYLE A hair style in the manner of those depicted by the painter Raphael (1483–1520).

RASTICK HENNA OR HENNA RASTICK A paste made from a combination of henna and another substance such as powdered gall nuts, salts of copper or iron, lucerne, rhubarb, catechu, etc. (*Savill*)

RAT (1) A tapered hair pad for dressing the hair over.
(2) A tangled bunch of hairs.

RAT, TO Vigorous backcombing, especially at the point end of a plait to prevent it unbraiding. (*Rohrer, Beauty Formulas*)

RATAPPENADY A Macaroni. (Recorded on an 18th century print of a Macaroni.)

RAT'S NEST (1) A dirty, touzled wig. 19th/20th century. West of England usage.
(2) The hair bun after the head hair has been dressed over a pad. Slang, American usage. (*B and B*)

RAT'S TAIL A thin, straight hanging lock of hair. 'on each side of his face a few straight locks hang down like, what are vulgarly called, "rats' tails".' (*Lambert, J Travels through Lower Canada*, 1810 Vol 1 p 162)

RAT TAIL COMB See Tail comb.

RATTING The action of back-combing to produce a 'rat' or puffed effect. American usage. (*Trusty*) See Rat and Back combing.

RAVEN BLACK A similative term denoting deep black.

RAVEN HAIR Deep black hair.

RAVE WIG A type of fashion wig, 1964. The name presumably infers that either the wearer or spectators will rave about it.

RAVIR Fr. See a Ravir

RAW CUTTINGS Human hair as cut from the head.

RAW HAIR Untreated hair. Hair as it is cut from the head.

RAZE To erase or scrape out. From the same Latin root as razor, ie *rasus*, participle of *rado*, to scrape. See Razor.

RAZOR (1) A sharp-edged implement for shaving the beard and hair, or cutting hair. See also Concave, Cut-throat, Electric, French, German, Hollow ground, Safety, Semi-Solid and Solid Razor. 87 (3) 108, 440
(2) Verb. To cut with a razor. 'The hairdresser razored the ends of the child's hair.'

RAZOR BLADE That part of a cut-throat or safety razor having the cutting edge.

RAZOR CUT Haircutting by means of a razor instead of scissors.

RAZOR EDGE A keen edge.

RAZOR FACE Lord and Lady Anglesea appeared under this name in the poem *The Morning Visit*, 1768. (*NFH*)

RAZOR PASTE Putty powder, 1 oz, oxalic acid ¼ oz, Honey enough to make into a stiff paste. A 19th century formula. (*Englishwoman's Domestic Magazine*, Vol 3) Also a mixture of tallow and jeweller's rouge.

RAZOR SCISSOR A haircutting scissor for hairdressers' use, made with very thin blades that did not require grinding, but could be set on a hone after the manner of a razor. Marketed by R Hovenden, (Adv in *Creer's Lessons in Hairdressing*) 19th century.

RAZOR SETTING The honing of a razor to produce a sharp edge. See Hollow ground Razor and Solid razor.

RAZOR SETTING STONE See Hone.

RAZOR SHELL The shell of a mollusc shaped like a cut-throat razor blade.

RAZOR'S TOOTH The cutting edge of a razor. 'A keen toothed razor.' A very sharp razor. Bristol usage.

RAZOR STROP See Strop.

RAZOR WIPE A shallow, circular, rubber cup, on the rim of which the lather and shaven whiskers are removed from the razor.

RAZOR WIPER See Razor wipe.

READY, TO To comb (the hair). Northern usage. (*Grose, Prov Glos*)

READYING COMB A wide toothed comb. See also To Ready. Northern usage. (Grose, *Prov Glos*)

REAGENT (1) A reactive substance.
(2) Any substance used in the permanent waving process to effect the necessary change in the hair structure to ensure a permanent curl.

REBROUSSER (Les cheveux) Fr. To turn up the hair.

RECAMIER CHIGNON A coiled chignon worn at and extending below the crown towards the nape. As worn by Madame Récamier (1777–1849).

RECAMIER COIFFURE A hair style similar to that worn by Madame Récamier (1777–1849).

RECEPTIONIST A person whose duty it is to receive clients, book appointments and often, to act as a cashier. 20th century.

RECHERCHE Fr. Choice, exquisite.

RECOLOURATION The dyeing of bleached hair.

RECONDITION (Hair (1) Verb. To restore hair by means of suitable substances and/or treatments to its normal condition.
(2) Subs. The action of restoring hair to its normal condition.

RECONDITIONER Subs. A preparation to recondition or restore the hair to a healthy condition.

RECONDITIONING Adj. Having the quality of being able to recondition, eg 'A reconditioning cream will improve the condition of your hair madam.' 20th century.

RECORD CARD A card on which details are recorded, such as colours, timing, strength, etc of dyes, solutions for permanent waving, etc which are used on individual clients, and which will act as a guide for future attention.

RECTILINEAR Taking the course of a straight line, bounded or formed in or by straight lines.

RE-CUT (1) Verb. To cut suitably a head of hair in preparation for a new style.
(2) Verb. To cut the hair to preserve an existing style.
(3) Subs. The action of cutting a head of hair to accomplish either (1) or (2) above.

RED (1) A red-haired person. Slang. (*B and B*)
(2) A jocular nickname for an auburn haired person. 'Red Nicoll, the Guernsey turf accountant.'

RED BEARD (1) Frederick I (1121–1190), Kaiser of Germany. See Barbarossa.
(2) Horush Horuc (1474–1518), Sultan of Algiers.
(3) Khair Eddin (1510–1546), Sultan of Algiers. (*Brewer*)

RED COMYN Sir John Comyn of Badenoch, stabbed by Robert Bruce, 1306; so called from his red hair. (*Brewer*)

REDD To untangle. Southern usage. (*Grose, Prov Glos*)

REDDIE A red-haired person. Slang. (*B and B*)

REDDING COMB An ordinary hair comb. The word redding has the meaning of tidying, separating, etc. (*Wilson*)

REDESIGN CUT A foundation cut when a hair style is changed.

RED HAIR Should anyone with red hair first foot a house in the New Year, this is regarded by many persons as an unlucky omen. One reason for the prejudice against red hair in many parts of Britain is that Judas Iscariot was red-haired. There is a Shakespearean reference to this in '*As You Like It*', Act III, Scene 4.

Red hair is also said to be a sign of fiery temper and of a passionate diposition in matters of love. In Cornwall the red haired are believed not to be able to make good butter. In Dumbartonshire red haired men are said to make unfaithful husbands. In the classical theatre of ancient Greece and Rome, red hair was a characteristic of the dishonest slave of comedy. (*Haigh*)

Famous historic and mythological figures who were red haired: Sampson, Apollo, Venus, Juno.

RED HAIRED PERSON At one time the fat of a dead red haired person was in demand as an ingredient for poisons. (Middleton, '*The Witch*', v ii). Chapman in *Bussy d'Ambois*, 1613, wrote that – flattery, like the plague 'Strikes into the brain of Man, and rageth in his entrils when he can, Worse than the poison of a red-haired man.'

RED HEAD An auburn-haired person.

RED HEADED JOB A red haired woman. Slang. (*B and B*)

RED HEADER A red haired person. Slang. (*B and B*)

RED THATCHED ROOF Auburn haired. American slang, 20th century. (*B and B*)

REDUCER See Colour reducer.

REDUCING AGENT A chemical that deprives another of oxygen.

REDUCTION DYE Colour produced on the hair by the chemical reduction of a metal salt to the metal.

REDUCTION OF COLOUR See Colour reduction.

REEDY HAIR Yellow hair. From the reed used for thatching.

REEL STICK See Spool stick.

REFINED CHINESE HAIR See Refined hair.

REFINED HAIR Oriental hair that has been bleached, coloured and prepared for use in wigmaking.

REFLECTED COLOUR Colour from an outside source which is reflected onto the hair.

REFRESHER CUT A hair trim.

REFRIGERANT WASH A cooling rinse for hair and scalp.

Two examples used in the 19th century were:
(1) Lactic acid 1 part, rose water 8 parts.
(2) Citric acid 1 part, distilled water 14 parts. (*Gurney*)

REGENCY PUFF A lightly dressed artificial front of hair, c 1892. *336*

REGENCY WIG Early name for Bag wig, *qv*. This wig was first worn (after 1730 – during the Regency of Duc d'Orleans, hence the name. (*Cox p 24*)

REGENT, THE English hair style for men. 1930s. (*Foan*) *101V*

REGENT DIP A pin wave, *qv* dressed in a cheek dip.

REGRINDING The process of grinding a new cutting edge on a razor or scissors as a result of their edges being dropped or damaged beyond the power of the honing process to put a cutting edge on them.

REGROWTH The new hair growth of natural colour and form. The word *regrowth* strictly is a misnomer. The hair does not regrow; it continues to grow. The better term would be new growth.

REGULAR HAIRCUTTING SCISSORS See Haircutting scissors.

REHABILITATION RINSE An acid rinse, usually acetic or citric acid.

RELAX HAIR To de-frizz hair. To weaken or remove frizz or curl from hair.

RELEVE Fr. Raised, high, lofty.

RELISLE WIG A man's wig. 18th century. Ms receipt of Richard Thomson, Edinburgh, June 1742. 'A relisle wig, £1 1s 0d'. (In possession of S C)

REMINDER BOWL (Barber's Basin, *qv*) In the 17th and 18th century clients often paid their barbers quarterly and the barber would remind them of their quarterly due by holding out their bowl and saying, 'Sir your quarter is up'.

REMOVER See Dye remover.

RENAISSANCE HAIR STYLES Hair styles developed in and characteristic of the Renaissance period, 14th to 16th century.

RENAISSANCE STYLE OF VEIL A veil attached to the back of the hairdress and hanging down the back of the head and body. (*Mallemont*)

RENG See Henna reng.

REPAIR (1) Verb. 18th century equivalent of cleaning and dressing a wig. To renovate a wig.
(2) Verb. To mend and effect reparations to a piece of postiche. 19th/20th century. (*Elegant Arts*)

REPEAT HAIR DESIGN A hair design composed of recurring motifs.

REPELLENT That which repels.

REPENTIR CURL (Magdalen curl, *qv*) A long ringlet or spiral curl of hair. Repentir is French for a penitentiary and les repentiers were the girls that were sent there for reformation.

REPENTIRS Ringlets, Curls.

RESERVOIR COMB A dressing or setting comb incorporating a receptacle for fluid, and so constructed that it will release the fluid onto the comb's teeth as required.

RE-SHAPE (1) Subs. A haircut to restore a style change. 'Madame needs a re-shape.'
(2) Subs. A haircut to change the hair foundation for a style.
(3) Verb. To cut hair to effect (1) and (2) above.

RESIDUE That which is left; the remainder.

RESISTANCE Subs. The impeding or stopping effect exercised by some hair that makes penetration by dye, bleach, permanent waving or other lotions, difficult.

RESORCINOL ($C_6H_6O_2$) White needle-like crystals which become pink on exposure to air and light. Soluble in ether and glycerol. It is an antiseptic, astringent and antipruritic agent, used in hair tonics and anti-dandruff lotions.

RESTORATIVE A preparation capable of restoring or renewing the normal condition of the hair or its colour, or inducing a new growth on a thinning head of hair.

RE-STYLING The action of designing a new style of hairdress.

RETICULATED HEADDRESS See Nebuly headdress.

RETOUCH (1) Subs. An application of bleach or dye to the new growth of hair.
(2) Verb. To apply bleach or dye to the new growth of hair.
(3) Verb. A going-over of a process already completed. 'Come back in two days and have your Marcel wave retouched.'

REVEREND BEARD A long flowing beard reaching the chest, 17th century. (*Cleveland, Poems*, 1687)

REVERSE CURLING Winding a row of curls in a clockwise direction and the next row in an anti-clockwise direction. (*Morris*)

REVERSE KNOTTING Knotting in the opposite direction to that in which the hair will be combed in the dressed postiche. This raises the hair from the foundation and gives fullness to a dressing.

REVERSE PERMANENT WAVE To take curl or frizz out of the hair by permanently straightening curled hair.

REVOLVING SLEEVE A plastic tube which surrounds the handle of the Marcel-waving irons. Each handle of the irons is covered with a tube or sleeve that readily revolves. It facilitates the rolling of the irons during the Marcel waving process and affords a degree of insulation and protects the hand if the irons become uncomfortably hot. Also called cheating irons because for students it makes waving easier.

RE-WAVE To wave over again (emphasizing the original waves) a head of hair previously waved.

REWAVING The action of permanently re-curling (rewaving) hair already subjected to the process of permanent curling, which presumably, had insufficient curl; or Marcel waving over an existing Marcel wave to strengthen it.

RHINOCEROS Name for a man's 18th century wig style (*London Mag*)

RHINOCEROS MARROW Unctuous concoctions of uncertain content sold by barbers in the 18th and early 19th century. (*Chambers Journal*, 1866 p 709)

RHUBARB Used in hair dyes to brighten blonde hair. An alkaline extraction from the roots imparts golden-red tones to hair. (*Wall*)

RHUSMA An oriental depilatory consisting of orpiment and unslaked lime, made into a paste with water. Dangerous and not employed in Europe. (*Poucher*)

RIBBON Galloon, *qv*.

RIBBON BANG A fringe of hair combed across the forehead, simulating a ribbon.

RIBBON PIN CURL A 1″ (approx) wide curled tress of hair.

RICHMOND A man's hair style created in the 1930s by Paul Glaus of the London Gentlemen's Academy of Hairdressing.

RIDER A jockey, *qv*.

RIDGE CURL A pin curl that is formed behind the ridge or crest of a wave and within the wave's curve. (*Wall*)

RIDGE PIN CURL See Ridge curl.

RIDING WIG A wig suitable for wearing when horse-riding, 18th century.

RIG, TO To prepare the weaving sticks by arranging the silks ready for weaving. 'Rig the weaving sticks with two silks and a middle wire ready for weaving a 25″ weft for a diamond mesh chignon.'

RIGHT-GOING WAVE A wave of which the trough is directed towards the right as looked at by the waver.

RIGHT-HAND STICK See Spool-stick.

RILL, TO (1) To over-process hair in permanent waving and produce small diameter curl.
(2) To set hair in narrow waves.

RILLING Setting hair in narrow waves. West Country usage. From 1920s.

RIMMERS A narrow band of whiskers around the face and chin. 19th century. American usage.

RING COMB A hair comb consisting of two toothed semi-circles, hinged at one end and used to secure the root ends of pony tails.

RING CURL A narrow curl of any diameter.

RINGED HAIR (Pili annulati) A type of canities in which the hair shaft shows alternating zones of light and dark when viewed in reflected light.

RINGLET (1) A curled lock or tress of hair, 1667.
'Her . . . tresses . . . in wanton ringlets wav'd.' (*Milton, P L*)
(2) A bubble curl.
(3) A spiral curl.

RINGLET BUNCH Side curls made of ringlet hair, irrespective of the length of hair or quantity wefted, and sewn up closely or in diamond shaped contours.　　　399

RINGLET CURL A tautological term, as in ringlets (curls).

RINGLET FRONT A front of hair dressed in ringlets (curls).

RINGLET WEFT See Once in weft.

RINGLET WIND Spiral-wind, *qv*. (*Smith*)

RING PAD A bun pad, *qv*.

RINGWORM A contagious skin disease caused by a vegetable parasite which appears as circular lesions. When affecting the scalp it is called *Tinea Tonsurans*.

RINOX-ERROS See A la rinoxerros.

RINSE (1) Verb. To pour liquid over or swill lightly.
(2) Subs. Liquid preparations to bleach, dye or recondition etc the hair by pouring the rinse over and through the hair hanging over the shampoo basin.

RITCHIE, DAVID A celebrated hairdresser and perfumer who practised his craft *c* 1772. Author of *Treatise on Hair*. (*Fairholt*, pp 386, 395).
A fashionable 18th century hairdresser, wigmaker and dentist of Rupert Street, London. His shop was two doors from Coventry Street. Ritchie was one of the principal popularisers of the very high coiffure in 1772. (*Smith, J T*)

ROACH A roll of hair dressed away from the forehead or ears. American usage. (*B and B*)

ROCOCO (*c* 1730–1770) or Louis quinze style. A type of decoration based on asymmetrical shell ornaments and is reflected in some hair styles of the period.

ROGERIAN A variety of wig. The word may have been derived from a 16th century wigmaker named Roger.
'The sportful wind, to mock the headless man,
Tosses a pace his pitched Rogerian,
And straight it to a deeper ditch hath blown –
There must my yonker* fetch his waxen crown.'
*A lusty young man. (*Hall*, 1598)
From this reference to wax it is probable that was the adhesive used to secure the wig to the head.

ROIS CHEVELURES, LES Fr. See Long haired.

ROLL (1) The hair turned up above the forehead. 'The heare of a woman that is laied over her forehead, gentylwomen did lately calle theim their rolles.' (*Elyot, Dictionaire*, 1548)
(2) A tress of hair rolled in a cylindrical form: Sausage-like in shape. (*Fairholt*)
(3) Verb. To wind hair around a cylindrical curler.

ROLLED BANG A fringe which is dressed in a long roll curled under towards the forehead – a curled under band; or dressed curled outwards away from the forehead – a curled outwards bang.

ROLLED EDGE The turned-under edge of the wig net sewn like a hem.

ROLLER (1) A curler of large diameter (¾" to 2"). See Roller curler.

(2) Verb. To wind strands of hair around rollers preparatory to setting or permanently waving it.

'Mary will roller the client's hair.'

(3) A hollow pad used as a support in a hairdress. (*The Ladies Treasury*, 1859)

ROLLER COMB A tail comb with a cylindrical tail for rolling hair on to form curls.

ROLLER CURL (1) A curl that has been formed on a roller or cylindrical curler.

(2) Barrel – Spring curl.

ROLLER CURLER A hair curler of plastic, metal, foam rubber, etc on which hair is wound from the points towards the roots on the head.

ROLLER HAIRDO A hair style fashioned from straight, naturally curly, or permanently curled hair, that has been rolled and set on rollers. 20th century American usage.

ROLLER NET A fine mesh, cap-shaped net with an elastic surround used on a head of roller-wound hair.

ROLLER PICK A plastic pin, 2½" to 3½" in length, used to hold a hair roller in position on the head during a hair set.

ROLLER PIN A plastic or metal hair grip similar to a "Kirbigrip", 3" to 4" long and used for securing a hair roller in position on the head during a hair set. This differs from a Roller pick, *qv*.

ROLLER SETTING Hair setting on rollers, *qv*.

ROLLER STAND (Roller trolley, etc) The stand or trolley, positioned near the client, on which the hair rollers are stacked ready for immediate use.

ROLLER TWIRLER A contemptuous term for a ladies hairdresser of limited capacity, whose ability just includes winding hair on a roller, but who has no real knowledge of the hairdressing craft.

ROLLING-UP CORD See Macrame.

ROLLING-UP MACHINE See Winding machine.

ROMAN CAMOMILE (Chamomile) *Anthenius Nobilis*. Also called Garden Camomile. See Camomile.

ROMAN GLADIATOR Man's hair style of the 1960's inspired by the film Cleopatra.

ROMAN POMADE A pomade for the hair incorporating vanilla, etc, also called Vanilla pomade. 19th century. (*qv*)

ROMAN T A short, straight moustache worn with a narrow, but long beard. Taylor, the water poet, wore a variant of this, with the beard twisted like a screw. Fashionable in the reign of Charles I. '. . . strokes his beard which now he puts i' the posture of a T. The Roman T. Your T beard is the fashion.' (*Beaumont and Fletcher, The Queen of Corinth*, 1647, Act 4, Scene 1) *188*

ROMANTIC HAIR STYLE A hair style in which the imagination is allowed full freedom. The opposite of the Classical Hair Style, *qv*. See also Fantasy hair style.

RONALD COLEMAN A moustache style similar to that worn by Ronald Coleman, the English film star. (*Foan*) *101Z*

RONDELETIA A perfume of exquisite odour invented by Hannay and Dietrichsen in the 19th century. Formula for Essence of Rondeletia: Spirit (60 over proof) 1 gallon; otto of Lavender 2 oz; otto of Cloves 1 oz; otto of roses 3 drachms; otto of Bergamot 1 oz; extract of musk, vanilla, ambergris of each ¼ pint. Excellent rondeletia may also be made by adding ¾ drachm otto of cloves to a pint of lavender millefleur, these being the potent ingredients of this perfume. (*Piesse*)

ROOT That part of a hair which is imbedded in the follicle.

ROOT AND POINT HAIR See Combings.

ROOT AND POINT MACHINE See Rooting machine.

ROOT END PROTRUSION That part of the root ends of a hair wisp that hangs free in weaving.

ROOTER See Root turning.

ROOTING See Root turning.

ROOTING MACHINE A device of one, two or three rows of closely set steel needles. A small strand of hair is impaled on the teeth and then drawn through. The points pass between the needles but the roots are unable to pass; also called a Root and Point machine, Turning machine, Rooter. *462*

ROOT SINGE A singe confined to the short hairs near the scalp.

ROOT TURNING The process of re-arranging the hairs of a bunch of hairs in which the roots and points are intermixed, by removing by means of a rooting machine or other method all the hair roots which are propinquent to the other hair points, and then reversing them so that all roots lie together.

ROOT WIND Spirally winding hair around a curler from the root end towards the hair points.

ROPE DESIGN Two tresses passing over and under each other. A twist. See also Cable twist.

ROPY Sticky and stringy.

ROSE A man's 19th century wig style. See Rose bag. (*London Mag*)

ROSE BAG An 18th century wig style for men, the name being derived from the rose-like bow tied to and securing within the bag, the ends of the back hair. *258*

ROSE-BLONDE A red or pink blonde.

ROSE HAIR POWDER A starch hair powder scented with Rose perfume, 18th/19th century. (*Lillie*)

ROSEMARY *Rosmarinus Officinalis*. A popular ingredient of 19th/20th century hair restorers.

ROSEMARY HAIR WASH Cold water ½ gallon; spirit of rosemary 10 ozs; Eau de Cologne, 10 oz; Glycerine 2 ozs; salts of Tartar 1 oz; Liquid ammonia ½ oz; Colour with burnt sugar. (*Creer*)

ROSEMARY OIL A volatile oil obtained by distillation from the flowers of Rosemary (*Rosmarinus Officinalis*) used in hair tonics.

ROSETTER'S HAIR RESTORER See Plumbiferous hair wash.

ROSE-WATER (1) Liquid distilled from Roses.

(2) Distilled water impregnated with essence of Roses.

ROSS TRI-SIDE STROP A three-sided strop invented by Robert Milton Ross. The sides are: (1) Red abrasive for keening the edge;

(2) Green chromic on fine granulated cork for protecting the razor's edge;

(3) A rich grained leather matured in oil on a resilient base, for finishing. 1930s.

ROTARY HAIR BRUSHING MACHINE A large, round brush with a handle at both ends geared by a leather band to a handle turned by an apprentice. This rotated the brush which was held by the hairdresser and applied to the client's head. The last one known to the writer, to have been used in Bristol, was discarded in the 1920s. There may well have been later survivers.

ROUGHING Backcombing. American usage.

ROUGH SCRATCH See Scratch wig.

ROULEAU A hair curler. A roller, *qv*, on which hair is wound to produce a curl. (*Art of Hairdressing*, 1770)

ROULEAU BANDEAU HAIR FRISETTE A hair frisette for dressing a rolled bandeau on. (*Waller*)

ROULETTE Fr. The same as Bilboquet, *qv.*

ROUND BEARD A beard style trimmed to a semi-curcular shape. (*Mitchell*)

ROUND CURLING Curling hair around a circular object in contrast to flat curling for papillotes.

ROUNDED BOB A bobbed hairstyle in which the middle sections of the back and the side hair stand out from the neck and temples, and the ends of this hair hug the neck and cheeks, producing a round silhouette.

ROUNDEL A small, flat curl.

ROUND-HEAD The name applied to a Puritan and supporter of Parliament against Charles I in the Civil War, which began in 1642. So called because they wore hair cropped short, the supposed method of cutting being by placing a round bowl on the head and cutting off the hair to the bowl's edge. See also Basin cut.

'What creature's this with his short hairs,
His little head and huge long ears,
That the new faith hath founded.' (*The Character of a Round-head*, 1641)

The Royalists wore long, curled hair (usually wigs) covering their shoulders.

ROUND TOP BUTCH A hair style for men in which the hair is cut very short to a round contour. (*Jones*)

ROUSSEAU Red haired. (*Creer*)

ROYAL See Churley.

ROYAL BIRD An 18th century woman's wig style. (*London Mag*)

ROYALE (1) Fr. See A la Royale.
(2) A tuft of beard just below the under-lip. Also called an imperial. (*Creer*)

ROYAL LIQUID A concoction for thickening the hair, made of 8 oz burdock root, sliced; 4 oz onions, cut. Boil them for ½ hour in 2 pints water, then add ½ pint rum, 1 pint sweet oil, and 2 oz pearlash dissolved in an ounce of warm water. 19th century. (*Lillie*)

ROYAL WHISKERS A small chin beard and inverted moustache, *c* 1650.

ROYAL WIG WEARERS The following Kings of England wore wigs: James I?, Charles I, Charles II, James II, William III, George I, George II, George III, George IV. William IV did not wear false hair. (*Notes and Queries*. 3 Series, Vol XII, 30 November 1868)

ROYAL WINDSOR HAIR RESTORER See Plumbiferous hair wash.

ROYER'S BEARD PRODUCING POMADE A 19th/20th century 'secret' preparation which consisted of 1 part of red cinchona powder and 1½ parts of wax hair pomade. (*Koller*)

ROYER'S BEARD PRODUCING TINCURE A 19th/20th century 'secret' preparation which consisted of 10 parts common salt, 130 parts of imitation French brandy (containing fusel oil) and 2 parts tincture of mace. It was innocuous. (*Koller*)

RUBBER GLOVES Used to protect the operator's hands in hair dyeing and waving processes.

RUBBING DOWN The abrasion of the rough cut wig spring ends on a rubbing stone.

RUBBING STONE A flat slab of abrasive natural stone, at least 6″ square on which the ends of wig springs are rubbed down smooth and rounded.

RUBEFACIENT A substance that reddens the scalp by vigorous local stimulation. Examples are glacial acetic acid, tincture of cantharides, glycol salicylate, nicotinic acid derivatives, tincture of capsicum, etc. (*Lubowe*)

RUCKING The sections of loosely wound hair which can appear when the process of point winding on a curler is unskillfully performed.

RUFF (1) A postiche composed of a 9″ row or rows of sewn curly weft attached to a narrow elastic band or ribbon to secure it to the head, and worn at the neck. '1 ruff from combings hair added 5/-,' 1898. (*Stevens Ms*)
(2) The pubic hair of a woman, 18th century slang.
'Tis said, that all the ladies there,
(By some who best pretend to know 'em)
Had brought their Ruffs, but did not care,
In such a publick place to show 'em:
And wisely judg'd; for well I ween,
A Ruff is better felt than seen.' (*Ballad*, 1727)
(3) A band of whiskers around the face. 19th century Dorset usage.
(4) The hair that grows low on the neck.

RUFFING Similar to Back-combing, *qv.*

RUFFLE A group of loose, haphazardly arranged curls.

RUFFLE LOOK A hair style for women in which the hair is left in a state of controlled disarray. 1963.

RUG An American slang term for a large wig or toupee. (*Berrey*)

RUM FLASH Slang for a fine long wig. 18th century. (*Grose*)

RUM STRUM A fine large wig. See Strum. 18th century. (*Grose Prov Glos*)

RUM TOPPING A woman's headdress. A slang term, 18th century. (*Grose, Lex Bal*)

RUNNING SPRING A coiled spring encased in galloon and used at the sides or the nape to hold a wig firmly on the head.

RUNNING STITCH See Stitching.

RUNNING-UP The winding of the weft on the macramé core in the manufacture of a switch. See Twisting.

RUN OVER A re-wave on a Marcel wave. Waving over an existing Marcel wave to strengthen it and prolong its life. In use before 1918 and until the mid 20th century.

RUN-UP See Running-up.

RUSMA A depilatory. (*EDM Vol 3*)

RUSSET A reddish-brown colour.

RUSSET PATED Grey headed. 16th century. (*Onions*)

RUSSIAN BEARD A long beard having the bottom cut straight. See Square cut beard.

RUSSIAN SHELL A razor strop made of horsehide from the horse's rump. (*Trusty*)

RUSSIAN STROP A cowhide strop tanned in the manner of Russian leather.

RUSTIC HAIRCUT (1) A crude haircut.
(2) Hair cut in steps.
(3) A Basin cut, *qv.*

RUSTY A red haired person. Slang. (*B and B*)

RUSTY ROOF Auburn haired. American slang. 20th century. (*B and B*)

SABLE (Heraldic) Black.

SABOT Fr. Wooden shoe; a name given to the large rolls worn behind the ears in women's hairdresses. 19th century. (*Creer*)

SABOURAUD-ROUSSEAU TEST See Skin test.

SACHET (1) A rectangular object of flannel, aluminium foil or other suitable material for holding the permanent waving lotion in contact with the hair, or by enclosing the wound hair and retaining the heat.

(2) A scent bag. 19th century. (*Creer*)

(3) Small plastic bags of shampoo, setting lotion, etc 1930s.

SACKERS COMB A fine toothed comb used for removing nits from hair.

SACULAR Bag-like.

SAFA Gold ornaments worn in the hanging hair braids of Egyptian women. (*Lane*)

SAFETY RAZOR A razor incorporating a guard to protect the skin from accidental cuts.

SAFFRON An extract of the plant used by Roman women, according to Galen, to obtain golden tints in their hair. (*Speight*)

SAGE An infusion of sage was used in the 18/19th century as a vegetable dye to darken the hair.

SAGE TEA RINSE An infusion of sage leaves to darken the hair, applied by pouring it over the hair with the subject's head held forward or backward over the shampoo basin.

SAILOR WHISKERS A full set of whiskers, but with the top lip clean shaven. Worn by sailors in the 19th and early 20th century. Sometimes, but incorrectly, called Galways, *qv*.

SAKKOS HEADDRESS An ancient Greek headdress for a woman. (*Rimmel*)   341

SALON A French word meaning reception room of a lady of fashion; often used by English hairdressers for Saloon. Presumably the good English word Saloon, owing to its association with shaving, ie Shaving Saloon, is felt by some to bear a derogatory undertone, so the French Salon is used instead. Both Salon and Saloon mean the same thing. Saloon, the English form, was used originally for a spacious and lofty room used to receive guests and, by extension, an apartment to which the public had access for a specific purpose; ie dancing saloon, shaving and haircutting saloon. In England the use of saloon for both ladies' and gentlemen's hairdressing establishments was common throughout the 19th century and at the beginning of the 20th century, but since the 1940s it has increasingly lost ground in the ladies' craft and has reverted to Salon.

SALOON (1) See Salon.

(2) A private cubicle within a large room, in which women and sometimes men receive attention to their hair. 'Show the lady to the Saloon.'

SALOON COAT An overall worn by hairdressers when working in the saloon.

SALOON JACKET A short overall worn by male hairdressers when working in the saloon.

SALOON NAMES The types of business name of hairdressing establishments have changed considerably over the period 1700–1983. In the period:

(1) *c* 1700 to *c* 1900 hairdressers traded under their real names, eg William White, Norwich, 1729; James Irvine, Edinburgh, 1786; William Scott, Bath, 1792; J Dalling, Barnstaple, 1800; William Davis, London, 1804; H P Trufitt, London, 1819.

(2) 1900–20 the name of the owner prefixed by Maison or House of, eg Maison Stephens, Bristol; The House of Hyman, Brighton.

(3) 1920–1975 Christian name of owner or an assumed Christian name and an affix, eg Charles of the Ritz; Alphonse of Paris; Arlette Hair Fashions; Janine; Adolphus.

(4) *c* 1945–83 gimmick names, eg A Cut Above the Rest; A Head of Time; Beyond the Fringe; Cheveux Chic Salon; Clip Joint; Clippers; Crowning Glory; Cut 'n Curl; Curl 'n Cut; Guys and Dolls; Hair; Hair Flair; Hair in Place; Hair

we are again; Hairport; Hair's Paradise; Head of Time; His and Her; House of Curls; Just Hair; Lady's Hair; Love of Hair; Marcels; Part Hair; Razors; Scissors; Sham-poo; Shapes and Shades; She and He; Short and Curly; Snips; The Hair Cut; The Hairy Ones; The Perm People; Tops; Tresses; Trims, Twirl and Curl; Unisex Hair Fashions; Vanity Fair; Wavy Line; Wagahead; Wigerama; Wiggery; Wigwams.

There was much overlapping of the types and there are still hairdressers who trade under their own names as in period (1) and one still finds examples of periods (2) and (3), but to find a saloon called Clip Joint in periods (1) or (2) or any other of the names found in period (4) is impossible.

SALOON OVERALL A kind of coat or jacket worn as a protective garment by hairdressers when working in the saloon.

SALT AND PEPPER HAIR A head of hair in which the hairs are of at least two different colours, one of which is white.

SALTED HAIR Grey hair. (*Lethbridge, T C, A Step in the Dark*, 1967).

SALT OF TARTAR See Potassium carbonate.

SALT OF WORMWOOD See Potassium carbonate.

SALT-WATER SOAP See Marine soap.

SAMSON or SAMPSON A judge in Israel of fabulous strength, who had freed his nation from the Philistines. He was betrayed by his lover, Delilah, who robbed him of his great strength by cutting off his hair. (*O T Judges* XIII–XVI)

SAMSONESS A female Sampson, 18th century. 'A female Sampsoness . . . my strength lies in my hair.' (*Stevens, J* (Trans) *Quevodo's Works*, 1709)

SAMSON HAIR A long and luxurious head of hair.

SAND SOAP Curd soap 7 lb, marine soap 7 lb, sifted silver sand 28 lb, otto of thyme 2 oz; otto of Cassia 2 oz; otto of Caraway 2 oz, otto of French Lavender 2 oz. (*Piesse*)

SANDY (1) A person with light yellowish brown hair. Modern English usage.

(2) A red-haired person. Slang. American usage. (*B and B*)

SANDY PATE A red-haired man or woman. 18th century. (*Grose, Lex Bal*)

SANITARY Free from the conditions, especially dirt and bacteria, that affect the health.

SANITATION The use of measures, such as disinfectants, that will improve the sanitary conditions.

SANITIZE To disinfect or make sanitary.

SANITIZER An apparatus to disinfect objects.

SAPO HISPANICUS Castile Soap. (*PPB*)

SAPONACEOUS SHAVING COMPOUND Shaving soap manufactured by H P and W C Taylor, New York, in the mid-19th century. Pots for this soap, similar to the bears-grease pots of Victorian England, have been excavated at Fort Kearny (occupied 1848–1871), Nebraska, USA. There are specimens in the museum at Lincoln, Nebraska.

SAPONACEOUS WASH See Egg julep.

SAPONIFIED BLEACH Similar to simple bleach, *qv*, but with a little soap solution added to prevent running.

SAPONIFY To convert into soap.

SAPONIN A glucoside derived from *Saponaria Officinalis* and *quillaia saponaria*; also other plants. Used in foam shampoos and as an emulsifying agent.

SAPO VIRIDIS See Green soft soap. (*PPB*)

SAPPHO The famous Greek poetess of Lesbos (*c* BC 600) was reputed to have had red hair.

SAPPHO COIFFURE A woman's hair style of 1863.

SARTORY, P Peter Sartory (1881–1951), born Amsterdam,

was one of the significant pioneers in the development of permanent waving. He was the first person to perfect a system of exothermic permanent waving, marketed as the Va-per-Marcel system, which as its name suggests relied on exothermic pads to supply the heat to a chemically saturated wound hair.

SATURN A Roman deity. Depicted by the ancients with hair of his head and beard milk white. (*Salmon*)

SATYRIC TUFT (1) The beard tuft of the Satyr, who was half man, half goat.

(2) A tuft of hair on the chin.

SAUCER BEARD A narrow band of whiskers around the face and below the chin, the upper lip and chin being shaven.

SAUSAGE CURL A wide, croquignole wound curl. Not to be confused with a spirally wound drop or hanging curl.

SAVAGE BLACK Man's theatrical wig style, 18th century. (*Encyc Brit*)

SAVIN The Juniper Savin (*Sabina*) or Saffern, a small evergreen shrub, once known as the 'Devil's Tree' and 'Magicians Cypress' because it was used by witches when working their spells. Possesses stimulating virtues for curing baldness. (*Fernie*)

SAVINIANUS The martyr. He was red bearded.

SAVON Fr. Soap.

SAVONET The same as a Savonette, *qv*. 18th century. (*Stewart*)

SAVONETTE The same as Washball, *qv*. 'Moulded into spherical forms also known as washballs.' (*Pears*)

SAVONETTE TREE A West Indian tree, *Pithecolobium Micradenium*, the bark of which can be used as a substitute for soap.

SAVOY POMPADOUR See Pneumatic roll.

SAW CUT COMB A comb manufactured by cutting a series of slits with a fine circular saw in order to form the teeth. The comb is then finished with a grail, *qv*.

SBP SPIRIT Used for cleaning wigs.

Special boiling point spirit No 1. Specific gravity (at 60°F) 0.675–0.695; flash point below 73°F; normal distillation range 35/115°C.

No 2 SG 0.695–0.715; flash point below 73°F; normal distillation range 70–95°C.

No 3 SG 0.730–0.750; flash point below 73°F; normal distillation range 100/120°C.

No 4 SG 0.690–0.715; flash point below 73°F; normal distillation range 40–150°C.

These four spirits are used for cleaning postiche.

SCABIES A contagious disease of the skin caused by the parasite *Sarcoptes Scabiei*. 'The scabies, or itch is an eruption of pustules.'

SCALD HEAD Eczema of the scalp. (*Wheeler*)

SCALLOP SHELL Also called Italian Curl, *qv*. An 18th century name for a curl that was dressed back from the face. (*Stewart*)

SCALP (1) The skin covering of the head.

(2) A part-wig for a man, similar to a Scalpette, *qv*, 19th century. (*Stevens* Ms) 'An artificial covering for the bald head of a man, but not a wig.' (*Creer*)

SCALP BATH A shampoo. (*Wheeler*)

SCALP BRUSH A long, narrow, stiff-bristle brush, used for scalp and hair brushing. (*Smith*)

SCALP CEMENT An adhesive for sticking toupees, etc, to the scalp.

SCALP COLOURING Colouring the scalp with a suitable tint to conceal thinning hair.

SCALP DOILY A slang American term for a wig. (*Berrey*)

SCALPETTE (1) An artificial covering for concealing a

deficiency of hair, or to cover a bald place upon the female head – but not a wig. Referred to by Edward Creer in his *Board-Work*, 1887, as a comparatively new word.

(2) The word later (19th century) became transferred to an artificial covering (toupet) for part of a man's head, and since *c* 1900 has been used only in reference to a man's postiche.

SCALP FOUNDATION The net or gauze and galloon foundation for a scalp. See Scalp (2).

SCALPING The removal of the scalp from the skull. Some of the North American Indian tribes habitually scalped their enemies. An instance of a scalping by Comanches of an old woman, and her subsequent complete recovery is given by G F Von Tempsky in his work *Mitla*, 1858, but recovery was very unusual.

SCALP LOCK The hair tuft left on the otherwise bald head of the North American Indian, and seized by a conquering enemy when he tore off the scalp.

SCALP MAKER A manufacturer of scalps for bald heads. A wig maker. 'Peruke and scalp makers.' (*Pigot*, 1832)

SCALP MASSAGE Digital or mechanical massage of the head and scalp, usually to tone the flesh and promote the growth of hair.

SCALP MOULD A mould of the head on which the scalp foundation was mounted.

SCALP SNAP A small metal grip which snaps shut. Sewn on a small postiche, it is used to secure it to the remaining head-hair.

SCALP STEAMER A hooded apparatus that emits hot water-vapour upon the hair and scalp.

SCARF KNOT Folded hair in the fashion of the knot used on a scarf.

SCARF SKIN The outer layer of the skin, the epidermis.

SCAUP Variant form of scalp; a part wig similar to a scalpette.

SCENT A perfume; an odoriferous liquid prepared by distillation from flowers; an odour. Formerly 'sent', from Latin *sentio*, to feel, hence to feel by the sense of smell.

SCENT SPRAY A bottle or other suitable container complete with an apparatus for distributing the scent in the form of a spray of finely atomized drops.

SCHED, also Shed, *qv*. Verb. To part the hair. Scottish usage. (*Brown*)

SCHNECWEISS'S RAPID HAIR DYE A 19/20th century 'secret' preparation which contained copper and could have been dangerous. (*Koller*)

SCHNURBARTBINDE German. See Moustache trainer.

SCIENCE That body of systematized observations from which scientific laws are deduced. 'Science is the application of experience from observation.'

SCIPIO AFRICANUS The first recorded Roman to shave regularly.

SCISSOR Verb. To cut with scissors. 'I shall scissor her hair.'

SCISSOR BILL A nagging or gossiping woman.

SCISSOR SHEER A scissors' sheath. 19th century. Somerset usage.

SCISSORS An implement for cutting, consisting of a small pair of handled shears or blades, moveable on a pivot. The handles when brought together, at the same time cause the cutting edges of the blades to pass each other and simultaneously to cut the hair or other substance that lies within the scissors' crutch. Scissors of iron first came into use during the La Tène period of the early Iron Age. (*MacCurdy, G G The Coming of Man* p 86, illus) See also Shears.

106, 107

SCISSORS CUT Haircutting by means of scissors.

SCISSORS PERM A Wave cut, *qv.*

SCISSORS TEST Wet cotton wool or tissue paper is cut without any lateral pressure, holding the scissors between the first finger and thumb. If this wool or paper is cut cleanly, without any tearing or distortion, the scissors are regarded as sharp and in condition for haircutting.

SCOLDING CURL A curl that will not remain in position. Slang, American usage. (*B and B*)

SCOLLOP SHELL CURL Large diameter wide curls, shaped like a scollop shell, and tapering at each side. 18th century. (*Stewart*)

SCOTCH BEAVER Slang term for a ginger-coloured beard. 20th century. (*Mitchell*)

SCOTTISH TONSURE See John (Apostle), Tonsure of.

SCOURING SOAP Soap, liquid or solid, with an admixture of powdered pumice and very fine sand. Used as a saponaceous abrasive for removing hair dye from the skin.

SCRAPE To shave, 18/19th century. Slang. (*Vulg Tong*)

SCRATCH BOB See Scratch wig.

SCRATCHING STICK A long, thin stick of ivory or bone used for scratching the head when high, elaborate hair styles were fashionable. The end of the scratching stick was sometimes in the form of a human hand or pointed or broad for killing lice. 18th century.

SCRATCH WIG (1) A short, natural looking wig resemblir the wearer's own shockylocks, just large enough to cove the baldness. Much worn by tradesman in the 18th century.
'Spruce was the barber shop,
Wigs decorated every block
From Scratch to Tyburn Top.' (*Sportsman's Slang etc*, 1827 by *J Bee – John Badcock*)
A smooth scratch was one in which the hair was dressed smoothly and tidily. When the hair was in a dishevelled condition the wig was said to be a rough scratch.
(2) A short bob wig that covered only the back part of the head; the wearer's own front hair was brushed over it in front. (*Cunnington*)

SCREW BEARD A narrow, twisted tuft of beard on the centre of the chin from the lower lip to one or two inches beyond the chin. 17th century.   *100 (29)*

SCREW CURL A helical-shaped curl; a spiral curl.

SCRINT Verb. To singe. Ilchester, Somerset usage.

SCROFF (1) Downy neck hair. Ilchester usage.
(2) The short hairs and detritus which are discarded when getting-out combings. Also called leftings, *qv.* Bristol usage, 19th/early 20th century.

SCROLL A deep roll. American usage.

SCRUBBING BRUSH BEARD A short, bristly beard. (*Mitchell*)

SCRUFF Short, untidy hairs, especially on the neck; also a beard of a few days growth. Expression: 'To take by the scruff of the neck'.

SCRUFFY Covered with scurf.

SCULL THATCHER A peruke maker, 18th century. Slang. (*Grose, Lex Bal*)

SCULPTURE CURL See Sculptured curl.

SCULPTURE CUT A clubbed haircut in preparation for a sculptured hair style. When dressed will display a sculptured effect with a definite form as opposed to a loose or free-flowing style.

SCULPTURED CURL A firmly and smoothly formed curl showing the comb-teeth lines.

SCULPTURED HAIR STYLE A hairdress with hard, firm, definite lines in its constituent parts; not fussy, light or tapered.

SCURF A morbid condition of the scalp characterised by dry, branny scales. See Pityriasis.

SCURF COMB A fine toothed comb for removing scurf from the hair.

SCURF ESSENCES 19/20th century 'secret' preparations compounded of scented ammonia soap with alcohol and glycerine. (*Koller*)

SCURF POMADE An emollient for the cure or relief of a scurfy condition. A 19th/20th century formula comprised: white petroleum oil 30 oz; white wax 8 oz; oil of Bergamot 1 oz; oil soluble vegetable green, a trace.

SCURLOCK A surname. Scur – an early form of shower. Probably so called because of a lock of hair falling over the forehead. Jonathan Scurlock of Carmarthan County, 17th century. (*Addisoniana*)

S-CURVE Two waves and one wave crest.

SEA BREEZE BOB A short hair style for women, similar to the Wind-blown bob, *qv.* ((*Wilson, K*)

SEARCHING BRISTLE The long bristle in one of the bunches of bristles inserted in the pad of a hair brush.

SEBACEOUS Of or relating to the sebum, *qv.*

SEBACEOUS GLAND Oil secreting gland found in the skin on all parts of the body except the palms of the hands and soles of the feet. They open onto the skin surface as pores, secrete sebum and lubricate skin, scalp and hair shaft.

SEBORRHOEA A disease of the sebaceous glands characterised by excessive oil excretion.

SEBORRHOEA FLAVESCENS Yellow dandruff. (*Wheeler*)

SEBORRHOEA NIGRICANS A very rare condition of scalp, characterised by dark or black sebaceous matter. (*Wheeler*)

SEBORRHOEA SIMPLEX Scurf. (*Wheeler*)

SEBUM The fatty (semi-liquid) secretion which lubricates the skin and hair and is secreted by the sebaceous glands, *qv.*

SECOND DEGREE BURN These burns affect the deeper layers of the skin and involve the nerves. See also First and Third Degree Burns.

SECOND PLI See Pli.

SECRETAGE A method of crisping or curling hair or fur. See next entry.

SECRETAGE LIQUID A permanent curling fluid of: quicksilver 1 drachm, aqua fortis 2 oz; dissolved. Before use this compound was diluted with half its volume to an equal volume of water. It was poisonous and dangerous. The hair was moistened and wound in greased hair papers and left for several hours in a hot atmosphere to 'set', then washed in tepid water with no soap. None of the liquid was allowed to touch the skin. This permanent waving process was practiced on the growing hair of human heads before 1866. (*Cooley*)

SECTIONING Also Blocking (American usage). The dividing of the hair into suitably sized sections (a) To wind the hair on curlers for a permanent wave; (b) to apply a bleach or dye; (c) Preparatory to hair cutting; or (d) To facilitate the application of oil or other substance for a treatment.

SECTIONING CLIP A long-fingered, spring clip to grip and control sections of the hair during the process of sectioning, styling, or cutting.

SEEBOLD'S HAIR TINCTURE A 19th/20th century 'secret' hair tonic, consisting of 40 parts of resorcin; 0.6 parts of caramel; 2.5 parts of lemon oil; 1.5 parts of Peruvian Balsam and 92 parts of spirit. (*Koller*)

SEEBOLD's TINCTURE A 19th/20th century 'secret' preparation for preventing scurf and falling hair. It consisted of fresh orange peel in dilute alcohol, with 5% of resorcin and 3% of Peruvian Balsam. In many instances this produced a reddening of the skin and pustules and it could therefore have been injurious. (*Koller*)

SEEDY WIG (1) A round cake sprinkled with caraway seeds. Sussex usage. (*Gale*)

(2) An old rough wig, 'gone to seed'. Slang. West Country usage.

SEEGAR'S BLONDE HAIR DYE A 19th/20th century 'secret' preparation compounded of 1% pyrogallol and 1% cupric chloride. This preparation could be injurious to health. (*Koller*)

SEEING GLASS Mirror or looking glass. Northern usage. (*Grose, Prov Glos*)

SEE-THROUGH BANG A thin fringe which reveals parts of the forehead beneath. American usage.

SELLOTAPE A type of sticky tape used to hold the ends of set hair (especially in the neck and on the forehead or cheek) in position during the drying process. From *c* 1950.

SEMI A Semi Transformation, *qv*.

SEMICIRCULAR CURL See Crescent Curl.

SEMI-COVERED STEM See Inverted Stem. (*Creer*)

SEMI-PERM A permanent wave to strengthen weak, natural curl. 'For naturally curly hair, which is not curly enough to stay put.' (Brochure published 1936 by J F Ray Ltd, 326 Oxford St, London W1)

SEMI-PERMANENT DYE A regrettable misnomer. There can be no such dye. A permanent dye means one that lasts for the life of the hair; any dye that lasts less than this is a temporary dye, either long-lasting or short-lasting. The expression 'semi-permanent is as meaningless as the equally common, but also incorrect 'very unique' and 'very complete' and it is to be hoped it will be replaced by the more accurate *temporary* dye, long or short lasting.

SEMI-POMPADOUR A woman's pompadour hair style in which four waves dip forward, two over one side of the forehead and one over each temple.

SEMIRAMIS (*c* 800 BC) Queen of Assyria, wife of Ninus; famous for, among other matters, her wigs and hair styles. 'Semiramis, the Assyrian Queen,
Perukked like Bully Rake was seen.' (*Gent's Mag* v 8, p 157, 173)

SEMI-SHINGLE A woman's hair style from *c* 1924 and later, which was intermediate in length at the back of the head, between a bob, *qv* and a shingle, *qv*.

SEMI-SOLID RAZOR See Solid razor. A razor with its blade slightly concave.

SEMI-TRANSFORMATION An artificial covering of hair for the front, top and sides of the head When dressed, the hair of the semi-transformation mingles with the natural hair of the head. Measurements required: 1 Circumference, 2 Front (ear to ear across the front of the head), 3 Parting length, 4 Parting position. 253

SEMI-TRANSFORMATION RIBBON The loose galloon with hook and eye attached that extends from the ear points of a semi-transformation and secures it to the head.

SEMI-WIG A three-quarter transformation with caul net filling the open space behind the stiff foundation.

SEMI-WINDBLOWN Rather less than Windblown, *qv* or, put differently, 'Semi-windblown is to windblown as zephyr is to gale.'

SENIOR HAND A fully qualified assistant hairdresser.

SENSITIVITY Subs. A positive reaction in the form of redness or irritation by a chemical or treatment that touches the scalp.

SENSITIVITY TEST Skin test, *qv*.

SENTIMENT PUFF A puff constructed of, or incorporating, the hair of persons dear to the wearer. In 1774 the Duchesse de Chartres had a puff made of the hair of her father, the Duc de Penthierre; and her father-in-law, the Duc d'Orleans. (*Corson*)

SEPIA HAIR DYE A 19th century animal dye composed of the ink fluid of a cuttlefish the *sepia officinalis*, also spirit and essence of musk. It gave brown to black colours. (*Cooley*)

SEPSIS Putrefaction due to pathogenic bacteria.

SEPTIZONIUM HAIRDRESS A tower hairdress of the Roman period and 17th century, named after the very high tower in Rome built by the Emperor Severus, which consisted of seven ranks of pillars set one upon the other, and diminishing to the top, which was described by Juvenal in his sixth *Satire:*
'Such rows of curles press'd on each other lyre,
She builds her hair so many stories high,
That look on her before, and you would swear,
Hector's tall wife Andromache she were,
Behind a Pigmy . . .' (*Evelyn*)

SERJEANT-AT-LAW'S WIG A frizzled wig with three rows of seven curls then one row of four curls, with one perpendicular curl between them and two tails, and a round black patch on the crown, called a 'coif'. Apart from the coif this was similar to a Barrister's wig.

SERLO (12th century) A Norman Bishop who preached before Henry I against long hair. See Serlon, D'abou. (*Speight*)

SERLON D'ABOU Bishop of Séey on Easter Day 1104, preached such an eloquent homily against beards before Henry I, King of England, that the King there and then had his beard cut off before the whole court and this example was at once followed by all the bearded ones present.

SERPENT (1) A hanging plait or coil of hair looped with its points secured near its roots. An 18th century style usually worn as part of a head-dress for Court balls, and actresses.

(2) Thin, loosely waved, straggling tress of hair, the end hanging free from the hairdress, 19th century.

SERPENTINE KNOT A long plait, coiled and twisted as a serpent.

SERRATED CUT The point ends of hair strands cut in notches like the edge of a saw.

SERRATED SCISSORS Scissors with the cutting edge of one blade serrated to prevent the hair slipping when cutting fringes, etc.

SERVERY A room or section of a hair-dressing establishment in which materials are stored and prepared for use in the saloon. 20th century.

SET (1) Subs. Hair dressed or set, 17th century. (*R Percivale, A Dictionary in Spanish and English*, 1623)
'Instead of well-set hair, baldness.' (*Isiah Ch 3, v 18–24*)
(2) Subs. Wet hair arranged into waves, curls or other devices basic to the required style. 'I am going to have a hair set.'
(3) Verb. The action of arranging wet tresses of hair into waves, curls or other hair movements basic to the required style.

SET KEEPING (1) Adj. Having the power to hold a hair-set in position. 'The set-keeping quality of a tragacanth lotion is high.'
(2) Subs. Hair that will hold a set.

SET OF WHISKERS The beard. A full set of whiskers is the beard and moustache. See also Whiskers.

SETTEE The double pinner. (*Evelyn*)

SETTING Subs. The same as Set, *qv*. Set is the English usage, setting the American usage. 'She needs a hair setting.'

SETTING (A RAZOR) See Razor setting.

SETTING COMB Curved combs of non-inflammable material, 4″ to 5″ long, used to hold the set waves in position during the drying process. From *c* 1925. Since *c* 1945 the term 'Setting comb' has been applied to the comb used by the hairdresser to set or wave the hair. See also comb.

SETTING GEL A semi-solid, colloidal solution used for setting hair.

SETTING LOTION A liquid preparation with which to moisten the hair to facilitate setting it in position, and to help retain the strength and position of waves and curls or other hair movements.

SETTING NET A silk or synthetic net used to cover a hair set and prevent the hair dryer disarranging the positioned tresses.

SETTING PATTERN The disposition of the rollers on the head for a projected hair style. (*Greene*)

SETTING STICK Curling Stick. A polished, cigar-shaped, wooden stick used to form or set curls. They vary in length from 6″ to 15″ or more.
'Irons, Combes, bodkins, setting stickes.' 17th century. The *OED* also gives 'a rod used for stiffening the plaits or "sets" of ruffs', etc. But in Burton's context they are directly associated with other hair accessories. The term was used for curling stick by my grandmother and parents in their hairdressing saloon at Bristol.

SEVEN BASIC FACE SHAPES See Face shape.

SEVEN STRAND DOUBLE PLAIT See Plait. (*Creer*, p 94)

SEVEN SUTHERLAND SISTERS' HAIR GROWER A popular American cure for baldness in the 1880s. (*Advert, Brochure*)

SEVIGNE COIFFURE A hair style in the fashion of that worn by the Marquise de Sévigné. See Sévigné curl. *355*

SEVIGNE (OR SEVIGNY) CURL (1) Plump drop curls worn at the side of the coiffure over pads.
(2) Spiral curl. So called after Marie de Rabutin-Chantal, Marquise de Sévigné (1626–86) who affected this type of curl. (*Creer*)

SEWING SILK Strong, fine silk used for sewing postiche mounts.

SEWING STITCH See Stitching.

SEWN PARTING A wig parting with the hair sewn directly on the foundation.

SHADE (1) Hair lying plain and straight on either side of the forehead (shading it). 17th century. (*Holme*)
(2) Dark degree of a hue; eg 'the darker shades of Auburn'.
(3) Verb. To part the hair. (*Scot*)
(4) Sub. A hair parting. North country usage.

SHADE CHART A named collection of wisps of hair, each being of a different colour or hue.

SHADE RING See Shade Chart.

SHADOW An English moustache style, thin and short. (*Foan*) *101x*

SHADOW MARCEL WAVE A Marcel wave that has shallow troughs and low unaccented crests.

SHADOW WAVE A very shallow wave, the merest indication of a wave.

SHAFT (1) That part of a hair between the root and point.
(2) The solid rod of a curling or waving iron.
(3) The grooved or concave shaft of a curling or waving iron.

SHAG Subs. Rough, matted hair.

SHAGGY Adj. Having long, coarse, bushy hair; unkempt hair.

SHAG STYLE A hair style in studied disorder, shaggy. USA, *c* 1970.

SHAITTEL A wig worn by married Jewesses. (*Jewish Encyc*) See Wig, Jewish.

SHALLOON (CHALON) A wigtie made of shalloon which was a closely woven, woollen material. The tie was made in the draw-string at the neck part of the wig. 17th–19th

century. From the French *chalon*.

SHAMPOO The word shampoo originated from the Hindi word *champo*, the imperative form of *champna*, to press, knead, thrust in, etc. The first introduction of the word to England was through the Anglo-Indian community in the 18th century and its meaning then, in its Anglicized form, was to subject a person's body or limbs to massage; but before 1856 the word shampoo had also assumed its modern meaning of rubbing and washing the hair and scalp with a cleansing agent, such as soap and water.
'Smart, cheery places, brilliant with gas, and redolent of rich perfume, are the modern shampooing saloons.' (*Procter*, 1856). R W Procter's *The Barber's Shop*, Manchester, 1856, was the first edition of that work and this apparently had escaped the Editors of the Oxford English Dictionary, which gives the earliest printed reference as 1860.
(1) Subs. The process of cleansing the scalp and hair by washing and rubbing with the fingers.
(2) Subs. A preparation in powder, liquid, cream or solid form which will absorb, dissolve or emulsify grease and act as a carrier in the removal of dirt and debris from the scalp and hair, without any deleterious effect. A satisfactory shampoo must enable the hair to be cleansed thoroughly without removing an excessive amount of the natural oil from the hair shaft, and should leave the hair clean, lustrous, fragrant and manageable. Shampoos may be named and classified according to –
A Their physical consistency, ie powder, liquid, cream, solid, etc.
B Their ingredients, ie Pine-tar, camomile, egg julep, sulphonated, henna, spirit (at one time called a dry shampoo), etc.
C One or more of their properties, ie brightening, medicating, deep cleansing, etc. There are other acceptable classifications. For adequately descriptive definitions, combinations of the above classifications would be necessary, such as: 'camomile liquid green soft soap shampoo'; a combination of A and B.
(3) Verb. To rub the scalp and hair with the fingers in the presence of a detergent such as soap and water.
(4) The shampoo: 1965 jargon for the *Twist*, a contortive dance. (*Daily Express*, 15 July 1965)

SHAMPOO, DEEP CLEANSING A shampoo or detergent used for greasy hair which not only removes surface grease and adherent dirt, but also degreases the cuticle of the hair shaft.

SHAMPOO BASIN A large basin over which a client's hair is shampooed. *467*

SHAMPOO BLEACH A shampoo solution incorporating a bleaching agent, usually hydrogen peroxide.

SHAMPOO BOTTLE A bottle with a small neck to hold warm shampoo to be sprinkled on the head. (*Ogee*, 1905)

SHAMPOO BRUSH A stiff-bristled hairbrush used to disentangle and remove loose debris before shampooing the hair.

SHAMPOO CAPE A protective covering placed over the shoulders of a client during a shampoo.

SHAMPOO CHUTE A kind of metal gutter about 18″ wide and 2′ 6″ long with a semi-circular end to fit the neck and on which a woman's long hair rests during a backward shampoo, allowing the water to run down into a drain or a bucket, 19th/20th century.

SHAMPOO COMB A Rake, *qv*, used to disentangle hair before a shampoo.

SHAMPOO CONTAINER A jug, ewer, flask, carafe or other type of container from which shampoo is poured onto the head. *168*

SHAMPOO DYE A shampoo solution incorporating a penetrative dye that cleanses and dyes the hair during the process of the shampoo. See also Soap cap.

SHAMPOOER One who shampoos, a shampoo girl, *qv*.

SHAMPOO GIRL A girl employed in a hairdressing saloon whose sole task is to shampoo heads of hair, ready for the hairdresser's or hair stylist's attention. This is an undesirable development which has occured since *c* 1945. Shampoo girls are often paid less than hairdressers although they are themselves specialists in one important branch of the hairdressing craft. The division is artificial, unjustifiable and unbecoming.

SHAMPOOING MACHINE Invented by Ralph O'Toole and his brother, M O'Toole, Guernsey, 1960. It consisted of a helmet that emitted warm shampoo and water for rinsing and vibrating rubber fingers that massaged the head.

SHAMPOOING SURGEON One who performed shampooing (massage) on the body, in conjunction with the Indian medicated vapour bath. Sake Deen Mahomed in an advertisement in *Pigot's London and Provincial Commercial Directory*, 1832, claimed to have introduced the practice into England in 1784.

SHAMPOOIST The same as shampooer, *qv*; one who shampoos. This form first noticed by editor in 1966.

SHAMPOO LIQUID The liquid preparation, usually a soap solution, used to effect a shampoo, 1866.

SHAMPOO POT A container of glass, china or metal from which shampoo is poured onto the head. Guernsey usage.

SHAMPOO POWDER (Wet shampoo). A 19th/20th century formula is: Borax 4.6%, powdered soap 24.4%, sodium carbonate 71.0%, Perfume to taste.

(Dry shampoo). A 19th/20th century formula is: Starch 50%, orris-root powder 30%, sodium sesquicarbonate 15%, borax 5%. Perfume to taste.

SHAMPOO SHIELD A plastic brim worn outside the hairline to protect the eyes from the shampoo, 20th century.

SHAMPOO SPRAY A sprinkling-nozzle or rose attached to the flexible water pipe to distribute the water in the form of a diffused spray. 19/20th century.

SHAMPOO SPRINKLER A container with a sprinkler top for the application of shampoo to the head in controlled quantities.

SHAMPOO STAND A stand with a metal basin attached over which heads are shampooed. The back of the client's head rests over the basin and the face looks upward. Excellent for those who suffer from claustrophobia.

SHAMPOO TINT See Shampoo dye.

SHAMPOO TRAY See Shampoo chute.

SHAMPOO WAVE A method of fixing (temporarily) a wave in hair that lacks curl, by the incorporation in the shampoo of substances conducive to this result, and then either water-waving the hair or curl setting it on rollers. (*H and B*, Nov 1964)

SHAMROCK KNOT A wire hair frame with three 2″ wide marteaux fixed beneath and pulled through the frame's centre hole, combed over it in three directions and the ends of the marteaux secured beneath the frame. (*Foan*)

SHAPE Subs. The head shape moulded in plaster of Paris, papier mâché or wax to provide for the manufacture of a hair-piece foundation. Also called mould.

SHAPER A razor with an attached guard used for cutting hair.

SHAPING Hair-cutting to a desired contour.

SHAVE (1) Subs. The action of removing the beard close to the skin by means of a razor or implement that has a similar effect.

(2) Verb. To remove the whiskers, beard, moustache, head or other body hair by means of a razor, etc. See (1).
'He was shave al newe.' (*Chaucer*, 1386)
(3) To fleece, 18th century slang.

SHAVEE The person receiving the shave. (*G of L M*)

SHAVER (1) One who shaves with a razor or other implement with the same result. 'Under the shaver's hand.' (*Ford, Lover's Melancholy*, 1628)
(2) A small boy.
(3) (Scottish) Humorous wag.
(4) (Scottish) A barber.
(5) A plunderer or trickster using immoral but legal means. A cunning shaver – a swindler. A mad shaver – a roysterer.
(6) A shaving machine.
(7) A close fisted, huckstering fellow; a miser.
'He's a proper old shaver.' West Somerset. (*Elworthy*)
(8) John MacGowan, 1726–1780, a baptist minister.

SHAVE-GRASS See Shave-Rush.

SHAVE RUSH *Equisetum Hiemale*. A type of American grass with sharp-edged leaves.

SHAVING The action of removing hair from the face, head or the body by means of a razor.

SHAVING CUP A shaving mug.

SHAVING BASIN See Barbers' bowl.

SHAVING BOX A small, round wooden container with a lid filled with a block of shaving soap. By *c* 1756 the old English hard lather and soap-ball that frothed in the pewter or pottery barber's basin began to give way to the French fashion of shaving box and brush for lathering the beard.

SHAVING BRUSH (1) A small, circular brush (the best are of badger hair) by which the lather is applied, preparatory to razoring the beard. 'Shaving brushes for applying lather to the face were introduced into England in 1756, previously the lather was rubbed in with the fingers.' (*Pulleyn*)
(2) Underarm hair. Slang.

SHAVING BRUSH PALM *Rhophalostylis Sapida*; a native palm of New Zealand. (*Muirhead*)

SHAVING CHAIR See Barber's chair.

SHAVING CLOTH A cloth thrown over the shoulders to protect the clothes of the shavee during the shave. (*Clerk*, 1602)

SHAVING COMPETITION There were popular contests among barbers in the 19th to early 20th century. The objective was for the barber, with the help of one lather boy, to shave as many faces as possible, without drawing blood, in one hour. At Bristol the record was 60 faces shaved in the hour (but not with me in the chair! *JSC*)

SHAVING CREAM A preparation of a creamy consistency by means of which the beard is softened preparatory to shaving, either by brushing the soap type into a lather or, with soapless types, applying them lightly by means of the fingers.

SHAVING EDGE A very sharp edge on a razor.

SHAVING HAT A hat made of finely plaited wood shavings, 1723. (*Cunnington*)

SHAVING IN CHURCHYARDS In the 14th and early 15th centuries it was a custom in England for the barbers to shave parishioners in the churchyard before matins on high festivals such as Easter, Whitsuntide, etc. The observance of this custom was prohibited by Richard Flemyng, Bishop of Lincoln in 1422. (*The Olio*, vol 1 1828)

SHAVING MACHINE An electrically stimulated apparatus whose blades either by oscillation or rotation will cut hair as short as a razor will cut.

SHAVING MIRROR A round, double-sided mirror, one side being a normal mirror, the other a magnifying mirror.

SHAVING MUG A handled china or earthenware container consisting of two divisions, the upper one in which the soap was kept and a lower, entered through a protruding lip, which contained water and received the shaving brush.

SHAVING PAPER A soft toilet paper onto which the shaven bristles and lather are deposited from the razor's blade.

SHAVING PAPER VASE A vase-like container which held the shaving paper upon which lather and whiskers were wiped from the razor blade. 19/20th century.

SHAVING POT See Shaving mug

SHAVING RAG A cloth for shaving. 'May the 10th, 1796: Wash given out to Mrs Wheeler . . . 1 pair under stockings, thread, 3 shaving wrages.' (*Wale*)

SHAVING REST A head-rest upon which the shavee could comfortably lay his head during a shave.

SHAVING SOAP Soap of a gentle nature suitable for lathering the face daily, to soften the beard preparatory to shaving. It often contains rosin to increase the lathering properties of the preparation.

SHAVING URN A small water boiler to supply hot water for shaving.

SHAVOMAT An establishment that offers a complete gentleman's hairdressing service and ancillary services such as showers, coffee and shoe shine facilities. (*Hair and Beauty*, Feb 1971)

SHEARS Large haircutting scissors used for bobbing and shingling from long hair, *cf* Tapering scissors.

SHEATH COMB A dressing comb and sheath to protect it.

SHED (1) Subs. A parting in the hair of the head. 'Haire divided at the sheade.' (*Cooper*, Under *Dividuus – coma dividua*)
(2) Verb. To part or divide hair. 'The Combe . . . is of most use with women for shedding and trimming their haire and head-tires . . .' (*Guillim*, p 291)

SHE-DRAGON A man's 18th century wig style. (*London Mag*)

SHEEN (1) Subs. Brightness, lustre, gleam, radiance.
(2) Brilliantine, 20th century.
(3) Hair lacquer, 20th century. 'Spray my hair with the new sheen,' 1960.

SHEEPDOG COIFFURE See Veronica Lake coiffure.

SHEEPDOG HAIRCUT A man's long hair style worn over the face, ears and neck, 1950–1967.

SHEEP'S HEAD Used in the 17/19th century by barber's apprentices for shaving practice.

SHEE-SHAVER A woman barber, 17th century.
'A little woman barber, a shee-shaver.' (*Clerk*)

SHELL Loosely knotted hair forming a bow, 18th century. (*Cunnington*)

SHELLAC A brittle, yellowish, transparent resinous excretion of the insect *Laccifer* (*Tachardia*) *Lacca*. Resiniferous trees of India serve as hosts for the sucking insects. Soluble in alcohol, ether and benzene; not soluble in water. Used in hair lacquers. For a comprehensive review of shellac, including its chemistry, see the monograph by Gardner in Mattiello, *Protective and Decorative Coatings*, New York, 1941. (*Merck*)

SHELL CURL A part curl or curve of hair resembling a shell.

SHENANDOAH BEARD See Spade beard. American usage. (*Trusty*)

SHEPHERDESS, THE A woman's hair style of the time of Louis XVI. (*Bysterveld*, p 63)

SHERMANIC MOUSTACHE A moustache style as worn by the American General W T Sherman (1820–1891). (*Trusty*) *101K*

SHIELD See Finger shield.

SHIMADA The formal hairdress of a Japanese woman, so called from the name of the town where it first came into fashion. (*Inouye*)

SHIMADA MAGE The oldest known form of Japanese coiffure for women. Depicted on Haniwa figures of women. (*Hashimoto*)

SHINGLE (1) Subs. A woman's short hair style of 1924 and later, in which the back hair was cut to a taper from the back of the head to the nape and the side hair was cut to the level of the ear.
(2) Verb. To cut a woman's hair to the style described in (1) above.

SHINGLE BOB See Semi-shingle.

SHINGLE CAP See Shingle net.

SHINGLE CHIGNON A chignon for wear on a shingled head to transform its appearance to a long-haired dressing. (*HWJ* 2 June, 1928).

SHINGLE GRIP See Hair grip.

SHINGLE NET A net of silk, cotton or other suitable material, worn over the head and secured under the chin with a ribbon. Used to keep the coiffure in position whilst sleeping.

SHINGLE SEMI A semi-transformation worked with 9″ hair for wear on a shingled head that lacks sufficient front hair. From 1924.

SHINGLE WIG A short-haired wig, dressed like the shingle style on the natural head.

SHINGLING Cutting hair at the back of the head short at the nape and leaving it longer as the hair is cut towards the crown, but showing no visible line of demarcation. See also Shingle.

SHIP TIRE A woman's head-dress of extravagant construction resembling a 16th century high prowed ship. Fashionable in the Elizabethan period. 'Thou hast the right-arched beauty of the brow, that becomes the ship-tire.' (*Shakespeare*, *Merry Wives of Windsor*, 1602)

SHOCK A thick mass of hair. 'She puts her shock in papers nightly.'

SHOCK HEAD Subs. A head of thick, coarse, stand-up hair. 'A shock head of auburn hair.'

SHOCK HEADED Having a rough looking thick head of hair, especially standing up hair.

SHODE A parting in the hair of the head, *cf* Shed.
'His herte blode hath bathed all his here,
The nailey driven in the shode.' 14th century. (*Chaucer*, *Knight's Tale*)

SHOOSTER A non-tipper. Used in hairdressing saloons, West Scotland and London from the early 1920s. Presumably derived from the verb to shoo = to hasten away, first used in this sense in 1851; so a shooster became one who hastened away without awarding the customary tip. Not noticed in Partridge's Dictionary of Slang. (*F Austin*). But compare the word shyster = a twister.

SHOP WORK A well executed hairdress, suitable for the saloon, but lacking the creative originality of the hair artist is spoken of as shopwork.

SHORT BOB (1) An 18th century wig style for men.
(2) A 20th century short hair style for women. See Bob.

SHORT CURL also SHORT FILLET Hair lying the whole breadth of the forehead; a wide, short curled fringe. 17th century. (*Holme*)

SHORT FILLET See Short curl.

SHORT HAIR (1) A sign of submission to a superior. Caesar obliged the Gauls to cut off their hair in token of submission. The Goths regarded short hair as a mark of thraldom. A monk's tonsure is the sign of his submission to religious authority.
(2) The genital hair.

SHORT QUEUE An 18th century wig style for men. Dressed rather flat on top and at sides, fuller at back with short queue.

SHORT TERM RINSE A colour applied to the hair in the form of a rinse, which lasts for only a short period – days or weeks.

SHORT TIME RINSE See Short term rinse.

SHOU CHANG See Hsüan wên-hua.

SHOVEL, SIR CLOWDISLEY (1650–1707), Admiral of the Fleet. A 17/18th century wig style named after him. See Sir Clowdisley Shovel.

SHOW BLOCK A plush covered, faceless model of a skull on which the wigmaker can display postiches. These blocks are sometimes solid, but more often hollow and the hollow ones are also called wig shells.

SHOW STAND A metal, glass or wooden stand for the display of postiches.

SHREDDING Hair cutting from beneath in long, narrow, vertical sections. See also Slithering. (*Trusty*)

SHRUBBERY A false beard; also the natural beard. Slang American and English usage. (*B and B*)

SHYLOCK WIG An 18th century wig name for the characterisation of Shylock in *The Merchant of Venice*. (*Stewart*)

SICKLE (1) A crescentic tress of hair. 19th century.
(2) A crescentic hair ornament. 19th century.

SIDE BANG A fringe at one side or the other of the forehead.

SIDEBARS See Sideburns.

SIDEBAR WHISKERS See Sideburns.

SIDEBOARDS Side whiskers; once regarded as slang, but now common English usage.

SIDEBORDS See Sideboards.

SIDEBURN A short side whisker, one on each side of the face, worn with a smooth chin. Name derived from the American General Burnside, *c* 1875, who favoured this style. In America they are called Burnsides.

SIDEBURN CURL A curl placed adjacent to and in front of the ear. American usage, 20th century.

SIDEBURN WHISKERS See Sideburn.

SIDE COMB A curved comb with teeth on one side of the spine only, equidistant from each other, but shorter than the teeth of a backcomb. Used to secure the dressed hair on the head.

SIDE CURL A postiche of curls on weft with or without a loop or loops for attachment to the hair at the side of the head by means of hairpins or a hair grip.

SIDE FRISETTE A small frisette for use at the side of the head, usually sold and used in pairs – one at each side.

SIDE LOCK The lock on a peruke that covers the ears and neck and keeps them warm, being a degree shorter than the Bottom Lock, *qv*. 17th century. (*Holme*)

SIDE LOCK OF HAIR A lock of hair worn against the side of the face; often regarded as a symbol of intuition. (*Gaskell*)

SIDE PIECE See Side curl.

SIDE STITCHING See Stitching.

SIDE WAVELET Sewn wefts of short, waved hair, worn over the ears and side of the cheek, somewhat similar to a pin wave, but sewn as a marteau.

SIDE WHISKERS Face hair on the cheek extending from the ear down towards the chin.

SIDIES Side whiskers. Slang. (*Daily Telegraph*, 22 May 1969)

SILHOUETTE A figure or object filled with solid colour. A monochrome outline of a hairdress, without other detail such as colour, tone, texture, wave or curl detail. Originally a portrait of a person in profile, the inside of the outline being black on a white background. Named after Etienne de Silhouette, a Frenchman (1709–1767).

SILK (For weaving) Strong silk string of colour to match the hair being woven.

SILK BOLTING CLOTH A finely woven white or flesh-coloured cloth used for drawn-through partings.

SILKEN BEARD Sictryg, son-in-law of Brian, King of Dublin, 11th century.

SILK NET A wig net of silk. See Soft foundation net.

SILK RIBBON Gallon, *qv*.

SILKS See Weaving silks.

SILK STICK See Spool stick.

SILK WIG A theatrical wig for which strands of silk are used in place of hair.

SILVER BLONDE (1) Bleached hair that approximates to white.
(2) White hair.

SILVER BLONDING Bleaching hair to lightest blond and rinsing with suitable chemicals to obtain a silvery appearance. See Platinum blonde.

SILVER DYE Silver dyes are still used. The basis is silver nitrate, a salt which is soluble in water and is decolourised by light. *It is poisonous, caustic and blackens the skin.* Silver nitrate with ammonium hydroxide first forms silver hydroxide (AgOH) which precipitates. As more ammonia is added the silver hydroxide redissolves to form the silver ammonia complex (Ag+NH$_3$). This complex is reduced by pyrogallol to granular metallic silver which is deposited on the hair. This dye is applied in two solutions. *Pyrogallol is a tri-hydric phenol and is poisonous and has to be used with great care.* Solutions over 5% strength make hair brittle. (*Moodie*)

SILVERHEAD (1) A silver blonde.
(2) A white head of hair.

SILVERING A hair rinse of suitable chemicals, on white hair that produces a silvery appearance.

SILVER TIP A blonde or grey haired person, especially a blonde Swede. American slang. (*B and B*)

SIMONIZE Verb trans. To use Brilliantine on the hair. American slang, 20th century. Originating from the high-gloss car polish of that name. (*B and B*)

SIMON MAGUS'S TONSURE A semi circle shaved from ear to ear above the forehead, but not extended to the back of the head. (*Brewer*)

SIMPLE BLEACH A mixture of 20 volume hydrogen peroxide and .880 ammonium hydroxide. Proportions, ¼ pint H$_2$O$_2$ and about 5 drops of ammonium hydroxide. Too much of the latter is likely to produce brassy tones.

SIMPLE HAIR DYE A hair dye that is effective as a result of one application of a single liquid.

SIMPLE-M An 18th century name for once-in-weaving on two silks. (*Garsault*)

SINCIPUT The head from forehead to crown.

SINGE (1) Verb. To burn off the tips of hair as a hairdressing process.
(2) Subs. The process of burning the hair tips.

SINGEING The burning of the hair ends by means of a lighted taper. A popular service in the hairdressing saloon in the 19th and early 20th century, now less used. It was supposed to: (1) Seal the ends of the hair and prevent them bleeding; (2) Effectively get rid of split ends; (3) Prevent the client catching cold. The practice had no beneficial effect whatsoever to the client, except as a disinfectant, but it was monetarily beneficial to the hairdresser.　　*301*

SINGEING MACHINE An electrical device consisting of a red hot wire secured between two insulated prongs by means of which the hair could be singed.

SINGLE KNOTTING Tyeing a wisp of hair to a wig net foundation by means of a single knot at the root ends of the wisp.

SINGLE STEM SWITCH A switch or tail with only one stem or core.

SINGULIERE See A La singulière.

SIR CLOWDISLEY SHOVEL (Also spelt Cloudesley). An 18th century wig style, similar to a full-bottomed wig, *qv.* See Shovel, Sir Clowdesley. 257

SIRENE HEADDRESS A woman's hair style of 1866. (*Bysterveld*, p 80)

SITIL A metal hanging basin with a tap, used by Turkish barbers.

SIX TIER BOB WIG 18th century man's style. 255

SKAP The pate or head. Scottish usage. (*Scot*)

SKEIN A folded coil of thread.

SKELETON WIG (1) A light-weight wig in which the hair is knotted on a foundation of silk or net having several large apertures. 19th century. 'Making a skeleton wig for old Mrs Taverner 42/-.' 1891. (*Stevens Ms*)
(2) A full transformation made in the form of a complete band of foundation without hooks and eyes at the back. 19th century.
(3) A transformation or border of hair (with no crown) that encircles the circumference of the scalp. 19th and early 20th century.
(4) A wig, the foundation of which consists of gallons radiating from a central point at the crown to the perimeter galloon, with similar galloons encircling the head at regular angles to the radiating galloons. Foundation net only between alternate encircling galloons.

SKIMMED MILK Used as a setting lotion on fine hair. Early 20th century.

SKINHEAD A young man who followed a 1969 cult of very short hair or a shaven head.

SKIN TEST A test on the skin to determine the individual's reaction to a chemical preparation such as a hair dye or permanent waving lotion. It consists of cleansing a patch of skin 1″ in diameter on the hairline behind the ear, applying the chemical which it is proposed to use in the treatment, allowing it to dry and covering it with collodium to prevent its removal by the subject when washing. It is left in contact with the skin for from 24 to 48 hours and if no inflammation or other evident ill effect can be seen it may be safe to proceed with the treatment. This test is obligatory by law in the United States of America, but not in England, although it is morally obligatory in England on every hairdresser who intends to dye a head of hair to make this test. If it is not made and the client contracts dermatitis, she or he could succeed in a court action as it would be held that the hairdresser had not used the care and skill, or taken the reasonable precautions, necessary to avoid damage to the client which would be expected by the public from one claiming to be a qualified hairdresser.

SKIP WAVE A combination of finger waves and pincurls. The pincurl is formed in alternate finger wave troughs. Suitable only when setting medium to loose curl on hair four or five inches long.

SKUFT Back of the neck. Northern usage. (*Grose, Prov Glos*)

SKULL BLOCK A small, head-shaped, malleable block for putting inside a hollow display shape when dressing postiche for a window display. It is positioned on a block stand to facilitate the dressing of a postiche. After dressing the hair the skull-block is removed and the display shape put on a stand.

SKULL CAP A toupée.

SKULL THATCHER Facetious name for a wig maker. (*Hone, Table Book*, 1827)

SLAB CURL A long, lank curl. 18th century. (*Lady's Mag*, 1776)

SLEEKED HAIR Hair that has been brushed straight and flat. (*Coiffeur Européen*, 1865)

SLEEPING CAP See Sleeping net.

SLEEPING NET A bonnet-type cap of silk net to cover the head and prevent the hair becoming disarranged during sleep. Also called Shingle Net, Beauty Cap, etc.

SLIDE A kind of brooch, fastener or clasp to secure and/or decorate hair, composed of two parts, the decorative which rests on the top of the hair, and hinged to it, a wire loop arm which slides beneath the hair tress. The two parts are then pressed together and the wire loop arm engages a knobbed protrusion fixed to the underside of the decorative part. 'Plain and inlaid tortoiseshell slides for ladies Braids, of all patterns.' (*Morning Herald*, Dec 13th, 1787)

SLIDING DISTANCE In Marcel waving the distance that the irons are slid or dragged along the hair to form the trough of the wave. (*Zentler*)

SLIP, THE A strip of coarse, brown paper 10″ × 2½″, folded three times to form a rectangle of 1¼″ × 2½″, is known as 'the slip'. One slip is required for each of the three grooves of the spool stick around which the weaving silks are wound in a clockwise direction. The slip facilitates the turning of the wound silk on the stick when the tension is adjusted.

SLIP KNOT A knot that can be easily slipped or untied.

SLIP STITCH See Stitching.

SLITHER CUT The same as Taper cut, *qv.* American usage. (*Reno*)

SLITHERING A cutting movement used in thinning hair with the hair-cutting scissors by slithering the scissors up and down a strand of hair and at the same time slightly opening and closing the scissor blades to cut one or two hairs at a time, thus producing a tapered effect in the hair strand.

SLOCKSTER A hairdresser who entices away another hairdresser's assistant. 19/20th century.

SLOPING BOX CAR MOUSTACHE A 20th century moustache. American usage. (*Trusty*) 101E

SLUMBER HELMET See Sleeping net.

SLUMBER NET See Sleeping net.

SMALL BACK Man's 18th century wig style.

SMALL SIDE That side of the parting opposite the large side, *qv.*

SMALL TOOTH COMB A small, fine-toothed comb for drawing through the hair to remove dandruff and loose scales. Also called Dandruff comb, dandriff comb, dust comb, and flea comb.

SMEGMA A sebaceous secretion.

SMOCKING A method of sewing weft to form a pattern of diamond or triangular shapes. See Diamond mesh. American usage.

SMOOTH FACE CUT A close shave. (*Rowlands*)

SMOOTH SCRATCH See Scratch wig.

SMOOTHING PIN See Winding needle. American usage.

SMYRNA SOAP A bastard sort of Joppa Soap, *qv*, from Smyrna. 18/19th century. (*Lillie*)

SNAIL BACK A man's 18th century wig style. (*London Mag* 1753)

SNAIL BUCKLE, THE See En-escargot.

SNAIL CURL A small curl, 20th century. Name suggested by the spiral shell of the common garden snail. *Helix Aspersa,* 219

SNAKE (1) A long curl at the back of a wig, often worn draped over the shoulders and called a love lock. 'And this the yard long snake he twirls behind.' (*Sir G Etherege, The Man of Mode*, 1676)

(2) A curved lock of hair usually terminating in a frond curl, *qv*.

SNAKE CURL When the locks turn round many times and hang down as the dildo or Pole lock does. 17th century. (*Holme*)

SNAKE OIL An early cure for baldness and recorded as such by Pliny the elder, AD 23–79. Rattlesnake oil is used by the women of the Nahuatl in Mexico to promote a luxuriant growth of hair for which they are famous. It was also a standard remedy offered by itinerant salesmen in the United States of America in the 19th century.

SNAKE OUT (1) Subs. Diswound hair that has been left curled at the points, and curved near the roots.

(2) Verb. To diswind hair leaving the ends curled and the stem curved. 'Snake out the rollers and leave the diswound hair casual.' To arrange strands of curly hair into sinuous shapes.

SNAP A barber, 17th century. (*Braithwaite*, ed 1641)

SNAP SPRING A spring that will cause the arms of a hair clip to close suddenly with a snap. Used for securing postiches to the head hair.

SNARL A tangle in the hair. See also Knot, Mat, Tangle, Tug, etc.

SNED, TO To cut or form by cutting. 18th century.

SNIP (1) Verb. To cut off by scissors.

(2) Subs. A barber. Slang. Bristol usage. 19th/early 20th century.

(3) Subs. A tailor. Slang.

SNIPPERS Scissors. 16th century.

SNIPS See (2)

SNODDED Adj. Trimmed, made straight. Scottish usage. (*Brown*)

SNOOD (1) Subs. The band or ribbon or string for tying up a woman's hair. 17/18th century. Scottish usage. (*Ramsay*) By the 20th century its meaning in English usage had been extended to a bag-shaped net to contain the hair on the head, or some part of it.

(2) Verb. To tie up or enclose the tresses in a band or filet. Scottish usage. See Veronica Lake Coiffure. (*Companion*)

SNOT A vulgarism for thick, slimy hair setting lotion. South of England usage. 1920s.

SNOW CURLING Strands of hair very loosely crimped. 19th century.

SNOW HEADDRESS A woman's hair style of 1866. (*Bysterveld*, p 90)

SNOW PIN A very fine, silver coloured hairpin, an 'Invisible' pin, *qv*. (*Coiffeur Européen*, 1867)

SOAP (1) Subs. A substance formed by the combination of particular fats and oils with alkaline bases. Used for the manufacture of shampoos for cleansing the hair and scalp. Soft soaps are manufactured from vegetable oils and caustic potash; and hard soaps from animal fats and caustic soda.

(2) Verb. To smear, rub or cover with soap.

SOAP BALL A ball or round cake of soap.

SOAP BARK See Quillaia.

SOAP BERRY The fruit of a tropical American plant, containing Saponia, which can be used as a substitute for fine soap. (*Verrill*)

SOAP BRUSH The same as shaving brush. American usage.

SOAP CAP A mixture of shampoo and a dye by means of which the hair is coloured at the same time as it is shampooed. To permit longer developing time the client is sometimes allowed to resume her normal sitting posture for a few minutes, the soapy dye-impregnated head being covered with a plastic cap. See also Shampoo dye.

SOAP CLAY Earth or clay mixed with natron used by the ancient Egyptians and other peoples of the East instead of soap. (*Verrill, Hist Tech*)

SOAPLESS DETERGENT A detergent that contains no soap. The synthetic detergents are commonly manufactured from ammonium lauryl sulphate, sodium lauryl sulphate or triethanolamine lauryl sulphate. Sulphonated vegetable oils are also used in another type of soapless detergent. (*Sagarin*)

SOAPLESS OIL SHAMPOO A shampoo mostly consisting of sulphonated oils, *qv*.

SOAPLESS SHAMPOO See Soapless detergent.

SOAP LOCK Curl on the forehead held in position by soap.

SOAP PLANTS There are several plants, such as the soapworts, the juices of which can be employed for washing. (*Piesse*)

SOAP POWDER MACHINE (Container) A globular metal container which when inverted released a small quantity of soap powder for shaving.

SOAP SCUM See Scum

SOAPSTONE OF MYLOS In the 19th century this mineral was imported from Turkey and Russia. An analysis showed: Silex 63, alumina 23, water 12 and sesquioxide of iron 1.25%.

SOAP SUDS Water that is impregnated with dissolved soap.

SOAPSUDS SCULPTURE The fashioning of soap-sodden hair into a sculptured style in order to decide upon the suitability of the style. (*Vito*)

SOAP TREE See Quillaia.

SOAPY Silly, effeminate, 20th century slang.

SOCRATES Athenian philosopher (469–399 BC). The ancients depicted him with whitish bright hair. (*Salmon*)

SODIUM CARBONATE Na_2CO_3. An alkali commonly used in hot permanent waving solutions. The crystalline sodium carbonate $Na_2CO_31OH_2O$ is used in bath crystals and the crude product is common washing soda. Another use is for softening hard water.

SODIUM PERBORATE $NaBO_34H_2O$. A white crystalline substance containing approximately 10 per cent available oxygen. It is readily activated by acids when it will behave like 10 volume hydrogen peroxide solution. Employed as a bleaching agent, deodorant and antiseptic, and used in freckle lotions, toothpaste and the paste bleach for the hair, euphemistically called 'white henna'.

SODIUM PEROXIDE Na_2O_2. Containing 20% of available oxygen, is a powerful bleaching agent, freely soluble in water, forming sodium hydroxide and hydrogen peroxide. In contact with organic materials ignition and explosion can take place. Has been used, suitably diluted and compounded with an inert carrier, to produce a platinum blonde effect.

SODIUM SULPHATE $Na_2SO_4\ 1OH_2O$. Glauber's Salt. See also Sodium sulphite.

SODIUM SULPHITE $Na_2SO_37H_2O$. An unstable colourless efflorescent crystalline substance, oxidising in the air to sodium sulphate. A reducing agent used in hot permanent waving solutions, especially for white hair, which it did not discolour.

SOFT BLOCK See Malleable block.

SOFT-COILED-KNOT A back-combed, lightly dressed coil formed from a single-stemmed switch and worn as a chignon.

SOFTENING AGENT (1) A substance that will soften hard water.

(2) A substance that will soften hair to make it more absorbent for successful hair dyeing, eg hydrogen peroxide.

SOFT FOUNDATION NET See Soft wig net.

SOFT HEAD A malleable block.

SOFT PRESSING See Hair pressing.

SOFT SOAP Soap made from vegetable oils and caustic potash. See Soap.

SOFT WATER Water which readily produces with soap a lather that will remain for a minimum of two minutes is regarded as soft water.

SOFT WIG NET A soft, close mesh net of silk, cotton or nylon, used as part of the foundation, the crown and back area of a wig, to which hair is knotted or weft sewn. Also called wig net, silk net, soft foundation net.

SOIREE COIFFURE See Evening hairdress.

SOL The Roman sun god. Depicted by the ancients, beardless with long, curled, golden hair, crowned with a laurel, but the Assyrians depicted him with a long beard. (*Salmon*)

SOLANA Large brimmed straw hat with no crown worn by Italian women to protect their complexion when exposing their hair to the sun to bleach it. (*Rimmel*)

SOLDIERS' POMATUM A piece of tallow candle. (*Grose*, ed, 1823)

SOLID BRILLIANTINE The consistency of solid brilliantine varies from a kind of soft pomade to a firm wax. Three typical formulae are: (1) Paraffin wax 20%, mineral oil 50%, petrolatum 30%, perfume and colour to taste. (2) Castor oil 80%, beeswax 20%, perfume and colour to taste. (3) Rosin 25%, white oil 20%, paraffin wax 25%, ceresin 30%, perfume and colour to taste.

SOLID HYDROGEN PEROXIDE Made in tablet form of peroxide and urea; or a mixture of sodium perborate and tartaric acid. They are dissolved in distilled water immediately before use. Neither of these preparations should be allowed to come into contact with metal.

SOLID RAZOR A wedge-shaped razor tapering from the back to the cutting edge. When slightly hollow ground it is called semi-solid or half hollow ground; the French razor is this type, of soft steel. (*Foan*)

Many men preferred the solid razor to the hollow-ground razor, as it glided over the face silently, whereas a hollow ground razor made a rasping metallic sound as it cut the beard hair.

SOLUBLE Capable of being dissolved in fluid.

SOLUTE The substance dissolved in a solution.

SOLUTION (1) A liquid or semi-liquid resulting from the combinaiton of a solid with a solvent. A dissolved condition.

(2) The action of dissolving from a gaseous or solid to a liquid state by means of a solvent.

SOLVENT Subs. A substance having the power of dissolving another substance or substances.

SORE FINGER The same as Fish Hook, *qv*. 'Stuck out like a sore finger.' Northampton usage. (*Mrs J Savage*)

SORREL Yellowish red. A sorrel pate; one having red hair. (*Grose, Lex Bal*)

SOUBRETTE, THE A woman's hair style of the time of Louis XV of France. (*Bysterveld*, p 61)

SOUBRETTE BOB 1920s style.   *268*

SOUFFLE LOOK A light, fluffy look. A head of loose, fluffy curls.

SOUP-STRAINER Slang. A long moustache over the upper lip; a walrus Moustache, *qv*. (*Mitchell*)

SOUTHERNWOOD (Southern wormwood, *Artemisia Abrotanum*). A decoction of the leaves promotes the growth of hair. (*Fernie*)

SOUTHEY, ROBERT Southey, the poet, said of himself that he carried shaving to its *ne plus ultra* of independency,

inasmuch as he performed that operation *sans* looking-glass, *sans* shaving brush, *sans* soap or substitute for soap, *sans* hot water, *sans* cold water, *sans* everything except a razor. (*Southey, The Doctor*)

SPADE BEARD A beard, cut to the shape of a pointed or broad spade blade, but not cut straight across in the Russian fashion. 16th/19th century. 'Long spade beards and matted hair.' (*Dryden*, 1693)   *97d*

SPANIEL EAR See Bouffon.

SPANISH BEARD Similar to the Cathedral beard, *qv*, 'The ugly long Spanish beard.' (*Wycherley*, 1673)

SPANISH COIL CHIGNON Constructed with three cable twists. (*Creer*)   *226*

SPANISH COMB A decorative hair comb with a deep wide top which stands out from the head when fixed in position.

SPANISH CUT (Spanish manner) (1) A 16th century hair style for men. (*Stubbes*). Long at the ears and 'curled like to the two ends of an old cast perriwig.' (*Repton*)

(2) The sideboards cut to a forward point. 20th century.

SPANISH FLY (1) An 18th century man's wig. (*Stewart*)

(2) A popular name for Cantharides, *qv*.

SPANISH LOCKS Disordered hair. 16th century. (*Kendall*)

SPANISH MANNER See Spanish cut.

SPANISH SOAP Olive oil soap. (*PPB*)

SPANISH STYLE OF VEIL A veil arranged mantilla fashion and fixed to the coiffure at the crown of the head, then draped over both shoulders and the back. (*Mallemont Illus* p 65)

SPANISH WHITE Prepared chalk, used in the surface preparation of wax models. (*PPB*)

SPATULA A flexible, blunt, knife-shaped implement of metal, horn, bone, ivory, plastic or shell, used for mixing cream, etc, also with one end covered with cotton wool, for applying bleach cream (white henna) and dyes.

SPEAR A coarse, single-pronged hairpin, used in first pli, to hold a wound curler in position. 1950.

SPECIALIST A hairdresser who specially or exclusively studies and practices one particular branch of his art, eg a hair-dyeing specialist.

SPENCER PERUKE See Spencer wig.

SPENCER WIG A kind of man's wig (1742). From the family name Spencer and probably after Charles Spencer, Third Earl of Sunderland (1674–1722). Richard Morrison, Edinburgh, Ms receipt in collection of writer, 'June 1742, Spencer Wig £1.'

SPERMACETI White, brittle, fatty substance from the sperm whale, used to give substance to toilet creams.

SPERRYWIG Pixie. Devon usage. (*Elworthy, Devonshire Verbal Provincialisms*, 1898)

SPICED HENNA See Henna.

SPIDER DRYER A type of hood dryer with adjustable, holed-fingers, through which the hot air is blown onto the head.

SPIKE COMB A tail or needle comb, *qv*.

SPIKE HAIR A style worn by Punk Rockers. Hair standing up in spikes, held in position by hair lacquer. From late 1960s. See Spiky style.

SPIKE ROLLER See Spiky roller.

SPIKY ROLLER A hair roller of plastic or rubber, incorporating bristle or plastic spikes.

SPIKY STYLE (1) Hair cut short, ¼" to ½", over the whole head. From 1950s.

(2) Hair well tapered and dressed in high cones (3" to 8"), standing away from the head and held in position by hair lacquer. From late 1960s.

SPILL The hard, flexible rod of woven and wound hair that forms part of a switch or tail. There are two in a two-spill tail and three in a three-spill tail. See One-stem switch. For elaborate plaiting designs tails may be constructed of more than three spills.

SPINACH A false beard; also the natural beard. Slang, American usage. (*B and B*)

SPINACH SEED, THE A hair style. See En-Grain-d'Epinard.

SPINAGE SEED A man's 18th century wig style. (*London Mag*, 1753)

SPINDELHAARE See Monilethrix.

SPINDLE-SHAPED CURLER A rounded rod, tapering towards each end. When hair is wound spirally on these curlers a hanging curl which is loose in the middle and tight at the root end and point end is produced.

SPINDLE TREE (*Celastraceoe*) Its fruit was applied to children's heads to destroy lice (hence its other name, louseberry tree) and its powdered bark to kill nits and remove scurf. 19th century. (*Fernie*)

SPINDLE WINDING See Spiral winding.

SPINNER A winding machine for winding spills for a switch. (*Symonds*)

SPIRAL BRUSH A hairbrush with the bristles set spirally down and around the base.

SPIRAL CURL A hanging curl shaped like a corkscrew; also called Drop curl and Corkscrew curl, *qv*. 325

SPIRAL POWDERING MACHINE Carrot-shaped powder puff constructed from a spiral spring covered with fabric or thin leather and used for puffing powder onto the hair. 18th century. (*Pyne*)

SPIRAL SPRING See Tension spring.

SPIRAL WAVING Waving by breaking a spirally wound curl into waves.

SPIRAL WIND Subs. A wisp of hair wound round a cylindrical object forming a succession of curls arranged like the thread of a screw.

SPIRAL WINDING (also called Helical Winding and Spindle winding). The method of winding hair around a curler in a spiral manner from the root end towards the point or tip of the hair. From 1920 to 1940 there were two methods of spiral winding commonly used: (1) The hair strand wound flat and obliquely down the curler, and (2) The hair strand was first twisted and then wound obliquely down the curler. See Twist Wind. (*Smith*)

SPIRIT GUM A quick-drying preparation used by actors to secure false hair to their faces. A useful formula is: Mastic 5.5%, ether, sp gr 0.720, 5.5%, Rosin 33.5%, sandarac 11%, alcohol 44.5%. (*Redgrove and Foan*)

SPIRIT SOAP A solution of soft soap in 50% alcohol and 50% distilled water. A popular shampoo in the late Victorian and Edwardian periods.

SPIRITS OF ACID Glacial acetic acid. (*PPB*)

SPIRITUS COLOGNE Eau de Cologne, *qv*.

SPIT CURL A small curl on the forehead, positioned by human spittle.

'I'm an only daughter young girl,
A spit curl and frizzes young girl.'

(*Brooklyn Eagle*, c 1900)

SPITTOON A round, earthenware or metal vessel with a funnel-shaped or open top, used to spit into and a ubiquitous utensil in the 19th century barber shops, English and especially American. Several were in use in Bristol barber's shops as late as 1937. There may still be a few in use today, 1983.

SPLIT ENDS The point of a hair which, through ill treatment or neglect, has split into two or more ends.

SPONGE COMB A dual purpose tail comb with a sponge fixed to the tail end, used for dyeing and in permanent waving processes to apply solutions and comb hair strands.

SPONGE SHAVE A shave which follows the application of a softening agent to the beard by means of a sponge.

SPONGY Porous like a sponge. Compressible and absorbent.

SPOOL STICK (Reel stick, Silk stick, Right-hand stick). The right-hand weaving stick with three grooves on which the unwefted silks are wound.

SPOT BLEACHING The application of bleach to selected strands of hair, either because they are darker than the bulk of the hair and need lightening to produce an even colour throughout the head, or to make selected strands lighter than the bulk of hair.

SPOT DYEING The same as Spot bleaching except that the hair is dyed instead of bleached.

SPRAY (1) Subs. An instrument that will diffuse scent, hair lacquer or other liquid for application to the hair.
(2) Verb. To diffuse in the form of minute droplets.

SPREKELIA FORMOSISSIMA (Aztec Lily; Jacobean Lily) A deciduous bulb, native of Mexico. The bulb produces the alkaloid amarilliana which is used in Mexico, by applying it to the scalp to prevent hair fall. (*Pesman*)

SPRIG See Sprig wire.

SPRIGGY Frizzy hair that stands up is said to be spriggy. West of England usage.

SPRIG WIRE The wire from which slender headless nails (sprigs) were cut. Sprigs were used to secure wig ribbons to the wooden blocks. 18th century. (*Earle*, p 264) See also Block point.

SPRING Two kinds of spring are used in boardwork: (1) Positional spring, *qv*, and (2) Tension spring, *qv*.

SPRING CREPON A front of hair worked on a spring and crêpe pad, worn around the front of the head. (*HWJ* No 1991)

SPRING CURL A corkscrew curl.

SPRING FOUNDATION A foundation for a pompadour front worked on a clock spring shaped to conform to the contour of the front of the head.

SPRINGING Bleeding resulting from a too close shave.

SPRING OF LIFE See Plumbiferous hair water.

SPRUNKING A Dutch term for pruning, tissing, trimming and setting out, by the glass or pocket mirror. 17th century. (*Evelyn*)

SPURGE (Euphorbioe) The juice of the wood spurge, mixed with honey and rubbed on the skin, in the sunshine will cause the hair to fall out of the annointed part. (*Gerard*)

SQUARE BEARD A beard cut straight across at the bottom. Russian style.

SQUARE BUTTON MOUSTACHE A small, square cut moustache. (*Trusty*)

SQUARE CUT BEARD See Square beard.

SQUARE CUTTING The same as Club cutting, *qv*.

SQUARED WIG A man's wig style, 18th century. (*Garsault*) 92 (3, 4)

SQUARE ROOT Woman's hair style. 19th century (*HTATH*) 288

SQUEAKY CLEAN Very clean. The hair when thoroughly clean after a shampoo squeaks when rubbed between the fingers.

SQUIGGLE A 16″–18″ length of weft of 6″–8″ curled hair worked on a wire and worn as a halo, bun, chignon, etc. 1974.

SQUIRLING Delousing a living head of hair by picking out the pests by means of the fingers. 19/20th century.

ST AGNES Depicted in paintings as stripped of her clothing, but hidden by her long hair. (*Roeder*)

ST ANSELM St Anselm when Archbishop of Canterbury

pronounced sentence of excommunication against all who wore long hair.

ST ANTHONY'S BALDNESS See Erysipelas Alopecia. (*Wheeler*)

ST APOLLONIA Depicted as dragged by the hair. (*Roeder*)

ST BARBARA Depicted in paintings as being dragged by her hair by her father. (*Roeder*)

ST CYPRIAN Died 258. He made twelve objections to hair dye, including: (1) The act of staining the hair is worse than adultery.

(2) To blacken the hair argues a detestation of that whiteness which belongs to the head of the Lord.

ST GALLA Died 546. The Patron saint of widows. Depicted in paintings as a widow with a long beard. (*Roeder*)

ST JAMES A 20th century beard style. (*Gents Acad*) After the district of St James, London. See Regent.

ST JOHN'S TONSURE A semi-circular tonsure worn by priests.

ST JOHN'S WORT (*Hypericum Perforatum*) The Venetians collected the dew which fell from it onto vegetation before daybreak on St John's morning, believing it to renew the hair roots on bald heads. (*Fernie*)

ST JULIANA OF NICOMEDIA d 305. In paintings she is depicted as being hung up naked by her hair. Her name was invoked against infectious diseases. (*Roeder*)

ST LOUIS Louis IX (1214–1270), King of France, canonized in 1297; patron saint of barbers, hairdressers and wigmakers.

ST MARY MAGDALENE Depicted in paintings with long hair and a jar of ointment. (*Roeder*)

ST MARY OF EGYPT In paintings she is depicted with long hair and three loaves. (*Roeder*)

ST ONUPHRIUS In paintings he is depicted as an old hermit, clad only in long hair and a loincloth of leaves. Patron saint of weavers. (*Roeder*)

ST PAUL'S TONSURE Having the whole head shaved. (*Brewer*)

ST PETER'S TONSURE A shaven circle right round the head to indicate the crown of thorns, worn by priests and preferred to St John's Tonsure, *qv*, in England, Germany, Italy and Spain. (*Brewer; Speight*)

ST RAINELDIS Depicted in painting as being dragged by her hair. (*Roeder*)

ST UNCUMBER See St Wilgefortis.

ST WILGEFORTIS (known in England as St Uncumber). She is depicted as a bearded woman being crucified. Invoked by maidens who wished to rid themselves of unwanted suitors.

ST WULSTAN Bishop of Worcester, vehemently declaimed against the luxury of long hair and when anyone with long tresses bowed for his blessing he cut off a lock with a sharp knife which he carried for this purpose and ordered that as a penance the rest of the hair should be cut off in the same way. (*Speight*)

STACKING Backcombing hair to produce volume (bouffance). American usage.

STAGGER KNOTTING See Cross knotting.

STAININGER, HANNSS Burgemeister of Branau (d 1567), possessor of possibly the longest recorded beard.

STAIRCASE A man's 18th century wig style. (*London Mag* 1753) See En-escalier.

STALK See Stem.

STANDAWAY PINCURL A pincurl which is formed on a strand of hair that is combed towards the crown of the head. (*Vito*)

STAND-UP PINCURL A pin curl which is set at right angles to the head; a pin curl standing out from the head.

This type of setting facilitates a finished dressing with movement away from the head, and induces fullness.

STAR, THE A woman's hair style of 1866 for wear at a fancy dress ball. Derived from a style of the 16th century. (*Bysterveld*, p. 96)

STARCH Made in the 18/19th century from unrefined wheatmeal. (*Lillie*)

STARCH POWDER Often adulterated by rice which, for this purpose, was ground by a horse mill. Used in some hair powders. 18/19th century.

STARTING KNOT The first knot in a length of weft.

STARTING WEFT See Fly weft.

STASH Moustache. Slang.

STATE BARBER LAWS (*USA*) Minnesota in 1897 was the first American State to pass legislation controlling the barber's craft. (*Trusty*)

STATIC BLADE The lower blade in a pair of hand clippers, which is in contact with the face or neck, and over and against which the upper mobile blade moves.

STATIC HAIRDO A hair style in which the hair is firmly secured by hairpins, clips, etc, or by lacquer, *cf* Flowing style.

STATIC HAIR STYLE A style that will hold fast in wind or excessive head movement.

STAY A position spring or wire for holding the edge of a postiche firmly against the scalp. They are positioned at the centre of the forehead at the temples, at the ears and two in the neck.

STEAMER An apparatus which produces steam and directs it onto the hair through holes in a hood placed over the head. Used in conjunction with massage and the application of various substances, such as oils, to the hair and scalp.

STEAMING TIME The length of time the wound hair is subjected to the application of steam in a hot permanent wave.

STEAM MARCEL A method of strengthening a Marcel wave. After the hair has been Marcel waved in the normal manner, the surface hair is slightly dampened by an atomized spray of water and then rewaved in the original conformations. (*Wilson*)

STEAM TOWEL A towel heated by steam and applied to the face after a shave.

STEATORRHEA See Alopecia Seborrheica.

STEATOSIS Excessive oil on the hair. (*Wilson*)

STEEL STAY A positional spring, *qv* American usage. See also Stay.

STEM (1) The woven and wound hard core of a hair switch or tail. See Spill.

(2) The straight length of hair near the scalp, before the hair curl starts.

(3) A tail or switch of hair. 'Mrs Rogers has ordered an 18″ two-stem.' (*Stevens MS*, 1892)

STEM CORD Macramé, upon which the woven hair is wound to form the stem of a switch.

STEP CUTTING Cutting hair in distinct steps.

STEPHENS An eccentric Bristol barber of the 19th century who, among other unusual activities, shaved a man in a lion's den; made an excursion in a balloon; drifted over Niagara Falls in a barrel made by Bristol coopers and exhibited at Avonmouth before his fatal voyage over the Falls. (*C Stephens*)

STEPPED HAIRCUT See Steppered Haircut.

STEPPERED HAIRCUT Hair cut in steps.

STERILE Free from from living germs.

STERILIZATION The process of destroying bacteria by chemical or physical means:

(1) Chemical means: disinfectant and fumigants.

(2) Physical means: Boiling, steaming, baking (dry heat) and irradiation.

STERILIZER An apparatus or container used to sterilize by freeing from harmful bacteria. There are wet sterilizers for use with liquids and dry sterilizers for use with vapour for fumigation.

STERILIZING CABINET An apparatus for sterilizing by fumigation.

STERLING'S AMBROSIA See plumbiferous hair water.

STICK OF HAIR A gathering of cut hair clubbed at the root and and tied. (*Baker and Wade*)

STICK PIN A plastic pin about 2½″ long, consisting of one shaft and point only, used to hold rollers and hair against the head during the setting process.

STICKS A pair of weaving sticks, ie the anchor stick and the spool stick.

STICK WAVING Spirally winding hair on a round stick and when 'set', breaking the curl into waves. (*Mallemont*)

STIDDEN, Thomas A Swedish barber-surgeon of the 17th century who played a part in the settlement of America, where he landed in 1654.

STIFF WIG NET (Also called Foundation net, Hoc net, Vegetable net) Stiffened cotton or silk net with hexagonal holes 1/16″ diameter. The net is stiffened by immersion in a solution of acacia gum and dried. Used for closely knotted postiche foundation such as transformations.

STILETTO BEARD A 16th century pointed beard style as worn by the Earl of Southampton. (*Repton*)

'The steeletto beard –

O, it makes me afeard,

It is so sharp beneath.' 1660 (*Rudyerd*)   *100 (22)*

STIMMIGE A Greek household slave who coloured or painted hair or eyebrows. (*Forbes*)

STITCHING The passing of the needle through the material in sewing. The following stitches have been used in the manufacture of postiches:

(1) Running stitch or slip stitch: The needle is run into the material in front of the stitch just formed.

(2) English stitch: The needle is passed in an upward direction on the cross. The strongest of all the stitches.

(3) Back stitch: Done in two ways; First by sewing from right to left, the needle stitches into the work behind where it has been drawn out, in order to take a stitch of the same size in front. Passing from left to right, the needle is inserted in front of the stitch last formed, this caused the stitch to appear on the reverse side of the material. Useful for turned-down seams.

(4) Hem stitch: The needle is placed under the material and drawn out about two threads above the edge.

(5) Side stitch: The stitch is made on the slant in the opposite side to that which is held towards the sewer.

(6) Sewing stitch: Used to join two edges together, the needle directed over the edges, passes through the outer fold and comes under that which is held nearest to the sewer.

(7) Overcasting or oversewing: Sewing with very wide stitches to prevent the edges of material ravelling out.

(8) Herringbone or cross stitch: Used to join two edges of material, which, instead of being folded together, are laid one over the other, and worked from left to right, making alternately a stitch below and one above. The cross stitch is made by the thread being drawn-out each time above the stitch which has just been made.

(9) Buttonhole stitch: The stitches are taken from left to right in the slit of the buttonhole, to be drawn out behind the tracing at the upper end, and making the thread form a

species of knot. Blanket stitch is similar, but longer.

(10) Chain stitch: These stitches are like rings chained together. The needle is held straight and always placed in the last ring or stitch, to be drawn out an equal distance to the length of the following ring; the cotton is held below the needle.

STIVER Subs. Bristly hair. Somerset usage. (*Williams*)

STOIC BEARD A long beard, as worn by the ancient philosophers.

STOP BLOCK A small strip of wood fixed to the bench to hold the drawing brushes in position when drawing off hair. See Adjustable block holder (and block).

STOP WEFT The starting knot and finishing knot in weaving. So woven that they will not loosen, but provide a secure holdfast to prevent the weft unravelling.

STORAX An aromatic gum from India and Turkey, used in perfumery. (*Lillie*)

STORY WIG A wig dressed in rows of curls. The earliest portraits of Dr Johnson show him wearing a five-row story wig. (*Smith*) Mr Saunders Welch, the father-in-law of Nollekens, the painter, wore a story wig with nine rows of curls. (*Smith*)

STRAIGHTENING COMB A metal comb with fine teeth and an insulated handle: used for straightening kinky hair. See Hair pressing.

STRAIGHT HAIR BANDEAU A bandeau constructed of straight hair. (*Creer*)

STRAND A tress or filament of hair. See also Bunch, Filament, Lock, Tress and Wisp.

STRAND TEST A dyeing, bleaching or permanent waving test on a small strand of hair before the full treatment is embarked upon in order to determine the correct strength of lotion, the timing, and the reaction of the hair to the proposed treatment.

STRAP A length of leather upon which the razor's edge is stropped to maintain its 'sweetness'. See also Strop.

STRAP, HUGH The barber in Smollett's *Roderick Random*, 1748. His real name was Hugh Hughson and he died, aged 85, in the parish of St Martin-in-the-Fields where he had kept a barber-shop for some forty years.

STRAPPING The act of correcting a razor's edge by rubbing on a strap. See also Strop and Stropping.

STRATUM BASALE A layer of cells in the epidermis situated beneath the stratum spinosum. (*Montagna*)

STRATUM CORNEUM The outer, horny layer of the skin. (*Montagna*)

STRATUM GRANULOSUM A layer of cells with granules forming part of the epidermis and situated between the stratum lucidum and the stratum spinosum. (*Montagna*)

STRATUM LUCIDUM The layer of cells beneath the stratum lucidum in the epidermis. (*Montagna*)

STRATUM SPINOSUM A layer of cells in the epidermis, situated between the stratum granulosum and the stratum basale. (*Montagna*)

STRAWBERRY BLONDE (1) Red blonde in colour.

(2) A red haired woman. Slang. (*B and B*)

STREAKING The bleaching of a few strands of hair in the coiffure.

STREAKING CAP See High-light Cap, also Tipping cap.

STREAKING HOOK A kind of crochet hook used for pulling small strands of hair through the apertures of a rubber or plastic streaking cap, *qv* preparatory to bleaching the strands.

STREAKS (1) Light or dark patches or strands in the hair, often caused by incorrect dyeing or bleaching applications.

(2) Light strands of hair deliberately contrived to enhance the appearance.

STREET WIG A wig worn in the course of a person's daily vocation.

STRETCH BASE (FOUNDATION) A wig foundation made of elasticised material that enables the wig to be fitted to most heads.

STRETCH WIG A wig made on a foundation of elasticized material. See Stretch base.

STRIATED Marked with parallel bands.

STRINGS See Weaving silk.

STRIP To remove dye from a head of hair.

STRIPPER A chemical which can be used for removing or stripping colour from the hair.

STRIPPING (1) The process of removing colour from the hair.
(2) Tapering. American usage.

STRIP-TEASE COIFFURE See Veronica Lake Coiffure.

STRIP-TEASER MOUSTACHE A very narrow moustache, midway between the upper lip and nose, with slightly upturned ends. American usage. (*Trusty*)   *101G*

STROMMEL 18th century slang word for hair. (*Carew*)

STRONTIUM SULPHIDE (SrS) A commonly used and rapid dehairing ingredient in depilatories. A common formula is: strontium sulphide 30%, zinc oxide 3%, glycerol 8%, methylcellulose 2.5%, methol 1%, water 50.5%.

STROP (1) Subs. A strip of canvas or leather, preferably horse-hide, or a strip of wood covered with leather or any other suitable material and used for setting the edge on razors. Other sources include: pig, bullock, sheep, bear and seal. 'Strops for setting razors.' 1702.
(2) Verb. To sharpen or set the edge of a razor on a strop.

STROP FUNGUS A tree fungus that grows on old birch trees and was formerly used as a strop powder for stropping cut-throat razors.

STROPHOS HEAD-DRESS An ancient Greek head dress for a woman. (*Rimmel*)   *341*

STROP PASTE (Also called razor paste.) Paste used on strops to facilitate the setting of the razor's edge. One formula contains: blacklead, tin oxide, lard, soft paraffin, lavender and rosemary oils.

STROPPING The act of setting the edge of a razor on a strop. The process of smoothing both sides of a razor's edge on a strop to produce an acute shaving edge.

STROPPING MACHINE An apparatus having a slow revolving leather-covered wheel on which a razor's edge can be stropped.

STRUM A perwig. Rum strum, a fine, large wig. 18th century slang. (*Grose, Lex Bal*)

STRUMMEL Hair, 18/19th century slang. 'With my strummel faked in the newest twig' With my hair dressed in the first fashion. (*Life of Jack Sheppard*, 1840)

STUBBLE (1) Short, spiky hairs which stick up from the scalp. Usually caused by inefficient hair thinning.
(2) Short beard bristles. Slang.

STUBBLE BEARD A short, spiky beard covering the whole of the hair-growing area of the face. (*Taylor*)   *99 (7)*

STYLE (1) Subs. The mode, style or way of dressing the hair. See also Mode and Fashion.
(2) Verb. To dress hair to a style.

STYLE CUT A haircut that reduces hair to the length and thickness needed to dress a given hair style.

STYLE WIG The same as fashion wig, qv. c 1960.

STYLERAMA Hair styling saloon. USA. 1964.

STYLING The act of dressing a head of hair to a particular style.

STYLING BRUSH A narrow brush for brushing the hair to a style after the set has dried.

STYLISH Adj. Of a person's appearance; being in conformity with the contemporary fashionable standard of elegance.

STYLIZATION In conformity with a conventional style.

STYPTIC A substance which stops bleeding by contracting the skin tissues.

SUBCARBONATE OF POTASH See potassium carbonate.

SUB-CUTANEOUS Beneath the skin.

SUB-CUTIS The third layer of the skin below the epidermis and corium.

SUBDERMAL Beneath the skin.

SUBERCHE The hair on the lower part of the face and neck; also suboscoe; 16th century. 'His suberches taken away with a rasor.' (*Green, R Quip for an Upstart Courtier*). See also Bosco.

SUBOSCOE See Suberche.

SUBSTANTIVE DYE A hair dye that colours without the use of a mordant.

SUB-TEEN STYLE A hair style suitable for a child under thirteen years of age. American spelling: Subteen. See Teenage style.

SUD-DISH A shaving pot for holding soap-suds. 'Barbers' sud-dish hanging from a pendant in front.' (*Jasmin*, p. 32)

SUDORIFEROUS GLAND Sweat gland.

SUDS (1) Water impregnated with soap.
(2) The frothy mass of soap bubbles that collect on the surface of soapy water. 'A Barber's suds.' 'Barbers . . . throwing all the suddes out of their learned Latin Basons.' (*Dekker, Seven Deadly Sinnes*, 1606)

SUEDE HEAD A man's hair style, August 1970. Slightly longer hair than the skin head, qv.

SUETT, RICHARD (1755–1805) Actor and comedian, made a large collection of old wigs, including a wig of Charles II, which Suett bought at the sale of Rawle, the Antiquarian. The collection was destroyed by fire. (*Caulfield*)

SUFFLOPLIM See Dildo. 17th century. (*Holme*)

SUGAR LOAF A 16th century beard style affected by the Protector Somerset, the first Protestant ruler of England.   *99 (12)*

SUGDEN, EDWARD BURTENSHAW Baron St Leonards (1781–1875), Lord Chancellor; Tory MP for Weymouth and Melcombe Regis, 1828–30, etc. Famous lawyer. Son of a barber in business near Lincoln's Inn, London. (*Procter*, p 41)

SUICIDE BLONDE An artificial blonde. Slang. (*B and B*)

SULPHIDE DYE A hair dye that relies on the formation of an insoluble sulphide coating the hair's surface by means of the action of sodium sulphide on a metal salt, copper sulphate, lead acetate or silver nitrate, etc. (*Kilgour*)

SULPHONATED OIL Sulphonated vegetable oils used in soapless shampoos.

SULPHUR SOAP See Medicated soap.

SULTANA A 19th century proprietary soap. (*Piesse*)

SULTANE A kind of small aigrette worn upright like a pompon on the hairdress and composed of decorative hair drawn from the dressing or added feathers or other suitable decorative device stiffened by wire. 'The only feather permitted is a black or white sultane perched up on the left side', 1766. (*Lennox*) The name probably originated from an upright decoration worn in the 18th century on a sultan's turban.

SULTONE A variant (probably a printer's error) of Sultane qv. (*Guide to Health, Beauty and Riches*)

SUNDAY BARBER (1) 17th/18th century term for a barber who practiced his craft on a Sunday. (*Hamersley*)
(2) A person who cut hair on a Sunday, but practised another craft during the rest of the week.

SUN GOD (of Egypt) The ancient Egyptians composed the statue of the sun in the shape of a man with his head half shaven. (Salmon)

SUNNY RAYS A 19th century 'secret' hair preparation for bleaching the hair was an aqueous solution of hydrogen peroxide. This was made and extensively sold in the West Country by the writer's grandfather, John Stevens.

SUNNY TIPS Bleached ends of hair.

SUNTIPPING The bleaching of the hair at the front hair-line.

SUPERCILIA ATROPHY Eyebrow hair diminishing in size. (Wheeler)

SUPERCILIUM Eyebrow hair.

SUPERFICIAL COMBING Combing only the surface hair, not allowing the teeth of the comb to penetrate the scalp.

SUPERFLUOUS HAIR Unwanted hair.

SURFACE COLOURING Dye deposited only on the surface of the hair cuticle.

SURFACTANT A soapless detergent.

SURGICAL SPIRIT Industrial methylated spirit containing 2.5% castor oil, 2% diethylphthalate and 0.5% methyl salicylate.

SURNAMES Many surnames derived from the hair, head or beard, such as: Downyhead, Coxhead, Rufhead, Hardhead, Whithead, Redhead, Flaxenhead, Shavenhead, Goldenhead, Weaselhead, Greenhead, Whitelock, Silverlock, Blacklock, Shakelock, Whitehair, (William Whiteheare was Dean of Bristol, 1551), Fairhair, Yallowhair, Fairfax, Beard, Copperbeard, Greybeard, Blackbeard, Whitebeard, Redbeard, Leatherbeard, Eaglebeard, Wirebeard, Brownbeard, Lovelock, Curle, Crispe, Locke, Stykebeard, Callow, (Calewe 1313 – bald-headed), Bald, Chauf, Chaufyn, Le Pele, Le Pyl, Peile, Peel and many others. Some of these surnames, common in the middle ages, are now obsolete. (Bardsley)

SUSCEPTIBLE SUBJECT A person who is sensitive to a para dye and reacts positively to the skin test.

SUTTON'S FLY WEFT The hair wisp is woven on three silks as follows: through the bottom space, away from the weaver, forward through the top silk, over the top silk, forward through the top space, under the bottom space, over the top silk, forward through the top space.

SWALE, TO See Sweal, to.

SWALLOW'S TAIL BEARD Also Swallow Tail Beard. A long beard, forked and pointed like a swallow's tail. 16th century. *99 (17)*

SWATHE (1) Subs. A postiche, the hair of which is dressed to encircle the head. In making, the hair is secured to the centre of a large or double marteaux foundation. A switch can be worn as a swathe. *314*
(2) Subs. A band of material or marteau of long, straight hair to encircle the head.
(3) Verb. To encircle with a swathe.

SWATY or SWATTY A fast cutting razor hone. (Moler, p 16)

SWEAL, TO To singe. (Grose, Prov Glos)

SWEDISH RAZOR A thin bladed razor consisting of a strip of steel fitting into a grooved nickel back. (Foan)

SWEDISH RAZOR POINT An open razor blade with a bulging, rounded point. Some had detachable blades. (Chalmers)

SWEDISH SHAMPOO A shampoo incorporating a bleach.

SWEATING The process of arranging wetted tresses of hair on a wig into curls or other hair formations to achieve the required style, then drying the wet hair in front of a fire or in an oven. 18th century. 'Thomas Barker, peruke-maker

. . . maketh all sort of perukes . . . and having obtained the greatest art that ever was found out, for sweating of wigs, though never so much out of curl, causing them to hold a strong and lasting curl little inferior to new wigs, . . . : His prices are two shillings and six pence each Bob, three shillings and sixpence a Tye, and three shillings a Pig Tail . . . His days of sweating are Tuesdays and Thursdays, and he sends them home fit for wear the next day.' (From a broadside $4\frac{7}{8}'' \times 7''$, London, c 1740-)

SWEENEY TODD A character in the play *Sweeney Todd, the Demon Barber of Fleet Street*. This drama set in the reign of George II was written by George Dibdin Pitt (d 1854/5), a Victorian dramatist of prolific output. Pitt described Sweeney Todd as a 'legendary drama', presumably implying that there still lingered in the old courts of Fleet Street a legend of a demon barber, and this he used as a foundation for his drama. The year 1842 appears to be the earliest date of record of this 'barbarous' character, Todd. The Sweeney Todd legend concerns the cutting of clients throats when being shaved by the barber, their precipitation through a trap door into the cellar, and subsequent transformation into succulent 'veal' pies. (see *Sweeney Todd* by G D Pitt, edited by Montaga Slater, 1928, for a full account of Pitt, his production and Sweeney Todd)

SWEET BALL Soap balls perfumed with camphor musk, etc to make hair wash. 17th century (Comenius)

SWEETHEART BOB A child's style similar to the Buster Brown, qv, but the fringe is cut in a V shape. From c 1922. (Rohrer)

SWEET SOAP Soap perfumed with musk, camphor, etc. A kind of toilet soap. (Ms account book in collection of writer)

SWING CURL A ringlet on the face. (B and B)

SWINGING HAIR Hair of a length that permits it to swing loosely with the natural movement of the head.(WO, 10. 10. 64)

SWINGING MANE A long, thick strand or mane of hair in a woman's hair style that is left loose and pendant. (Dell, Hair Do, April, 1965)

SWIRL (1) Subs. A tress of hair wound around the head. 1909.
(2) Subs. A twist or convolution of hair, c 1900.
(3) Subs. A curl of hair, 1844.
(4) Verb. To twist or wind hair and give it a twisted or convoluted form.

SWIRL CURL A curl with a very large diameter. See Swirl. (Morris)

SWIRL LINE A hair style in which swirls form the major feature of the contour.

SWIRL WAVE A very large diameter wave with little depth.

SWITCH A postiche consisting of a long bunch of hair, the root ends of which are secured by weaving on silks and winding on macramé stem cord. Also called a tail, qv. Worn by women to supplement their natural hair, 19/20th century. 'I might wear a switch too.' (Bret Harte, 1887)

SWITCHCRAFT The art of dressing heads of hair using switches or tails.

SWITCHERY See Switchcraft.

SWITCH TORSADE See Torsade.

SWITHER, TO To singe. Northern and Midlands usage. 17/18th century. (Derham)

SWITHER-ROD A glass rod used to mix liquid hair preparations. West Country usage.

SWIZZEN, TO To singe. Northern usage. (Grose, Prov Glos)

SWIZZLE-ROD A glass rod used for stirring liquids. See also Swither-rod.

SWOB (SWAB) Cotton wool or other absorbent material

used as a pad to apply chemicals to the hair. Bristol and West of England usage.

SWORD KNOT A hanging lock of hair, straight except at the end which was dressed in a spiral curl. (*Legros*)

SYCOSIS BARBAE Barbers' rash, Barber's itch, etc. A skin disease of the bearded part of the face, or scalp.

SYMMETRICAL STYLE A hair style with such proportions between its constituent parts that a balanced or harmonious style is the result.

SYMMETRY The harmonious arrangement of material producing aesthetic balance. The opposite to Asymmetry, *qv*.

SYNTAX WIG A wig similar to the bob periwig worn by the fictional Dr Syntax and depicted by T Rowlandson in W Combe's *Tours of Dr Syntax*, 1819–21. Also called the Wig of Fame.

SYNTHETIC An artifical production of compounds from their constituent elements, as opposed to their extraction from natural substances.

SYNTHETIC DETERGENT A detergent built-up from chemical elements.

SYNTHETIC HAIR Any artifically made hair. It may be manufactured from a great variety of man-made fibres. Two commonly used types are: (a) Nylon-Savan, which has a high sheen but looks artificial; (b) Nylon-Savan-Dynel, with less sheen, but more nearly resembles natural human hair.

SYNTHETIC NET Net for wig-making that is made from man-made substances, such as nylon, etc.

SYNTHETIC ORGANIC DYE See Dye.

SYNTHETIC WIG A wig that is made of synthetic hair. (*Shaw and Stockton*)

SYPHILITIC ALOPECIA Loss of hair from the effects of syphilis, either direct or by inheritance from infected ancestors. (*Wheeler*)

SYRIAN HAIR A mixture of Angora and Yak hair. The relative quantities can be adjusted to the needs of the hair worker. (*AH*, 1915)

T

TABBING See Eye tabbing.

TACHE Also Tash. Early 20th century slang word for a moustache. (*Partridge*)

TAFFETA A kind of thin, glossy silk of plain texture used by the wigmaker in the manufacture of theatrical wigs. 19th century.

TAFFLE To tangle. 19th century South Somerset and Dorset usage. 'Her hair be taffled.' (*Barnes*)

TAIL (SWITCH) (1) A postiche constructed of hair woven on silks to form weft which is then spirally wound round a central stem of macramé and secured to it by stitching at both ends of the stem. So named because of its similarity of appearance to a horse's tail. See also Switch.

(2) A gathering of unworked hair tied at the root end.

TAIL BRUSH A hairbrush with a long, pointed handle. See also Tail comb.

TAIL COMB A haircomb with teeth at one end and a handle tapering to a point at the other. Mainly used for dressing curls and putting the finishing touches to a hairdress. 1773. (*Earle*)

TAIL CORD Macramé, *qv*.

TAILED COMB A Tail comb, A Curl comb, *qv*.

TAIL LOOP (TAIL EYE) The loop of macramé or tail cord worked at the head-end of a tail of hair by which the tail is secured to the head by means of a hairpin.

TAIL WINDER The same as Winding Machine, *qv*.

TAKE-APART WIG See Three-part wig.

TANGLE A confusedly interwined mass of hair. See also Knot, Mat, Snarl and Tug.

TANGLE-COMB A Rake, *qv*.

TANGLEHAIR Something that tangles the hair. 'My new straw hat is a veritable tanglehair.'

TANGS (also TAINGS) Tongs. Scottish usage. (*Brown*)

TAPE (1) A narrow, woven strip of cotton or linen used to hold the hair of a set postiche on a malleable block in position during the drying process.

(2) Verb. To position tape along the trough of the waves on a set postiche and pin it to the malleable block. This keeps the set of the coiffure in position during drying.

TAPE-MEASURE A measuring tool consisting of a strong, flexible, but non-elastic, strip of tape, marked in centimetres (formerly inches), used by the wig maker for measuring heads.

TAPER (1) Subs. A wax rod consisting of a central wick, encased in wax, and used for singeing hair.

(2) Verb. To singe hair with a taper. 19th century.

(3) Verb. To diminish a strand of hair gradually towards the points by cutting. 'I will taper the ends of your hair.'

(4) Subs. The condition of being tapered (by cutting). 'The taper was not too extreme.' 19/20th century.

(5) Adj. Diminishing gradually towards the hair points. 'Taper hair is easily curled.'

TAPER CURLED HAIR See Curled taper hair.

TAPER CUT A hair cut in which the strands of hair are cut so that the bulk diminishes gradually towards the points.

TAPERED HAIR (1) Hair that has been tapered. 19/20th century. See Taper (3).

(2) Singed hair. 19th/early 20th century.

TAPER HAIR A quantity of hair that tapers towards the points.

TAPER HOLDER A metal or earthenware vase for storing tapers.

TAPERING (1) The action of singeing.

(2) The action of cutting hair to a taper.

TAPERING CLIPPERS See Thinning clippers.

TAPERING SCISSORS (1) Small haircutting scissors, used for tapering hair.

(2) Notched scissors. See Thinning scissors.

TAPING The action of placing tape along the troughs of the waves of a set postiche and pinning it to the malleable block to hold the waves in position during the drying process.

121

TAPOTEMENT Fr. Tapping. The percussion part of a massage treatment consisting of tapping with the finger pads to stimulate the blood in the area being treated.

TAR SHAMPOO See Pine-tar shampoo. Only tars of vegetable origin are used in shampoos, never coal tar.

TATE (1) Also Tête, *qv*. A wig or covering postiche, 18th century. From the French *tête*; a head. 'William Johnson . . . makes all sorts of Perukes and Ladys Tates in the neatest manner . . .' (18th century advert)

(2) Also Tait. Small lock of hair. 18th century. Scottish usage. (*Ramsay; Brown*)

TAURE Subs. Fr – Bull. Curled hair on the forehead, standing out. Also called Bull Head, when the forehead curls were much larger than the Taure. 17th century. (*Holme*)

TAYLOR, GEORGE The boxing barber who beat Stack in 1750. (*Boxiana*)

TAYLOR, JEREMY (1613–1667). Bishop and writer; son of a hairdresser. Among his published works was *A Discourse of Auxiliary Beauty*, 1656.

TAYLOR, JOHN Ll D (1704–1766). Philologer and classical scholar. Son of a barber. Sizar at St John's College, Cambridge.

TAZZ A rough head of hair. Midlands and West Country usage. (*Sternberg*)

TAZZLE Tangled and tousled. 'Her hair be all of a tazzle.' Midlands and West Country usage. (*Dartnell*)

T BEARD See Roman T.

TEA HAIR WASH An infusion of tea was said to be very useful in preventing hair falling out. (*EDM* Vol 3)

TEASE TO To comb or card hair or wool. From teasel or teazel, a kind of thistle which is used for raising the nap on woollen cloth. See also Card and Vex.

TEASE BRUSH A small hair brush with hard bristles for:
(1) Teasing hair,
(2) Backcombing hair.

TEASING (1) Disentangling matted hair by means of the comb's tip.
(2) Combing-out tangled hair by means of a brush or comb. See Tease brush.
(3) Backcombing to produce a puffed effect. American usage.

TEASING BRUSH See Tease brush.

TECHNIQUE The disciplined mastery of methods and materials in an art or craft. The manner of performance in relation to practical details in an art or craft.

TEENAGE STYLE A hair style for youths and girls of thirteen to nineteen years of age, cf Subteen Style.

TEEN HAIRDO A hairdress suitable for a teenager. (*AH* 1963)

TEE PIN A T-shaped pin used to hold set hair in position on a malleable block. See also T Pin.

TEINT Fr. Dye, colour, tincture.

TEINTURE Fr. Dye, dyeing.

TELOGEN The state of rest in the growth cycle of a hair follicle.

TEMPLATE Variant of templet, *qv*.

TEMPLE A man's 18th century wig style. (*London Mag* 1753). See Temple tie wig.

TEMPLE CURL (1) A postiche of curls mounted on a hairpin and used to thicken thin hair at the temples.
(2) A small curl, natural or a postiche, worn at the temple.

TEMPLE HAIR The hair that grows in the region of the temple.

TEMPLE MOUNTED FRONT (Semi-transformation). A postiche for the front of the head, shaped at the temples. (*Creer*)

TEMPLET (1) A guide or pattern used in wigmaking, shaped to correspond to the desired shape of the foundation.
(2) An ornament worn on a woman's head. 16th century.

TEMPLE TIE WIG A man's 18th century wig style with a cluster of curls at the temples. Mainly a military and naval style and usually worn with a pig tail. Also known as Fox Ear. (*Colman*)

TEMPORAL Relating to the temple.

TEMPORARY COLOUR A dye or colour rinse, the effect of which will last only for a limited time.

TEMPORARY RINSE A rinse, the effect of which will last only for a limited time.

TENDRIL (1) Subs. A slight strand of hair delicately dressed.

(2) A wispy narrow curl.
(3) A Poker curl, *qv*.

TENDRIL CURL A very narrow curl like a string. See also Filament curl.

TENNIS BALLS In the 16th and 17th century these balls were hand stuffed with human hair to give bounce. 'They may sell their haire by the pound, to stuffe Tennice balles.' (*Nashe, A Wonderful Strange and Miraculous Astrological Prognosication*. 1591) 'Thy beard shall serve to stuff those balls by which I get me heat at Tenice.' (*Ram Alley*, 1611) 'The old ornament of his cheek hath already stufft tennis-balls.' (*Much Ado About Nothing*, 1600)

TENSILE Capable of being stretched.

TENSILE STRENGTH OF HAIR An average, healthy, virgin hair will break at about a 7 oz pull. The tensile strength of dyed, bleached and permanently waved hair is lower than healthy, virgin hair.

TENSION SPRING A spirally wound and flattened wire spring which, when stretched, returns to its original length. Used in boardwork at the necks of wigs and transformations to hold them firmly on the head. The tension spring is sometimes replaced by elastic.

TENTERDEN, CHARLES ABBOTT 1762. Son of a barber from Canterbury; he entered the law, was raised to the peerage and became Baron Tenterden of Hendon and Lord Chief Justice.

TEPID CURLING Low temperature permanent waving.

TEPID WAVE A permanent waving system using a minimum degree of heat to effectively curl the hair.

TERMINAL HAIR (1) Hair situated at the end or boundary of an area of hair growth.
(2) The ends of the hair.

TERMINAL KNOT The first or last knot on a weft. See Starting knot and Finishing knot.

TERRY TOWEL A thick cotton towel composed of closely woven loops of thread to give a high degree of absorbency.

TEST CURL A small strand of hair that has been permanently waved in order to determine before undertaking the complete head, how the hair will react to the process proposed. The result will indicate if the solution, diameter of curler and timing are correct for the type of hair to be treated.

TEST MIXING In boardwork, the mixing of two or more hair strands of differing shades to ascertain if a desired shade can be produced and the relative quantity of each that will be needed when the head is prepared. See Head (7).

TETE (Also Tate, *qv*) (1) A head of false hair. A wig. 18/19th century. (*Stewart*)
(2) A wooden block upon which wigs were made or displayed. 18th century. (*Stewart*)
(3) A head of hair. 19th century. (*Creer*)
(4) A quantity of prepared hair sufficient for the manufacture of a wig.
(5) All the cut hair taken from one head by the hair collector, kept together until sold to the wigmaker. Also known as a Head.

TETE DE MOUTON Fr. Sheep's head. An 18th century style of coiffure dressed in small frizzy curls, reminiscent of the short, tight curls on a sheep's head. (*Stewart*)
'Perhaps on Palfry pace along,
With ruffled shirt and tête-moutton;' (*Barber*)

TETE-MAKER Wig maker, 18th century.

TETTER Psoriasis. (*Wilson*)

TEXTOMETER An apparatus for measuring the texture of hair. (*Nessler*)

TEXTURE The characteristics of the hair surface such as: rough, gritty, smooth, silky; also descriptive of the fineness or coarseness of the hair shaft itself.

TEXTURIZE To effect an alteration in the hair texture by the use of suitable chemicals. 20th century American usage.

THALLIUM ACETATE A deadly poison used in the 19th century in a proprietary depilatory. It caused disability to and the death of many women who used it on their armpits and legs. (*Phillips*)

THANKSGIVING BEARD The beard of Philip Nye (1596?–1672) divine, so called because it was said to have secured him his appointment at thanksgiving services. (*Butler*)

THATCH A head of hair. Slang.

THEATRICAL WIG A wig for use in the theatre by actors and actresses.

THEATRICAL WIG HAIR In the 19th and early 20th century second quality human hair and mohair were used. Since c 1950 synthetic hair also used.

THEATRICAL WIGMAKER A wig maker who manufactures wigs for theatrical wear. See also Mechanical Wig maker and Private Wigmaker.

THERMAL Pertaining to heat.

THERMAL PAD Heat pad.

THERMO-CURL A hair curl formed by the use of hot curling irons.

THERMOSTAT An automatic device to regulate temperature.

THESAUROSIS The accumulation of hair-spray products in the lungs. This word was coined in 1958 by an American doctor.

THICK CLUB A man's 18th century wig style. (*Colman*)

THICKENING AGENT A substance, such as magnesium carbonate or soap, that can be added to a liquid bleach or dye to thicken it and reduce its tendency to run.

THIGH LACE Hair of the thighs and legs. Slang. South Coast of England usage.

THIMBLE A metal or hard plastic sheath for covering the thumb or finger tip and used to push the needle in sewing. Originally called the Fingerlinge, diminutive of thumb. Earlier than the 14th century it was made of leather. (*Draper's Dictionary*)

THIN, TO To reduce the bulk or thickness of a head of hair by cutting. 'The hairdresser will thin your hair and it will be more comfortable in the hot weather.'

THINNING The reduction or decrease in the thickness, or numbers of hairs on the head. See Thin.

THINNING CLIPPERS (Tapering clippers) Hair clippers having serrated blades so that when opened and closed only a few hairs of a strand are cut.

THINNING COMB A vulcanite comb with a metal top which slides off. A small blade fits into the fine end of the comb, the teeth of which are spaced to enable the hair to be tapered by drawing the comb firmly through the hair.

THINNING SCISSORS Scissors in which the blades are so notched that when closed only a few hairs are actually cut, the scissors, due to the notching, harmlessly closing on most of the hair without cutting it.

THINNING SHEARS American term. See Thinning scissors.

THIOGLYCOLLIC ACID (Thiogylcolic acid) HS.CH$_2$COOH. A liquid with a strong unpleasant odour, readily oxidized by air. Miscible with water, alcohol, benzene and many other organic solvents. The ammonium and sodium salts are commonly used in cold permanent waving processes and the calcium salt as a depilatory. Liberates hydrogen sulphide gas on decomposition. This gas is flammable and poisonous with the characteristic odour of rotten eggs. See also ammonium thioglycolate.

THIRD DEGREE BURN This type of burn penetrates the skin and involves the subcutaneous layers, affecting the muscles and sometimes the bones. Such burning is very serious and often causes death.

THIRD PLI See Pli.

THOLIA HEAD DRESS An ancient Greek head dress for women. (*Rimmel*) *341*

THREAD A twisted filament of a fibrous substance used by the wig maker.

THREAD FOR TYING HAIR A strong, linen thread used to encircle tightly the root ends of hair some twenty to thirty times, and hold them firmly together during storage.

THREAD FOR WEAVING For crêpe weft strong linen thread is used and for weft for wigs, marteaux or switches a strong, fine silk thread is employed.

THREE-CABLE TWIST Similar to a plait but the hair of the three stems is first twisted in a clock-wise direction or, if preferred, in an anti-clockwise direction. (*Creer*)

THREE-FOLD PLAIT A plait of three stems.

THREE-PART WIG A wig made in three separate sections – the front, the crown and the back, which together make a complete wig. These sections can also be used separately or in combinations.

THREE POINTED BEARD A characteristic of the ancient Israelite.

THREE-QUARTER POMPADOUR FRAME A concentric hollow hair frame of wire and mohair or other suitable material used to form a foundation over which to dress a pompadour style. Shorter than a full pompadour frame. See also Pompadour pad.

THREE-QUARTER TRANSFORMATION A transformation, *qv* which encircles about three-quarters of the circumference of the head, including the whole of the front but, except for the galloon to complete the encirclement, not the whole of the nape.

THREE-QUARTER WIG (A Three-quarter transformation). A wig foundation that covers the front and sides of the head.

THREE-SILK FLY WEFT Fly weft worked on three silks. See Fly Weft.

THREE-STEM SWITCH A hair switch composed of three stems or spills. See Switch. *416 (7)*

THREE-TIER Name of an 18th century wig style for men, characterised by three rows of rolled curls.

THRICE-IN-WEAVING See Thrice-in-Weft.

THRICE-IN-WEFT Wig weft, *qv*.

THRIXALINE A transparent fluid for fixing the moustache in any position. A proprietary substance marketed by John Caster, Hairdresser, Fleet Street, London, in the 1890s. (*The Idler* 1893)

THROAT WHISKERS A narrow band of whiskers from ear to ear and beneath the chin, the remainder of the face being shaven.

THROWN-IN-WAVE The same as Forgotten Wave, *qv*.

THRUM The short fringe ends of woven hair in a weft.

THYMOL C$_{10}$H$_{14}$O. Obtained from the essential oil *Thymus Vulgaris* and some other volatile oils; also produced synthetically. It comprises colourless, translucent crystals, a pungent odour and is volatile at 100°C. A valuable fungicide and germicide, less toxic than phenol.

TICKER A false beard. Slang. American usage. (*B and B*)

TICKLER A moustache. Slang. (*B and B*)

TIER CUTTING See Step cutting.

TIE-UP COIFFURE A hair style in which a significant part is tied. (*Greene*)

TIFF (1) Subs. The manner in which the wig or hair is dressed. 'The beautiful tiff of his wig.'

(2) Verb. To dress or titivate the hair, etc 13th to 18th century.

TIFT Verb. To dress or set in order, especially the hair; to put the finishing touches to a hairdress. From 15th to 19th century.

TIGNASSE Fr. An old, scrubby wig or mop of hair.

TIGNOMER Fr. To curl the hair behind the head (of women).

TIGNON Fr. A roll of hair twisted behind the head; also Chignon, *qv*.

TILE BEARD A long, square-cut beard; 16th/17th century. (*Repton*) 99 (14)

TILLOTSON, JOHN (1630–1694) Archbishop of Canterbury, credited with being the first English prelate to wear a wig. (*Creer*)

TIMOTHEUS (d 353 BC) The poet and musician who wore an excessively long beard.

TINCTURE Colouring matter, pigment or dye.

TINCTURE DE LEYTENS A 19th/20th century 'secret' preparation which was claimed to be a vegetable hair dye but was in fact, a liquid chemical dye consisting of a solution of silver nitrate coloured with aniline blue, and a dilute solution of calcium pentasulphide. (*Koller*)

TINE The metal rod of a Marcel waving, curling or creoling iron. Also called prong.

TINEA CAPITIS Ringworm of the scalp. (*Lubowe*)

TINEA SYCOSIS Ringworm.

TINEA TONSURANS Ringworm of the scalp. (*Wheeler*)

TINGE Verb. To impart a slight trace of colour to hair. To tint or modify the existing colour.

TINSEL Excessively bleached and fragile hair.

TINSEL TOP (1) A girl with excessively bleached and fragile hair.
(2) A head of hair which has become brittle through excessive bleaching.

TINT (1) Subs. Light degree of a hue, eg the pale tint of a platinum blonde.
(2) Subs. A dye. See (3) below.
(3) Verb. To dye. The word tint, used for dye, is one of the many euphemisms employed in the hairdressing craft. A euphenmism is a mild, vague or woolly mode of talk as a substitute for a disagreeable truth or a precise statement of fact. For instance, to refer to 'the dead' as the 'dear departed' or a concubine as an 'unmarried mother' would be euphemisms. Many of the unpleasant associations of the word *dye*, harshly indicative of greyness, old age and artificiality, are thought to be less noticeable to a client if the mild, discreet term, *tint*, with its suggestion of only slight 'touching up' or 'helping' the natural colour, is used. The word is employed as a synonym of dye.

TINT BLEACH A process of hair dyeing in which the solution incorporates strong hydrogen peroxide in addition to the dye. Used to lighten the dark hairs and darken the white of a head in one operation.

TINTILLATED HAIRDO A hair set in which the hair is also coloured or tinted. Tintillated is a 'made' word and appears to have been suggested by Tint and Titivate. (*HS 1963*)

TINTING (1) Imparting a tint to, or colouring hair, especially with delicate shades.
(2) Effecting slight colour changes by means of colour rinses, temporary or permanent.
(3) A euphemistic misnomer for dyeing, *qv*. See also Tint (3).

TINTING BRUSH A small brush for the application of dye to the hair.

TINT RINSE See colour rinse.

TINT SHAMPOO See Shampoo tint.

TIPPING (1) The same as Frosting, *qv* but applying bleach only to the hair strands within 3″ of the front hair line.
(2) Bleaching the tips of small strands of hair.
(3) The cutting of the hair tips only.

TIPPING CAP A cap with holes in it through which strands of hair are pulled with a metal hook. The strands can then be bleached without the chemical coming in contact with the scalp. Similar to a Streaking Cap.

TIRE (= **ATTIRE**) A headdress. 16th century. 'I like the new tire within excellently, if the hair were a thought browner.' (*Shakespeare, Much Ado About Nothing*, 1600)

TIRE-BOUCHON A corkscrew curl. (*Ménard*)

TIRED RAZOR Barbers have found that razors get tired, but that they will recover if rested for a time. Microscopic examination has shown that a razor, much stropped by the same hand and in the same direction, has the edge fibres all arranged in that direction, like the edge of a piece of cut velvet. After a few weeks' rest the fibres rearrange themselves heterogeneously, crossing each other and presenting a saw-like edge, each fibre supporting its fellow and enabling the razor's edge to cut the beard instead of the steel fibres being forced down flat, without cutting cleanly.

TIRE WOMAN See Tiring Woman.

TIRING Dressing; probably an abbreviation of attiring. 18th century. (*Grose, Lex Bal*)

TIRING-WOMAN A woman who cut or dressed ladies' hair, and assisted with the toilet generally. 18th century. (*Grose, Lex Bal*)

TIT BRUSH A man's chest hair. Air Force slang. (*Symonds*)

TITIAN (1) Bright golden auburn, a colour favoured by the Venetian painter Titian (Tiziano Vecellio, 1477–1576). 'Titian-tinted tresses', 1896.

TITIAN TOP A red haired woman. Slang. (*B and B*)

TIT MAT A man's chest hair. Air Force slang. (*Symonds*)

TITTLEBAT TITMOUSE The hero in Samuel Warren's *Ten Thousand A Year*, 1841, who, wishing to modify a head of red hair, bought a substance with a long name and after treating his locks, rose next morning with pea-green hair. He reduced this result by means of a pair of blacking brushes.

TITUS A woman's hair style in which the hair of the head is cut very short, *c* 1882. 295

TITUS CUT See A la Jacobin.

TITUS STYLE See Titus.

TITUS WIG A short, untidy wig. (*Cunnington*)

TOADSTOOL A woman's hair style of the 1960s, so named on account of its resemblance to the shape of the fungus.

TOILET (1) Subs. A cloth or towel worn over the shoulders whilst being hairdressed or shaved. From the French *Toilette*, dim of Toile – cloth. (1684, *J Phillip's* trans of *Plutarch's Morals*)
(2) Subs. The process of washing, hair-dressing and dressing. Originally the term was applied to the cloth or cover of a dressing-table.
(3) Verb. To perform one's toilet. 'I had toiletted and gone below.' 1893.

TOILET CAP (1) A cap worn by men of fashion whilst making their toilet. 19th century.
(2) A silk cap worn by women to protect their hairdress during their toilet. See Shingle net, Sleeping net, etc.

TOILET CLUB A barber's shop which, in the 19th century, offered reduced charges to clients who paid a regular quarterly or yearly subscription. As late as 1924 Bristol had at least one toilet club extant. (Gaiety Toilet Club, Strand, London: shampooing 4d, Haircutting 4d; Advert, *c* 1870)

TOILET PAPER (1) Soft paper used for hair cutting.

(2) Paper to wipe the razor in shaving, etc.

TOILET PARLOR (*sic*) A hairdressing saloon; a beauty parlour, a saloon which offered hair, beauty, manicure facilities, or chiropody. Sometimes spelt Toilette Parlor. American usage. (*AH*, 1915)

TOILETRY (1) The performance of one's toilet.

(2) The things appertaining to the toilet.

TOILET SALOON A hairdressing saloon; a barber shop. Weston and Cheal, Hairdressers, Turl Street, Oxford, 1963, advertise their establishment as a 'Toilet Saloon'.

TOILETTE Fr. Toilet, dress, dressing-table.

TOILET VINEGAR (1) Aromatic vinegar, *acetum odoratum*, *BPC*.

(2) An alcoholic preparation containing vinegar and perfume, used as a skin cleanser and after-shave lotion.

TOILET WATER A perfumed liquid for the toilet.

TOKE See Toque.

TOM JONES COIFFURE A woman's hair style *c* 1963, popularized by the film *Tom Jones*, after Henry Fielding's novel *The History of Tom Jones, a Foundling*; 1749. It is a straight, short hair style with a short centre parting, heavy fringe, the crown hair back-combed and surface smoothed to form a half sphere high on the crown, the side hair drawn back and secured at the nape, the ends being flicked up.

TON Fr. Manner, style, taste.

TONE (1) Subs. The prevailing effect of the general scheme of colouring with the play of light and shade, descriptive of the general effect, eg 'The bright tone of an auburn head of hair'; 'The dull tone of over-peroxided hair'; 'The silvery tone of greying hair'.

(2) Verb. To change or modify the general colouring or tone of a head of hair.

TONER A substance which when applied to the hair effects a change of tone or an accentuation of an existing tone.

TONG, TO To curl or wave hair with curling or waving irons.

'She will tong the hair'.

TONGS An implement with two 'legs' connected by a pivot or a hinge used for curling hair. See Curling irons.

TONIC SHAMPOO A shampoo incorporating a substance that has an invigorating effect on the scalp.

TONING DOWN The application of dye or a colour rinse to overbleached hair to add colour, or to tone down a too harsh or brilliant dye.

TONQUIN BEAN (= **TONKA BEAN**) The black, fragrant seed of *Dipterix Odorata*, a leguminous tree of Brazil, used as an ingredient of perfumes and for scenting snuff.

TONQUIN POMADE Tonquin beans ½ lb, fat or oil 4 lb. (*Piesse*)

TONSOR An 18th century barber.

TONSORIAL Adj. Of a barber or his barbering. 'Of grave tonsorial preparation', 1813.

TONSORIAL PARLOR (**TONSORIAL SALOON**) A barber shop. American usage. 19/20th century.

TONSORIAL TOPIARIST A haircutter skilled in cutting hair into fantastic or ornamental shapes. West Country badinage.

TONSORIAN Adj. Tonsorial, *qv*.

TONSORIOUS Adj. Tonsorial, *qv*.

TONSURATE The state of being tonsured, *qv*.

TONSURE (1) Subs. The act of clipping or shaving the hair.

(2) Subs. The rite of shaving the crown of the head (Tonsure of St Peter – Catholic Church), or the whole head (Greek Church – Tonsure of St Paul) of a novice entering a monastic order. In the ancient Celtic church the tonsure consisted of the head shaven in front of a line drawn from ear to ear, (Tonsure of St John).

(3) Subs. The shaven part of a priest's head.

(4) Verb. To shave or clip the head of hair. To confer an ecclesiastical tonsure.

(5) Verb. To make bald-headed.

(6) The hay crop. Somerset usage, 18th/19th century. (*Britten*)

TONSURE CAP A cap or covering for the tonsure.

TONSURE (1) One who has received the tonsure; who is in priestly orders. 'The Tonsured'.

(2) Cut or clipped.

TONSURE OF ST PAUL A shaved head.

TONSURE PLATE A round, thin plate, slightly convex, to fit the top of the head, used to mark the line of the tonsure according to the Roman rite. (*Century Dictionary*, 1891)

TONY CURTIS A hair style for men similar to that worn by, and named after the American film star of that name, *c* 1950. Medium length style, combed back at the sides, and the top front hair worn curled and dressed forward on the forehead.

TOOTHBRUSH MOUSTACHE A small, square moustache similar to that worn by the film comedian, Charlie Chaplin, and German Nazi, Adolph Hitler.

TOP See Toupet.

TOP, TO To cut the hair. 'The barber will soon top you.' Slang.

TOP COMB A small, curved comb for holding a fringe forward.

TOPEE An 18th century form of Toupee, *qv*.

TOPETTE A toupet. 1960s.

TOP KNOT, THE (1) A woman's hair style of 1865. (*Bysterveld*, p 58)

(2) An arrangement of hair on top of the head. See also Pompon.

TOPPEE See Toupee. American usage.

TOPPER A toupee, *qv*. From USA, introduced into Britain by 1960. Used on BBC, May 1963.

An extension of top or top piece; cf Topper = Top hat. (*N and N*)

TOPPETTE A top-piece or toupee, *qv*, of artificial hair for a woman. American usage.

TOP PIECE West Counry term for Toupee, used from before 1925 to date (1983).

TOPPING (1) Club cutting the hair ends when holding the strand at right angles to the head, between the first and second fingers of the left hand, or when holding the hair in the teeth of the comb. (*Jones*)

(2) Also forelock, *qv*. A lock of hair from the foretop to the crown of the head, commonly worn by young children, 17th century. (*Holme*)

(3) Any hair arrangement on the top part of the head. 20th century. (*Hanle*)

TOP ROW The top row of the weaving silks, the two top silks.

TOP ROW WEFT Weaving on the top silk and the middle silk. Also called Fly Weft.

TOQUE (1) 'A sort of triangular cushion or edifice of horsehair called, I believe, a toque or a system, was fastened on the female head . . . over this system the hair was erected and crisped and frizzed.' (*Edgeworth*, 1817; *Stewart*, 1782)

(2) Since *c* 1800 a cap or small hat without a brim, or with a very small brim, often made of swathed material.

TOQUET Fr. Head-dress.

TORCH THATCH Auburn haired. 20th century American slang. (*B and B*)

TORMENTED COLOUR See Drowned colour.

TORSADE (1) Twisted hair.

(2) A small postiche dressed with twisted or plaited hair.

(3) A twist made with two pieces of hair, either 2 marteaux or 2 switch stems. They can also be dressed from knotted hair on a net.

(4) A twist made from a two-stem switch. (*Creer*)

TORSADE COIL A coiled torsade, ie two separate tails of twisted hair that are twisted around each other in the opposite direction to their individual twisting and then coiled. (*Nicol*)

TORSADE DONDEL A puffed cable twist, dressed on a 2-spill switch in which each spill is frizzed upon the inner side, the hair spread out and twisted upon itself and then both spills are twisted upon each other.

TORSADE GOUFFREE See Torsade dondel. (*Creer*)

TORSADE REPOUSSEE See Torsade dondel. (*Creer*)

TORTOISE COMB (TORTOISESHELL COMB) A comb made chiefly from the shell of the hawkbill or imbricated turtle (*Chamber's Journal*, 3 Feb 1866). Counterfeit tortoise-shell combs were made of horn stained to the colour of tortoise-shell. 17th century. (*Holme*)

TORTOISESHELL The shell, especially the carapace (upper shell) of a tortoise, used for the manufacture of combs and other hair ornaments since as early as the 17th century. 'A great tortoise-shell comb'. (*London Gazette*, 1683)

TOTEMISTIC COIFFURE A hair style indicative of a profession, social class or other social or economic grouping with which the wearer wishes to be identified.

TOTEMISTIC HAIRDRESS See Totemistic coiffure.

TOUCH-UP (1) A euphemism for either hair colouring or bleaching.

(2) Bleaching or dyeing of new hair-growth on a bleached or dyed head.

(3) A superficial tidying of a hair-dress.

(4) A temporary comb-press treatment between regular shampoo-press treatments. See Hair pressing.

(5) Strengthening Marcel waves by re-waving them in the same waves a short time after the original Marcel.

TOUCH-UP CRAYON A crayon of colour used between dyes to cover the new growth of hair at the roots.

TOUFFE Fr. Tuft, bunch.

TOUFFEE Fr. Tufted, bushy.

TOUPE See Toupee.

TOUPEE (Toupée, Toupet, Tupee, etc) From Fr. Toupet = a tuft of hair.

(1) An artificial lock of hair or curl, especially as the crowning feature of a wig, 18th century.

(2) A wig in which the front hair was dressed into the form of a top-knot, 18th century.

(3) The growing hair dressed at the front into the form of a top-knot; a tuft of hair sticking up; a forelock. 18th century. (*Creer*)

(4) A postiche patch or scalpette, 1731.

(5) A small wig, 1753 (Fairholt) or artificial covering of hair on a foundation, seemingly natural, worn on the front and top of the head; 18th/20th century.

(6) A wig, early 18th century.

'To a feather or powder'd tuppee

Her heart soon a captive wou'd be.'

(*John Hippisley, Flora – an Opera*, 1729)

(7) A person who wears a toupee.

'Here a bright Redcoat, there a smart toupee.' (*Pope, Art of Sinking*, 1727)

(8) Nickname of General Pattison, 18th century. (*Fenton*)

(9) A very thick head of hair.

'inhabitant of congo made a secret fob in their woolly toupet.' (*Southey, The Doctor*, 1862)

(10) An artificial front for a woman. (Adv 1910)

TOUPEE ARCHITECT Facetious appellation for a wig-maker. (*Hone*, 1838)

TOUPEE CRAMBER COMB A wig comb. Cramber = a double-sided comb? 'Fine dandruff combs and Tupee Cramber combs.' (*Boston Evening Post*, 1763) (*Earle*)

TOUPEE LIQUID A liquid adhesive for securing toupees to bald heads. (*AH* 1915)

TOUPEE PLASTER See Toupee tape.

TOUPEE TAPE Tape with adhesive on both sides, used for securing toupees and other types of hair pieces to the scalp. See also Diachylon.

TOUPET See Toupee.

'Think we that modern words eternal are?

Toupet, and Tompion, Cousins and Colmar

Hereafter will be call'd by some plain man

A wig, a watch, a pair of stays, a fan.' (*Bramston*, 1729)

TOUPET COMB A hair comb to dress a toupet. 1763. (*Earle*)

TOUPETTE Any small piece of postiche or added hair for a woman's coiffure. American usage. (*Hairdo*, Jan 1965). See also Toupee, Toupet, etc.

TOUPET TITMOUSE The crested titmouse.

TOUPET WIG A wig of which the front hair was dressed into the form of a top-knot. 18th century.

'I'd deck out Bandy-legs with gold-clock't Hose,

Or wear a toupet-wig without a nose.' (*Bramston, Art of Politicks*, 1729)

TOUPILLON Fr. Little tuft of hair.

TOUPY (Toupee, Toupet, etc.) Tuft of hair on the head. (*Woodforde*)

TOUR (1) Artificial curls of hair on the forehead. (*Evelyn*, 1690)

'This tour must come more forward, madam, to hide the wrinkles at the corners of your eyes.'

(2) A tower or high hairdress.

TOUR DE TETE See Tour of Hair.

TOUR OF HAIR A part-wig, tress or border of hair round the head which added length and thickness to the natural hair. 18th century. Similar to a 19th/20th century transformation. (*Chambers*)   *202*

TOUSEY HAIR (1) Untidy hair.

(2) A person with untidy hair. Slang.

TOUSLE To disorder or dishevel the hair.

TOUSLETOP (1) An untidy head of hair.

(2) A person with untidy or disordered hair.

TOUSSAINT, PIERRE A famous coloured ladies' hairdresser of the Caribbean and later New York. (*Sheehan, A and E Odell. Black Pearl, the hairdresser from Haiti*. 1956)

TOUZLE See Tousle.

TOUZLETOP See Tousletop.

TOWEL A cloth of linen, hemp or other suitably absorbent material used for drying the hair after a shampoo, and other purposes.

'They with their fine, soft, grassy towels stand,

To wipe away the drops and moisture from the hand.'

(*Drayton*, 17th century)

TOWEL DRYING The removal of surface water from the hair by means of absorption in a suitable towel by rubbing and pressing with it.

TOWEL SHAMPOO A method of cleansing the head hair by spraying with a suitable liquid to loosen dirt and foreign bodies and then by brisk rubbing of the hair and scalp with a towel carrying the dirt away in the towel.

TOWEL STEAMER An oven designed to steam-heat towels for application to the face after a shave.

TOWEL URN See Towel steamer.

TOWER (1) A high headdress. See also Tour. (*Fairholt*)
(2) A Half wig, *qv.* 18th century. (*Fenton*, XIV)

TOWHEAD A blonde woman. Slang. (*B and B*)

TOWPEE See Toupee.

TOWZIE Shaggy, rough, touzled. 18th century Scottish usage. (*Burns*)

TOXIC Poisonous.

T PIN A pin in the shape of the letter T, claimed to be kinder to the finger nails when extracting it from a block. Also called a Banker's Pin. American usage (*N and N*) See also Tee pin.

TRACTION ALOPECIA Baldness induced by pulling of or continued movement of the hair, or friction at the point where the hair emerges from the follicle. (*Lubowe*)

TRADE CARD A small advertising card with the name and address of the shop-keeper and a brief description of the services which he offers to the public. In the 18th/19th century they often carried illustrations of the goods offered, also used by other categories of persons.

TRAGACANTH A mucilaginous substance obtained from several species of the spiny shrub *astragalus*. Gum tragacanth, in a solution of spirit and water, prepared and coloured, is used for hair dressings such as thick setting lotion.

TRAGEDY HEAD 18th century man's theatrical wig style suitable for the portrayal of a tragic character. (*Stewart*)

TRAGUS Ear hair.

TRAIN OIL Whale oil; the oil from the blubber of Balaena.

TRAMLINES Very tight, narrow waves produced by a permanent waving process. From *c* 1925.

TRANSFER A transformation, *qv.* Bristol usage.

TRANSFORMATION (1) An artificial covering of hair, the narrow foundation of which encircles the head, but lacks a crown. When dressed, the hair of the transformation completely covers the crown and can blend with any hair the wearer may have. *464*
(2) In American usage any postiche can be referred to as a transformation, but in Britain the word usually carries the meaning described in (1), although the writer has seen 'transformation' used as a euphemism for 'wig' in advertisements to the public.

TRANSFORMATION BLOCK See Malleable transformation block.

TRANSFORMATION MEASUREMENTS (1) Circumference,
(2) Front (ear to ear across the front of the head),
(3) Parting length,
(4) Distance of parting from centre line.

TRANSFORMATION NET Stiff, waterproof wig net. See also Hoc net.

TRANSFORMATION SPRING A flat positional spring for transformations, etc. Made from narrow clock-springs in lengths of (usually) 3, 5, 7 and 9 cm or any other required length.

TRANSIENT DYE A temporary dye. (*SDP*)

TRANSVERSE PARTING A parting across the head from one side to the other. Not a parting from the front of the head towards the back.

TRAVELLER'S HAIRBRUSH See Military hairbrush.

TRAVELLING HEADDRESS A hair style suitable for wear during a long journey.

TRAVELLING WIG Similar to a Campaign Wig, *qv.*

TREE OF HAIR See Capillaris Arbor.

TREFOIL A three-lobed grouping of hair.

TRENCHER BEARD See Saucer beard.

TRESS (1) Subs. A plait or braid of the hair on the head, especially a girl's or woman's. 14th century. A woman's 'tress' is composed of three locks or portions of her hair braided together. The word is derived from the Greek word implying threefold.
(2) Subs. A long lock of hair, not necessarily plaited or braided, 13th century.
(3) Subs. A hanging lock of hair, 17th century. (*Phillips*)
(4) Subs. A plait or braid of hair off the head. 15th century.
(5) Verb. To arrange the hair; to dress the hair. 'The hair has been carefully tressed.'

TRESSER Fr. To weave; to plait; to form into tresses.

TRESSEUR Fr. Plaiter or weaver.

TRESSEUSE Fr. A female hair weaver. *212*

TRIANGLE BEARD A 16th/17th century beard style, cut to the shape of a triangle. (*Taylor*).

TRIANGULAR NET A silk or nylon hair setting net, shaped in the form of an isosceles triangle.

TRICHAESTHESIA A form of paraesthesia with the sensation as of hair touching the skin.

TRICHANGIA The capillary blood vessels.

TRICHANGIECTASIA Dilation of the capillaries.

TRICHANGIECTASIS See Trichangiectasia.

TRICHASTHENIA Weak hair. (*Wheeler*)

TRICHATROPHIA Atrophy of the hair-bulbs, including brittleness of the hair.

TRICHAUXIS Excessive or abnormal growth of hair.

TRICHIASIS OF THE EYELASHES Introverted growth; also growth of an extra row of eyelashes beneath the normal ones.

TRICHLORETHYLENE Non-flammable fluid used for cleaning wigs. Dissolves most fixed and volatile oils. Use with adequate ventilation, store in light-resistant glass tubes, avoid exposure to heat. Symptoms of industrial poisoning include epileptiform seizures, trigeminal nerve paralysis and optic neuritis with permanent blindness.

TRICHOCARPOUS Having hairy fruit.

TRICHOCLASIA Brittleness of the hair.

TRICHOCLASIS See Trichorrhexis Nodosa. (*Wheeler*)

TRICHOCRYPTOSIS Disease of the hair follicle.

TRICHODAL Hair-like.

TRICHOGENOUS Promoting or producing the growth of hair.

TRICHOID Hair-like.

TRICHOKINESIS A rare hair condition in which the hair shaft is twisted throughout its entire length. This kind of hair has a shimmering appearance because of the reflection of light from the twists. (*Savill*)

TRICHOKRYPTOMANIA (1) The habit of breaking off hairs of the head.
(2) The condition of broken off head hairs.

TRICHOKRYPTOMANIAC A person affected with trichokryptomania.

TRICHOLOGIST A person qualified in the science of trichology.

TRICHOLOGY The scientific study of the structure, function and diseases of human hair.

TRICHOMA A disease of the hair. See Plica Polonica.

TRICHOMANIA Excessive enthusiasm and obsessive involvement with hair.

TRICHOMANIAC One who has excessive enthusiasm for hair. A persistant hair fusser, for example one who habitually picks at or twists his hair, or is forever combing it.

TRICHOME An outgrowth of the epidermis.

TRICHONODOSIS A rare condition of the hair in which it forms knots and loops. Excessive brushing, combing or singeing can produce the condition. (*McCarthy*)

TRICHONODOSIS LAQUEATA See Trichonodosis.

TRICHONOSIS VERSICOLOR See Ringed hair.

TRICHONOSUS Diseases of the hair.

TRICHOPATHIC Relating to diseases of the hair.

TRICHOPATHY The treatment of diseases of the hair.

TRICHOPHAGIA The eating of hair. *(Wilson)*

TRICHOPHAGIST A hair eater.

TRICHOPHAGY The habit of eating, chewing or biting hair. A word I have heard used in hairdressing circles, but for which I can find no authority. It is included here as a curiosity.

TRICHOPHOBE A person who has a morbid fear of touching hair.

TRICHOPHOBIA Fear of hair.

TRICHOPHOROUS Bearing hairs.

TRICHOPHYTIC This term denotes vegetoid or fungoid parasitical diseases of the hair. *(Wheeler)*

TRICHOPHYTINA Ringworm.

TRICHOPHYTON A vegetable parasite which causes ringworm.

TRICHOPHYTOSIS Ringworm of the scalp and skin.

TRICHOPTILOSIS A longitudinal swelling of the hair resulting in its splitting at the distal end or for a distance along its shaft.

TRICHORRHEXIS NODOSA The breaking off of the hair at nodular swellings along the hair shaft. *(McCarthy)*

TRICHORRHOEA Falling of hair accompanied by fluid discharge *(Wheeles)*

TRICHOSIS Abnormal growth of hair.   *432*

TRICHOSIS DISTRIX Forky hair; hair that is weak, withered and split at the points.

TRICHOSIS PLICA Matted hair. *(Winter)*

TRICHOTAPH (1) One who hoards hair by preserving it locked in a cabinet or box.

(2) One who buries hair for magical purposes.

TRICHOTILLOMANIA A mania for tearing out hair. *(Lubowe, p 68)*

TRICHOTILLOMANIAC A person who tears out hair. (See *Helen Temple* in an article *'What can be done for fine hair'*, in the magazine *Woman*, 26 May 1962)

TRICHOTOMIST A hair cutter.

TRICHOTOMY The art and craft of haircutting. (Andrew Marvell, 17th century)

TRICOSIAN FLUID An 18th century proprietary hair dye and tonic. *(P and T p 370)*

TRIFID Divided into three.

TRILBY FRINGE A full, straight, severe looking fringe, similar to the fringe of Trilby in George du Maurier's novel *Trilby*, 1894.

TRIM (1) Subs. A cutting operation performed on the hair with scissors with the object of shortening the hair of an existing hair style; a gentle haircut. See also Re-style, Style cut.

(2) Verb. To slightly shorten hair by cutting.

To trim, in barber parlance, originally meant, to cut the beard, 16th/17th century; to poll being the verb used for cutting the hair of the head. Hence poller = a barber. To be trimmed also meant shaving, cutting and curling the hair in the 16th/early 18th century.

TRIMMER One who trims.

TRIMMING (1) Subs. The action of slightly shortening hair by cutting.

(2) An ornamented addition to a hairdress.

(3) A hairdressing or boardwork accessory. 'Human hair merchant, toilet requisities, tools, trimmings, etc.'

(4) See trim for another meaning in the 16th/18th century.

TRISKELE A three-legged whorl. See also whorl.

TRIXOGENE HAIR RESTORER A 19th/20th century 'secret' preparation that contained small quantities of alcohol, ammonia, boric acid, salicylic acid and glycerine; the great bulk, however, having been merely water. *(Koller)*

TROJAN BEAD A full, medium-length beard of spiral curls cut straight at the bottom. 'And eke their beards cut Trojan wise.' *(Phillips, J Maronides, 1678)*

TRONCHIN See A la Tronchin.

TROPHY-LOCK A lock of hair cut from the head of a slain enemy, used to adorn a weapon or shield. *(Cent Dictionary)*

TROPHYISTICAL HEADDRESS A hairdress incorporating an object or objects taken from a vanquished enemy.

TROUVILLE HEAD-DRESS A late 19th century hair style for which the hair is divided into two parts; the back is sub-divided to form a loop or loose catagon. A wide plait forms a thick coronet. The front hair is parted at the side and is waved, some locks falling as a fringe on the forehead. *(The Queen, 12 Aug 1876)*

TRUNK DRYER A pedestal hair dryer having a long, flexible, leather-covered tube like an elephant's trunk, which was held in the hand and its hot-air steam directed on to the hair of the head to dry it, c 1910.

TRYING IRON PAPER A portion of paper about $4'' \times 12''$, of the consistency of common newsprint on which Marcel waving irons and curling irons are tested after heating and before use on the hair. This ensures that no damage is inflicted on the hair. When waving white hair, tissue paper is used instead of newsprint or its equivalent.

TUBULAR GALLOON See Tubular ribbon.

TUBULAR RIBBON A type of binding used in wigmaking, for covering positional springs, stretch springs and elastic.

TUCK (1) Subs. A flat fold sewn in wig net to dispose of spare material when shaping the net to a curved wig block. See also Dart.

(2) A plait of hair, 17th/18th century.

'Her tresses in tucks, braided with silver.'

(3) Verb. To gather with flat folds for stitching.

TUCKER (1) To backcomb hair. 19th century.

(2) A strand of backcombed hair.

TUCK-UP WIG A wig with dressed plaits. See also Tuck wig. *(KP May, 1739)*

TUCK-WIG 18th century wig style incorporating a plait. In the 17th/18th century a tuck in addition to other uses, also meant a plait of hair. See Tuck.

TUFF See Tuft.

TUFFE OF HAIRES Tuft of hairs, 1570.

TUFF OUT To backcomb hair and fluff it into a loose bouffant cushion. *(Percival)*

TUFT (1) A small group of hairs growing together. In the 17th century the men of St Croix of the Mount, shaved their heads except for a tuft at the front. *(Bulwer)*

A bunch of hairs (1523); a small patch of hair on the face or head (1601). A lock of hair.

'No tuft, moustache, nor whiskers trace,

Can show, the dandy, the hussar!' *(Geary)*

(2) A side piece or curl, the weft wound round a side comb instead of being sewn upon it. In the 19th century in the English provincial towns, the word tuft was applied to almost any small piece of postiche, whether upon a comb or a hairpin, as pincurls are made. *(Creer)*

(3) A goatee beard. Slang. *(B and B)*

(4) See Invisible tuft.

TUG Subs. A tangle or knot in hair. Slang.

'You must comb all the tugs out first.'

TULIP CUT A woman's short hair style. 1950s.

TULLE A fine silk bobbin-net named after the town of Tulle in France, where it was first made. From 1812.

TULLE IMPERMEABLE A waterproof wig net marketed by the firm of Ledanois, 20th century. (Hairdressing 1924)

TULLE YAK A postiche foundation of lace or tulle made of yak hair. Between 1870–1890 a considerable amount of this tulle–yak was manufactured in the mountain villages of Saxony and Bohemia. (*Creer*)

TULLOID NET A patented net for postiche mounts. Also called Hook or Hoc net, *qv*.

TUMP Chignon. Somerset usage. 'Her's got a tump on her's head.'

TUNISIAN HENNA See Henna.

TUPEE A wig. See Toupee.
'With smart Tupee
Fort Bien Poudree.' (*The Cambro Britain Robb'd of his Bauble*, 1727)

TURBAN (1) A headdress of paper, cloth, plastic or other suitable material, wound round the head to retain heat in bleaching, dyeing, hennaing, permanent waving, etc. (*Foan*)
(2) A hair style in which the hair is swathed like a turban.

TURBAN SWIRL An early 1900 hair style for women, in which the hair covered the head like a smooth helmet, almost down to the eyebrows. (*Wall*)

TURBINATOR DRYER A hairdryer in which the hot air is blown around the inside of the hood and over the surface of the set hair.

TURKEY RED OIL Sulphated (sulphonated) castor oil.

TURKEY STONE A fine-grained, hard, siliceous stone imported from the Levant for the manufacture of whetstones.

TURKISH COSMETIQUE A solid pommade type of dressing for the hair. First marketed in 1876 in USA, a proprietary product. (*Smith*)

TURKISH DEPILATORY This consisted of 5 oz of quicklime, 1 oz of orpiment, made into a paste with warm water. (*Francis*)

TURKISH DYE A hair dye manufactured by roasting powdered gall nuts with oil and adding iron or copper oxide. (*Wall*)

TURKISH TOWEL A towel with a long nap of cut or uncut loops used for drying the hair after a shampoo.

TURKISH WHISKERS (1) Long whiskers. (*Dulaure*, p 80)
(2) A henna'd beard.
(3) A red beard. (*Nicolay*; *Dulaure*)

TURNED-HAIR Hair such as combings where the roots and points are mixed, has to be so divided that all the roots are together and all the points taper away at the other end of the bunch. This process is called Turning, *qv* and the hair which has been processed is known as turned-hair. (*Creer*)

TURNED-UP MOUSTACHE A moustache, both ends of which are inverted. Similar to that worn by the German Emperor, William II (1859–1941).

TURNED-UP PART The hair at the front of a barrister's wig.

TURNER JMW (1775–1851) Famous painter, son of a London Barber.

TURNING The process of separating the roots from the points in a strand of hair where the roots and points are mixed at both ends of the strand.

TURNING-MACHINE Also Root and Point machine; also Rooting machine, *qv*.

TURNINGS Hair combings that have had the roots and points separated so that all the roots are at one end of a strand of hair and all the points the other end. (*Symonds*)

TURNIP PATED White or fair haired. 16th century slang. (*Grose, Lex Bal*)

TURNOVER-WAVE A Marcel or water wave widely drawn-out and turned over in a half roll, but not forming a crest.

TURN UNDER Subs. That bottom part of a fall of hair which is dressed turning under towards the head.

TURN-UNDER STYLE A hair style in which the hair ends are turned under as in a Page Boy style, *qv*.

TURN-UP An outward turning half curl at the ends of hanging hair; A flick-up.

TURRET TOP A bald head; or bald-headed man. Slang. American usage. (*B and B*)

TURTLES' MARROW A 19th century proprietary soap. (*Piesse*)

TUSHE OF HEYRES Tuft of hairs. (*Levens, 1570*)

TUSSLE Touzled. A dialect word drawn from Dorset and Somerset. Phrase – 'Her hair be all tussled.'

TUSSOCK A tuft or bunch of hair. 16th/19th century. 'Bushy tussocks of grey eye-brow.' 1893

TUTULUS An early Roman hair style for women.　　*341*

TWEEZE, TO Verb. To use tweezers, *qv* for removing unwanted eyebrows. American usage.

TWEEZERS Small pinchers or nippers for plucking out hairs from the face, etc. 17th/20th century.

TWEEZLE Verb. To loosen hair with the fingers. Bristol usage. 19th/early 20th century. 'She is tweezling the wet hair with her left hand and playing the hand-dryer on it with her right hand.'

TWICE-IN WEFT Similar to Once-in Weft, but with an additional interlacing of the hair strand. (*Botham and Sharrad*)

TWICE OVER SHAVE See Close shaving.

TWINE String of two or more strands of hemp or other suitable material twisted together. Used in various hair processes such as dressing, to secure a tress; in permanent waving to hold hair on the curlers, etc; in postiches to secure a hand of hair or smaller groupings.

TWINE PEG A wooden peg similar to a weaving peg on which twine is wound. Used to tie strands of hair.

TWIN TRESS Any double form of small tress postiche such as two switches joined together.　　*204*

TWIRL To twine, coil or curl.

TWIRLIGIG A twirly or spirally twisted motif in a hairdress. 20th century.

TWIRLY TAIL See Twirligig.

TWISERS Tweezers. 17th century usage. See Pincers. (*Comenius*)

TWIST (1) Subs. A switch of hair. 19th century. (*Sutton*)　　*385*
(2) Subs. A one-spill or two-spill tail, dressed in a twist.
(3) A torsade, *qv* (*Walker, 1837*)
(4) Subs. A way of dressing the growing hair – in a twist. (*Mallemont*)　　*451*
(5) Verb. To coil or twine together about or around.

TWISTED WAVE A wave produced by twisting strands of hair and then winding the twisted hair around the prong of a heated curling iron.

TWIST HAIRBRUSH A brush with bristles set in the brush head in a spiral twist; 20th century.

TWISTING The action of winding (running up) the weft around the macramé (tail cord) by means of the twisting machine (jigger) in the manufacture of a switch.

TWISTING MACHINE Also Jigger. A machine to wind or run-up weft upon the macramé stem in switch making. Kordal Machine　　*95A, 462*

TWISTING SILK Silken twine to form the stem or core of a switch spill and used in the same manner as macramé for winding the weft on.

TWIST-ON-SPRING See Plait-on-spring.

TWIST WIG A name for an 18th century wig style. (*Earle*)

TWIST WIND A method of winding a strand of hair obliquely on a curler, by first twisting it and spirally winding the twisted hair on the curler. (*Smith*)

TWIZZLE Small barrel curl.

TWO BOTTLE DYE See Paraphenylenediamine.

TWO CABLE TWIST Similar to a cable twist but with two stems, the hair of each stem being twisted in opposite directions and then each stem is twisted around the other. (*Creer*)

TWO SILK FLY WEFT See Top-Row weft.

TWO SILK WEFT Hair weft worked on two silks.

TWO STEM SWITCH A switch or tail having two spills or stems, used for coils.

TYBURN COLLAR (Also Newgate fringe) A beard growing below the shaven chin. (*Why Shave?*)

TYBURN SCRATCH A man's 18th century wig style. (*Colman*)

TYBURN TOP or FORETOP A wig style with the 'foretop combed over the eyes in a knowing style; such being much worn by the gentlemen pads, scamps, divers and other knowing hands.' (*Grose*) Also dressed on the natural hair, when it was combed over the forehead with a curl between the eye and ear. This style had fallen into disuse by 1827. Variant: Tyburn topped wig.

TYBURN TOPPED WIG. See Tyburn top.

TYE See Tye wig.

TYE CROWN A wig of which the crown part was tied. 18th century (*KP*, May 1739)

TYED WIG The same as Tye wig, *qv*. A propos, Mr St Andre's case, . . . published in the *London Gazette* of February 23, 1724/1725, London (*ND*) p 6, 'A man, middle-sized, having on a light tyed short wig . . .'

TYE WIG A man's wig with a tied queue which came into fashion early in the 18th century, during the reign of George 'The smart tye-wig with the black ribbon shows a man of fierceness of temper.' (*Guardian*, No 149, September, 1713)

TYFFEN To adorn. 16th century.
'For to tyffen heare fas.' (*Romance of Alisaunder*)

U

ULIGINOUS Slimy.

ULOTA CURLING FLUID A proprietary preparation marketed in the 19th century by Rouse Bros, Manufacturing Chemists, London.

ULOTRICHY Woolly hair. (*Webster*)

ULTRA-VIOLET RAYS The radiation from beyond the violet end of the spectrum. Ultra-violet ray treatment or artificial sunlight can be applied by means of a carbon-arc lamp or a mercury vapour lamp. These rays have powerful disinfecting qualities, but are harmful to the naked eyes. This treatment should not be used except under medical supervision.

UMBRELLA COMBING The combing of the hair from the crown in the directions in which it naturally grows – like the outward curving spokes of an umbrella.

UNCLE SAM American beard style in the fashion of the bearded Uncle Sam, the symbolic figure of the United States of America. (*Reynolds* p 280)

UNDER-COLOUR The colour beneath any applied colour such as henna that coats the surface of the hair. Henna can be scraped off the external surface of the hair shaft, revealing the original colour beneath.

UNDER-COMB A plain hair comb worn in the coiffure and positioned under a tress to hold it away from the head. (*Walker*)

UNDER-CURL (1) Subs. Curl that turns towards the face, ears or nape, instead of outwards.
(2) Verb. To curl hair as in (1) above.
(3) Verb. To curl hair too loosely for the required result. 'The hair hangs limply because you have under-curled it.'

UNDER-CURLING (1) Curling the hair ends adjacent to the face, ears or neck under, instead of outwards.
(2) Curling too loosely.

UNDERDRAWN KNOTTING Knots made by inserting the knotting hook from the underside of the foundation at the hairline edge and knotting the hair over the extreme edge of the mount.

UNDERKNOTTING Knotting on the hair-line edge of the underside of a wig or transformation foundation. The hair is brought forward and mingles with the top-surface knotting and softens the postiche's edge.

UNDER-PAD (1) A pad of hair worn beneath growing hair or as a foundation for a marteau or a weft.
(2) A weft of hair worn beneath the natural hair to give bulk.

UNDERPARTING A front or semi-transformation in which the parting is omitted and the wearer's own parting is used, the natural hair being combed over the cut-out front.

UNDER-PIECE A postiche patch for wear beneath some part of the growing hair.

UNDER-PROCESS Verb. To allow insufficient developing time in a dye, bleach or permanent wave. 'You have under-processed the front hair.'

UNDER-SILK See Lining Silk.

UNDER-WAVE (1) See Under-curl (3).
(2) Waves beneath the visible surface.

UNDER-WAVING The process of Marcel waving the hair beneath the visible top hair of the head.

UNDULATED HAIR Waved hair.

UNDULATION Wavy form. From Latin *unda*: wave, *cf* Fr ondulation.

UNFOLD Disentangle (hair). 17th century. (*Comenius*)

UNGUENT An ointment or salve.

UNGUENTUM GALENI Cold cream.

UNG. URSAE (UNGUENTUM URSAE) Bear's grease.

UNISEX WIG A wig suitable for wear by man or woman. 1968/9.

UNIVERSAL-FITTING WIG See Adjustable wig.

UNKEMPT Adj. Uncombed, untrimmed. 'He was unkempt, rough and ready.'

UNRAVELLING COMB A short comb with long, widely spaced and pointed teeth, used to unmat or unravel hair on or off the head. (*Cox*) (For illustration see Plate 2 – The Wigmaker's Art in the 18th Century)

UNSANITARY Unhealthy.

UNTHATCHED ROOF A bald head. 20th century slang.

UNTRIMMED A virgin. Shakespearean bawdy. (*Partridge, Shakespearean Bawdy*, 1968)

UNWIG To take off a wig.

UP-DO (Updo style) A hair style dressed up towards the crown and away from the face and neck. Updo – American spelling. (*Dell, Hair Do*, April, 1965)

UPPER BEARD Moustache. (*Olio*, 1828)

UPRIGHT SHAMPOO See Backward shampoo.

UPSWEPT A hair style in which the hair is combed away from the neck.   *320*

URCHIN HAIRDO A woman's hair style of the 1950s;

short, straight and wispy, like that of the street urchin of Victorian times.

URCHIN LOOK See Urchin Hairdo.

URN A metal or pottery vessel with a lid, in which hot water or shampoo is kept hot, and from which they are dispensed as required.

USTULATE To curl, 17th century. (*Cockeram*)

VAGABOND BOB A hair style for women similar to the Wind-blown Bob, qv. (*Wilson, K*)

VALLANCEY A man's 18th century wig style. (*Fairholt*)

VANDYKE BEARD A pointed beard usually without side whiskers, but with a waxed moustache. Named after the beards frequently depicted in Sir Anthony Vandyke's portraits, especially of Charles I. 17th century (*Fairholt*)
97L

VANDYKE CURL A long, flowing curl.

VANITY COMB A small dressing comb for the hair carried in the pocket or handbag.

VA-PER-MARCEL See Sartory.

VAPET A small square of metal foil and paper, incorporating a chemical which is activated by water, evolving steam and used in machineless permanent waving systems; an exothermic pad.

VAPOUR The gaseous form of a normally liquid or solid substance.

VARIEGATED HAIR Hair of diverse colours, irregular patches of different colours.

VASELINE See Petroleum Jelly. Vaseline is a proprietary name of Chesebrough-Ponds Inc.

VEGETABLE COLOUR A colour derived from henna, indigo, sage or other vegetable source. See also Hair dye, Vegetable.

VEGETABLE DYE See Hair dye, Vegetable.

VEGETABLE HAIR Hair made from the leaves of an Algerian dwarf palm tree.

VEGETABLE HAIR DYE A hair dye derived from a vegetable substance such as Henna. See also Dyeing.

VEGETABLE HAIR OIL The most commonly used included: Almond, apricot, avocado, castor, olive, palm, peach kernel, sesame and soya bean.

VEGETABLE NET Wig net made from sources other than animal or synthetic. Example: cotton. See Stiff wig net.

VEGETABLE OIL Oil derived from vegetable matter. Examples: olive, almond, coconut, etc. See Vegetable hair oil.

VEGETABLE SPONGE A sponge made from a vegetable product such as *Luffa Aegyptiaca*. See also Loofah.

VEHICLE The liquid or material in which is incorporated the active chemical; for instance in the case of certain colour rinses water is the vehicle which carries the correct dilution of colour molecules to the hair's surface.

VEIL, JEWISH See Jewish style of veil.

VELLICATE To pluck or tear by small points. 17th century. 'The Vellication of her eyebrows by means of tweezers improved her appearance.'

VELLICATED HAIR Plucked hair.

VELLICATION The process of pulling or plucking, 17th century.

VELLUS HAIR Hair which retains its foetal characteristics. Lanugo hair. (*McCarthy*)

VELOUTE Fr. Velvet, velvety.

VENICE SOAP A firm, white soap from Venice, 18th century. (*Lillie*)

VENT BRUSH Hair brush with apertures in the bristle base.

VENTILATED GOODS Postiches in which the hair is knotted on a net foundation. American usage. (*American Hairdresser*, 1915)

VENTILATED PAD See Vent pad.

VENTILATED WIG (1) A wig with several open circles in the foundation.
(2) A wig having a large mesh foundation.

VENTILATING Knotting hair on a net foundation. American usage. (*Nazarro and Norhaft*)

VENTILATING-BLOCK Wig block made of wood in the same shape as the human skull. (*Moler*)

VENTILATING-NEEDLE A Knotting needle, qv. American usage.

VENT-PAD (1) A hermispherical hair pad on a wire frame with a circular hole in the middle, often with hair weft sewn to the circumference. The hole allowed the wearer's own hair to be pulled through and mingle with the pad hair.
(2) An open mesh pad.

VENUS The goddess of Love who received the prize of Beauty from the hand of Paris, and the origin of words such as Venereal, from Latin *Venereus*. Depicted by the ancients with yellow hair. (*Salmon*)

VENUS' HAIR Spanish Moss. *Tillandsia Usneoides*.

VENUS'S HAIR The plant *adiantum capillus-veneris*. (*B and H*)

VENUS SOAP Synonym for Venice Soap; called Venus soap for its whiteness, after Venus, who, according to mythology, was born from the foam of the sea, 18th century. (*Lillie*)

VERBENA The scented species of the lemon verbena, *aloysia citriodora*. The otto, which can be extracted from the leaves by distillation with water, is rarely used by the manufacturing perfumer on account of its high price. Instead, it is successfully imitated by mixing the otto of lemon grass *andropogon nardus*, with rectified spirit.

VERBENA OIL Mineral oil perfumed by verbena or, more usually, by a substance resembling the scent of verbena.

VERITABLE Fr. Genuine, pure.

VERMICELLI Jellied hair caused by overbleaching. Slang.

VERMICULAR CURL A long, thin, sinuous curl. Vermicular = Vermiform or worm-like.

VERONICA LAKE COIFFURE A very long hair style for women, worn nearly straight and hanging loosely on the shoulders. Named after the American film star, Veronica Lake, who popularized this style. In 1941, during the War, for some months most young women affected this fashion, and, working among moving machinery in munitions factories, as many of them were, they were exposed to the danger of having their long, loose hair caught in it and being scalped. After a number of such fatal accidents had occurred an effort was made to encourage women to wear their hair in snoods. This was largely successful and the accident rate fell.

VERSICOLOUR PILARIS Variegated hair. (*Wheeler*)

VERTEX The top of the head. The crown.

VERTEX HAIR The hair that grows at the top of the head.

VERTICAL PAD WEFT One top loop and one bottom loop on two or three sides.

VEX To tease or vex hair or wool. From Latin *vexare*.

VIBRATION A massage movement in which a vibrator or the fingers are employed to transmit a trembling movement to the skin surface and its deeper structures.

VIBRATOR An electrically operated apparatus that transmits a vibratory motion to a rubber applicator and is used in massage of the scalp, face, etc.

VIBRATOR APPLICATOR The rubber attachment for a vibrator, *qv*.

VIBRATOR MASSAGER See Vibrator.

VIBRO See Vibrator, of which vibro is a commonly used, shortened form.

VIBRO-MASSAGE Massage by means of a vibrator, *qv*.

VIBRISSA The hairs growing in the nostril.

VICTORIAN CURL A curl or ringlet of spiral form, also called spiral curl; corkscrew curl; drop curl.

VICTORIAN HAIR STYLES Hair styles as worn in the Victorian period, 1837–1900. Historically the period is usually divided into early, middle and late.

VICTORIAN LOOK Having the fashion or appearance in hair and dress of a Victorian.

VICTORY A woman's hair style of 1865. (*Bysterveld*, p 62)

VIEILLARD Fr. Old person, See au Vieillard.   *458*

VIENNA COSMETIC (*Seegar's hair water*) A 19/20th century 'secret' preparation consisting of large proportions of iron, copper, pyrogallic acid and free hydrochloric acid. This could have been dangerous to health. (*Koller*)

VILLOUS (of animals) Hairy, furry. 'The hair is most villous.'

VILLUS In botany a long, slender, soft hair. In anatomy a minute projection forming one of numerous close-set projections.

VINEGAR A dilute solution of 5% acetic acid with traces of other substances such as mineral salts and sugars. Aromatic: Acid aceticum aromaticum. Distilled: Dilute acetic acid. Toilet: Acetum odoratum. White: Dilute Acetic acid. White wine: Vinegar prepared from red and white wine.

VINEGAR RINSE A dilute acetic acid rinse for the hair. See also Acid Hair Rinse.

VIOLET HAIR POWDER A starch hair powder scented with violet perfume. 18/19th century. (*Lillie*)

VIOLET OIL Liquid paraffin 80%; almond oil 20%, chlorophyll, *qv*. Violet perfume to taste. Used as a hair dressing.

VIOLET RAY See High frequency.

VIOLET RAY OUTFIT See High frequency machine.

VIRGIN BLEACH The first bleaching of hair.

VIRGIN DYE The application of a hair dye on virgin hair, *qv*. A first dye.

VIRGIN HAIR Hair that has never been touched by dye, bleach, permanent waving lotion or any other similar lotion or chemical that has any permanent effect on the hair.

VIRGIN HEAD A head of Virgin hair, *qv*. But see Virgin-head.

VIRGINHEAD The condition of being a virgin.

VIRGINIA POMADE White vaseline 12 oz, white wax 1 oz, powdered benzoin 1 oz, Peruvian balsam 2 drachms, bergamot oil and otto of rose as required. (*MacEwan*)

VIRGIN MILK (1) Tincture of benzoin and rosewater – a few drops of the former to an ounce or two of the latter. Massaged on the face it was found in the 17/19th century to give a beautiful ivory colour. (*Toilette*, 1832)
(2) Benjamin Water. (*Phillips*)

VIRGIN OIL Finest (aix) olive oil, or the oil which separates spontaneously from the paste of crushed olives. (*PPB*)

VIRGIN'S GREASE (1) The non-oily, white, thick, slimy dressing used on men's hair at the barber's. Slang. West of England usage, early 20th century. 'No oil, thank you. Just a touch of your Virgin's Grease.'
(2) Verdigris. Colloquial usage. This being the greenish-blue copper acetate that forms on brass and copper utensils in the hairdressing saloon. (*Dr B Jones*)

VIRGIN'S KNOT A small bow of ribbon worn in the hair by unmarried girls.

VIRGIN'S MILK See Virgin milk.

VIRGIN WAX (1) White beeswax; bleached beeswax. (*Merle*)
(2) Fresh, unused beeswax.
(3) The first wax produced by a swarm of bees.
(4) A fine quality, purified beeswax.

VIRICIDE A distinfectant substance which will destroy viruses. (*PPB*)

VIR PILOSUS The hairy man; Elias. (*Powell*)

VISCID Sticky, having a glutinous character.

VISCOSITY The quality of being viscous, *qv*.

VISCOUS (1) Having a glutinous character.
(2) Intermediate between liquid and solid.

VISITING BARBER A barber who calls on his clients and serves them in their homes. Today, 1983, most of them carry their implements and materials by van or motor car. There are several in the Channel Islands. See Flying barber.

VITAMINS, HAIR See Hair vitamins.

VITILIGO Congenital white streaks in hair. (*Wilson*)

VITILIGO BALDNESS See Morphoea Alopecia. (*Wheeler*)

VITTA An early Roman hair style for women. (*Rimmel*)   *341*

V-NECK V-shaped neck edge.

VOGUE The prevailing fashion.

VOLATILE OIL An essential oil obtained by the distillation of those parts of plants that afford essential oils.

VOLCANO A cone of hair dressed on a wire net foundation with a froth of curls at the top. USA 1972.

VOOGD'S RAZOR A 19th century hollow ground proprietary razor of high quality. Made with square, round or Irish points in five sizes – ½″, ⅝″, ¾″, ⅞″ and 1″, with black handles 30/- doz. Ivory handles 44/-doz. (Advert, 1887, *Creer*)

VOOGD'S SCISSORS A proprietary scissor with finger rest: 6½″, 7″ and 7½″ at 32/-, 38/- and 44/- per doz. respectively. With flat shanks 6½″, 7″ and 7½″ at 24/-, 30/- and 36/- per doz respectively. (Advert, 1887, *Creer*)

VOSS'S BARBER Isaac Voss, an eccentric Dutchman, who died a Canon of Windsor in 1689, wrote, 'Men (barbers) who could imitate any measure of song in combing the hair, so as sometimes to express very intelligibly iambics, trochees, dactyls, etc.' (*Isaac Voss, De Poematum Cantu*, Oxford, 1673)

VOTIVE HAIR Hair offered freely to the gods. A custom of greatest antiquity which implied that the worshipper placed himself in the power of the god. The long, youthful hair or the first down on the chin was offered at puberty. (*Rouse, GVO*)

VUZZ POLL A head of untidy hair. Devon usage. (*Hewett*)

W

WAFER RAZOR A thin bladed razor.

WAFFLE TOWEL The same as Honeycomb towel. The marked ridges and hollows of the weave expose more surface for absorption of water than a plain weave.

WAIF A straggling wisp of hair. Dorset usage.

WALKING HEADDRESS (Day dressing, *qv*.) A hair style suitable for outdoor wear. An informal style, *cf* Evening hairdress.

WALKING STICK CURL A stand-up curl forming three-quarters of a circle with a long straight stem similar to a stem curl. 1965.

WALLIS, JOHN, D D (1616–1703) A theologian and

mathematician, famed as probably the first divine to don the wig. See engraving by Burgher, pub Oxon, 1699. (*Smith H C*)

WALLRITZ'S CACTUS POMADE A 19/20 century 'secret' preparation for promoting the growth of the hair, prepared by crushing 125 parts of cactus (spines and all) in a mortar and boiling the result in a vessel (not copper), an addition of turmeric and indigo being made until a green colour was produced. The strained liquid was stirred until cold, with 750 parts of water, 60 of glycerine, 15 of tannin, 7½ of rosemary oil and 4 parts fennel oil. (*Koller*)

WALL RUE (*Ruta Muraria*) A white maidenhair fern. A decoction of this herb encourages the hair's growth. (*Fernie*)

WALNUT The roots, leaves, and rind of the walnut yield a brown dye which was used as a hair dye in England until the 1920s.

WALNUT HAIR DYE A hair dye composed of walnut juice, which is expressed from the bark or shell of green walnuts. A little rectified spirit and a few bruised cloves are usually added. The dye should be stored in a cool place. See also Walnut.

WALNUT HAIR STAIN See Walnut and Walnut hair dye.

WALNUT POMADE A pomade for dressing the hair and darkening it, incorporating walnut juice expressed from the bark or shell of green walnuts. 18th century. (*Brodie, Price List*, 1890)

WALNUT STAIN See Walnut hair dye.

WALRUS A film extra with a large moustache. American slang. (*B and B*)

WALRUS MOUSTACHE A large moustache which overhangs the lips, like that of a walrus. *101 i, 101 s.*

WARM COLOUR A colour of a warm hue such as red or yellow, as opposed to the cool colours such as blue or green.

WASH (1) Subs. Cosmetic water. 18th century. (*Grose*)
(2) Subs. Liquid shampoo, West Country usage, 19/20th century.
(3) Subs. The action of cleansing with soap and water. The action of shampooing. 'Your dirty hair needs a good wash.'
(4) Verb. To clean with soap and water; to shampoo. 'I shall wash my hair to-night.'

WASH BALL (Soap ball) A ball of soap, often perfumed, used by barbers. 16th/19th century. (*NBK*)
'The Barbar (*sic*) with his washball sweet,
With Bason, Towell, and all Things meet;
He cuts, and shaves with skilfull aime,
No cause to crie, fie, fie for shame.'
(*Looking-glass of the World*, 1644; Wing, 3037)
'I remember a wash ball that had a quality truly wonderful – It gave an exquisite edge to the razor.' (*The Idler*, No 40, 1759)
An 18th century formula for the composition of a common wash ball was: 40 lb rice in fine powder form; 28 lb flour; 28 lb starch powder; 12 lb white lead; 4 lb orris root. This was a dangerous mixture that must have caused grievous disorders to the users. A 19th century formula for 'best common wash balls' was: 40 lb oil soap (Castile, etc), 60 lb tallow soap.

WASH BARREL Wooden barrels of 5 to 10 gallon capacity, used in the 18th to early 20th century for holding the shampoo wash.

WASH BOTTLE See Shampoo bottle.

WASHED-OUT BLONDE A pale, insipid blonde head of hair.

WASHERWOMAN STYLE Hair drawn back from the forehead, ears and neck and dressed in a bun on top of the head. In Bristol in the 19th century, the washerwoman who attended families weekly for a day's washing, invariably dressed their hair this fashion.

WASH HAND BASIN The same as Lavatory basin, *qv*.

WASHING BALLES See Wash ball. (*Clerk*, 1602)

WASHINGTON, MARTHA General Washington's wife, née Dandridge, first married in 1749 to Daniel Parke Custis, married Washington in 1758. In 1754 James Kent, wigmaker at the Locks of Hair, against the Bolt and Tunn Inn, Fleet Street, London, made a wig for Mrs Custis, as she then was. The bill records:

To one best curl'd cutt wigg	£3 3s	0d
To a sett of curlls	12s	0d
	£3 15s	d

(*Procter*)

WASHITE HONE Made from a natural rock found in the Washite River area of Arkansas, USA. Used as ballast in ships returning to Bristol in the early 20th century. A good razor and scissor sharpener.

WASH URN A metal urn with a tap and heated by a gas ring beneath. Used in the 19th and early 20th century to keep the shampoo wash hot, ready for use.

WASP An 18th century hairpin decorated with insects, birds, etc, made of precious stones mounted on vibrating wire and attached to the hairpin. (*Smith, H C*) See also Butterfly.

WASTE HAIR When long hair was fashionable women were in the habit of rolling their hair combings over their fingers before putting them into a small piece of paper to prevent them flying about. In that state they were thrown away and later collected from the rubbish by the chiffonier in France, and rag and bone man in England. Waste hair was then sold to the wigmaker, who prepared it for use in the manufacture of cheap wigs. An article by M Alphonse Bouchard in *The Hairdressing Chronicle*, 1873, gives a full description of this waste hair trade.

WATCH SPRING Lengths of prepared watch spring are used for positional springs, *qv* in the manufacture of wigs and transformations.

WATER COSMETIC Water-soluble colouring block used for colour-coating new hair growth between applications of permanent hair dye; also used for the make up of eyebrows or eyelashes.

WATER CURLING Forming and setting wet hair in curls. Early 19th century.

WATERFALL A chignon bearing a likeness to a waterfall, loose and flowing. American usage. (*B and B*)

WATER HEATER A small geyser for the rapid preparation of hot water for use in the saloon.

WATER HONE A razor hone on which water is used as a lubricant.

WATER-MADE COIFFURE A water waved hairdress. Late 19th century. (*Mallemont*). See Water wave.

WATERPROOF NET Water repellent net used in wig-making.

WATERPROOF WIG NET See Hoc net.

WATER SETTING See Water waving.

WATER SOFTENER An apparatus for the conversion (by chemical media) of hard water into soft water.

WATER WAVING The formation of waves in wet hair by the use of a dressing comb and the fingers, the waves being subsequently dried in position. It was not until *c* 1865 or 1866 that this method was introduced. 'The waving represented in our engraving is performed with water; this new proceeding is coming more in practice every day, and we expect our fellow tradesmen will give it all their attention.' (*Le Coiffeur Européen*, 15th August, 1866) According to Creer, Eugène Ménard described water-waving in a lecture at the Academie International de Coiffure, 1884, and it must have been after this that the new method became common practice.

WATKINS, JOSEPH Born Richmond, Yorks, 1739. William Hogarth's barber. (*Smith, J T The Cries of London*, 1839)

WATTEAU STYLE A hair style in the fashion of those depicted in the paintings of women by Antoine Watteau (1684–1721), French Artist and Master of the rococo. He painted mock-pastoral idylls, depicting the aristocracy in court dress. *320*

WAVE (1) Subs. An undulating conformation of hair; each separate undulation of such a conformation. Half of an annulation of a curl. 'A mass of blond hair in wave fell on her shoulders.' 'The temple wave of her coiffure was too small for her features.' A wave consists of a crest or ridge, and the trough. It may be wide or narrow, deep or shallow, loose or tight, weak or strong, depending on the quality and diameter of the hairs, the difference in the lengths of the longitudinal sections of the hairs, and the manner in which the hair is set. (See *The Physical Reason for Hair Curl and Wave*, by *J Stevens Cox*, HRC 1964)
(2) Verb. To make wavy in conformation. To undulate in form. 'Her hair was waved with the Marcel waving irons.'

WAVE CLIP See Wave setter.

WAVE CUT A method of revealing by cutting and setting the latent wave in the hair. The method was widely commercialized in 1938 by Kenneth A Christy, an American, and quickly exploited by several British hairdressers, including the writer, who introduced their own versions to the hairdressing craft. (*HWJ*)

WAVED-BANDEAU COIFFURE A hairdress incorporating a waved bandeau, *qv*.

WAVED HAIR Hair that has been artificially waved.

WAVE-DO A hair setting of waves. Slang. 1950s.

WAVED MARTEAU See Wavy marteau.

WAVE FORM (1) The form or shape of a hair wave.
(2) The set style, order or arrangement of waves in a hairdress.

WAVELET (1) A weft of waved hair 1″ to 3″ or so wide and 4″ to 6″ long, with two loops to secure it to the head.
(2) A small wave.

WAVELETTE See Wavelet.

WAVE MOVEMENT The arrangement and direction of the waves in a hairdress. See also Wave form.

WAVE NET Setting net, *qv*.

WAVER (1) One who waves hair by means of Marcel irons, a permanent waving system, or by setting waves with fingers and comb.
(2) A contrivance for waving hair by rolling or twisting it in a hair-waver and leaving it to take on a wavy appearance.
(3) A permanent waving machine.
(4) A contrivance for waving hair, such as Marcel waving irons.

WAVESET (1) Subs. Setting lotion, *qv*. 'Waveset will help to hold the waves in position.'
(2) Adj. Having the quality of facilitating the formation or retention of waves in the finger-wave setting process. 'Waveset cosmetics sell readily.'

WAVE SETTER A curved, spring-operated, metal slip, 3″ to 6″ in length, with teeth, used to grip the hair and form the crest of a wave in wet or damp hair. See Wave.

WAVE-SETTING COMB See Setting comb.

WAVE WIDTH The distance between two consecutive wave crests.

WAVING (1) Subs. The action of imparting waves to hair. 'Hair waving is our speciality'.

(2) Adj. Of hair; ie undulating in form or outline. 'She had waving, flaxen hair.' 1848.

WAVING COMB A hair comb used to control the hair during Marcel waving or hair setting; also Setting comb.

WAVING IRONS Irons for waving hair, consisting of two prongs, one solid and rounded, the other, into which the solid round prong fits, concave. They are made in different diameters indicated by the letters A, B, C, and D. A being the smallest and D the largest diameter. *442, 443*

WAVING LIQUID (1) A permanent waving lotion.
(2) A liquid preparation, often incorporating an alkali, that was supposed to give a longer life to a Marcel wave.
(3) Brilliantine applied to the hair before Marcel waving helped, by protecting the hair from the moisture of the atmosphere, to hold the wave longer. 'Put a little waving liquid on before you Marcel me.' 19th/20th century.

WAVING LOTION See Waving liquid.

WAVING MACHINE An apparatus incorporating numerous small heaters by means of which wound hair, with a suitable chemical application, was heated and thus permanently waved.

WAVING ROD A metal hair curler used in permanent waving processes from 1906 to the 1950s, by which time the heat permanent waving process had been superceded by the cold processes.

WAVINGS (of curls) Loose drop curls that wave or move as the head moves. (*Le Coiffeur Européen*, Sept 1866)

WAVING STICK See Curl stick (2).

WAVING TONGS See Waving irons.

WAVOUS Full of waves. 'Her lovely wavous head.' 16/17th century.

WAVY HAIR Hair with a wave; but this term, as used by a wigmaker, refers exclusively to naturally wavy hair, not artificially waved hair, which is always referred to as 'waved hair'.

WAVY MARTEAU A marteau made of naturally wavy hair. A 'waved marteau' would indicate one made of artificially waved hair.

WAWKS The corners of the moustache. 17th/18th century Midlands usage. (*Derham*)

WAX (1) Beeswax used on wigmaking silks and threads.
(2) Artificial compounds having the qualities of wax.

WAX, MOUSTACHE See Moustache wax.

WAXED MOUSTACHE A moustache dressed with wax, usually in a style with two pointed ends. Popular from late 19th to early 20th century.

WAXED POINT MOUSTACHE See Wax pointed moustache.

WAX EPILATION The removal of unwanted eyebrow hair by means of an application of a prepared wax to the hair to be removed, and then, by a rapid firm motion against the direction of the hair growth the wax is ripped off, taking the hairs with it.

WAX FIGURE See Wax model.

WAX HAIR One of the long hairs growing on the body of the flea-louse. (*Psyllidae*)

WAXING The application of beeswax to the silks in the weaving process. This protects the silks and facilitates the sliding of the individual knots along the silks towards the anchor stick.

WAX MODEL A head or head and bust of wax, upon which the wig-maker displays his postiches, such as wigs and transformations. 18th/20th century.

WAX POINTED MOUSTACHE A moustache of which both ends are drawn to a hairy point and held in position by means of a wax.

WEARING COMB A decorative or plain comb for wearing in the hair. See Dressing comb.

WEAT, TO To search for lice. 'To weat the head.' Northern usage. (*Grose, Prov Glos*)

WEATHER-COCK The name of a beard. 20th century. (*Mitchell*)

WEAVE (1) Verb. To fabricate hair weft by interlacing strands of hair in weaving silks.
(2) Subs. Hair that has been woven. 'This is a very fine weave.'

WEAVER A boardworker skilled in the art of weaving hair on silks or threads for the subsequent manufacture of post-iches.

WEAVER'S KNOT See Hair Weaver's Knot.

WEAVING The operation of forming hair weft. 'Weaving was the invention of the Egyptians.'

WEAVING CARD See Drawing mat.

WEAVING CLAMP Screw clamp for securing a weaving stick to the bench.

WEAVING FRAME (Weaving loom) The right and left hand weaving sticks in position on the work-bench with the weaving silks affixed.

WEAVING LOOM See Weaving frame.

WEAVING PEG See Weaving stick.

WEAVING POLE A continental type of long weaving stick with six pegs.

WEAVING SCREW The screw-clamp secured to the work bench and into which the weaving stick fits.

WEAVING SET See Weaving frame.

WEAVING SILK The string of cotton or, more usually silk, upon which the hair is woven. There is a top (No. 1), middle (No 2) and bottom (No 3) silk (or, if more than three are used the numbers continue downwards consecutively) and they are attached to a left and right-hand weaving stick, peg, post, or rod and the whole constitutes the weaving-frame, loom or jigger.

WEAVING STICK A round peg (above 12″ long, 1″ diameter) that forms a part of the weaving loom. The left-hand weaving stick (plain with a small nail to hold the weaving silks) is the anchor stick; the right-hand stick is the spool stick, and has three 1½″ wide grooves on which the three spools of silk are wound.

WEAVING STRING See Weaving silk.

WEAVING WHISKERS The protruding short hairs that stand out irregularly from ill-woven weft.

WEAVING WIRE Thin, malleable wire used in place of a third silk in the weaving process for the production of diamond-mesh chignons, etc. (*Brodie, Price List*, 1890)

WEDGE RAZOR A razor with a solid wedge-shaped blade.

WEEDS The beard. Slang. American usage. (*B and B*)

WEEPERS See Piccadilly weepers.

WEEPING BILLY An 18th/early 19th century man's wig, as worn by The Hon Henry Grey Bennett. (*Spirit of the Public Journals*, 1824)

WEFT (1) Subs. A length of hair woven on silks. There are five principal types of weft: 1 Once-in-weft; 2 Twice-in-weft; 3 Thrice-in-weft; 4 Fly-weft on three silks; 5 Fly-weft on two silks; See also close-weft; crop-weft; flat-weft; ringlet-weft; top-weft; wig-weft, etc.   468

WEFT CLIP A jockey, *qv*. (*Symonds*)

WEFT FRINGE A 4″ to 10″ length of 4″–6″ long wefted, curled hair.

WEFT HAND A weft worker or weaver in the workroom.

WEFT PARTING A wig parting made of fine weft.

WEFT PINCHING The process of pinching the finished weft on the weaving-loom by means of hot pinching irons.

WEFT POMPADOUR A hair-weft sewn on a puff-pad and dressed as a pompadour.

WEFT PRESSING The process of pressing weft by means of a hot pressing iron after it has been removed from the weaving loom.

WEFT WIG A wig covered with hair woven into weft and sewn on the wig-net foundation from a pivot-point usually the crown, and encircling the foundation until it is entirely covered with hair.

WELCH WIG A worsted cap. 19/20th century. 'The sexton's Welch wig which he wore at rainy funerals.' (*A Smith, The Pottleton Legacy*, 1849, *N Q* 30.8.1862)

WELSH A man's 18th century wig style.

WELSH WIG See Welch wig.

WEST END, THE See Regent, The.

WET CUTTING The cutting of wet hair by a razor, occasionally by means of scissors.

WETTING AGENT A substance which will facilitate wetting by a liquid by breaking down or reducing the surface tension of the liquid. A detergent is an example of a wetting agent.

WET-WINDING PROCESS In permanent waving, the winding of a strand of hair, wetted with waving solution, onto a curler.

WHALEBONE BRUSH A hairbrush with bristles made from baleen, the elastic, horny substance that grows in the upper jaw of certain whales instead of teeth.

WHEELER-LEA ACT An Act of the United States Congress of May 1938, which gave the Federal Trade Commission power to protect the public against false claims for beauty products and other preparations, many of which had proved unsafe to use. (*Phillips*)

WHETSTONE A shaped stone for sharpening the edges of metal tools and implements after they have been ground. See Hone.

WHEY BEARD (1) Pale coloured beard.
(2) A person with a whey beard.
'An orchard may conduce to the green-sicknesse;
A Dayrie to a whey beard.' 17th century. (*Spinola*)

WHIG DRESSER, THE A weekly penny political paper published from Sat Jan 5 to Sat 9th March, 1833. A vignette under the title depicts a barber in his apron surrounded by seven identifiable heads on blocks.

WHIPPING (1) The binding with twine of the root ends of raw or prepared hair, consisting of numerous tight and close-lying encirclements of the hair by the twine, completed without a knot by drawing the loose ends down under the wound twine by means of a loop of twine or a hairpin. (*Ashley*)
(2) Loose, frothy-looking curls dressed on top of the head. 1960s.

WHIRL See Whorl.

WHISKER (1) The hair on the cheeks and chin of a man, or very exceptionally, a woman. At one time applied to the hair on the upper lip, now called the moustache; and to the hair on the chin, now the beard. 'My whiskers hanging o're the overlipp.' 1600. (*Timon of Athens*)
'His whiskers . . . cut to the old-fashioned . . . mutton-chop.' 1878.
(2) A great lie. 18th century. Slang. (*Grose, ed 1823*)
(3) A verbal blunder on the radio. American radio slang. (*B and B*)
(4) An uncommon surname. The same as wiskar, wisker and derived from wisgar and wiscar, which were corruptions of Visigardus – a daughter of Theodebert, King of the Franks and wife of Gregory of Tours. (*Charnock*)

WHISKERADE A display of whiskers. American slang. (*B and B*)

WHISKERETTE A feeble-growing or slight whisker. 20th century. (*Mitchell*)

WHISKER IRONS See Moustache irons.

WHISKERS Late 17th century name for curls that were dressed to hang down the cheeks as far as the bosom. (*Dulaure*)

'Servants and Citizens' wives who wore whiskers like ladies of fashion were attacked without mercy.' (*Dulaure*)

WHISKER SPLITTER A man of intrigue. 18th century slang. (*Grose*, ed 1823)

WHISKER WAX A dressing for the moustache and whiskers, 18th century. A kind of pomade incorporating beeswax. (*Dulaure*)

WHISP See Wisp.

WHISPERING HEADDRESS An early 18th century woman's headdress.

Scrape: 'I am not in my whispering head-dress.'

Snuff: 'Pray, madam, what headdress is that?'

Scrape: 'Why the newest fashion; cornets all back for the better conveniency of hearing.' (*Injur'd Love*, 1711)

WHISTLE AND WIG An 18th century Inn name, *cf* Pig and Whistle. (*Fairburn's Laughable Songster*, 1819)

WHITE BALM OF CONSTANTINOPLE The same as Balm of Mecca, *qv*.

WHITE BOLE See Kaolin.

WHITE COURT See Court wig.

WHITE DIACHYLON PLASTER Plaster of lead.

WHITE HENNA A euphemism. It has no possible connection with henna but it is a mixture of kaolin and magnesium carbonate or sodium perborate, etc. with hydrogen peroxide, which is the actual bleaching agent. This paste-form facilitates the application, as it does not run. The term White Henna arose as a mild deception at a time when hydrogen peroxide had earned a bad reputation, owing to misuse, for damaging the hair. Pure henna does no damage to hair. Usage from *c* 1920.

WHITELOCKS Silver-coloured hair. 18th century.

WHITE LOTION A 19th century hair restorer which consisted of: Distilled water 1 quart, glycerine ½ oz, glacial acetic acid 2 fl oz and tincture of cantharides 1½ fl oz. (*Stevens Ms*)

WHITENER A solution of up to 5% hyposulphite of soda applied as a hot oil application to white hair after a permanent wave to remove any yellow tinge.

WHITENING AGENT (1) A substance used to remove or disguise yellowing of white hair, eg methyl violet or methylene blue dyes, etc.

(2) A bleach, *qv*.

WHITE OF EGG SHAMPOO See Egg shampoo.

WHITE PERRUKE Voltaire lodged for three years at the sign of the White Perruke, Maiden Lane, London, near the birthplace of J M W Turner.

WHITE SYRIAN CROQUIGNOLE Croquignole curled *bleached* white hair (angora and yak); croquignole of white Syrian hair. Maximum length 18″. See Syrian hair.

WHITE VITRIOL Zinc sulphate.

WHITE WALLS The shaved scalp at the side of the head above the ears. American usage, mid-20th century.

WHITE WAX Bleached wax. (*Simmonds*)

WHITE WIG (1) Nickname of General Whitford, colonel of the 19th Regiment in the 18th century. (*Fenton*, p XIV)

(2) A local name (Dorset and Hants) for the men employed by Isaac Gulliver, the smuggler, *c* 1800. These smugglers had worn white wigs, but when hair powder was taxed they discarded the wig, powdered their own hair and wore it long. (*Oakley*)

WHORL (1) Curved wisps of hair radiating from a common centre, suggesting a whirling movement.

(2) A convolution of hair.

(3) A curl or spiral of hair.

WHORL PIECE The crown piece for a postiche, which is knotted to a whorl design.

WIDOW'S CURL A short lock of curly hair which cannot be disciplined into the head-dress, but falls in a curl on the forehead. It is said to indicate widowhood. (*Brewer*). Also called waif.

WIDOW'S LOCK A lock of hair which hangs apart from the rest. Formerly believed to presage an early widowhood.

WIDOW'S PEAK A V- or U-shaped growth of hair projecting onto the middle of the forehead; said by some to indicate widowhood, but in Devon, Somerset and Dorset it is the sign of a long life. (*Brewer*)

WIG (1) Subs. An artificial head of hair, from the French Perruque and through the forms, Peruke, Periwyk and Periwig, became wig by 1675, as a result of the elision of the first two syllables. See also Periwig. 'Beneath an ample wig he tucks his hair.' 1760. (*Woty*)

In *England's Vanity*, 1683, the three different spellings: wigg, periwigg and peruke appeared in the text.

Evidence of the use of wigs in remote ages is provided by an Egyptian bald-headed clay figure of *c* 2500 bc with a removeable wig of black clay hair over it. This also indicated that shaving of the head in Egypt had become a custom at a very early period. Used at a time before (in Egypt) the evidence of clothing. (*Flinders Petrie, The Making of Egypt*, 1939). Wigs were also worn, according to Xenephon, the historian (*c* 430–354 bc), by the monarchs of Persia, also by Astyages, King of the Medes. Other early allusions to wigs are found in Ovid, Plutarch and Suetonius.

Speight records the introduction of wigs into England as having been in the reign of Stephen (1135–1154). The peruke is recorded in a wardrobe account of the reign of Edward VI (1547–1553).

Stow informs us that women's periwigs were first introduced into England about the time of the Massacre of Paris, 1572. Many references occur to wigs worn by women in the 16th century.

'Her hair is auburn, mine is perfect yellow,

If that be all the difference in his love.

I'll get me such a colour'd periwig.' (*Shakespeare, The Two Gentlemen of Verona*, Act IV, Scene 4, 1594/5)

'But O, her silver-framed coronet,

With low-down dangling, spangles all beset,

Her sumptuous periwig, her Curious Curles.' (*Middleton, Micro-Cynicon*, 1599, STC 17154)

'That beaver band, the colour of that periwig. The farthingale above the navel all as if the fashion were his own invention.' (*Middleton, A Mad World, My Masters*. Act IV, 1608)

Men wore wigs of natural colours until *c* 1714, when it became fashionable to adopt bleached hair, but this soon faded and looked lifeless and powdered wigs became the vogue.

'Others who lay the stress of beauty in their face, exert all their extravagance in the periwig, which is a kind of index of the mind: the full-bottom formally combed all before, denotes the lawyer and the politician; the smart tye-wig with the black ribbon shows a man of fierceness of temper.' (*John Gay, The Guardian*, No 149, Sept 1713)

'March ye 30: 1748 Recd of Wm Chalmers esqr the sum of five pound five shillings in full for two Bob Wiggs.' 'John Franklin Recd for a Bob Wigg and a Brigadeair Wigg £4 10s 0d' (Ms diary in possession of JSC) From these receipts it appears that in Scotland in 1748, Bob wigs were £2 12s 6d each and Brigadier wigs £1 17s 6d.

1–15, 17–84, 233–239

(2) Verb. To fit and supply a wig. To put on a wig.
'Clarkson wigged three operas in one evening.' 1889.
(3) To rebuke severely.
(4) Verb. To site a scout with a hen pigeon on the route of a pigeon race to distract the opponents' birds. 19th century slang. (*Partridge*)
(5) Verb trans int. To enjoy any ecstatic experience. American 20th century slang.
(6) A head of hair. Slang. From *c* 1918.
(7) American slang for bobbed hair, *qv*, *c* 1920. (*Weseen*)
(8) An intellectual. American slang, *c* 1940. (*W and F*)
(9) A judge.
(10) A member of the white races. American Negro usage (20th century) in reference to the noticeable straighter and longer hair of the white races. (*W and F*)
(11) 'The Wig', a nickname of General Skinner, Engineer, who wore a large black wig at the siege of Belle Isle. 18th century. (*Fenton*)
(12) A fisherman's term for an old seal. (*Simmonds*; *Goodridge*)
(13) A beast of burden, a horse.
'What's that to you, old dead wig.[1] You won't
Come down with the brads, will you? Hold your slang,
Then, and sherry, morris, broom – cut the stick
With your set of raw-bones and heavy drag.'
[1] reference to a horse. (*Universal Songster*, v 3, p 314)
(14) A comestible bun. (*Gales*)

WIG, JEWISH It was once the custom for married Jewesses to cover closely their hair and heads with a cloth so that no hair was visible. Later, as a compromise, not wishing to cover the hair completely as in ancient times and yet not desiring to show her own hair, a wig called a Shaittel was worn. Publicly to exhibit the hair of a married Jewess was a mark of disgrace and when the infidelity of a Jewess was to be made public the priest uncovered the woman's head. (*Numbers*, v 13)

WIG-A-CALOTTE A wig with a coif, as though the tonsure had been regularly performed and the wig was natural hair. (*Doran*, p 155)

WIGANNOWNS A man wearing a large wig. 18th century. (*Grose, Lex, Bal,*)

WIGBAND A band of ribbon which covers the hair-line of a part-wig, and to which it is attached; hair mounted on a base of stretch material, worn around the circumference of the head.   *411*

WIG BAR A 1963 'with it' expression indicating the availability of ready-made style wigs in the shop.

WIG BATHING CAP A styled wig made on a waterproof foundation for wear when bathing.

WIG BEARD A beard, the hair of which is worked on a gauze or net foundation. 1895. (*Stevens Ms*)

WIG BIN A wig bin for storing clients' wigs, waiting for the cleaning and dressing process. American usage.

WIG BLOCK (1) A wooden head-shaped block of wood on which to make wigs or a malleable block on which to dress them.
(2) The head. 19th century slang, *cf* Block head.

WIG BONE A slightly curved, flat sliver of bone or synthetic material sewn between galloons in the foundation of a wig or transformation to hold the hair-line tightly against the scalp. American usage. See also Spring.

WIG BOX A box of wood or pasteboard to contain a wig. Some 18th century wig boxes had a Mushroom, *qv*, fitted within upon which the wig was placed; the boxes were also occasionally lined with newspapers. (*S N*)

WIG CAP The completed foundation of a wig, without the hair.

WIG CITY A shop or store that sells wigs. American usage, 1964.

WIG CLEANER (1) One who cleans wigs.
(2) A substance used for cleaning wigs such as carbon tetrachloride, naphtha, or petroleum spirit, SBP 1, 2 or 3.

WIG CLEANING The process of cleaning a wig.

WIG COMBER One who combs wigs – an 18th century division of the hairdressing craft. 'I have been in town but a few days, and am at present returned to my old trade of combing wigs.' (*Bentley*, 1775)

WIGDOM Judges, Barristers and Solicitors as a body, all of whom wear wigs in Court.

WIG DRESSER One who dresses wigs.

WIG DRESSING The arranging of the hair of a wig to a required style. 'Pay'd for curl of wigs. 16s' (*Wale*, 1701)

WIG DRYER A Postiche oven, *qv*. A small, plastic cabinet through which warm air is circulated. Used to dry in-pli wigs and other forms of postiche. 1960s.

WIGERAMA A shop or store that sells wigs. American usage, 1964.

WIG FAKER A hairdresser. Low London slang. 18/19th century. (*Partridge*)

WIGFALL A surname. Derbyshire.

WIG FASHION FORM A foam wig block. American usage.

WIGG (1) Wigg is a modern, facetious American spelling for wig, *qv*.
(2) A surname from the Anglo-Saxon wicga or wiga, a farrier. (*Charnock*)

WIG GALLOON See Galloon.

WIG GAME, THE Played by wigmakers children and apprentices. The game consisted of throwing an old wig to touch the ceiling and catching it on the head. A point was scored for each successful catch. Played as early as 1880 in the workrooms of the writer's grandfather, John Stevens.

WIGGED CHIMNEY SWEEP May Day was the sweep's holiday which they celebrated by walking in procession with blackened or whitened faces and large wigs, beating together their shovels and brushes. 'Chimney sweeps were dancing before Lord Bute's door . . . heads covered with enormous periwigs, clothes laced with paper, and faces masked with chalk.' (*Whitehall Evening Post* 26.5.1763)

WIGGEN TREE The Rowan or Mountain Ash.

WIGGER Strong. 'A wigger fellow.' 18th century Northern usage. (*Grose, Lex Bal*)

WIGGERY (1) A shop or store which sells wigs. American usage. 1964.
(2) The art and craft of designing, making, dressing, fitting, buying and selling wigs. 'The Art of Wiggery', American usage. 1964.

WIGGING Subs. A severe scolding; a rebuke.

WIGGLES Two pigtails. Slang. American usage. (*B and B*)

WIGGOMANIA A rage or mania for wigs. 1815. (*Fenton*)

WIGGOMANIAC A compulsive collector or wearer of wigs. 1815. (*Fenton*)

WIGGY (1) Bewigged.
(2) Looking like a wig. 'Her new hair style looked wiggy.'
(3) Nickname for a wig wearer.
(4) Nickname of a man with the surname Bennett. 'Wiggy Bennett', *cf* Nobby Clark. (*Partridge*)

WIG HAT A wig made of imitation hair in the form of a bonnet; a short-lived craze of 1963/4. 'Cheap and nasty-looking, disposable wig-hats.'

WIGLET A small 'top' wig for a woman that covers the crown and extends towards the hairline, without actually reaching it. A kind of toupet, *qv*.

WIGLETTE A small wig for a doll.

WIGLOMERATION Used facetiously for a ceremonial fuss

in the law court. 'The whole thing will be vastly ceremonious, wordy, unsatisfactory, and expensive, and I call it, in general, Wiglomeration.' (*Dickens, Bleak House*)

WIGMAKER (also **WIG MAKER**) One who makes wigs.

WIGMAKER'S HAMMER See Mounting hammer.

WIGMAKER'S TRIMMINGS Net, silk, gauze, thread, silks, elastic, galloon, springs, blockpoints, pins, etc.

WIGMAN A surname. From old German – 'Man of war'. See Wigg. (*Charnock*)

WIGMASTER (1) A master wig manufacturer as opposed to an employee wig worker.

(2) An expert wigmaker.

WIG MEASUREMENTS English wigmakers usually work to the following measurements:

1 Circumference (average 22″)

2 Depth or forehead to nape (av 13½″)

3 Front or ear to ear over forehead (av 11″)

4 Ear to ear over top (av 11½″)

5 Temple to temple round the back (av 14″)

6 Neck (av 4″)

Other details required are length and position of parting, colour, quality, length, type and texture of hair, straight or curled, and style.

WIG NET A close mesh, soft net of silk, cotton or nylon used as part of the foundation (the crown) of a wig, and to which the hair is knotted. See Soft wig net.

WIG-OF-FAME The wig worn by the fictional Dr Syntax in William Combe's book *The Tours of Dr Syntax*. 1819–21.

WIG-OF-NECESSITY A wig for a bald head or a sparse-haired head in contradistinction to a fashion wig, *qv*, or theatrical wig.

WIGOLOGIST One who studies wigs, or has a knowledge of wigs. (*Miami Herald* 17.11.68)

WIGOLOGY The study of wigs.

WIG OVEN A metal oven with internal trays and ventilation for low temperature drying of wet, dressed postiches on malleable blocks.

WIG PASTE An early name for grease paint.

WIG POINT Block point, *qv*. American usage.

WIG-POWDERING-CARROT (1) A carrot-shaped, wooden dredging canister.

(2) A powder-puffer of similar shape to (1), but composed of a soft, leather-covered, tapering, circular spring. The powder was ejected by compressing and releasing the spring.

WIG RIBBON Galloon, *qv*.

WIG RIG An outfit of clothing, such as that of a judge, which includes a wig. (*Mitchell*, v 2, No 4, 1964)

WIG RIOT By 1764 the fashion for men to wear wigs had so declined that the wigmakers who had been very numerous in London were thrown out of work and in great distress they drew up a petition to the King for relief and on 11th February, 1765, carried it to St James's to present it to George III. As the procession moved through the streets it was noticed that the majority of the wig makers who wanted to force the wearing of wigs on the public did not themselves wear wigs. The London mob, regarding this as monstrously unfair seized the petitioners and cut off all the wigmakers' hair by force. Horace Walpole alludes to this ludicrous incident in '*Letters to the Earle of Hertford*.' (*Book of Table Talk*, 1847)

WIGSBY (Mr Wigsby) A man wearing a wig. 18th century slang. (*Grose, Lex Bal*)

WIG SKIN Probably the bladder of pig, or sheep. Before 1861 the French Wigmakers achieved a remarkable imitation of the natural growth of hair on the head by threading human hair through an imitation skin with a needle. In this way false fronts were made that defied recognition. (*Temple Bar*, 3rd September, 1861)

WIG SPECTACLES Spectacles with extending arms for wear with wigs. Before 1780– *c* 1820. Examples in the Museum of the History of Science, Oxford and the writer's collection.

WIG SPRING (1) A flat, curved spring. See Postiche spring and Positional spring.

(2) A tension spring, *qv*.

WIG STAND (1) Made from at least the early 17th century to early 19th century. They were made from wood with a circular base, a pillar three or four feet high ending in a tapered finial on which the wig block fitted.

(2) See Mushroom.

WIG STEEL A thin, narrow band of steel 1½″ to 2″ long. Similar to, and often made from, a watch spring; used crosswise to hold the edge of the wig tight against the temples. 18th century. See also Postiche spring. (*Earle, p 264; Garsault, p 27*)

WIGSTER Wig maker. (*All the Year Round*, Vol IX *New Session*, p 450, 1873)

WIG STRETCHER An apparatus in the shape of a head divided down the middle with a screw between, which when turned forces the two sides of the head apart. Similar to a hat stretcher.

WIG TAIL (1) The tail of an 18th century wig.

(2) Name for a tropic-bird because of its long tail-feather.

WIG TREE (Rhus Cotinus) The sumach or Smoke tree.

WIG TURBAN A fashion wig, *qv* American usage.

WIG-WAG A danger signal. American usage. 20th century. (*Weseen*)

WIG WEFT Four top loops on three silks. See Thrice-in-Weft.

WIG-WITH-ONE-CURL A man's 18th century wig style. (*Tennent*)

WIG WOOD Nickname of an officer of the Artillery named Wood. 18th century. (*Fenton*)

WILD BOAR'S BACK A man's 18th century wig style. (*London Mag*, 1753)

WIMPLE A garment worn by women of the medieval period which covered the head, sides of the face, chin and neck, completely obscuring the hair.

WIMPLERS Tresses. Scottish usage. (*Scot*)

WIND See Wind-up.

WIND BLOWN The name of a short hair style originating in France late 1931 and introduced into England in 1932. Based on the shingle, but having the front hair cut and dressed to simulate a windblown appearance.

WINDBLOWN SHOCK An untidy long hair style for men. 1964. American usage.

WIND CHIMERS The beard. Slang. American usage. (*B and B*)

WINDING (1) The action of wrapping hair around a circular curler in the permanent waving process.

(2) Rolling hair on rollers.

WINDING BLOUSE Loose hair between a wound curler and the scalp caused by winding hair at an acute angle to the scalp surface, instead of winding at right angles.

WINDING JIGGER See Twisting machine and jigger (1).

WINDING KEY A device by means of which the wound hair on a curler can be tightened by turning the key of the curler within the wound hair.

WINDING MACHINE (1) See Twisting machine.

(2) A small device so constructed, that, by closing it around a long, metal curler and a strand of hair, the hair can be spirally wound by revolving the device on the curler, *c* 1926.

WINDING NEEDLE A thin, steel needle, 4″ to 8″ long, attached to a handle and used in point-winding methods of permanent waving to tuck neatly around the curler all the hair ends that protrude from the underside of the strand being wound.

WINDING PIN See Winding needle.

WINDSOR SOAP A tallow soap made at Windsor in the 19th century. (*Lillie*) 9 parts tallow, 1 part each olive oil and soda lye. The perfume is added while the soap is melting. (*E D M Vol 3*)

WINDSWEPT See Windblown.

WIND TORMENTORS The beard. Slang. American usage. (*B and B*)

WIND-UP (1) Subs. The winding of the hair on curlers preparatory to permanently curling it or when setting a head of hair.
'She has finished the wind-up.'
(2) Verb. To wind hair on curlers or rollers preparatory to permanently curling it or when setting a head of hair.
'I shall wind-up before having my tea.'

WINGAWAY BOB Bobbed hair with the ends turning slightly outwards, away from the head. 1950s.

WING FRONT Similar to the Diamond Front, *qv*, but shaped like a bird's wings, the narrow end towards the upper part of the head, the broader part towards the ears. 19th century. (*Creer*)

WING MOUSTACHE A small, flat-topped pyramidal moustache. (*Trusty*)   *101.O*

WINGS The strand of hair on either side of the head dyed a different colour from the top and back hair, *c* 1980.

WIRED CUSHION A high frame over which tall coiffures were constructed in the 18th century. (*Thornbury; Pyne*)

WIRE DRAWERS See Drawing card.

WIRE DRAWING BRUSH See Drawing card.

WIRE DRAWING MAT See Drawing card.

WIRELESS PERMANENT WAVING An exothermic permanent waving system that has no electric wires near the head.

WIRELESS WAVING See Wireless permanent waving.

WIRE MESH FOUNDATION A hair foundation incorporating a strand of wire such as a Diamond Mesh Foundation, *qv*.

WIRE WIG In the 18th and 19th century attempts were made to popularise wigs manufactured from wire. In 1758 the *Ipswich Journal* advertised a wig made of copper wire that would 'last for ever'.

WIRE WOVEN DIAMOND MESH A diamond mesh foundation incorporating weft interlaced on silks and a strand of wire.

WIRY HAIR Tough, flexible hair.

WISKE COMB A wide and slender comb with teeth on one side. 17th century. (*Holme*)

WISP (OF HAIR) A thin, narrow or slight strand of hair.

WISP BANG A short, slight, curved fringe. American usage. (*Trusty*)

WITCH HAZEL Extracted from the dried leaves of the shrub *Hamamelis Virginiana* and used in after-shave and other types of face lotion.

WITCH LOCKS Long, straight, straggly hair.

WITH-IT HAIRDO A fashionable hairdress. Usage from 1950s.

WOMAN'S KNOT A bunch of hair on the top and front of the head. See Greek hair styles.

WOOD COMB A comb made of close, light wood such as blackthorn. 17th century. (*Holme*)

WOODEN BLOCK See Wig maker's block.

WOODEN MOUNTING BLOCK A wooden, head-shaped block on which wigs and transformations are made. They are manufactured in sizes 18″ to 24″ in circumference. The 18th and early 19th century blocks often had carved faces.

WOOF Subs. The cuttings of a head of hair. 1850. (*Companion*)

WOOL Slang. A wig and by extension, human hair. 'Don't get your wool off.'

WOOL CREPE Crêpe hair.

WOOL FAT See Lanolin.

WOOLLEN WIG A letter dated 1833 refers to celebrations in 1832 following the passing of the Reform Bill, in which a procession at Tavistock, Devon, included persons representing St George, Moses, Joseph in a coat of many colours, Jason in a cocked hat, bearing the golden fleece, and Bishop Blaze in a woollen wig. (*Mrs Bray, Traditions of . . . Devonshire*, 1838)

WORK BENCH The wig maker's table at which he works hair.

WORKROOM The room in which the hair worker makes and dresses wigs and performs other tasks connected with wigmaking.

WORMWOOD (*Artemisia Absinthium*) A plant common on waste ground in England. An infusion of wormwood with a few drops of the essential oil of wormwood has been used as an astringent wash to prevent the hair falling out. (*Fernie*)
'What savour is better, if physic be true,
For places infected, than wormwood and rue.' (*Turner*, 16th century)

WORTLEY'S BERENIZON A 19th/20th century 'secret' preparation for stimulating the growth of the hair, which consisted of Peruvian balsam 3 parts; castor oil 3 parts; cantharides 4 parts; alcohol 35 parts and rosewater 40 parts. (*Koller*)

WOVEN HAIR Hair weft, *qv*.

WOVEN HORSEHAIR POMPADOUR PAD A long, hollow hair pad constructed of horsehair, light in weight and used to dress hair over for pompadour dressings, and to give height to the front.

WOVEN STEM A one-spill tail (switch).

WRAP A long strand of hair wrapped around a part of the dressing. If the strand is much wider than its thickness it is called a ribbon of hair. (*Greene*)

WRAPAROUND STYLE A woman's hair style incorporating a wrap, *qv*. (*Greene*)

WRIGGLY CURL A mobile curl that moves with the movement of the head in contrast to a static curl that remains firmly in position.

WRINKLING The doubled-back point of a badly wound curl in the permanent waving process, or in curling with the irons. Also called fishook, *qv*.

WRIST PINCUSHION A pincushion for hairpins worn on the left wrist and secured by an elastic band.

WRITHED CURL 18th century usage. The same as Corkscrew curl, *qv*. (*Stewart*)

WULFSTAN (ST), BISHOP OF WORCESTER (1012?–1095). Declaimed with vehemence against luxury of long hair as most criminal. He carried a small knife to cut off the locks. (*William of Malmesbury*)

WYCHERLEY COMBS Sets of large, beautifully engraved combs of finest tortoiseshell, named after William Wycherley (1640–1715), handsome, wig wearing playwright. These combs were carried in cases in the pockets of fashionable wig wearers and used to adjust their curls ruffled by the wind. (*Smith*)
'You might . . . praise the carvings upon a Wycherley comb, so carefully preserved by the collector of old china and such gimcracks.' (*Smith, J T*)

X

XANTHEIN The water-soluble part of the yellow colouring matter in yellow flowers. Used in colour rinses for hair.

XANTHOCHROI A subdivison of the leiotrichi or smooth-haired variety of mankind, having light-coloured hair and pale complexion.

XANTHOMELANOI In Huxley's classification of the types of mankind, is a subdivision of the leiotrichi or smooth-haired class, that has black hair and brown, olive or yellowish complexion.

XANTHOMELANOUS Having yellow, brown or olive skin and black hair.

XANTHOTRICHIA Blonde, yellow or golden coloured hair. (*Wheeler*)

XERASIA Excessive dryness of the hair.

X-RAYS A form of radiation that can penetrate many substances impervious to light.

XYSTER An instrument that was used by Barber-Surgeons to scrape and shave bones. 16/18th century. (*Bailey*)

Y

YAHOO HEAD An untidy, brutish-looking head of hair.

YAK HAIR Long, coarse, curly hair from the yak (*Poephagus Grunniens*), a wild and silky-haired, domesticated animal of the oxen family, indigenous to the uplands of Tibet, used as a beast of burden and for milk, meat and hair. The hair colours readily and is used for fantasy and theatrical wigs.

YAK TULLE FOUNDATION A tulle net of yak hair.

YARN A continuous strand of spun fibres. Distinguished from thread which is composed of two or more yarns united by twisting. Thread is used for sewing; yarn for weaving cloth.

YELLOW CAXON Man's theatrical wig style, 18th century. (*Encyc Brit*)

YELLOWING The discolouration of white hair, some of the chief causes of which are tobacco smoke and other atmospheric impurities, unsuitable detergents that contain traces of colouring matter, uric acid, iron waving at too high a temperature.

YELLOW-SOAP A soda soap of tallow, resin and lard, etc.

YELLOW WIG The characteristic wig of the Courtesan of ancient Rome. (*Juvenal*)

YLANG YLANG OIL An odoriferous oil derived from the tree *Cananginum Odoratum* of Malaysia.

YUL BRYNNER STYLE The head shaven. Named after the film star of that name, *c* 1957. *104F*

Z

ZAKEN Long-bearded. American usage.

ZAPATA MOUSTACHE The same as Mexican Moustache, *qv*. This name popularized in 1967 by Marlon Brando, the film star, in '*Viva Zapata*', a film of the Mexican Revolution.

ZAZZERA A 15th century frizzed, long, bobbed, man's hair style of Florentine origin. When this style reached London it was called *The Florentine*. (*Corson*)

ZEBEDEEAN One who shaves himself. (*Southey, The Doctor*, 1849)

ZEPHYR COIFFURE Hair styles that incorporated switches whose points were tapered and curled. In the dressing these curled ends became a prominent feature, *c* 1880.275

ZIBET A variant of civet, *qv*.

ZIBETHUM See Civet.

ZIGGURAT COIFFURE A high hairdress in which each section is smaller than that beneath it.

ZILLAH A celtic woman's name meaning 'made by ringlets'. (*Long*)

ZINCALO HAIRDRESS A gipsy hairdress.

ZITS (1) A film extra or an actor with an artificial beard. American slang. (*B and B*)
(2) A false beard. (*B and B*)

ZODIAC HAIR STYLE See A la Zodiaque.

ZOOMORPHIC HAIRDRESS Hair style incorporating or representing animal forms.

ZYMURGY The art and practice of fermentation in distilling, etc.

BIBLIOGRAPHY OF SOURCES

Original manuscripts

Bragge MS, Bragge family Devon and Dorset. 18th century Diaries

Chignon MS, The Chignon Attacked and Defended. Illustrated by CEF

Pickering MS, Pickering, Rev CF, An Illustrated Diary kept during his residence in Barotseland, Africa in the 1890s

Stevens MS, Stevens, John, MS, Work books 1860 to 1882
  Stevens and Co Work books 1882 to 1900
  Stevens, Mrs F MS Work books 1900 to 1937
  Stevens Hair Artists Ltd., Work books 1937 to 1948

Stukeley MS, Stukeley, Dr Wiliam, Of the Hair. Its History Civil and Natural, its uses and diseases, with remarks on the extravagant folly and ridiculous custom of cutting it off, and how far tis prejudicial to health. 1724. Original manuscript in possession of the editor.

Stukeley MS, Stukeley, W On the Use of Perukes. 1725. Original manuscript in possession of the editor.

Printed works

An Account of the Old Hairy Gentleman, 1679. (Not in Wing)

An act for granting to His Majesty a duty on certificates issued for using Hair Powder. (30 April 1795)

Addison, Joseph, *Works*, ed G Greene, NY 1856

Address, An, to the Worshipful Company of Barbers in Oxford; occasioned by a late Infamous Libel, intitled, *The Barber and Fireworks*, a Fable, highly reflecting on one of the Honourable Members, by a Barber. The second edition, Oxford 1749

Airola, Paavo, O, *Stop Hair Loss*, New Swedish Discovery, Phoenix, Arizona 1965. 2nd ed 1970, 3rd ed 1972

Akerman, J Y, *A Glossary of Words*, Wiltshire 1842

Alexandre, P, *La Beauté de la Chevelure*, Paris 1924

Alexis of Piedmont, The Secretes of, translated by W Warde. ed 1568

Almanach de la toilette et de la Coëffure des dames Françoises, 1777

American Hairdresser vol 38 No. 5, May 1915

Ames, R, *Islington-Wells*, 1691

Anderson, E, *Hair Care*, 1967

Andrews, A, *The Eighteenth Century*, 1856

Andrews, W, *At The Sign of the Barbers Pole*

Andrews, W, *England in the Days of Old*, 1897

Anstey, C, *The New Bath Guide*, ed 1832

Apologie des Dames, les jolies Françaises leur coiffures et habillemens, 1781

An Apology for the Beard by Artium Magister, 1862

Apuleius, L, *The Golden Asse*, 1566, trans by William Adlington

Archaeologia Cantiana

Arkell, W J and Tomkeieff, *English Rock Terms*, 1953

Arnold, J, *Perukes and Periwigs*, HMSO 1970

Art of Preserving, *The Art of Preserving The Hair*, 1825

Askinson, G W, *Perfumes and their Preparation*, 1892

Asser, J, *Historic Hairdressing*, 1966

Astbury, W T, *Fundamentals of Fibre Structure*, 1933

Aubrey, J (1626–1697), *Brief Lives*, ed A Clark, 1898

Aurand, A M, *The Amish and the Mennonites*, Harrisburg, Penna 1938

Aurand, A M, *Little Known Facts about the Witches in our Hair*, Harrisburg, Penna 1938

Austin, H H, *Old stick leg*, 1921

Austin, Alfred, *Poetical Works*

Auzary, J, *Notions de Technologie général pour L'apprenti Coiffeur pour Dames*. Illustrated, 4th ed Paris 1964

Badcock, J, *Sportsman's Slang by John Bee*, 1827

Bailet, G, Price List, Bailet et Cie, Court Hairdressers, New Bond Street, London *c* 1905

Bailey, N, *An Universal Etymological English Dictionary*, 4th ed 1728

Bajerus, John Jacob, *Dissertatio Medica Inauguralis de Capillis*, Jenae 1700

Baker and Wade, Price List, Manchester 1972

A Ballad: Occasion'd by some ladies wearing Ruffs at Court . . . London, 1727 (by courtesy of Dr Lois Morrison)

Balzac, *Annuaire et Liste de Messieurs Les Perruquiers et Coiffeurs de la Ville de Paris pour l'an 1827*, Paris 1827

Barber, Mary, *Poems on Several Occasions*, 1735

The Barbers Wedding, Broadside with plate by Cruickshank, 1 July 1791 by J W Fores, No. 3 Piccadilly

Bardsley, C W, *English Surnames*, 1875

Baret, J, *An Alvearie or Quadruple Dictionarie*, 1580

Barham, Rev R H, *The Ingoldsby Legends*, 1840/42/47

Barker, William (Hairdresser) *A Treatise on the Principles of Hairdressing*, 1785

Barnes, W, *A Glossary of the Dorset Dialect*, 1886

Barondes, R de Rohan, *China: Lore, Legend and Lyrics*, NY 1960

Barr, R A, *British Rugby Team in Maoriland*, Dunedin 1908

Barrow, J, *A New and Universal Dictionary of Arts and Sciences*, 1751

Barry, D, *Ram-Alley*, 1611 (Greg 292)

Bayan, R G, *Armenian Proverbs*, Venice 1909

Beaumont, F and Fletcher, J, *Comedies and Tragedies*, ed 1647

Beck, Thomas, *The Age of Frivolity*, 2nd ed 1807

Beck, S W, *The Draper's Dictionary*, ND *c* 1890

Behn, A, *The Younger Brother*, 1696

Beigel, H, *The Human Hair*, 1869

Belcher, N, *The Barbers' and Hair Dressers' Private Recipe Book*, Boston 1868

Belden, E P, *New York: Past, Present and Future*. 4th ed NY 1851

Benét, W R, *The Reader's Encyclopaedia*, NY 1963

Benham, W G, *Cassell's Book of Quotations*, ed 1914

Bentley, Mr *The Rural Philosopher*, 1775

Bentley, *Miscellany*, v 53, p 537 (False Hair)

Berg, C, *The Unconscious Significance of Hair*. 1951

Berrey, L V, and M Van Den Bark, *The American Thesaurus of Slang*, 2nd ed, NY 1952

Bickham, G, *The Ladies Toilet*, 1768
Le Bijou des Dames, 1779
Bisignano, F, *The Wig Story*, Torrance, California 1962
Blanc, Charles, *Art in Ornament and Dress*, ed 1877
Bland, R, *Proverbs . . .* 1814
Blondel, S, *L'Art. Capillaire dans L'inde, à la chine et au Japon*, 1889
Bold, Henry, *Anniversary to the King's Most Excellent Majesty Charles the II* (poem), 1661
Bombaugh, L C, *Gleanings for the Curious*, 1890
Bonnerjea, B, *A Dictionary of Superstitions and Mythology*, 1927
Bonomo, J, *How to wear your Hair*, NY 1954
Botham, M and Sharrad, L, *Manual of Wigmaking*, 1964
Boxiana (by Pierce Egan) 1818–24
Brachet, A, *An Etymological Dictionary of the French Language*. 3rd ed, 1882
Bramston, James, *The Art of Politicks*, 1729
Brand, J, *Observations on the Popular Antiquities of Great Britain*, ed 1849
Brathwait, R, *The English Gentleman and English Gentlewoman*, 3rd ed 1641
Bray, W, *Everyday Life of the Aztecs*, 1968
Brewer, E C, *Dictionary of Phrase and Fable*, *The Historic note-book*, *The Reader's Handbook*
Brighte, J, *The Book to keep the Spirits up*. Halifax 1867
The British Legacy, 1754 (p 122/3 The art of curling, dressing and colouring hair)
British Museum Handbook to the Ethnographical Collections
Britten, J, and Holland, R, *A Dictionary of English plant names*, 1878
Britten, J, *Old Country and Farming Words*, 1880
Brodie, J, 41 Museum St, London WC. Price List dated 1890
Brome, F, *Five new playes*, 1659
Brown, T, *A Dictionary of the Scottish Language*, 1845
Brown, T, *Letters from the Dead to the Living*, 1702
Browne, F, *Professor Browne's Toilet Almanack*, 1861
Prof Frederick Browne was appointed hair dresser to the London Rifle Volunteers
Browning, R, *Collected Works*, 1896
Brusonii (*L Domitii*) *facetiarum exemplorumque lib VII*, Rome 1518
Budge, E A, Wallis (ed) *Oriental Wit and Wisdom* collected by Mar Gregory John Bar-Hebraeus, 13th century, 1899
Buerlinus, J, *De Foeminis ex suppressione mensium barbatis: altdorfina*, 1664
Bullock, W, *Six Month's Residence and Travels in Mexico*, 1822
Bulwer, J, *Anthropometamorphosis*. 2nd ed 1653
Burchardus de Bellevaux, *Apologia de Barbis* (12th century treatise on beards) 1935
Burney, W, *A New Universal Dictionary of the Marine*, 1815
Burns, R, *Poems*, ed 1794
Burton, Robert, *Anatomy of Melancholy*, 1st ed 1621 4th ed 1632
Button and Button-Hole: *With a Character of the Drabs*, London 1723 (by courtesy of Dr Lois Morrison)
Bysterveld, Henri de. *Album de Coiffures historiques*. 5 vols 1863–67 (Colas 499)

Canadian Hairdressers' Manual, The, Anon, foreword by H Crisford, ND
Canel, Alfred, *Histoire de la Barbe et des cheveux en Normandie*. Rouen 1859
Carew, B M, *Life and Adventures of Bampfylde Moore Carew*, 1788
Carew, T, *Poems*, ed 1670
Carlow, J, *Carlow on Hairpieces*, Jersey City 1964
Carter, T, *Curiosities of War*, 1860
Carter, W, *Rhythmical Essays on the Beard question*
Cartwright, E R, *A Late Summer*, 1964
Caulfield, James, *Chalcographimania*, 1814
Caulfield, S F A and Saward, B C, *A Dictionary of Needlework*, 1882
Century Dictionary, The, ed W D Whitney, 1891
Chalmers, G, *The Life of Mary Queen of Scots*, 1818
Chambers, Ephriam, *Cyclopaedia*, 1746 (1st ed 1728)
Chambers's Mineralogical Dictionary, ed 1960
Chambers' Journal, 1866
v 44, p 657 – 'Artists in Hair'; v 36, p 65 – 'False Hair';
v 30, p 119 – 'Harvest of Hair'; v 46, p 465 – 'Real and False Hair'.
Chapman, R W, (editor), *The Novels of Jane Austen*, ed 1926
Champion, S G, *The Eleven Religions and their Proverbial Lore*, 1944
Charles, A and Delanfrasio, R, *The History of Hair*, NY 1970
Charnock, R S, *Ludus Patronymics*, 1868
Chatterton, T, *Poems*, 1777, *Miscellanies*, 1778
Chaucer, G, *The Complete Works* (Canterbury Tales 1387–1400) ed 1933
Child, T, *Wimples and Crisping Pins*, 1895
Children's Hair Care, Dell Pub Co Inc, N Y 1962
Christy, R, *Proverbs, Maxims and Phrases of all Ages*, NY 1907
Clerk, William (editor), A *Dictionarie in English and Latine for Children*, ed 1602. Originally written by J Withals, STC 25884
Cobbett, W, *Rural Rides*, 1823
Cockeram, H, *The English Dictionarie*, 1623
Coclès, Barthélemy, *Physiognomonia*, Strasbourg 1533
Cocroft, S, *The Art of Keeping Young*, ND *c* 1910
Codex, Azcatitlan, *Journal de la Societe des Americanistes*, Nouvelle Série, vol 38, Paris 1949
Le Coiffeur Europeen, Paris 1864–1874+
Colas, R, *Bibliographie Générale du costume et de la mode*. Paris 1933
Coleridge, S T, *Poetical Works*
Collier, John, *The Battle of the Flying Dragon*, ND (*c* 1740)
Colman, G, *Haut Ton*
The companion to a cigar: by a veteran, 1850
Colton, R, *Pedestrian and Other Reminiscences*, 1846
Coma Berenices; or, *The Hairy Comet*, (an exposure of the vanity of wearing long hair and perriwigs), 1676. (Wing, *c* 5434)
Comenius, J O, *Janua Linguarum Trilinguis*, 1662
Conference, The; or *Gregg's Ghost*, 1711
Connoisseur, 31 January, 1754–30 September 1756, ed George Colman and Bonnell Thornton
Cook, D, (editor J Stevens Cox), *Historical Notes on Wigs*, Guernsey 1980
Cooley, A J, *The Toilet and Cosmetic Arts*, 1866
Cooney, S and Harper, C, *Wigs*, New Jersey 1973

Cooper, T, *Thesaurus Linguae Romanae et Britannicae*, ed 1584

Cooper, W, *Hair*, 1971

Cordwell, M and Rudoy, M, *Hair Design and Fashion*, NY 1956

Corson, R, *Fashions in Hair*, 1965

Corson, R, *Stage Make-up*, 1961

Cortambert, R, *Essai sur la chevelure des différents peuples*, 1861

Coryate, T, *Crudities*, 1611

Cotgrave, R, *A Dictionarie of the French and English Tongues*, 1611

Cotton, Charles, *Poems on Several Occasions*, 1689

Coulon, Dr H, *La Communauté des Chirurgiens-barbiers de Cambrai* (1366–1795), Cambrai 1908

Country Gentleman's Vade Mecum, The by ES, 1699

Cowley, A, *Poems*, 1656

Cowper, W, *The Task*, 1784

Cox, J Stevens, *Romano-British Bone Hairpins and Needles found at Ilchester between 1948 and 1955*, Guernsey 1982

Cox, J Stevens, *The Hair-Pedlar in Devon*, Toucan Press 1968

Cox, J Stevens, *The Construction of an Ancient Egyptian Wig* (c 1400 bc) *in The British Museum*, 1st ed, Guernsey 1975; 2nd ed, Guernsey 1978 (reprinted from *The Journal of Egyptian Archaeology*, vol 63, 1977)

Cox, J Stevens, *Dorset Folk Remedies*, 1962

Cox, J Stevens, *A History of Ilchester*, 1958

Cox, J Stevens, (editor) *The Art of the Wigmaker*, 1961

Cox, J Stevens, (editor) *The Wigmaker's Art in the 18th Century*, 1965

Cox, J Stevens, *The Physical Reason for Hair Curl and Wave*, 1964

Crabbe, Rev G, *Poems*, 1807

Crashaw, R, *Complete Works*, 1858

Creer, E, *Lessons in Hairdressing*. 1st ed 1877

Creer, E, *Board-Work*; or the *Art of Wig-making*, etc, 1887

Croisat, *Méthode de Coiffure*. Paris 1831

Croisat, *Théorie de L'Art du Coiffeur*, Paris 1847

Croisat, (ed) *Les Cent – Un Coiffeurs de Tous les Pays*, Paris vol I, 1836 – vol 5, 1841

Crosby's Merchant's and Tradesman's Pocket Directory, 1808

Cunnington, C W and P, (with C Beard), *A Dictionary of English Costume*, 1960

Cunnington, C W and P, *Handbook of English Costume in the 18th Century*, 1957

Cunnington, C W and P, *Handbook of English Costume in the 17th Century*, ed 1963

Daily Express, London

Daily Mirror, London

Daily News, London

The Daily Telegraph, London

Dandymania; being a dissertation on modern dandies, N D c 1820

Dartnell, G E and Goddard, E H, *Contributions towards a Wiltshire Glossary*, (Wilts Nat Hist Mag vol XXVII, p 124)

Das Buch der Haare und Bärte, 1844

Davies, T L O, *A Supplementary English Glossary*, 1881

Davis, M A J, *Law and Hairdressing*, 1964 *Outline of Law for Hairdressers*, 1965

Day, John, *Workes*, 1881

De Navarre, M G, *The Chemistry and Manufacture of Cosmetics*. N Y 1947

Debay, A, *Hygiène Médicale des Cheveux et de la Barbe*, Paris 1854

A Defence of Shorte Haire. Entered on the Register of the Stationers' Company, 3 February 1592/3, by John Wolfe

Deguerle, J M N, *Eloge des peruques*, 1799

Dekker, T, *The Seven Deadly Sinnes of London*, 1606

Dekker, T, *The Wonderfull Yeare*, 1603

Dekker, T, *The Meeting of Gallants*, 1604

Dekker, T, *A tragi-comedy called Match mee in London*, 1631

Dekker, T, *Works*

Dekker, T, *The Guls Horne-Booke*, 1609

Denham, M A, *Proverbial Folk Lore of Newcastle upon Tyne*, Richmond 1855 *Supplement to the Local Rhymes . . . of Durham*, Durham 1859

Denny, G G, *Fabrics*, Chicago, 4th ed 1936

Dennys, N B, *The Folk-Lore of China*, Hong Kong 1876

Derham, W, (editor) *Philosophical Letters between Mr Ray . . . and correspondents*, 1718

Dickens, C, *Sketches by Boz* ed 1839

Dickens, C, (ed) *All The Year Round*, 1859–1895

Dictionary of National Biography

Dissertatio Historico . . . De Origine, usu et administratione aldificii e Capillis in fronte erecti, et vulgo Cacadou . . . Breslau 1772

A Dissertation upon head dress; together with a Brief vindication of high coloured hair, and of those ladies on whom it grows. By an English Periwig-maker, 1767. 8vo (Copy sold at Sotheby's, 2 July 1946, lot 1)

Dodsley, R, *Sir John Cockle at Court* (play), 1738

Doran, Dr, *Habits and Men*, 1854

Douce, F, *Illustrations of Shakespeare*, ed 1807

Dryden, John, *Works*, 1760

Duflos, L J, *Essai sur la culture des cheveux*, 1812

Dulac, E, *Physiologie de la Barbe et des Moustaches*, 1842

Dulaure, J A, *Pogonologia*, (translated from French), Exeter 1786

D'Urfey, T, *New Operas*, 1721

D'urfey, T, *The Plague of Impertinence*: or *A Barber a Fury*, 1721

Dussauce, M, *A Practical Guide for The Perfumer*. Philadelphia 1868

Dyer, A E R, (editor) *Hairdressers' Technical Encyclopedia*, 1949

Dyer, I, *Science of Shaving*, 1727

Earle, A M, *Costume of Colonial Times*, 1894

Edgeworth, M Harrington, a tale; and Ormond, a tale, 1817

Edwards, E, *Words, Facts and Phrases*, ed 1897

Edwards, C, *History and Poetry of Finger-Rings*, Redfield 1855

Edwards T J, *Military Customs*, ed 1961

Elegant Arts for Ladies. N/D c 1870, P Ward and Lock

Eliot, G, *The Spanish Gypsy*, 1868

Elliott, MB, *Rustic Excursions*, N/D c 1830

Ellman, E B, *Recollections of a Sussex Parson*, 1912

Elworthy, F T, *West Somerset Word-Book*, 1886

England's Vanity, 1683

English, L E F, *Historic Newfoundland*, 5th ed 1972

Enquire within upon Everything, 1856

Epigrams: Original and Selected, Anon, 1877

Esar, E, *The Treasury of Humorous Quotations*, (ed N Bentley), ed 1967

The Eugène Method of Permanent Waving, N Y 1928

Evelyn, J and M, *Mundus Mulieribus*, 1690

Every-Lady's Own Fortune-Teller, 1793

Eze, M G and Marcel, A, *Histoire de la Coiffure des Femmes en France*, 1886

Fairholt, F W, *Costume in England*, ed 1896

Fairholt, F W, *A Dictionary of Terms in Art*, N/D

Fangé, Abbe, *Memoires Pour servir a L'Histoire de la Barbe de l'Homme. Liege*, 1774

Farmer, J S and Henley, W E, *Slang and it's Analogues*, 1890–1904

Fashion, An Epistolatory Satire to a Friend, 1742

Fenton, Richard, *Memoirs of An Old Wig*, 1815

Ferguson, G, *Signs and Symbols in Christian Art*, N Y 1954

Fernie, W T, *Herbal Simples*, 2nd ed, Bristol 1897

Ferrario, G H, *Costume Antico e Moderno*, Florence 1823–1830

Fielding, I, *Select proverbs of all nations*, c 1830

Firor, R A, *Folkways in Thomas Hardy*, ed N Y 1962

Fisher, J L, *A Medieval Farming Glossary*, 1968

Fitzpatrick, P V, *Thaumaturgus*, 1828

Fleischmann, H, *Dessous de Princesses et Maréchales d'Empire*, Paris 1909

Flitman, S G, *The Craft of ladies hairdressing*, 1959
Hairdressing, Hairdressers and Disease, 1963
High Frequency and Vibration, 1964
The Scalp, Hair and Nails in Health and Disease, 1973

Foan, G A (ed), *The Art and Craft of Hairdressing*, new ed J Bari-Woollss, N/D

Forbes, R J, *Studies in Ancient Technology*, v 3, Leiden 1955

Forby, R, *The Vocabulary of East Anglia*, 1830–58

Forster, J, *Life of Goldsmith*

Fosbroke, T D, *Synopsis of Ancient Costume*, 1825

Francis, G, *The Dictionary of Practical Receipts*, 1848

Franke, Prof Dr, *Technological Dictionary*, Wiesbaden 1855

Franklyn, J, *A Dictionary of Nicknames*, 1962

Fraser, E and Gibbons, J, *Soldiers and Sailors Words and Phrases*, 1925

Frazer, J G, *The Golden Bough*, ed 1923

Frek, *Life, Journal of the Society for Folk Life Studies*

Fry, John (editor), *Pieces of Ancient Poetry*, Bristol 1814

Fuller, T, *Works*

Fuller, Thomas, *Gnomologia*. A Collection of English Proverbs, 1732

Gales, R L, *Dwellers in Arcady*, 1931

Gallery of Literary Morceaux. 3rd ed 1835

Gardner, A, *Hair and Head-dress*, 1050–1600. *Journal of the British Archaeological Association*. 3rd Series, vol XIII 1950 p 4

Garsault, F A P de, *Art du Perruquier*, 5 plts, Folio 1797 (Sotheby, 2 July 1957, lot 542)

Garsault, F A P de, *The Art of the Wigmaker*, 1767. English translation, ed J Stevens Cox, 1961

Gaskell, G A, *A Dictionary of the Sacred Language*, 1923

Gay, John, *Poetical Works*

Gayton, E, *Pleasant Notes upon Don Quixote*, 1654

Geary, Francis N, *Lay of the Red Moustache*, 1851

General Shop Book, The, 1753

Gents' Acad, London Gentlemen's Hairdressing Academy, *Beard Styles*, ND

Gentleman's Magazine, 1731–1907

The Gentleman's Magazine of Fashions, vol I, May to December 1828

Gerarde, J, *Herball*, 1597

Gilchrist, Peter, *A Treatise on the Hair; or Every Lady her own Hair Dresser*, London 1770–87

Gillray, J, *The Caricatures of Gillray*. N/D c 1825

Girl's Own Paper

Gissler, A, *Technologie de la Coiffure*. Illustrated, 3rd ed Paris 1963

The Globe (newspaper)

Glossographia Anglicana Nova or a Dictionary interpreting such hard words '. . . as are at Present used in the English Tongue . . .' 1707

Godey's Magazine, Philadelphia and N Y, vols I (1830) – Vol 131 (1898). Through the years the title was varied, at first it was *The Ladies' Book* and by 1898 it had become *Godey's Magazine*

Goldin, H E (editor), A *Dictionary of American Underworld Lingo*. NY 1950

Goldsmith, O, *She Stoops to Conquer*, 1773

Good, J M, Gregory, O, and Bosworth, N, *Pantologia*, 1819

Goodridge, C M, *Narrative of a Voyage to the South Seas*, ed 1847

Gosson, S, *Quippes for Upstart Newfangled Gentlewomen*, 1595 STC 12096

Gowing, T S, *The Philosophy of Beards*, Ipswich ND

Grand-Carteret, J, *Les Elegances de la Toilette*, 1911

Graves, Richard, *Lucubrations by Peter of Pontefract*, 1786

Graves, R, *The Spiritual Quixote*, 1772

Greene, R, *A Quip for an Upstart Courtier*, 1592

Greene, W, *Styles and Sets for Long Hair*, NY 1966

Greg, W W, *A Bibliography of the English printed drama to the Restoration*, 1939–59

Gregory, A T, *Devonshire Verbal Provincialisms*, 1909

Griffith, G B, *A Journey Across The Desert*, 1845

Griffith, S Y, *New Historical Description of Cheltenham*, 1826

Grose, F, *A Classical Dictionary of the Vulgar Tongue*, 1785

Grose, F, *A Guide to Health, Beauty, Riches and Honour*, 2nd ed 1796

Grose, F, *Lexicon Balatronicum*, 1811

Grose, F, *A Provincial Glossary*, 1787

The Guardian, ed 1797

Guasco, F E, *Delli ornatrici . . .* 1775

Guernsey Magazine, The, vol XII, 1884

Guevara, Anthony of, *Diall of Princess*, 1557. Trans by Sir Thomas North

Guillim, J, *A Display of Heraldrie*, 4th ed 1660

Gunn, F, *The Artificial Face*, 1973

Gurney, Thomas, *The Trichologists Pharmacopoeia*, 1889

Guske, F and Henschel, H, *Die arbeit in Friseursalon*, Leipzig 1965

Gussman, Paul, *Zeichenvorlagen für den fachschul-unterricht im peruckenmachergewerbe*, 1910

Haigh, A E, *The Attic Theatre*, Oxford 1898

Hair Fashion by 'Debra' Postiche, 1965

Hair and Beauty

Hair Styling (magazine), NY

Hair and Scalp, The, by a Doctor of Medicine, 1903

Hair in Motion, c 1965: Illustrated wig styles pub by Brentwood Imperial Wig Co, California

Hairdressers' Chronicle (founded 1866)

Hairdressers' Journal

Hairdressers' Weekly Journal

Hairdressing Trade Directory, ed 1963, (pub by *Hairdressers' Journal*)

Hairdressing, a monthly journal for hairdressers and beauty specialists, no. 3, vol III (new series). Pub July 1924

Hairdressing Illustrated, ed Gaston Emile

Hakluyt, Richard, *Principal Navigations*, ed 1599–1600

Halhed, N B, *Imitations of Some Epigrams of Mastial*, 1793

Hall, J, *Virgidemiarum*, 1597/8

Hall, R P, *A Treatise on the Hair*, Nashua, New Hampshire 1866

Hall, T, *The Loathsomnesse of Long Haire*, 1654

Halliwell, J O, *The Nursery Rhymes of England*, ed 1844

Halpine, C G, (1829–1868) *Janette's Hair*

Hamersley, R, *Advice to Sunday Barbers, against Trimming on the Lord's Day*, 1706

Hammond, J (1710–1742), *Love Elegies*, ed 1805

Hanle, D Z, *The Hairdo Handbook*, NY 1964

Hanle, D Z, (editor), *Hair Pieces and Wig Styles*, Washington 1965

Havighurst, W, *Proud Prisoner*, NY 1964

Harrison, G, *Theatricals and Tableaux Vivants for Amateurs*, 1882

Harvey, Gabriel, *The Trimming of Thomas Nashe Gentleman*, 1597 (STC 12906)

Hazlitt, W Carew, *English Proverbs*, 2nd ed 1882

Hearth and Home 17 Sept 1903

Harrison, M, *The History of the Hat*, 1960

Hartrampf's Vocabularies, ed 1938

Hashimoto, Sumiko, *Old Japanese Coiffure*, Tokyo 1967

Hastings, J (editor), *Encyclopedia of Religion and Ethics*, 1937

Henderson, A, *Scottish Proverbs*, Edinburgh 1832

Henderson, W (editor), *Victorian Street Ballads*, 1937

Hendricks, G D, *Mirrors, Mice and Mustaches*, Dallas, USA 1966

Henning, J, *Trichologia, id est De Capillis Veterum Collectanea Historico-Philologica*, 1678

Henningsen, H, *Crossing the Equator*, Copenhagen 1961

Hentzner, Paul, *Itinerarium*, 1612

Herbert, George, *The Temple*, 1633

Herbert, George, *Outlandish Proverbs*, 1639

Herbert, Thomas, *Some Years Travels into Diverse Parts of Africa . . .* ed 1677

Heron, Robert, *The Comforts of Human Life*, 1807

Herrick, R, *Hesperides*, 1648

Hewett, S, *The Peasant Speech of Devon*, 2nd ed 1892

Heywood, T, *The English Traveller*, 1633

Heywoode, John, *Works*, 1562

Hickeringill, E, *Reflections on a Late Libel*, 1680

Hill, Richard, *The Sky-Rocket*, 1782

Hippocrates, *Opera Ommia*. Venice 1526

Hiscox, G D (editor), *Henley's Twentieth Century Formulas, Recipes and Processes*. ed 1930

A History of Technology, ed by Charles Singer, E J Holmyard and A R Hall, vol. I, Oxford 1954

Holley, M A, *Josiah Allen's Wife, c* 1896

Holloway, W, *A General Dictionary of Provincialisms*. Lewes 1839

Holme, Randle, *The Academy of Armory*. Chester 1688

Home Companion, vol 3, 1853

Homer, *The Whole Works*, 1616

Hone, William, *The Every-Day Book and Table Book*, 1838 EDB

Hone, William, *The Every-Day Book*, 1826–7

Hone, William, *The Year Book*, 1832

Hook, T E (1788–1841), *Bon-Mots of Samuel Foote and Theodore Hook*, 1894

Horace, *All the Odes*, 1638

Horman, W, *Vulgaria*, 1519

Hotman, A, *Jucundus et Veré Lectu dignus de Barba et Coma*, 1628

Hovenden's Handbook, 1939

How to Arrange The Hair, by one of the Ladies' Committee of Almacks, 1857

How to do Better Hair Coloring, Pub by Clairol Inc Stanford, Conn 1962

Howell, James, *Epistolae*, 1645

Howell, James, *Lexicon Tetraglotton*, 1660

Hoyerus, G L, *De Foemina barbata* (see *Acta Physico-Medica Academiae . . .* Nuremburg 1737, IV

Hudibras, 1662–78 by S Butler

Hunter, J, *The Hallamshire Glossary*, 1827

Huxley, T H, *On a Hitherto Undescribed Structure in the Human Hair Sheath*, (Lond Med Gaz 1845) describes 'Huxley's layer' and 'membrane' of the root of the hair follicle.

Huxley, T H, *On the Methods and Results of Ethnology*, 1865. Includes Huxley's classification of mankind by means of the hair.

The Idler, (editor) S Johnson (April 1758 – April 1760) ed 1816

Ingels, M, *Willis Haviland Carrier, Father of Air Conditioning*, Garden City 1952

Ingeria, *Long Hair* (Book 2)

Inouye, J, *Home Life in Tokyo*, 1911

James, C, *Military Dictionary*, 3rd ed 1810

Jankow, J A, *How to fix your Electric Shaver*, NY 1956

Javrett, A, Spearman, R I C and Riley, P A, *Dermatology*, 1966

Jeameson, T, *Artificiall Embellishments*, Oxford 1665

The Jewellers' Book of Patterns in Hair Work. Containing a great variety of copper-plate engravings of Devices and Patterns in hair; suitable for Mourning Jewellery, Brooches, Rings, Guards, Alberts, Necklets, Lockets, Bracelets, Miniatures, Studs, Links Earrings, etc, etc, etc. Published by W Halford and C Young, Manufacturing Jewellers, 160 St John Road, Clerkenwell, London. (*c* 1860)

Jewish Encyclopaedia, 1901–6

Joch, J G, *Dissertatio de foeminis barbatis*. Jena 1702

Johnson, H, *Creative Hairdo Ideas*. Greenwich, Connecticut 1962

Jones, D H, *How to give Haircuts at Home*. Los Angeles 1954

Jones, Col W D, *Records of the Royal Military Academy*, 1851

Jonson, B, *Epicene*, 1610, Works 1616–1640

Juvenal, *The Satires*, 1693

Kaemmerer, L, *Chodowiecki*. Leipzig, 1897

Kelly, J, *A Complete Collection of Scottish Proverbs*, 1721

Kelly, W K, *Proverbs of all Nations*, 1852

Ken and Company Limited, *Catalogue of Hairdressers' Sundries* 87 Newman St, W1 N/D (*c* 1936)

Kendall, T, *Flowers of Epigrammes*, 1577

Kennett, R H, *Ancient Hebrew Social Life and Custom as indicated in Law Narrative and Metaphor*, 1933

The Kentish Post, no. 1, 1717 to no. 5281, 1768

Kibbe, C V, *Standard Text Book of Cosmetology*, NY

Kidd, W, *Direction of Hair in Animals and Man*, 1903

Kilgour, O F G and McGarry, M, *An Introduction to Science and Hygiene for Hairdressers*, 1964

Killigrew, Henry, *A Book of New Epigrams*, 1695

Kingsbury, B, *A Treatise on Razors*, 9th ed, 1821

Kirchmaier, G G, *De Gloria et Majestate Barba*

Knöss, C, *Der Friseur*. Illustrated, Giessen 1961

Koken-Chisholm Corporation. Illustrated Catalog Barbers' Chairs and Barber Shop Equipment. ND (*c* 1925) K-S Corp, 755 East 134th St NY

Koller, T, *Cosmetics*, 1902

Korf, F, *Art and Fundamentals of Hairdressing*, *c* 1923

Korf, F, *Artistic Hair Cutting*, NY 1923

Korf, F, *Scientific Care of Hair and Scalp*, vol 5, Blue Book Series of Hair and Beauty Culture, NY 1925

La Sauvegarde des Coiffeurs, 1899

The Ladies' Companion, July 1851 (Article 'The Hair' by Miss M A Youat)

The Ladies' Dictionary, 1694 by N H (writer not identified)

The Lady

Lady's Pictorial, 1905–6

Lafoy, J B, *The Complete Coiffeur*, NY 1817

Lambert, G, *The Barbers' Company*. A paper read before The British Archaeological Association (15 Oct 1881)

Lane, E W, *An Account of the Manners and Customs of the Modern Egyptians*, 1836

Larwood, J and Hotten, J C, *The History of Signboards*, ed 1898

Laughing Philosopher, The, Dublin, ND (*c* 1780)

Lancet, 1857

Lawall, O H, *Four Thousand Years of Pharmacy*, 1927

Lawrence E, *The Hair in Health and Disease*, 1936

Lawson, E M, *The Nation in the Parish* (Upton-on-Severn) 1884

L'Eguillard, P, *Enopogonérythrée*, Caen 1580

Le Moniteur de la Coiffure

Le Moniteur de la Mode

L'Illustration de la Coiffure. (no. 13, 2nd Year, 1903)

Le Journal de la Coiffure, no. 19, 1903

Le Coiffeur Européen. (1865 et seq)

Le Congres des Coiffeurs (no. 158, 1903)

Ledoux, H, *50 Lecons de Coiffure: coupe, Mise en plis, ondulation*, 1931

Le Fournier, A, *La Décoration d'humaine Nature et Adornement des Dames*, Paris 1530; Lyons 1537; Lyons 1540

Leach, M (editor) *Dictionary of Folklore*. NY 1949–50

Lean's Collectanea. Bristol 1902–04

Leather, E M, *Folk-Lore of Herefordshire*

Lee, G E (editor), *News from the Channel* . . . to which are added a few notes by Elie Brevit, Guernsey 1902. A reprint of a lost original, small 4to pamphlet, dated 1673. Not recorded by Wing.

Lee, James Zee-Min, *Chinese Potpouri* (chapter on the Queue) Hong Kong 1950

Lee, C M and Inglis, J K, *Science for Hairdressing Students*, 1964

Leftwich, R W, *The Preservation of the Hair*. 1st ed 1901, 2nd ed 1902

Legros, *L'Art de la coëffure des dames Françoises*, 1768

Legros *The Ladies' Toilet*, or *The Art of Head-dressing*, 1768 30 plates engraved by G Bickham

Lempriere, J, *A Classical Dictionary*

Lennox, Lady Sarah, *Life and Letters*. 1745–1826, ed Countess of Ilchester and Lord Stavordale, 1961

Levens, P, *Manipulus Vocabulorum*, 1570

Levin, O L, *Your Hair and Your Health*, 1926

Levin, O L, and Behrman, H T, *Your Hair and its Care*. NY 1945

Leyel, C F, *Elixirs of Life*, 1948

Lichtenfeld, J, *Principles of Modern Hairdressing* (*c* 1880)
Principles of Physiognomical Hairdressing (*c* 1881)

Liebaut, J, *Trois Livres d'Embellissement et Ornement de Corps Humain*, Paris 1582; Lyons 1595

Lillie, C, *The British Perfumer*. 2nd ed 1822

Ling, N, *Politeuphuia*, ed 1678

Little Gipsy Girl, The; or *Universal Fortune-Teller*, 1799

London Academy of Gentlemen's Hairdressing, Rules and Technical Hand Book of the Academy, 1928

London Chronicle from 1757 to 1823

London Magazine, 1753

London Magazine, v 33, 1764

London Society, v 15, p 547 (Trade in Hair)

Long, H A, *Personal and Family Names*, 1883

Longman, E D and Loch, S, *Pins and Pincushions*, 1911

Lubowe, J J, *New Hope for Your Hair*. NY ed 1961

Lubowe, J J and Huss, B, *A Teen-Age Guide to Healthy Skin and Hair*, NY 1965

Lucas, A, *Ancient Egyptian Materials and Industries*. 2nd ed 1934

Lydgate, J (1370?–1450?), The *Hystorye Sige and Dystruccyon of Troye*, 1513

Lyly, J, *Euphues*, 1578

MacEwan, P, (editor) *Pharmaceutical Formulas*, 1899

Macfadden, B, *Hair Culture*, NY 1943

Macneill, Hector, *The Poetical Works* 1801

Macramé Lace by the Silkworm N/D (*c* 1880). Pub. by Madame Goubaud. 39 Bedford St, Covent Garden

Malaparte, C, *The Skin*, 1952

Magister, A, *Apology for the Beard* 1862

Mahomed, S D, *Shampooing*, Brighton 1826

Mallemont, A, *History of Ladies' Hairdressing*. Translated by C Klein from the French, 1904

Mallemont, A, *Manual of Ladies' Hairdressing*, 1899

Marchand, J H, *L'Enciclopédie Perruquiere* . . . Par M Beaumont. Paris 1757

Maridat, *Petro De Tractatus de Pileo*, Lugduni 1655

Marinellà, Giovanni, *Gli Ornamenti delle Donne*, Venice 1562; 1574

Martial (ad 38–104) *Epigrams*, ed 1877

Martin, W, *The Hair Worker's Manual*. Brighton, 1852

McCarthy, Lee, *Diagnosis and Treatment of Diseases of the Hair*, 1940

McClintock, H F, *Old Irish and Highland Dress*. Dundalk, 1943

McColl, D S, *The Changes of Fashion*, 1818

Masters, T W, *Hairdressing in Theory and Practice*, 1966

Masters, T W, *An Introduction to Hairstyling*, 1969

Mather, J (Perfumer), *Treatise on the Nature and Preservation of the Hair*; in which the causes of its different colours and diseases are explained, London 1794 *8vo*

Matthews, L G, *The Antiques of Perfume*, 1973

McClintock, D, *The Wild Flowers of Guernsey*, 1975

McWhirter, N and R, *The Guinness Book of Records*, ed 1967

Meadows, C A, *Trade Signs and their Origin*, 1957

Mechi. Prices and List of Articles Manufactured and sold wholesale, retail, and for exportation, by Mechi, Cutter, Dressing Case Maker, and Inventor of the celebrated Razor, Strops and Paste, 4 Leadenhall Street, London. Manufacturing, 12 Cambridge Road, Mile End, *c* 1840. (Mechi's business was established in 1827)

Mee, A, (editor), *I see all*

Menander (342–292 bc), *Principal Fragments*, ed 1921

Ménard, Eugène, *What a ladies coffeur ought to know*, 1887

Men's Hairstylist and Barbers' Journal, March 1965, Baltimore, USA

Menestrier, *Dissertation sur L'usage de se faire porter la queue, nouvelle edition, avec des notes*, 100 copies only, Lyon 1829

Mennes, J, *Recreation for Ingenious Head-pieces*, ed 1667 (Wing M, 1717)

Meriton, G, *The Praise of York-shire Ale*, 3rd ed 1697

Merle, G, *The Domestic Dictionary*, 1857

Miami Herald, The, 2 Jan 1963

Middleton, T A, *A Mad World, My Masters*, 1608

Middleton, T, *The Works of*, ed A Dyce, 1840

Middlewood, J, *A Treatise on the Human Hair*, Liverpool 1814

Miege, G, *The Short French Dictionary*, 1690

Milton, John, *A Maske (Comus)*, 1637

Milton, John *The Works of*, ed 1697

Minister's Head Dress'd According to Law, or *A word of comfort to Hair Dressers in general respecting the Powder Plot of 1795*, 1795

Minsheu, J, *Ductor in Linguas (The Guide into Tongues)* 1617

The Mirror of Literature, amusement and instruction, no. 1, 1822 to 1849

Mitchell, E V, *Concerning Beards*. Hartford, Conn 1930

Mitchell, R W, *Castile Soap*, Boston 1927

Mitford, W B J O, *Dawn Breaks in Mexico*, 1945

La Mode Illustrée, no. 1. 1 Jan, 1860, Paris (Colas. 2082)

Moler, A, *The Barbers, Hairdressers' and Manicurers' Manual*. Chicago 1906

Mollett, J W, *An Illustrated Dictionary of words used in Art and Archaeology*, 1883

Moncrief, John, *The Poor Man's Physician*. 3rd ed Edinburgh 1731

Moniteur de la Coiffure

Monségur, P A, *Hair Dyes and their Application*, 1915

Montagna, W, *The Skin*, 1965 (reprint from *Scientific American* Feb, 1965 vol 212 no 2 pp 56–66)

Montagna, W and Ellis, R A (eds), *The Biology of Hair Growth*, NY 1958

Montagu, Lady, *Memoirs* (ref to Wire Wig)

Montague, P, *The Family Pocket-Book* or *Fountain of True and Useful Knowledge*, N/D (*c* 1760)

Monteg, L, *The Arts of Beauty*, NY 1858

Moodie, A M, *Hair Colouring and Bleaching*, 1964

Morris, A, *Creative Hair Styling*, 1948

Morris, A, *Water Waving*, 1938

The Most Excellent, Profitable, and pleasant Booke, of the famous Doctor and expert Astrologian, Arcandam. (Translated W Warde), ed 1617

Muirhead, D Palms, (*Globe*, Arizona 1961)

Müller, F, *Der Moderne Friseur und Haarformer in Wort und Bild*, 4th ed Berlin 1926

Murray, M A, *The splendour that was Egypt*, 1951

Nageles' Catalogue of Hairdressers' Sundries, 1934

Nares, R, *A glossary of words, phrases, names and allusions in the works of English Authors*, ed 1905

Nash, George C and Co, New Illustrated and Descriptive Catalogue of Theatrical and Private Wigs, 36 Chandos St, Charing Cross, London WC, N/D (*c* 1880)

National Proverbs, India 1916

Nazzaro, A and Nothaft, F, *Wig Techniques*, Jersey City 1963

Nazzaro, A and Nothaft, F, *Wig Techniques*, 2nd ed, Jersey City USA 1964

Nessler, C, *The Story of Hair*. NY 1928

A New Book of Knowledge, 1697 (Wing N 585)

A New and Complete Dictionary of Arts and Sciences, 2nd ed 1763

New Family Receipt-Book, The, 1811

The New Foundling Hospital for Wit, ed 1768

New Larrouse Encyclopedia of Mythology, 1968

Newcomb, W W, *The Indians of Texas*, Austin, Texas 1961

The New York Herald, 1904

Nicol, David (Court Hairdresser), *The Art of Hairdressing*, 1912 (published as a series of articles in *Every-woman's Encyclopaedia*, 1912)

Nicolai, F, *Uber den gebrauch der falschen haare und perrucken in alten und freuern Zeiten*, 1801 (French ed 1809)

Nicolay D'Arfeville. *The Navigations . . . into Turkie*, 1585

Niederlücke, E, *Fachkunde für Friseure*, Wiesbaden 1956

Niemoeller, A F, *Superfluous Hair and its Removal*, NY 1938 (Every device that has ever been used to remove hair is described)

Nivelon, F, *The Rudiments of Genteel Behavior*, 1737

Norman, A, *Glossary of Archaeology*, ND

Notes and Queries

Nouvelles etrennes curieuses des incroyables, merveilleuses inconcevables, et des raisonnables de Paris . . . la notice de 30 differentes perruques à la Mode . . . dans des pays divers. 1796

Oakley, E R, *The Smugglers of Christchurch*, 1942

O'Donovan, W J, *The Hair*, 1930

Okamoto, K S, *Ancient and Modern Various Usages of Tokyo, Japan*, Tokyo 1885

Old Testament

Oldenberg, H, *Buddha*

Olio, The , 1828 et seq

Onions, C T, *A Shakespeare Glossary*, 2nd ed 1922

Oppenheim, C, *The Wig-Maker and his Servants* (A Farce), Clyde, Ohio 1885

Ordini et Statuti Dell' Universita et Collegio de Barbieri, Della Presente Citta Di Milano. 60 pages. Engraving on title depicting The Virgin and Child between St Cosma and St Damiano. Printed by Lodovico Monza, 1652. (Milanese Trade Guild, Barbers)

Osborne, Garrett. Quarterly List. October 1936, and catalogues, 19th century

Ovid, *The Art of Love* (on painting the face). Loeb ed 1962

Oxford Classical Dictionary, 1949

Oxford Companion to Music, ed P Scholes, ed 1938

Oxford English Dictionary, The Shorter. 3rd ed 1950, ed C T Onions

Oxford Magazine

Oxford Sausage, The, ed 1777

Pacichelli, Giambattista, *Schediasma Juridico-Philologicum Tripartitum*, 1693

Pack, R, *New Collection of Poetical Miscellanies*, 1725

Packwood, G, *Packwood's Whim. The Goldfinches' Nest*, 1796

Pagenstecher, J F W, *De Barba, liber singularis*, 1746

Pall Mall Budget (30 May 1889)

Palladino, L, *The Principles and Practice of Hairdressing*, 1972

Palmer, K, *Oral Folk-Tales of Wessex*, Newton Abbot 1973

Palsgrave, John, *Les Clarcissement de la Langue francoyse*, 1530

Parish, W D, *A Dictionary of the Sussex Dialect*, Lewes 1875

Parr, A F, *The Techniques of Hairdressing*, 1969

Parry, E J, *The Raw Materials of Perfumery*, N/D (c 1930)

Peacham, H, *The Truth of our Times*, 1638

Pears, F, *The Skin, Baths, Bathing and Soap*, 1859

Pelegromius, S, *Synonymorum Sylva*, ed 1639

Pepys, Samuel. *Memoirs, Comprising his Diary*, etc (1660–1669), ed Lord Braybrooke 1825

Percivale, R, *A Dictionary in Spanish and English*, ed 1623

Percy Manuscript of Ballads and Romances, ed J W Hales and F J Furnivall 1867–8

Perrot, J J, *La Pogonotomie ou L'Art d'Apprendre a se Raser soi-meme*, Yverdon 1770

Perry, Bela C, *A Treatise on the Human Hair and its Diseases*, New Bedford 1859

Persian Proverbs, ed L P Elwell-Sutton, 1954

Pesman, M W, *Meet Flora Mexicana*, Arizona 1962

Peters, S, *A General History of Connecticut*, 1829

The Pharmaceutical Pocket Book

Phillippe, Adrian, *Histoire Philosophique, Politique et Religieuse de la Barbe Chez les Principaux Peuples de la Terre*, Paris 1845

Phillips, E, *The New World of Words*, 1st ed 1658, ed 1706

Phillips, M C, *More than Skin Deep*. N Y 1948

Phillips, M and Tomkinson, W S, *English Women in Life and Letters*, 1927

Philips, K, *Poems*, 1667

Phillips, J, *Maronides*, 1678

Phillips, S, *Herod*, 1901

Piesse, G W S, *The Art of Perfumery*, 3rd ed, 1862 (1st ed 1855)

Pigot, *London and Provincial Commercial Directory*, 1832

Pitt, G D, *Sweeney Todd the Demon Barber of Fleet Street*, ed M Slater, 1928

Planché, J R, *History of British Costume*, ed 1893

Platt, Sir Hugh, *Delights for Ladies, to Adorne their Persons*, . . . edn. 1602; ND (c 1605); 1608; 1609; 1611; 1615; 1628; 1630; 1635; 1636; 1647; 1651; 1654; 1656

Pliny, *The Historie of the World*. Translated P Holland, 1601

Poland, H, *Fur-Bearing Animals in Nature and in Commerce*, 1892

Poole, J, *English Parnassus*, 1657

Pope, A, *Rape of the Lock*, 1712

Porter, T, *The Carnival*, 1664

Porter, T, *The French Conjurer*, 1678

Potter, Eliza, *A Hairdressing Experience in High Life*. Cincinnati 1859

Potter, J, *Archaeologia Graeca*, ed, 1764

Poucher, W A, *Perfumes, Cosmetics and Soaps*, 6th ed, NY 1942

Powell, T, *Humane Industry*, 1661

Pratt, Ellis, *The Art of Dressing the Hair*. Bath 1770

The 'Preemo' Book of Simple Recipes, N D (c 1926)

Price, George, *Ancient and Modern Beards*, 1893

Price, R, *A Treatise of the Utility of Sangui-Suction*, or *Leech Bleeding*, 1822

Procter, R W, The *Barber's Shop*, 1883. 1st ed, 1856

Procter, B W (1787–1874), *The Pearl Weavers*

Prole, Lozania, *The Little Wig-Maker of Brent Street*, 1959 (fiction)

Pruner-Bey, F, *De la Chevelure comme Caracteristique des Races Humaines*, (Mem Soc Anthrop Paris 1865–1872)

Prynne, W, *Histrio-Mastix*, 1630

Prynne, W, *The Unloveliness of Love-Lockes*, 1628

Puckett, N N, *Folk Beliefs of the Southern Negro*, Chapel Hill, 1926

Pulleyn, William, *The Etymological Compendium*, 1828

Puzzle, The, 1745

Pyne, William Henry, *Wine and Walnuts* by Ephraim Hardcastle, 2nd ed 1824

Quaritch, Bernard, *The Vulgar Tongue*, 1857

Queens Closet Opened, ed 1671

Quevodo Y Villegas, F de, *Fortune in her Wits*. Trans J Stevens, 1697

Rachewiltz, B de, *Black Eros*, 1964

Radford, E and M A, *Encyclopaedia of Superstitions*, ed C Hole, ed 1961

Rambaud, René, *Les Fugitives*. Paris 1947

Rambaud, René, *Maitresses du Temps*.

Rambaud, René, *L'Ondulation Bouclée*

Rambaud, René, *Précis D'histoire de la Coiffure Feminine a travers les Ages*.

Rambaud, René, *La Psychologie du Coiffeur Pour Dames*

Ramsay, A, *Poems*, Edinburgh 1721

Rango, K T, *De Capillamentis sen vulgo parucquen*, 1663

Ranville, Guernon, *Essai sur la culture des cheveux, suivi de quelques reflexions sur l'art de la coiffure*, by M Duflos (Guernon Ranville), Paris 1812

Rapsodia, Akerlio (pseud), *Eusayo de una Historia de las Pelucas, de los Peluquinco y de los Pelucones . . .* 2 plates, 12mo. Madrid 1806

Rauchfuss, G, *Illustrated Catalogue and Price List of Human Hair, Hair dressers' Materials, . . .* NY 1861

Ray, J, *A Collection of English Proverbs.* 2nd ed, 1678

Rayner, J L, *Proverbs and Maxims*, 1910

Recueil géneral de coeffures de differents gouts, 1778

Redgrove, H S and Foan, G A, *Paint, Powder and Patches*, 1930

Reeson, G and Bedeman, C, *Common Sense about Hair*, 1949

Reno, R H, *Scientific Method of Blue Print Curly Cutting*

Repton, John Adey, FSA, *Some Account of the Beard and the Moustachio*, 1839

Revius, Jacobus, *Libertas Christiana circa usum Capillitii Defensa*, Lyons 1647

Reynolds, R, *Beards*, 1950

Rich, Barnaby, *Opinion diefied (sic) discovering the injins, traps and traynes that are set to catch opinion*, 1613

Richardson, F, *Whiskers and Soda*, 1910

Richard's Select Toilet Saloon, 1909

Richardson, Richard, *A Declaration Against Wigs or Periwigs*, ND (1682–3), (Wing, R 1393)

Rimmel, E, *The Book of Perfumes*, 1865

Risley, H, *The People of India.* Calcutta 1908

Ritchie, D, *Treatise on Hair.* (18th century)

Ritchie, David (Hairdresser, Perfumer, etc), *A Treatise on Hair*, London 1770, 8vo

Ritchie's Lady's Head Dresser, or *Beauties Assistant for 1772*, 1772

Robertson, W, *Phraseologian Generalis*, 1681

Robinson, T, *The Etiology, Pathology and Treatment of Baldness and Greyness*, 1882

Roeder, H, *Saints and their Attributes*, 1955

Rogers, A and Allen, F L, *The American Procession*, 1923

Rohrer, J, *Artistic Marcel, Water, Permanent Waving, and Hair Bobbing*, NY 1924

Rohrer, J, *Beauty Formulas*, NY 1925

Rohrer, J, *Scientific Modern Beauty Culture*, NY 1924

Rothe, A, *An Illustrated Catalogue of Theatrical Wigs*, Boston 1902. Another edition 1911

Rothe de Nugent, D, *Anti-titus ou Remarques Critiques sur la Coiffure des Femmes au XIX siecle*, Paris 1813

Rouse, W H D, *Greek Votive Offerings*, 1902

Rouse's Synonyms for the use of Chemists, their Assistants and Apprentices, 1898

Rowe, E, *The History of Joseph*, 1736

Rowland, *The Human Hair*

Rowlands, S, *The Letting of Humors Blood in the Head Vaine*, 1600

Rowlandson, T, *Characteristic Sketches of the Lower Orders*, 1820

Rowley, W, *All's lost by lust*, 1633

Rowley, H, *Puniana*, N/D (c 1885)

Rudyerd, B, *Le Prince d'Amour*, 1660

Russell, G, *Fragments*, 1888

(SDP) *The Ugly-Girl Papers*; or *Hints for the Toilet*, 1874

Sagarin, E (ed), *Cosmetics, Science and Technology*, 1433 pp Interscience Publishers, ed 1963 (Sagarin). The most comprehensive work on this subject

Sagarin, E, *The Science and Art of Perfumery*, NY 1945 2nd ed 1954

Saito, R, *Japanese Coiffure*, Tokyo 1939

Salmasius, Cl, *Epistola ad Andream Colvium super Cap. XI Primae ad Corinth. Epist. de Caesarie Virorum et Mulierum coma.* Lugd Batavor. Elzevier, 1644. (Controversy on the manner of wearing the hair. Louis XIII of France had introduced the long hair style for men)

Salmasius, etc, Dutch edition. *Overgeset uyt Latijn in de Nederlandsche Taal door Joh. Mich. Hornanum.* Dordrecht, Ambrullaert, 1645. 2 Engraved Portraits

Salmon, W, *The Family Dictionary.* 4th ed 1710

Salmon, W, *Polygraphice*, 1681

Sampson, William, *The Vow Breaker* or *The Faire Maide of Clifton*, 1636

Sanderson, S F, *Two Scottish Riddles*, (Folk Life, v 5, 1967)

Sandys, Edwin, *Sermons* 1585

Saunders, F, *Salad for the Solitary*, 1853

Savill, A and Warren, C, *The Hair and Scalp.* 5th ed 1962

Saxe, J G (1816–1887), *The Lover's Vision*

Schaefer, S, *All about Wigs*, Miami Beach, USA 1962

Schofield, W, *The Truth about Patent Medicines*, ND (c 1920), Portsmouth

Scientific Approach to Hairdesign, NP 1965

Scot, R, *Discovery of Witchcraft*, 1584

Scottish Tragic Ballads, 1781

Scultetus, J, *Trichiasis Admiranda*, Nuremburg 1658

Serventi, H (editor). *Album of Period Coiffures* (1928)

Settle, E, *Pastor Fido . . . a Pastoral*, 1677

Sexton, G, *The Hair and Beard* 1858

Shadwell, T, *The Humorists*, 1671

Shadwell, T, *The Virtuoso*, 1676

Shakespeare, W, *Comedies, Histories and Tragedies.* 2nd ed, 1632

Shakespeare, W, *Works*, ed 1785

Sharrock, R, *De officiis Secundum Naturae Jus.* (*De Habitu Crinis Dissertatio Singularis*), Oxford, 1660. (Wing, S 3014)

Shaw, R and Stretton, G, *The Art and Technique of Wiggery*, Cleveland, USA 1962

Shirley, J, *The Accomplished Lady's Rich Closet of Varieties*, 1687; 2nd ed 1687; 3rd ed (1688); 4th ed 1690; 5th ed 1699; 6th ed 1699

Shirley, James (1596–1666) *Works*

Short Title Catalogue of Books . . . 1475–1640. Pollard, A W and Redgrave, G R (1926)

Sidgwick, F, *The Shaver's Calendar*, 1906

Sidney, Sir P, *Works*, 1724–5

Simmonds, P L, *A Dictionary of Trade Products*, 1858

Simmonds, P L, *The Commercial Dictionary of Trade Products*, 1883

Simpson, S, *Curling Irons International*, Los Angeles 1969

Sinclair, R, *Essential Oils*, ed 1963

Skelton, J, *Magnyfycence*, 1533

Smiles, S, *Jasmin: Barber Poet*, Philanthropist, 1891

Smith, H C, *Hair Jewellery*, 1908

Smith, J, *The Burse of Reformation* (c 1655). Referred to by the Cunningtons in *Handbook of English Costume in the 17th Century*.

Smith, J T, *A Book for a Rainy Day*, 1845

Smith Bros, *Barbers' Supplies Catalogue*, May 1888, Boston 1888

Smith, H J, *The Beauty Specialists Manual*, NY 1925
2nd ed 1930; 3rd ed 1931

Smith, J T, *Nollekens and His Times*, ed 1949

Smith, R, *A Wonder of Wonders, or a Metamorphosis of Fair Faces*, 1662. (Wing, S 4149)

Somervile, W, *Occasional Poems*, 1727

Something New by Automathes, 1772

Sorbiere, S, *A Journey to London in the year*, 1698

Southey, R, *The Doctor*, 1834–1847

Southey, R, *Omniana*, 1812 (ed) *Letters from England*, 1808

Sparrow, W S, *Hirsute Adornments and their lore.* (*Magazine of Art*, 1902)

Speight, A, *The Lock of Hair*, 1872

Spenser, E, *Works*, 1679

Spinola, G, *Rules to Get Children By*, 1642. (Wing, S 4983)

Standen, G, *Shakespeare Authorship*, 1930

Statute des Maitres Barbiers, Perruquiers, Baigneurs, etuvistes – de la ville de Marseille. Marseille 1762

Statuti, Ordini, e Privilegii Concessi . . . Alla Ven (erata) Scuola del glorioso annacorita . . . S. Onofrio de SS. Peruccari di . . . Milano. 24 pages. No printer nor date, but not before 1704. Engraving of St Onuphrius, patron of the Order, on title. Milanese Trade Guild, Wigmakers.

Stecklyn's Catalogue of Hairdressers' Sundries. ND (c 1936)

Steiner, *Crowning Glory*, 1955

Stellartius, P, *De coroms et tonsuris paganorum, Judaeorum, Christianorum*, 1625

Stephane, *L'art de la coiffure féminine*, 1932

Sternberg, T, *The Dialect and Folk-Lore of Northamptonshire*, 1851

Stewart, A, *Art of Hair Dressing*, 1788

Stewart, A, *On The Natural Production of Hair*, London 1795, 8vo

Stewart, J, *Plocacosmos, or the Art of Hair Dressing*, 1782

Stewart, W G, *Highland Superstition and Amusements*

Stone, Mrs, *Chronicles of Fashion*, 1846

Stow, John, *The Annales of England*, 1592. *Summarie of the Chronicles*, 1598

Stubbes, P, *The Anatomie of Abuses*, 1583

Stubbs, S G B and Bligh, E W, *Sixty Centuries of Health and Physick*, 1931

Styles and Sets for Black Hair, NY 1968

Styles and Sets for Long Hair, NY 1972

Sutton, A M, *Album of Historical Coiffures*, 1911

Sutton, A M, *Boardwork*, ed 1921

Swift, J, *A Complete Collection of Genteel and Ingenious Conversation*, 1738

Swift, J, *Poetical Works*, 1736

Sylvia's Family Management. ND (c 1890)

Symonds, N G S, *Modern Broadwork*. Pt 1 Weft Working, 1965

Symonds, N G S, *Modern Boardwork*, Pt 2 'Knotted and Drawn-through Work' new ed 1973

Tacitus, *Germania.*

Tardini, J, *Disquisitio Physiologica de Pilis*, Turnoni 1609

Tasho, Ernest, *Hair Styling for Women*, 1969

Taylor, J, *Ralph Richards, the Miser*, 1821

Taylor, John, *Superbiae Flagellum*, 1621. (Description of beards)

Teetgen, John, *My Razor and Shaving Tackle! As it Ought to be! and as it Ought Not. How to Shave without (illustrated with) Great Pains and Little Cuts.* Woodcuts including numbered diagram of the face, 1845

Tennyson, A Lord, *Works*, 1907–8

Thackeray, W M, *The History of Pendennis*, 1849/50. (Advertisements in original parts)

Theophrastus, *Concerning Odours*, ed. A Holt. Loeb Library, 1916

Thiers, J B, *Histoire des Perruques*, 1690. (Other eds 1702, 1722, 1724, 1777)

Thomas, G, *The Art of Modern Hair Dressing.* NY 1946

Thomas, William, *An argument wherein the apparaile of women is both reproved and defended.* Printed in black letter, title within a woodcut border enclosing the date 1534. (McKerrow, 30). T Berthelet, 1551. Sm 8vo. Not in STC (Sotheby, lot 363, 31 Jan. 1956. £230)

Thomas, Dylan, *Collected Poems*, 1952

Thompson, Edward, *The Courtesan*, 3rd ed 1765

Thompson, C J S, *The Cult of Beauty*, c 1900

Thornbury, W, *The Life of J M W Turner, RA*, 1862

Thornton, B, *The Battle of the Wigs* (A poem published 1774 in v 2 of *Miscellaneous and Fugitive Poems*)

Thornton, T, *Oriental Commerce*, 1825

Thornton, B, *The Battle of the Wigs*, 1768

Thorpe, S C, *Practice and Science of Standard Barbering*, NY ed 1964

Thurston, J, *The Toilette*, 1730

Timbs, John, *Things to be Remembered*, 1872

Todd, F P, *The Ins-and-Outs of Military Hair.* (*Infantry Journal* March/April 1940)

Todd, J M, *Sixty-two years in a Barber Shop.* Portland, USA 1906

The Toilet: a Dressing-table Companion, 1839

The Toilet of Flora, ed 1775

The Toilette . . . embracing . . . Beard, Eyebrows, Hair, etc, 1832

Tongue, R L, *Somerset Folklore*, 1965

Toone, W, *A Glossary*, 2nd ed 1834

Tottel, *Miscellany*, 1557

Treatise upon the Modes, or *A Farewell to French Kicks*, 1715

Treves, F, *The Tale of a Field Hospital*, 1900

The Trichologist. The official organ of the Institute of Trichologists, 1937 *et seq*

Trimmer Trimm'd (The); or *The Washball and Razor used to Some Purpose.* By a Real Barber. Printed in the Year 1749

The True Briton (newspaper)

Truefitt, H P, *New Views on Baldness*, 1863

Trusty, S, *The Art and Science of Barbering*, revised ed, 1962

Tuer, A W, *Old London Street Cries*, 1885

Tuke, T, *A Treatise against Painting and Tincturing of Men and Women*, 1616

Turkish Proverbs Translated into English, Venice 1880

Ulmus (Marc. Ant.). *Physiologia Barbae Humanae, in tres sectiones divisa, hoc est de fine illius philosophico et medico.* Bologna 1601
Title in red and black, with woodcut arms of Cardinal Aldobrandini. (The earliest work on beards)

Uzanne, V, *Coiffures de Style. La parure Excentrique, epoque Louis XVI*, Paris 1895

The Van Dean Manual. NY, ed, 1963

Van Holsbeck, Dr, *L'Art de conserver les Cheveux*. Bruxelles, N/D (*c* 1890)

Van Schaack and Sons. Price Current and Illustrated Catalogue (Chemicals and Toilet articles), 1887

Vanity, Catalogue of an Exhibition at Brighton, 9 May–31 August 1972

Vasco, T, *Coiffeur de Dames*, illustrated, priced brochure, *c* 1900

Vassetz, De, *Traite Contre le luxe des coiffures*, 1694

Vaughan, W, *The Golden Grove*, 1600

Verrill, A H, *Perfumes and Spices*, Boston 1940

Villaret, P, *Le coiffeur de la cour et de la ville*. Paris 1829

Villaret, P, *L'Art de se coiffer soi-même enseigné aux Dames*, Paris 1828

Villermont, Contesse Marie de, *Histoire de la Coiffure Féminine*, Paris, 1892

Virgilius Maro (Publius), *Opera*, 1492; *Works*, Birmingham 1757

Vito, Victor, *At home with your hairdo*. NY 1962

Vito, V, *Top Secrets of Hair Styling*, NY, 1954

Von Boehn, Max, *Dolls*, NY 1972

Vogue

The Vulgar Tongue; Comprising two glossaries of Slang, Cant and Flash Words and Phrases, principally used in London at the present day. By 'Ducange Anglicus' 1857

Wager, Lewis, *The Life and Repentance of Mary Magdalene*, (written 1550–66), 1567 ed Tudor Facsimile texts, 1908

Wale, Rev H J, *My Grandfather's Pocket-Book*, 1883

Walker, A, *Female Beauty*, 1837

Walker, O, *Vulgar Errours*, 1659

Walker, T, *The Wit of a Woman*, 1715

Wall, F E, *The Principles and Practice of Beauty Culture*, 4th ed

Wall, F E, *Canities*, NY 1926

Waller, W, Court Hair Dresser, 90 Great College Street, Camden New Town, Single sheet price list, N/D (*c* 1845)

Walsh, W S, *Handy Book of Literary Curiosities*, Philadelphia 1900

Ward, Ned, *Democritus: The Laughing Philosopher's Trip into England*, 1723

Ward, E, *Female Grievances Debated*, 2nd ed 1707

Ware, W P, *Price list of Occupations and Society emblems. Shaving Mugs*, Chicago 1949

Watson, G, *The Roxburghshire Word-Book*. Cambridge 1923

Webster's New International Dictionary, 2nd ed 1950

Weekley, E, *Something About Words*, ed 1936

Wells, S R, *New Physiognomy*. NY 1896

Wentworth, H, and Flexner, S B, *Dictionary of American Slang*. NY 1960

Wentworth, G, *The Poetical Note-Book*, 1824

Werner, E T C, *A Dictionary of Chinese Mythology*, ed, NY 1961

Weseen, M H, *A dictionary of American slang*. 3rd ed, NY, 1936

Whatley, Robert, *Characters at The Hot-Well*, Bristol in September and at Bath in October 1723, 1724

Wheeler, G H, *Head Washing by New Methods with*

Nature's Remedies, ND (*c* 1911)

Wheeler, G H, *Handbook of Hair and Scalp Diseases*, St Leonards-on-sea 1888

Whetstone, The, 1745

Why Shave? or *Beards v Barbery* by HM, ND (*c* 1890)

Wickenden, L, *Our Daily Poison*. NY 1955

Wilcox, R T, *The mode in Hats and Headdress*, NY 1948

Willich, A F M, *The Domestic Encyclopedia*; or *a Dictionary of facts*, 1802

Williams, W P and Jones, W A, *Glossary of Provincial Words and Phrases in use in Somersetshire*, 1873

Wiloringold, M, *Sauce for the Wedding Dinner*, 1742

Wilson, K, *The Successful Hairdresser*, Omaha, Nebraska, 10th ed 1945 (1st ed 1923)

Wilson, T, *The Swastika*, 1894

Wilson, K, *The successful hairdresser*. Omaha, ed 1945

Wing, D, *Short-Title Catalogue of Books printed in England: 1641–1700*. NY 1945–1951

Winick, C, *Dictionary of Anthropology*, Ames, Iowa 1958

Winter, A, *Trichologia*, 1869

Wit a-la-Mode by Jasper Quibble, 1745

Woestyn, E, *Le Livre de la coiffure*, Paris. N/D (*c* 1855)

Wolcot, John, *The Lousiad*, 1785–1795

Wolff, John, *A defence of short hair*, 1593 (Ret. p 205 vol 2 Fairholt Costume in England). In register of Stationers' Company for 1593

Wolley, H, *The Accomplish'd Ladies Delight*, 7th ed 1696

Woman's Own 3 March 1962

Woodforde, Rev James, *Diary of a Country Parson*, 1924–31

Woodforde, John, *The Strange Story of False Hair*, 1971

Wooton, E, *Toilet Medicine*, 1882

Wordsworth, W, *Poetical Works*. Oxford 1940–9

Woty, William, *The Shrubs of Parnassus*, 1760

Wraxall, L and Wehrhan, R, *Memoirs of Queen Hortense*, 1862

Wright, L, *A Display of dutie dect with sage sayings* (1st ed 1589) ed 1614

Wright, T, *Caricature History of the Georges*, 1867

Wycherley, W, *The Gentleman Dancing-Master*, 1673

Wykes-Joyce, M, *Cosmetics and Adornment*, 1961

Yeats, John, *The Technical History of Commerce* (Pt III *Modern Industrial Art*). Section VII 'The Hairdresser and the Combmaker' of Chapter 3 (arts relating to clothing) devotes 3½ pages to this subject, London 1872

Young, S, *The annals of the barber-surgeons of London*, 1890

Youths Behaviour, 8th ed 1663 (Wing Y 208)

Zentler, W F, *The technique and art of Marcel Waving*, NY 1925 ed 1963

Zöttl, H, *Das tachwissen des Friseurs. Bayerischer schulbachverlag*

The Illustrations

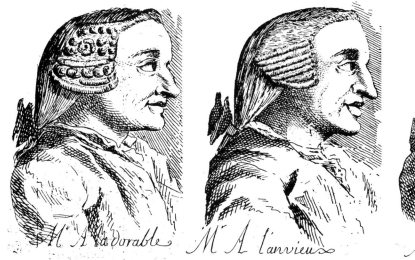

1 A l'Adorable peruke

2 A l'Anvieu peruke

3 A l'Aventure peruke

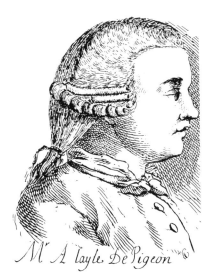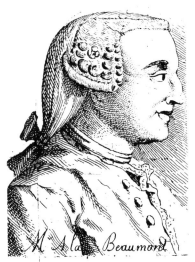

4 A l'Ayle de Piegeon peruke

5 A la Beaumont peruke

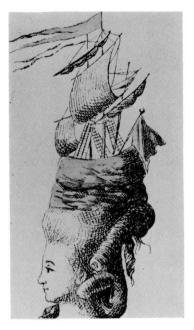

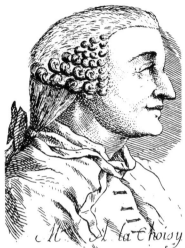

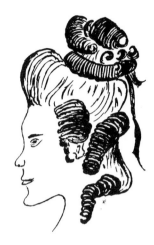

6 A la Belle Poule coiffure

7 A la Cabriolet peruke

8 A la Candeur coiffure

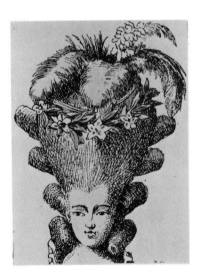

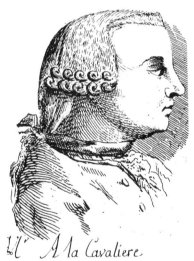

9 A la Capricieuse coiffure

10 A la Cavaliere peruke

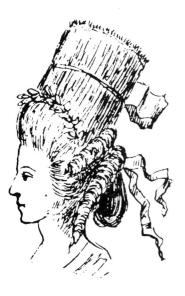

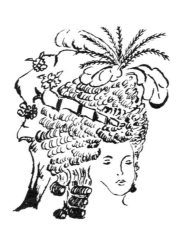

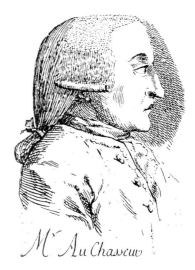

11 A la Cérès coiffure

12 Aux Charmes de la Liberté coiffure

13 Au Chasseur peruke

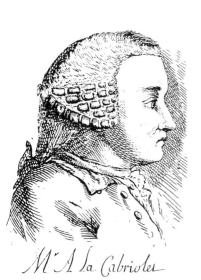

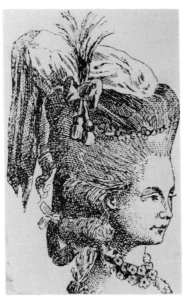

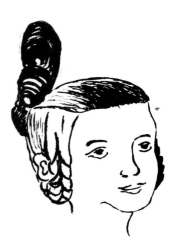

14 A la Choisy peruke

15 A la Circassienne coiffure

16 A la Clotilde coiffure

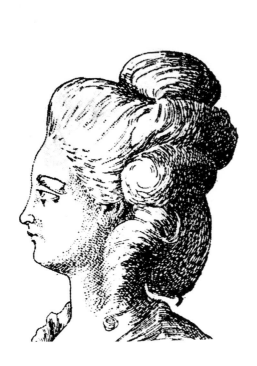

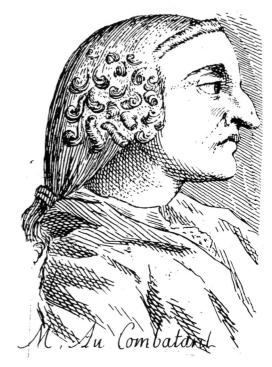

17 A la Colombe coiffure

18 Au Combatant peruke

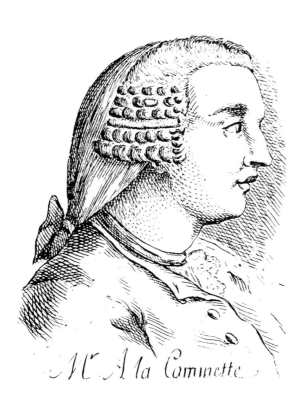

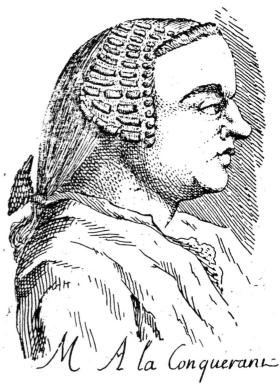

19 A la Commette peruke

20 A la Conquerant peruke

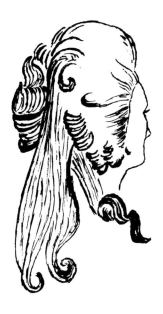

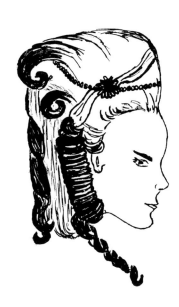

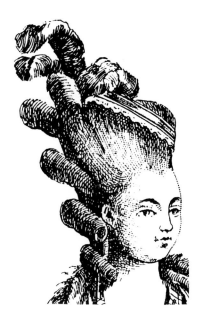

21 A la Conseilleur coiffure

22 A la Dauphine coiffure

23 Au Desir de Plaire coiffure

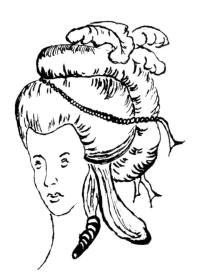

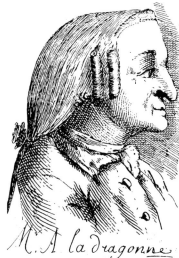

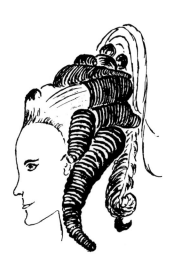

24 A la Distinction coiffure

25 A la Dragonne peruke

26 A la Driade coiffure

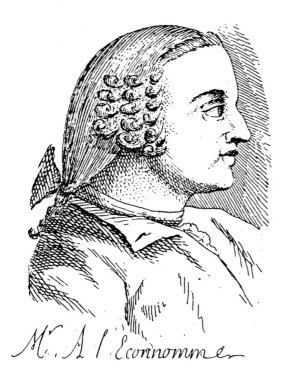

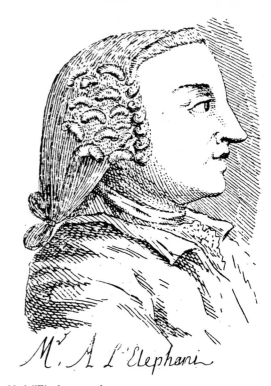

M. A l'Econnomme

M. A L'Elephant

27 A l'Econnomme peruke

28 A l'Elephant peruke

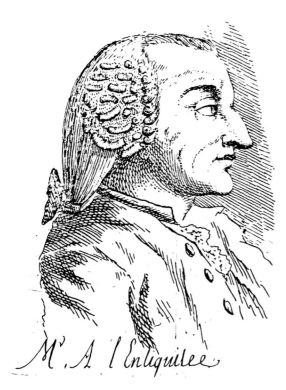

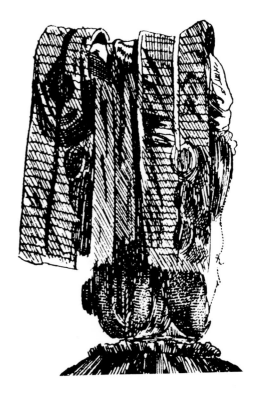

M. A l'Entiquitée

29 A l'Entiquitée

30 A l'Espagnole coiffure

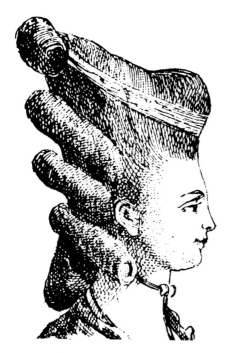

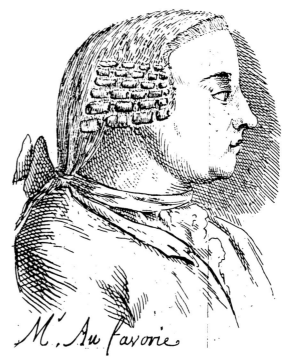

31 A l'Euridice coiffure

32 Au Favorie peruke

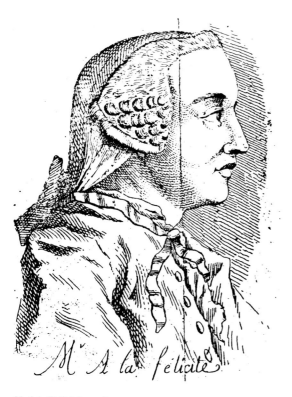

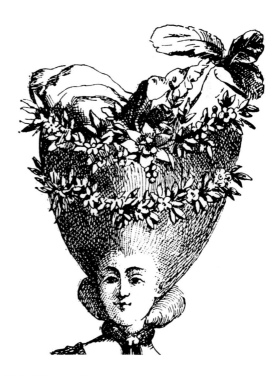

33 A la Felicité peruke

34 A la Flore coiffure

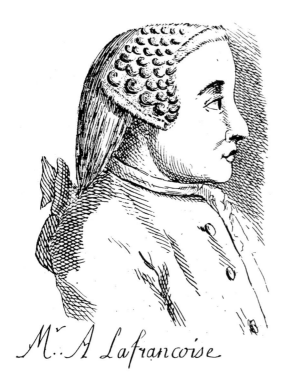

Mᵉ A Lafrancoise

35 A la Francoise peruke

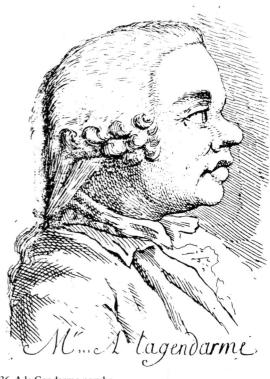

Mˡˡᵉ A la gendarme

36 A la Gendarme peruke

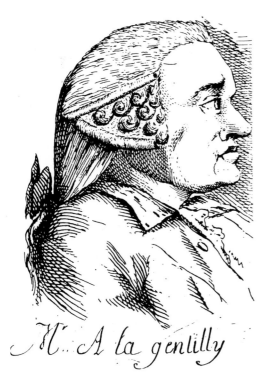

Mᵉ A la gentilly

37 A la Gentilly peruke

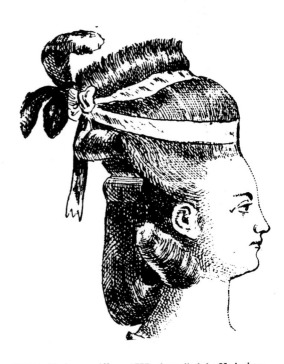

38 A la Herisson coiffure, 1777, also called the Hedgehog Hairdress

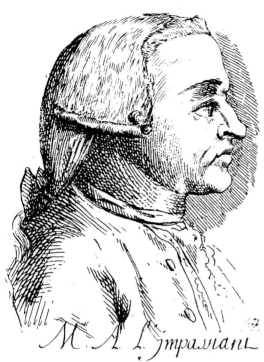

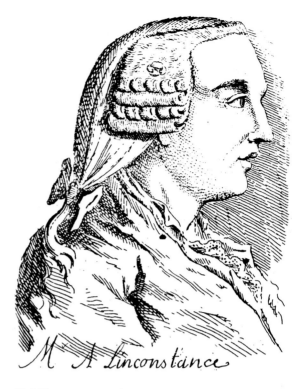

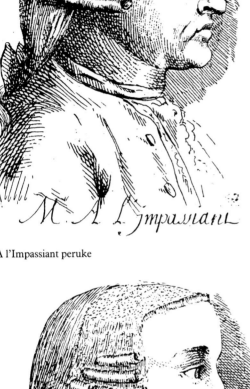

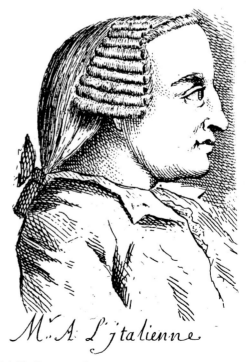

39 A l'Impassiant peruke

40 A l'Inconstance peruke

41 A l'Indiference peruke

42 A l'Italienne peruke

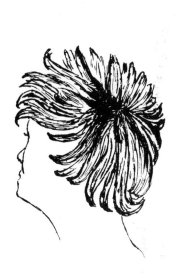

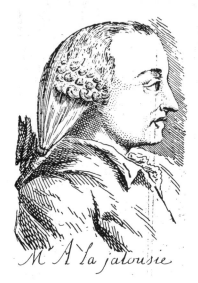

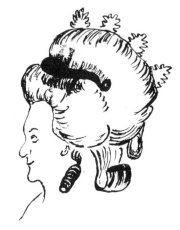

43 Titus cut à la Jacobine

44 A la Jalousie peruke

45 A la Janot coiffure

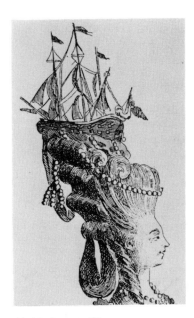

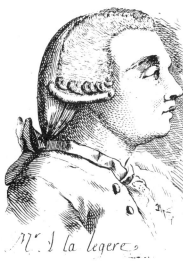

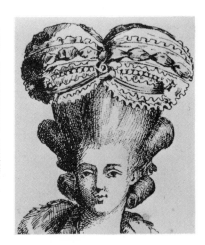

46 A la Junon coiffure

47 A la Legere peruke

48 Au Lever de la Reine coiffure

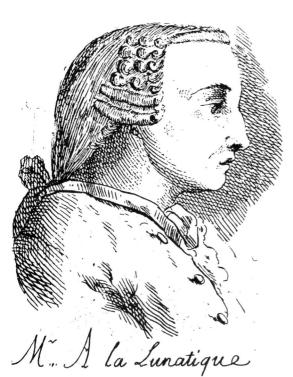

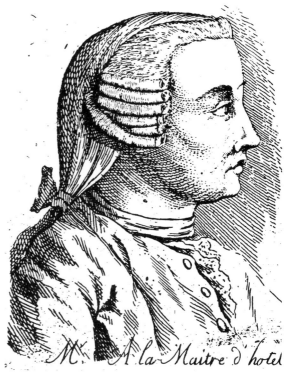

49 A la Lunatique peruke

50 A la Maitre d'Hotel peruke

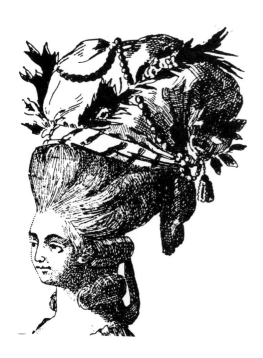

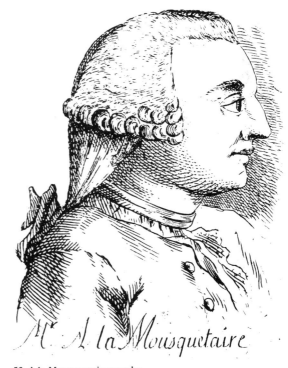

51 A la Mauresque coiffure

52 A la Mousquetaire peruke

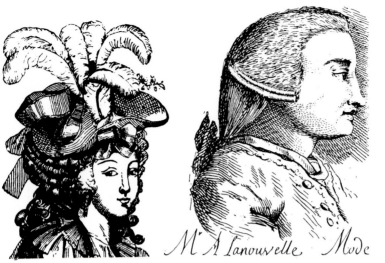

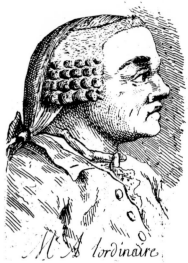

53 A la Nation coiffure, 1790

54 A la Nouvelle Mode peruke

55 A l'Ordinaire peruke

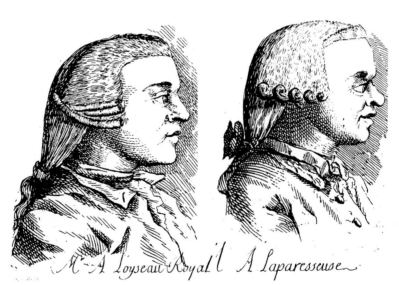

56 A l'Oyseau Royal peruke

57 A la Paresseuse peruke

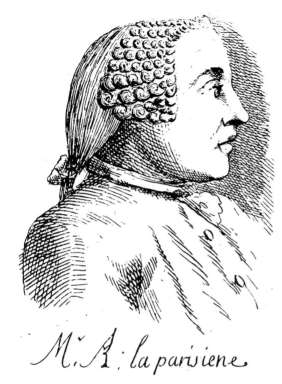

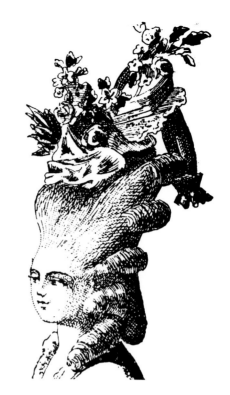

58 A la Parisiene peruke

59 Au Parterre Galant coiffure

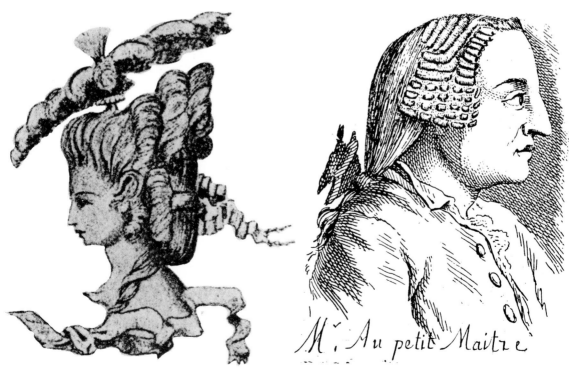

60 A la Persane Coiffure, 1777

61 Au Petit Maitre peruke

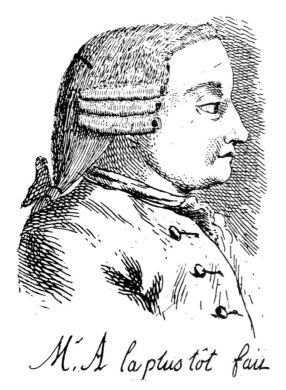

62 A la Plus Tôt Fair peruke

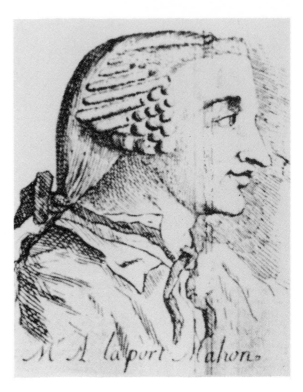

63 A la Port Mahon peruke

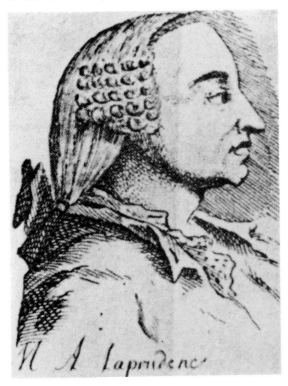

64 A la Prudence peruke

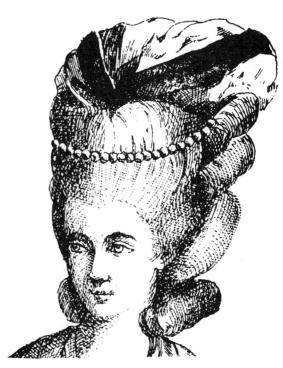

65 A Quatre Boucles avec une Barriere de Perles coiffure

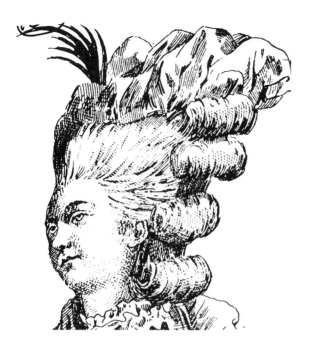

66 A Quatre Boucles Droites Séparées coiffure

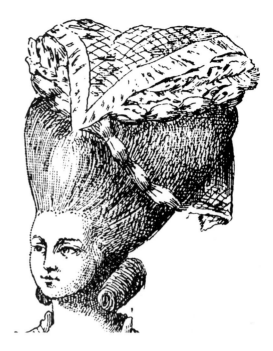

67 A la Quinot coiffure

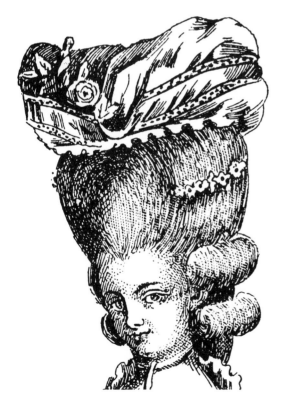

68 A la Rancour coiffure

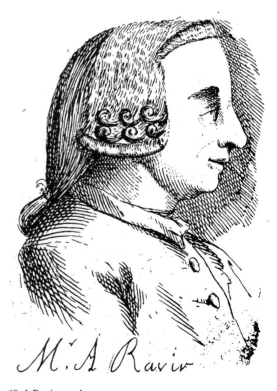

69 A Ravir peruke

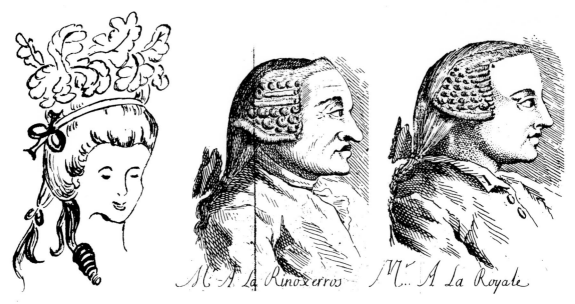

70 A la Reine coiffure

71 A la Rinoxerros peruke

72 A la Royale peruke

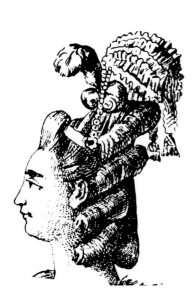

73 Aux Sentiments Repliés

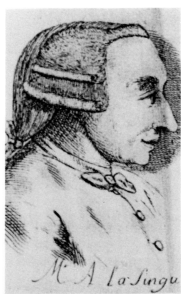

74 A la Singulierre peruke

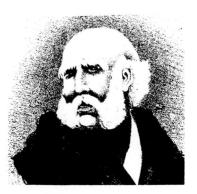

75 A la Souveroff whiskers, *c* 1839

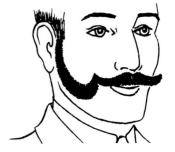

76 A la Souvaroff whiskers. American
version, 20th cent

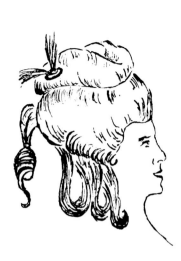

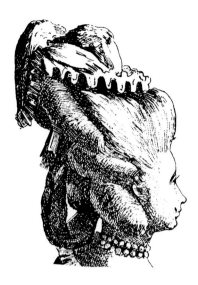

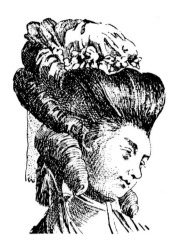

77 A la Sylphide coiffure

78 A Trois Boucles en Arrière coiffure

79 A Trois Grandes Boucles Lâches coiffure

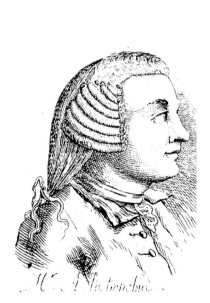

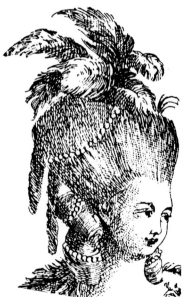

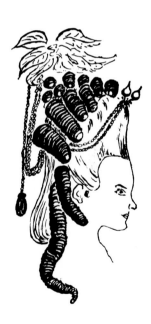

80 A la Tronchin peruke

81 Au Val d'Amour coiffure

82 A la Venus coiffure, c 1777

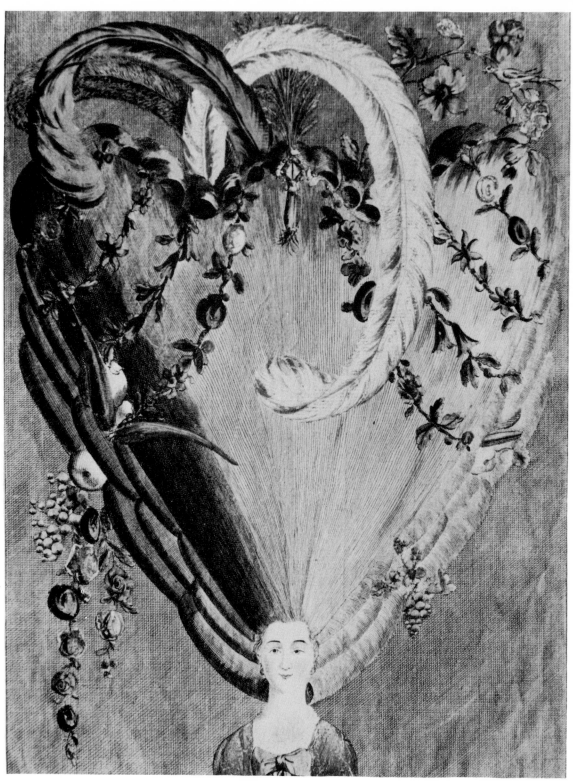

83 The Extravaganza coiffure, 1776

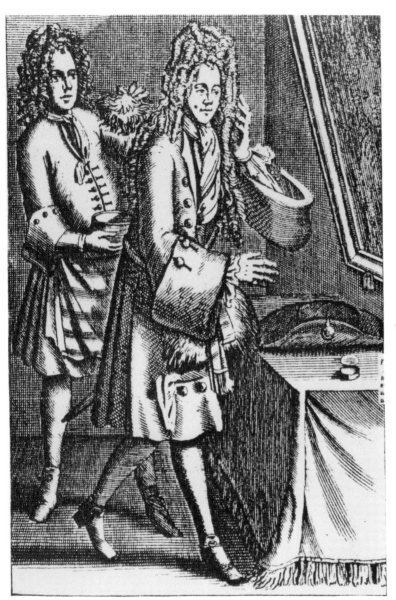

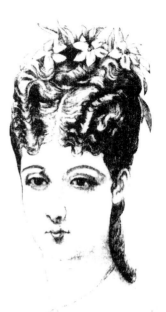

85 Full-dress coiffure, 1876
This style of headdress is suitable to a young lady. The hair is divided into four, and forms a large plait at each side a little higher than the ear, and which crosses on the neck. The strand that falls in a thick curl is false. The front is waved and arranged in bandeaux on the forehead and temples. The flowers are sprays of convolvuli

84 A gentleman of the late 17th century receiving the finishing touches to his wig by his man servant. (From *An Essay in Defence of the Female Sex*, 3rd ed, 1697, by Mary Astell)

85A A Morning coiffure, 1876
This is suitable either for a young lady or for a youthful married woman. The hair is combed up from the nape of the neck, and plaited; these plaits are crossed at the top of the head, and allowed to fall low at the back, where they join. When there is but a small quantity of natural growth, it is all used for the plaits at the top of the head. The pendent tresses are false

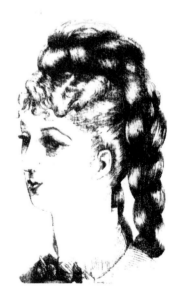

86 Wigmaker's workroom and appliances, 18the cent (After *Diderot*)
The top of this plate depicts a wig-maker's workshop or shop where several boys are engaged in different aspects of this art; one in (a) is busy shaving a beard; one in (b) is fitting a wig; a woman in (c) is weaving; two workers in (d) are mounting wigs; another in (e) heating the frizzing irons, while an individual in (f) is removing the powder from his face.

Bottom of the plate

1 Beard basin made from pewter or faience. A the hollow which the chin occupies during the shaving
2 Beard basin made from silver or silvered. A the hollow
3 Kettle to heat water. A the handle; B the handle, C the cover
4 Boiler. A handle; B the stopper or cover
5 Tin bottle for carrying water to town when one is going to shave there. A the bottle; B the spout; C the stopper
6 Another tin bottle for the same purpose. A the bottle, B the stopper
7 A strop with two faces for sharpening razors. A the strop; B the handle
8 Four-sided strop for sharpening razors. These sides are prepared in such a manner as to make the razors more and more sharp. A the strop, B the handle
9 Stone hone to grind razors
10 An inset hone for grinding razors. A the hone; B the frame; C the handle

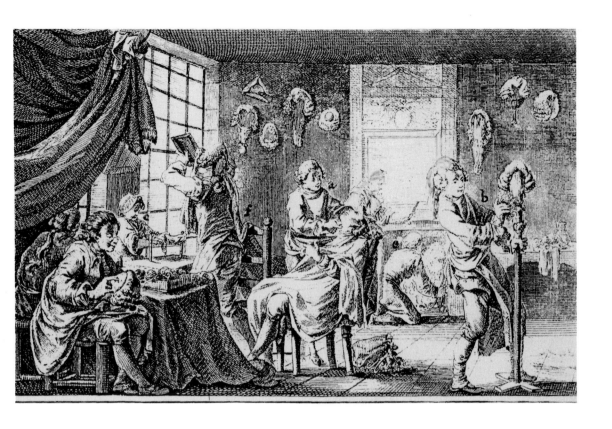

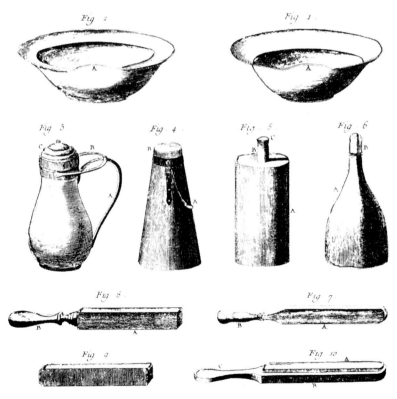

87 Wigmaker's tools and appliances, 18th cent (After *Diderot*)

1 Shaving soap box. A the box; B the lid
2 A the box; B the soap
3 Razor. A the blade; B the handle
4 Lid of the razor box
5 The razor box. A the box; BB the razors
6 & 7 Soap and sponge in their boxes
8 Razor pocket. A the pocket; BB the cords; CC the razors
9 & 10 Curl paper – ordinary and for crisping
11 & 12 Combs for dressing the tail. AA the teeth; BB the backs; CC the tails
13 Twisted curl paper on which one rolls the hairs
14 & 15 Small brushes for cleaning the combs. AA the bristles; BB the handles
16 Pinch of hair, half in curl paper. A the hairs; B the curl paper
17 The same placed in curl papers. A the pinch; B the completed curl paper
18 & 19 Elevation and section of a two ended dressing comb with a flat back. AA the teeth; B the flat spine
20 & 21 Elevation and section of a two ended dressing comb with a rounded back. AA the teeth; B the rounded spine
22 Scissors with no point for cutting hair. AA Blades; B joint; CC the finger rings
23 Iron for curling the toupet. Called toupet iron. AA the prongs; BB the finger rings; C the joint
24 Pistol shaped compass for rolling hair. AB the legs; B the handle; C the thumb stall; D joint; E spring
25 Another jointed compass for rolling hair. AA the legs; B the joint
26 Pinch of hair ready to be frizzed. A the tip
27 The same twisted since it is wished to place some split curl-papers there. A the tip; B the twist
28 The same pinch at the tip. A the tip pinched
29 The same curled
30 Ivory comb with two side for unravelling. AA the teeth; B the spine
30 & 31 Unravellers. AA the teeth; BB the spines
32 Banded chignon comb. A the teeth; B the banded spine
33 Curl-paper iron called a pinching iron. AA the pinches; B the joint; C the handle; D thumb stall
34 Another iron. AA the pinches; B the joint; C the handle; D thumb stall
34 (No. 2) Powder box. A Powder box; BB boxes for liquid and solid pomade; C the handle
34 (No. 3) Pot for liquid pomade
35 Box for liquid pomade. A the lid; B the box
36 Stick of solid pomade
37 Powder bag for carrying into town. AA the strings
38 Powder bellows. A the box; B the bellow
39 Powder puff of Swans down for ladies toilet. A the puff; B the handle
40 Headless puff
41 Puff with a head. A the head
42 Mask to place on the face when powdering
43 Mask made for the same purpose

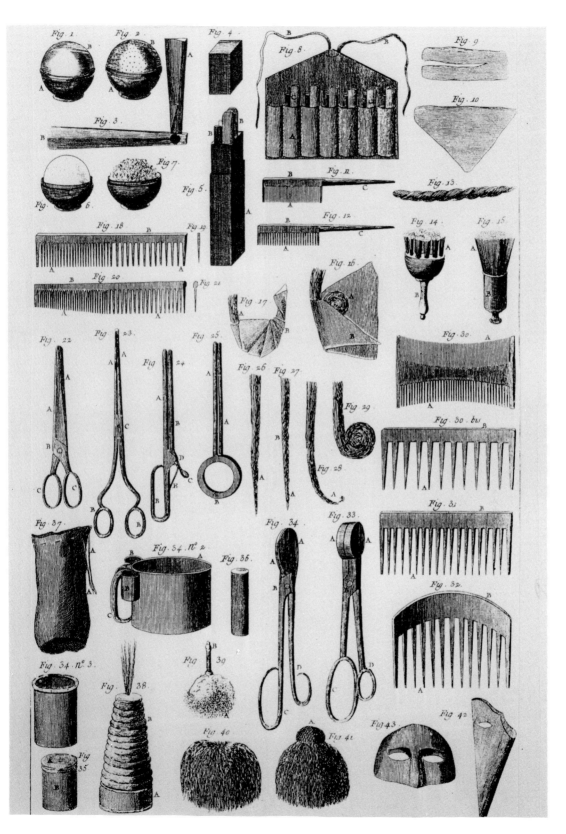

88 Wigmaker's tools and appliances, 18th cent (After *Diderot*)

1 Wig measure. AB, 1st measure from top of forehead to nape of neck, AC, 2nd measure from one temple to the other passing behind the head, AD, 3rd measure from one ear to the other passing over the top of the head higher for wigs to ear – lower for plain wigs, AE, 4th measure from the middle of one cheek to the middle of the other passing behind the head, AF, 5th and last measure from the middle of the top of the forehead to one of the temples

2 Iron comb or card. AA the teeth; B plate; CC holdfast

3 Double Cards, placed one on the other for drawing off hair. AA the points or tips; BB plates

  4, 5 & 6 Curlers. A larger number are employed than shown and are of differing thicknesses. They are used to roll the hair

7 Card for unravelling. AA the tips; BB the plate

8 Large card. AA tips; B the plate

9 Fine card. AA tips; B the plate

10 Preparation cards. AA the tips; BB the plate

11 & 12 Cards with tips similar to those of mattress cards. AA the tips; BB the plates; CC etc, the holdfasts

13 Finecard. AA the tips; B the plate; C holdfast

14 Wisps of hair arranged on curlers

15 Wisp of unravelled hair

16, 17, 18 & 20 Labelled and numbered hair wisps of different sizes

19 Wisp of hair ready to be thinned at the points

21 Weaving bench. AA the weaving sticks (rods); B base; CC woven hairs, DD the stretched strands; EE cards around which are rolled the strands

22 & 23 Thick paper for rolling the strands

24 & 25 Irons for pressing the hair of the wig. AA iron; BB the handles

26 Measure

27 & 28 Stages of different wefts. ABC the plain M of several kinds on two silk threads;

  D the M doubled on two silk threads

  E the simple N on three silk threads

  F The simple M

  G half the N

  H the M with a single twist

  I   the M and half

  K the M redoubled

  L final strand

  M first strand

29 & 30 graduated rulers

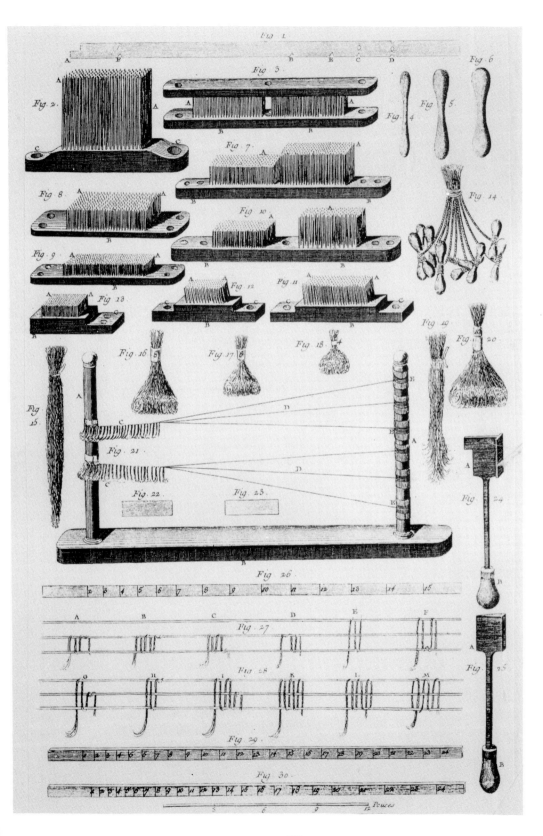

89 Wigmaker's tools and appliances, 18th cent (After *Diderot*)

1 Carpentry stove to dry the hair. A lid; B the inside grill; C the door for the entry of a charcoal fire

2 Copper for boiling the hairs

3 & 4 Angles which are employed for the blocks of dressed wigs

5 Hair. Method of distinguishing the tip end from that of the block end when one has lost it; it is by rubbing it between thumb and finger and making it slip which makes the tip approach as it is made up of an infinite number of little branches that are slim and pointed and stick to the trunk

6 & 9 Needles for sewing the wig. AA the heads

8 & 7 Tacks to hold the threads or ribbons. AA the heads

10 Another tip or crochet tack

11 Knot for catching up the strands of the tresses when they break. A the strand whose end is broken; B the strand carrying the ring

12 Ball of silk

13 Winding machine for hair strand. 1, Vice; A the moveable grip; B the stationary grip; CC side beams; D holdfast; E screw; F screw crank; G, H cord to tighten the screw

13 No. 2. Double spring of the vice

14 Wooden stove – A the cover; B interior grill

15 Fully prepared mount. AA the peripheral mount ribbon; BB the net work; CC covering ribbon; DD crossed ribbon

16 The same view from the front. AA etc the strands stopped at the tips

17 Mounting to the ear. AA the ribbon; B the hollow; CC the threads; D buckram of the ear; EE the garter or strap to secure the wig; F the net work; G buckram plaque

18 Full view of mounting from behind. A net-work; B buckram plaque; C the buckle and strap; DD the threads (or strands)

19 Full mounting for a plain head. A edge of forehead; BB small turns; CC big turns; D top of head, EE small rows of wefts; FF large rows of wefts; GG the plaque

20 & 21 A the strap (or garter), the buckle. (these nos omitted in original plate)

22 Hammer. A head; B claw foot; C handle

23 Lead plaque for ears

24 Spring of temples

25 Iron for wigs

26 Pinchers. AA pinches; BB handles

27 Pair of compasses. A head; BB legs

28 Copper or cauldron. AA legs; B handle

29 Oil-can

30 Work bench. A table; BB legs

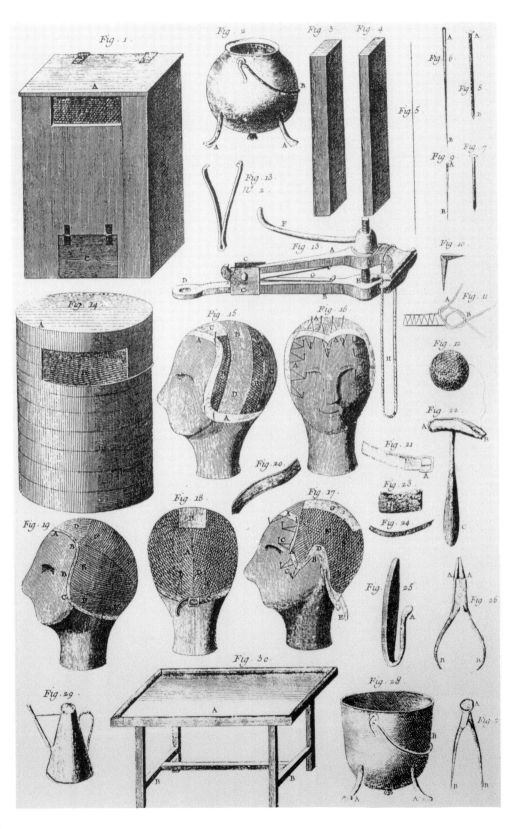

Fig. 1.
Fig. 2.
Fig. 3.
Fig. 4.
Fig. 5.
Fig. 6.
Fig. 7.
Fig. 8.
Fig. 9.
Fig. 10.
Fig. 11.
Fig. 12.
Fig. 13. N° 2.
Fig. 13.
Fig. 14.
Fig. 15.
Fig. 16.
Fig. 17.
Fig. 18.
Fig. 19.
Fig. 20.
Fig. 21.
Fig. 22.
Fig. 23.
Fig. 24.
Fig. 25.
Fig. 26.
Fig. 27.
Fig. 28.
Fig. 29.
Fig. 30.

90 Wigmaker's weft patterns and appliances, 18th cent (After *Diderot*)

1 Rows of wefts of ladies wigs, frizzed chignons. AB small rows of wefts; BC big rows of wefts; CD the *tournans*

2 Rows of wefts of raised chignon. AB small rows of wefts; BC big rows of wefts; CD the *tournans*

3 Rows of wefts *de tour de* face. AB small rows of wefts; BC big; CD the *tourans*

4 Rows of wefts of hair cap. AB small rows of wefts; BC big rows of wefts; CD the *tourans*

5 Tip to hold the wigs on the blocks during fitting

6 Brush of couch grass

7 Mobile wig block. A block; B shaft; C cylinder in which shaft is elevated or lowered to place at desired height; D screw to secure shaft; E base comprising 3 feet, more secure than crossed feet

8 & 9 Hooks to keep the wigs on the blocks during fittings. AA the hooks; BB cords which are knotted beneath the nose of the block

10 Wig box for carrying to town. A the box; B the lid; C the mushroom on which one places wig; D the stalk of the mushroom; E the tip to secure the wig; F the handle

11 Another wig box. A handle; B box; C lid

12 Powderer, made to powder wigs in such a way that the powder does not spread in the room. A wicker powderer; B wig block that it contains; C foot of block; D portion of the work bench on which everything is placed

13 Another base to carry wig block. A shaft; B crossed foot

14 Mushroom with a base. A mushroom; B shaft; C tip; D crossed foot

15 Simple mushroom to carry wigs. A the mushroom; B shaft; C tip

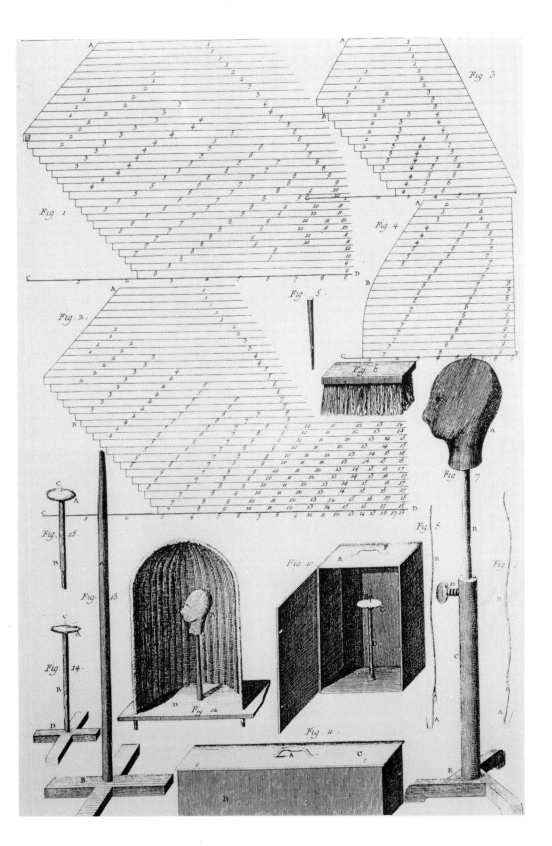

91 Types of 18th cent wigs (After *Diderot*)

1 & 2 Interior and exterior of a bonnet wig
3 & 4 Interior and exterior of bag wig. A the bag; BB buckle and strap
5 & 6 Interior and exterior of knotted wig. AA the knots; B spiral curl.
7 Knot of same wig
8 Spiral curl of same wig
9 Bag. A Rosette; BB cords
10 & 11 Exterior and interior of natural wig
12 & 13 Exterior and interior of Abbés wig. AA the tonsure
14 & 15 Interior and exterior of Brigadier wig. AA spiral curls; B rosette
16 Spiral curls of same wig
17 Rosette of same wig. AA cords

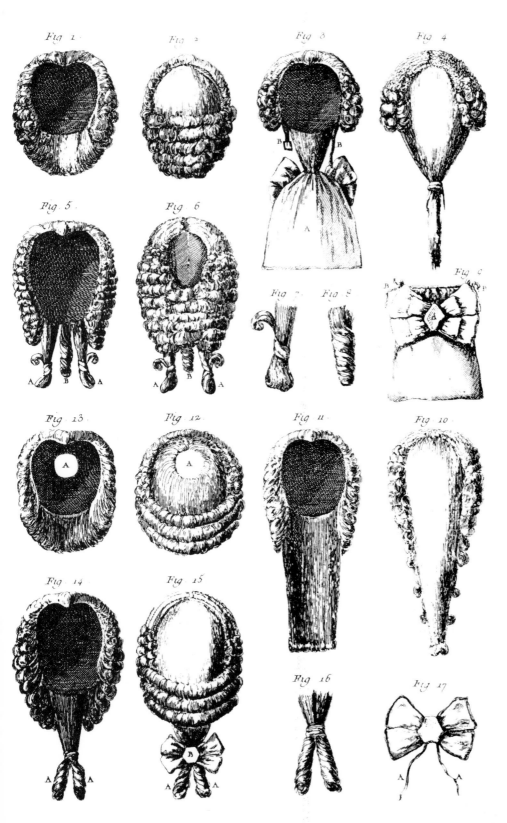

Fig 1.   Fig 2.   Fig 3.   Fig 4.

Fig 5.   Fig 6.   Fig 7.   Fig 8.   Fig 9.

Fig 13.   Fig 12.   Fig 11.   Fig 10.

Fig 14.   Fig 15.   Fig 16.   Fig 17.

92 Types of 18 cent wigs (After *Diderot*)

1 & 2 Exterior and interior of wig with two tails. AA tails; BB rosettes

3 & 4 Exterior and interior of squared wig. AA spiral curl

5 & 6 Interior and exterior of Catogan wig. AA Catogan

7 & 8 Ladies wig with frizzed chignon, side and back view. A crêpe; B frizz; CC cords

9 & 10 Interior and exterior of lady's wig with raised chignon. A crêpe; BB side curls; CC spiral curls; D hair cap; E comb; F chignon

11 Transformation, AA cords

12, 13 Hanging spiral curls (ringlets)

14 Hair employed as false plait (or tail)

15 Hair cap

16, 17 & 18 Curls of varying forms

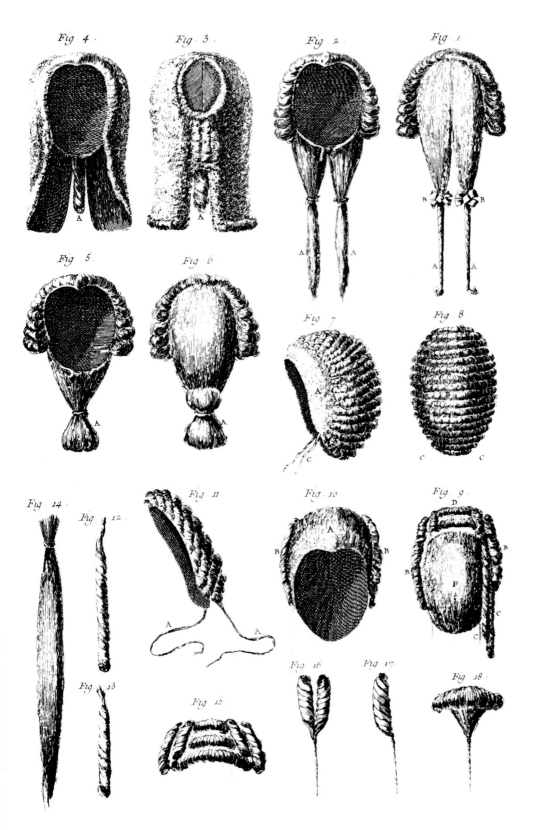

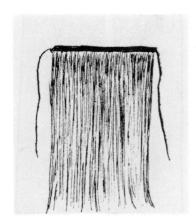

93 Adaptor. From the late 1920s

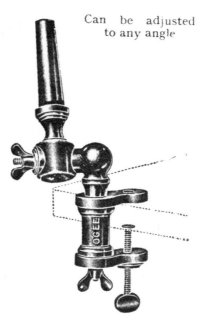

Can be adjusted to any angle

95 Iron block holder and clamp to secure to the work bench, 19th and 20th cent

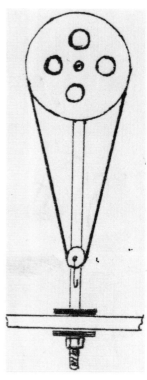

95A Jigger or winding machine, early 19 cent

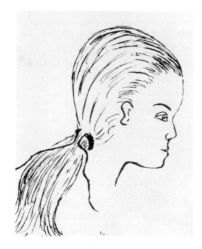

94 Adaptor in position

96 Letterhead of W Gibbs, Hairdresser and Peruke Maker, Dorchester, Dorset, c 1850

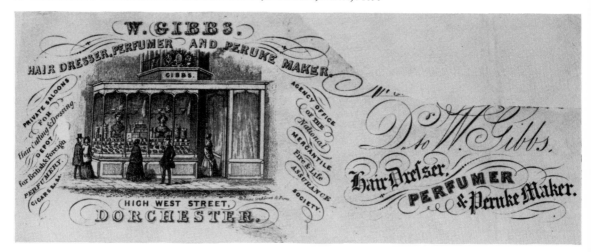

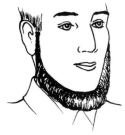

A Chin curtain beard

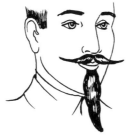

B Napoleon III or Imperial beard

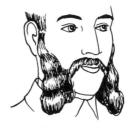

C Friendly mutton chops

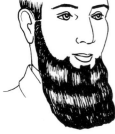

D Spade or Shenandoah beard

E à la Souvaroff whiskers (American version)

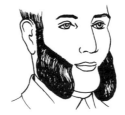

F Mutton chop whiskers

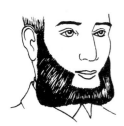

G Old Dutch beard

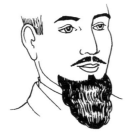

H Modified goatee beard

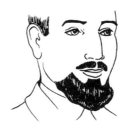

I Balbo beard

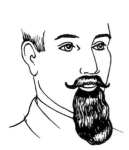

J Goatee beard

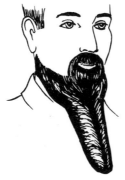

K Ducktail beard

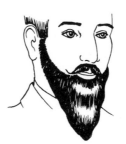

L Van Dyke beard

97 19th and 20th cent beard styles (After *Trusty*)

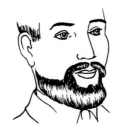 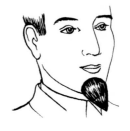 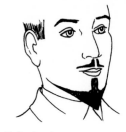

A Hollywoodian beard   B Petit goatee beard   C Anchor beard

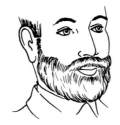 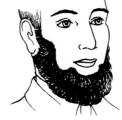 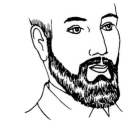

D Medium full beard   E Lincolnic beard   F Short beard

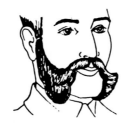  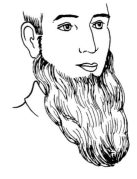

G Hulihee beard   H Handlebar and chin puff   I Jumbo junior beard

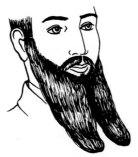 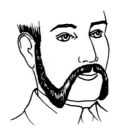 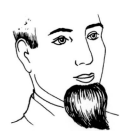

J French fork beard   K Franz Josef beard   L Norris skipper beard

98 19th and 20th cent beard styles (After *Trusty*)

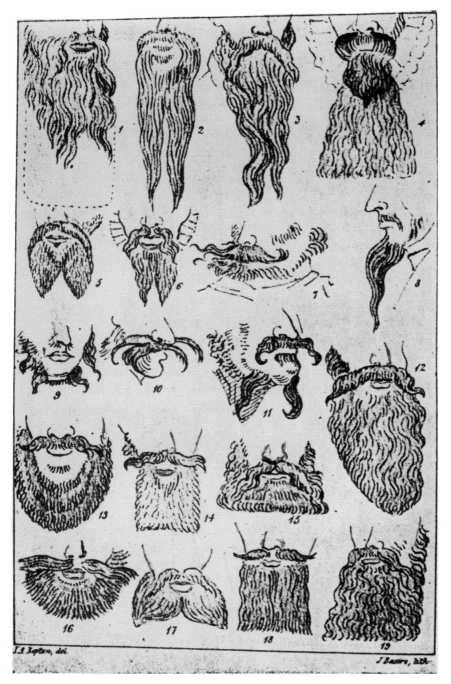

99 16th and 17th cent beards (After *Repton*)
(1) Bushy forked beard. (2) Forked beard. (3) Forked beard. (4) Long spread-out
beard. (5) Forked beard. (6) Forked beard. (7) Fools beard or stubble beard. (8) Pisa
beard. (9) Fools beard. (10) Fools beard. (11) Fools beard. (12) Sugar loaf beard. (13)
Circular or round beard. (14) Tile beard. (15) Broad spread-out beard. (16) Circular or
Round beard. (17) Swallow's tail beard. (18) Tile beard (similar to 19th cent miner's
beard). (19) Tile beard

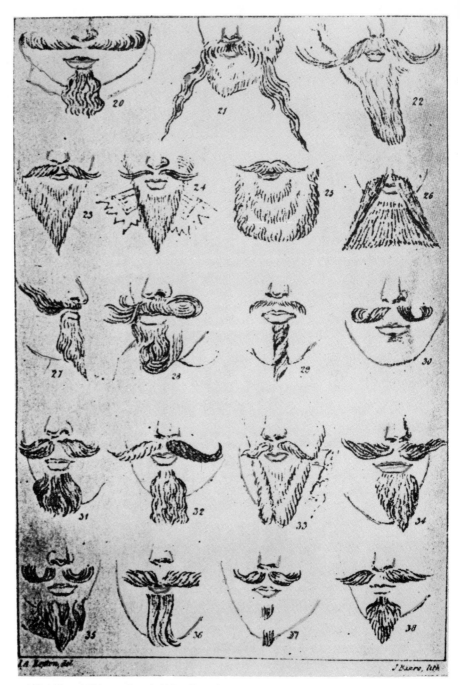

100 16th and 17th cent beards (After *Repton*)
(20) Chin tuft (barbula or pick-a-devant. (21) Bodkin beard with drooping ended
moustache. (22) Stiletto or bodkin beard. (23) Stiletto or bodkin beard. (24) Stiletto or
bodkin beard. (25) Spade beard. (26) Swallow's tail beard. (27) Stiletto or bodkin
beard. (28) Medium beard. (29) Screw beard. (30) Single tuft or barbula. (31) Round
chin tuft or round barbula. (32) Square chin tuft. (33) Triangular beard. (34) Stiletto
or bodkin beard. (35) Stiletto or bodkin beard. (36) Roman T beard or hammer-cut
beard. (37) Double tuft or double barbula. (38) Stiletto or bodkin beard

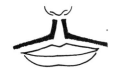  

A Pencil line moustache   B Handlebar moustache   C Howie moustache

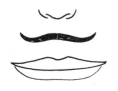 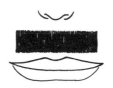 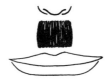

D Chevron moustache   E Sloping box car moustache   F Square Button, Hitler or
                                                                Charlie Chaplin moustache

 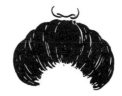

G Strip-teaser moustache   H Box Car moustache   I Walrus moustache

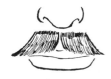  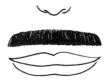

J The General (*Foan*)   K Shermanic moustache   L Painter's Brush moustache

101 A to L 19th cent and 20th cent. moustache styles (After *Foan and Trusty*)

(*continued overleaf*)

M Adolph Menjou moustache

N Mistletoe moustache

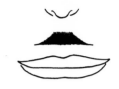

O Wing moustache

P Pyramidal moustache

Q The major (*Foan*)

R The guardsman (*Foan*)

S Walrus or Old Bill
moustache

T The Consort (*Foan*)

U The Captain (*Foan*)

V The Regent (*Foan*)

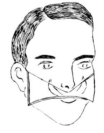

W Moustache trainer or
Schnurbart-binde

X The Shadow (*Foan*)

Y The Military (*Foan*)

Z The Coleman (*Foan*)

101 M to Z 19th cent and 20th cent moustache styles (After *Foan and Trusty*)

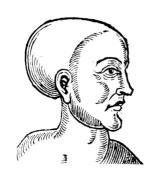

A Artificial baldness

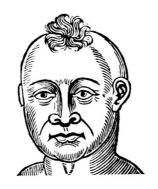

B Tuft of St Croix

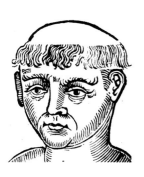

C Aetolian tonsure

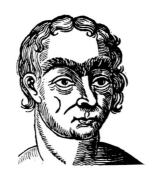

D Beetle brows

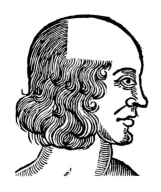

E Brazilian tonsure

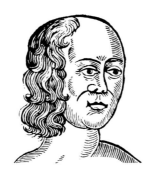

F Maxie hairdress

102 Men's hair styles A-F, 17th cent (After *Bulwer*)

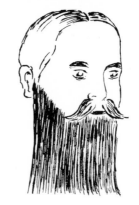

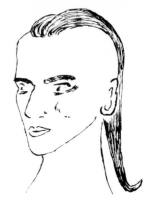

G Miner's beard (French) *c* 1912

H A celtic warrior wearing a glib or gleebe

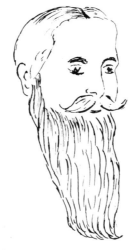

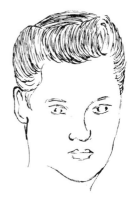

I Olympian beard (French) *c* 1912

J Elvis cut

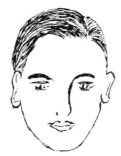

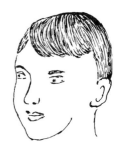

K English cut

L Caesar cut

102 Men's hair styles G-L, 19th and 20th cent (After *Bulwer*)

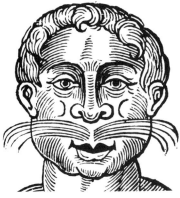

A Cat moustache; worn by men of mancy, India 17th cent (*Bulwer*)

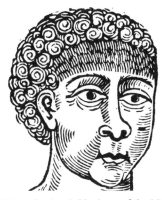

B Low forehead. Mexicans of the 16th/17th cent regarded a low forehead as being a mark of beauty. (*Bulwer*)

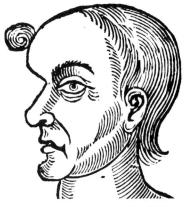

C Stoole-Ball hairdress. Italian 17th cent man's style (*Bulwer*)

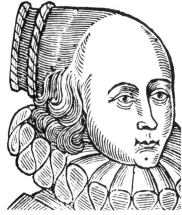

D Spanish woman of the 17th cent with plucked forehead. Italian women of the 15th cent affected high foreheads as a mark of beauty and plucked the hair from the front part of the head. Spanish women of the 17th cent adopted a similar style (*Bulwer*)

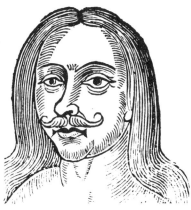

E A man of Comata. Comata was a district in the French Alps so called because of the long hair worn by men and women there in the 16th/17th cent (*Bulwer*)

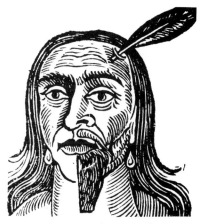

F Half beard. The native males of Virginia in the 16th/17th cent wore half of their beards shaven, and the other half long. The hairdressing was performed by women who shaved the men with shells (*Bulwer*)

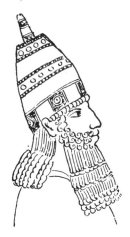

G Assyrian Beard. 1000 BC (After *Villermont*)

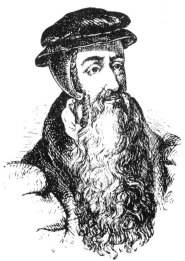

H Full, patriarchal or Olympian beard, as worn by John Knox, 16th cent (After *Proctor*)

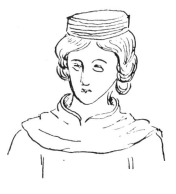

I Barrette headdress, 13th cent (After *Villermont*)

103 Hair styles A-F, 16th/17th cent (After *Bulwer*)

227

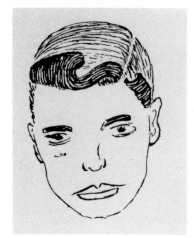

A The coif (*Foan*)

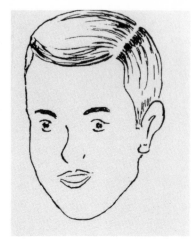

B Regular English cut

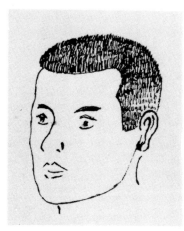

C Crew cut

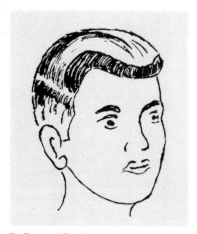

D Forward Boogie cut

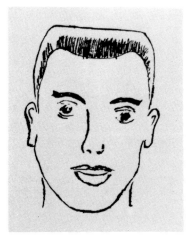

E Flat-top cut

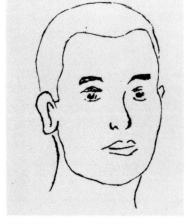

F Yul Brynner cut (*Bald*)

104 Men's hair styles, 20th cent A-F

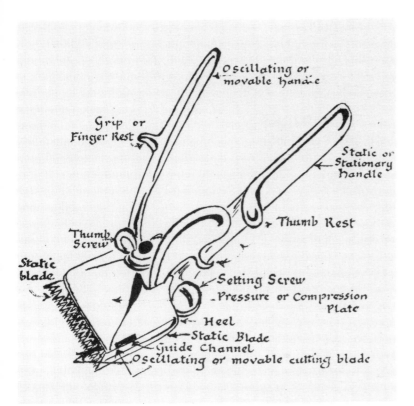

105 Hand clippers, 20th cent

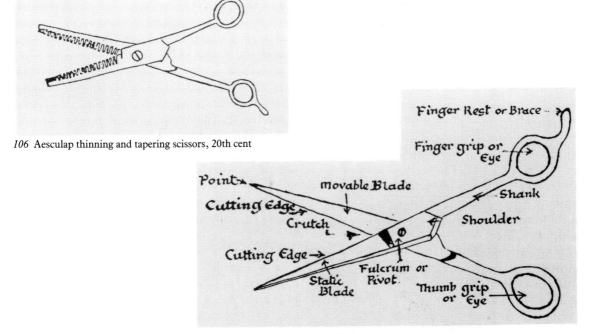

106 Aesculap thinning and tapering scissors, 20th cent

107 Constituent parts of a pair of scissors

229

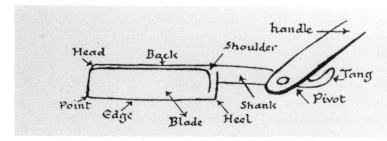

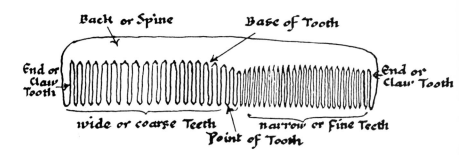

108 Constituent parts of a cut-throat razor, 19th/20th cent

109 Constituent parts of a hairdressing comb, 19th/20th cent

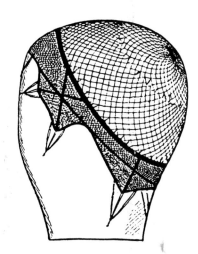

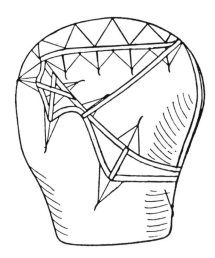

110 Transformation foundation with caul net, but when the caul is knotted with hair it constitutes a wig foundation – 19th/20th cent

111 Gentleman's wig foundation, 1887 (After *Creer*)

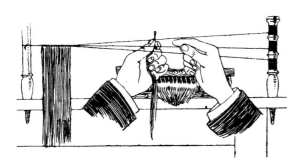

112 The process of weaving

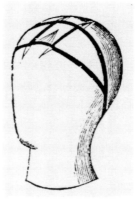

113 Temple mounted front.
(After *Sutton*)

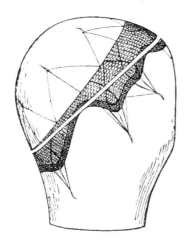

114 Hair net transformation mount,
showing gallon bind also bracings
(After *Sutton*)

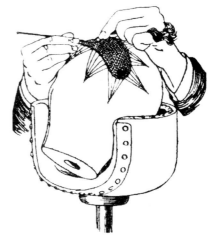

115 The process of knotting a front.
Wooden block resting in a cup-
shaped block holder, 19th cent

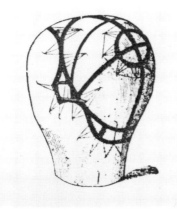

116 Gentleman's weft wig foundation,
19th cent (After *Sutton*)

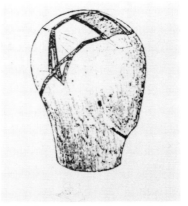

117 Gallon mount for a bandeau (before
the addition of the net foundation),
19th cent

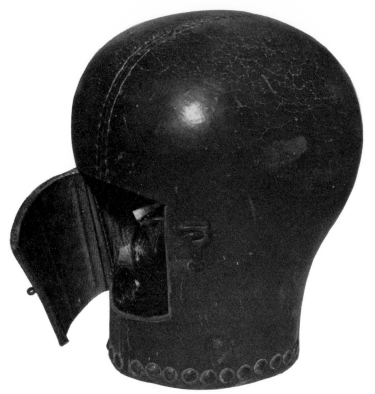

118 Portable hollow leather wig block, with door for access to interior where tools could be carried. Early 19th cent. Used by the writer's grandfather, John Stevens

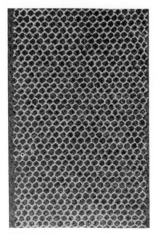

119 Medium-mesh stiffened foundation net

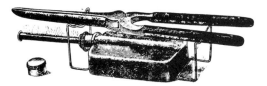

120 Travelling spirit stove for heating curling irons, c 1880

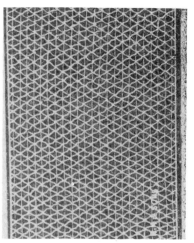

123 Diamond-barred-mesh hair net for postiche partings, 19th cent

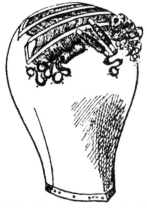

121 Postiche front taped and in-pli on a malleable block

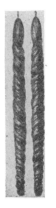

122 Alexandra curl

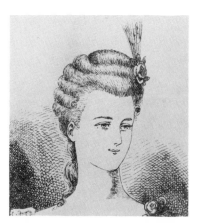

124 Marquise coiffure, time of Louis XV. Notice aigrette

232

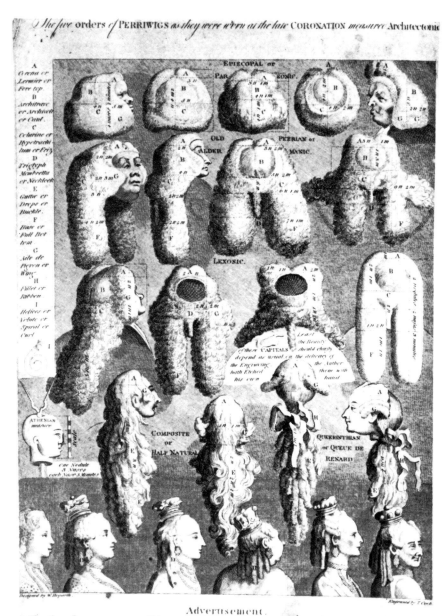

125 The Five Orders of Periwigs as they were worn at the Coronation (of George III, 1760) (After a print by William Hogarth)
Top row: Episcopal or parsonic wigs
2nd row: Aldermanic Wigs
3rd row: Lexonic wigs
4th row: Left-hand side, composite or half-natural
next the *Right-hand side,* queerinthian
or queue de Renard
5th row: Ladies wigs

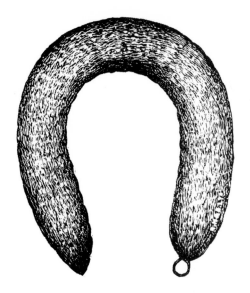

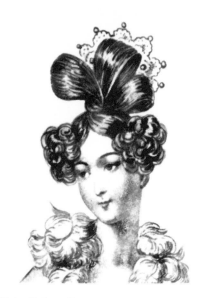

126 All-round frisette pad

127 Apollo knot (from *Le Beau Monde*, October 1831)

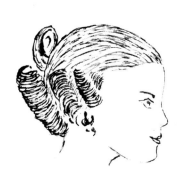

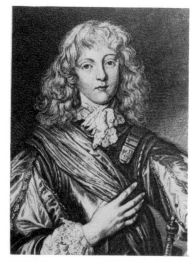

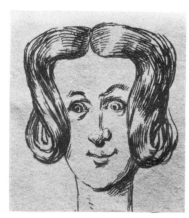

128 Antoine Bob

129 Natural hair flowing style, *c* 1660.
Philip, Earl of Pembroke

130 Architectural style, 1857

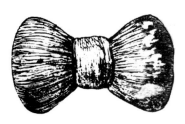

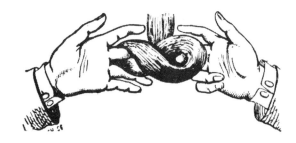

131 Apollo bow, also called Cravat bow and Coque d'Appolon

132 Apollo bow, method of formation

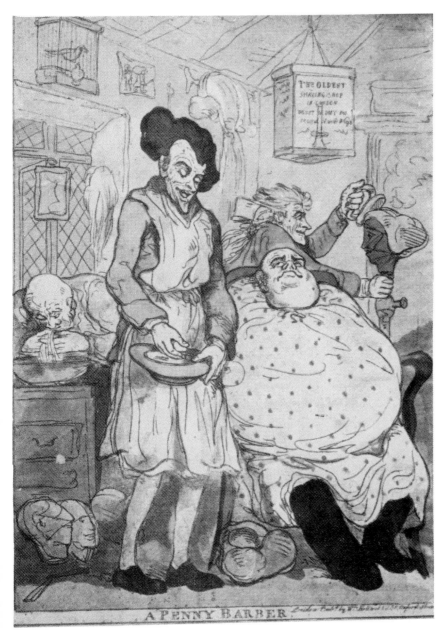

133 'At The Chair', a penny barber, late
18th cent (After a print by
W. Holland). Notice the barber
pressing the front hair of the wig
with a smoothing iron (flat-iron from
1810), also the caged bird. Birds
were kept by most barbers until the
1914-18 War. Linnets, goldfinches
and canaries were the popular choice

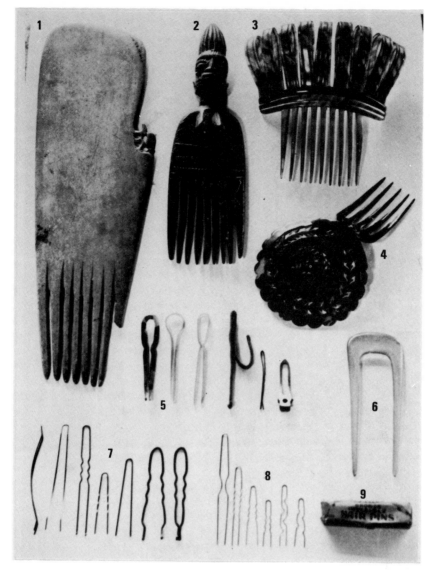

134

1 Maori hair comb of whalebone, early
  19th cent
2 African hair comb of carved wood,
  early 19th cent
3 Back comb, *c* 1900
4 Comb with hinged decoration, *c* 1900
5 Three shell pins a lead curler, a
  kirbigrip and curl clip
6 A shell comb
7 Hairpins of different designs, *c* 1920
8 Invisible pins of different designs
  c 1920
9 Packet of hairpins *c* 1920

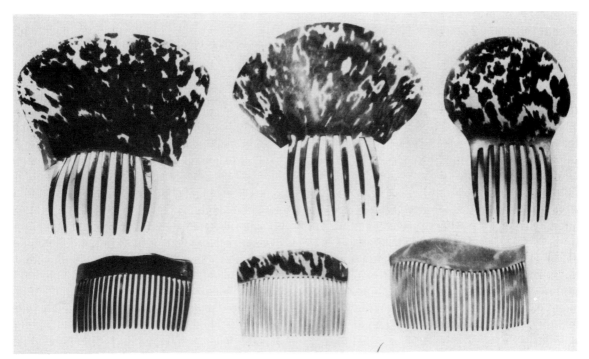

135 Top row: Spanish combs. *Bottom row:* Back combs

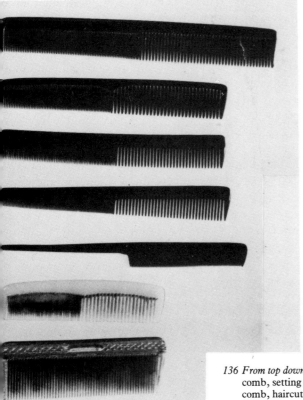

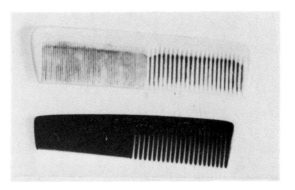

137 Two dressing combs for long hair, *c* 1900

136 From top down: Dressing or setting comb, setting comb, hair-cutting comb, haircutting comb, tail comb, pocket comb, pocket comb

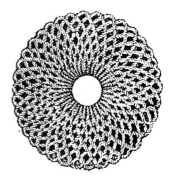

138 Expanding circular braid mount

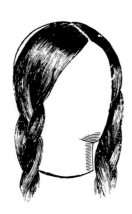

139 Bandeau

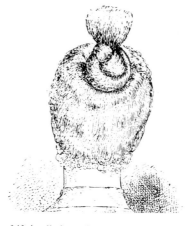

140 Apollo knot, late 19th cent (After *Mallemont*)

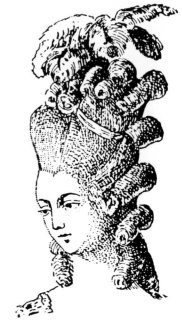

141 Bandeau d'Amour coiffure, *c* 1780

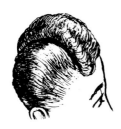

142 Bandeau Grecque, 19th cent

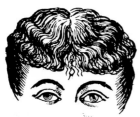

143 Bandeau Russe, 19th cent

144 1 Grecian style coiffure, 1867
2 Artificial chignon composed of long spiral curls mounted as a cachepeigne
3 Bandelette waved for wearing as a fringe. Made on a weft
4 Curled cachepeigne covered with an invisible net. The longest hanging curls are made of 36" curled hair
5 Chignon composed of a frizzed plait
6 Chignon composed of puffed curls
7 Frizzed loose coil

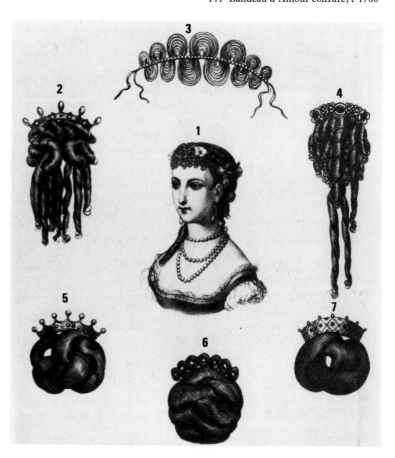

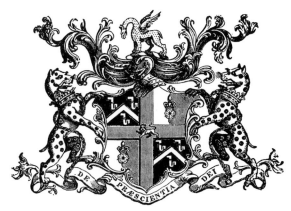

145 Arms of the Barbers Company. (After *Lambert*)

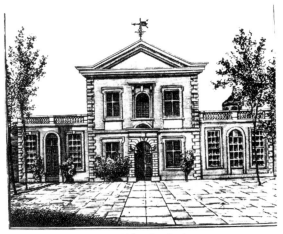

146 Barber's Hall, 1881. (After *Lambert*)

147 A Gallant being prinked (After *La Serre,
Le Breviere des Courtisans,* 1645)

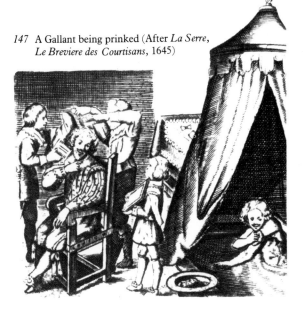

The OATH of a Freeman of the Company of
Barbers and *Surgeons* of *London.*

YOU shall Swear that you shall be True and
Loyal to our Sovereign Lord King GEORGE,
and faithful and true in all lawful things unto
the Corporation and Company of the Mystery
and Commonalty of the Barbers and Surgeons of
London, Whereof you are now made free, and accordingly be
obedient to the Masters or Governours thereof, and, as
much as in you lieth, maintain Amity and Unity therein,
and obey observe and perform all the lawful Rules, Sta
tutes, and Ordinances thereof, and be proportionably con
tributory to the best of your power to all lawful or reasonable Charges, Contributions and Payments belonging or
necessarily appertaining to you to bear and pay as other Bre
thren of the same Company do, and also you shall obey all
manner of lawful Summons or Warnings done or to be
made by the Clerk, Beadle or other Officer of the said Company thereunto assigned, in the Name of the Masters or
Governours having no lawful or reasonable Excuse or Im-
pediment to the contrary. All these Articles you shall duly
truly, fully and faithfully observe, perform and keep to the
best of your power. So help you God.

God save the KING.

148 Oath of a Freeman of the Company of Barbers and
Surgeons of London, *c* 1720

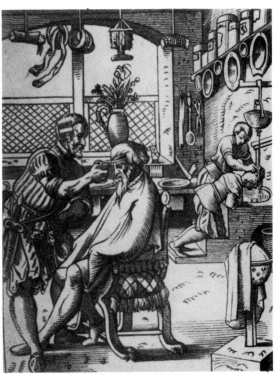

149 Interior of a 16th cent barber-surgeon's shop

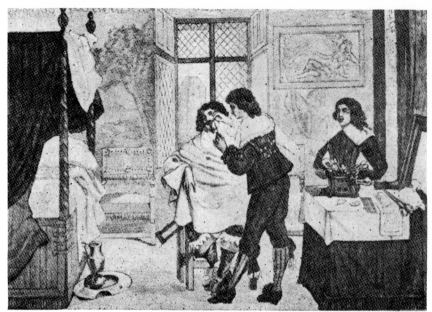

150 A French barber cutting a
moustache, 1642 (After *Abraham Bosse*)

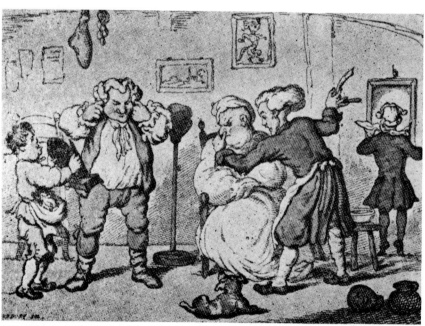

151 18th cent barber's shop (From a
print after *Bunbury*)

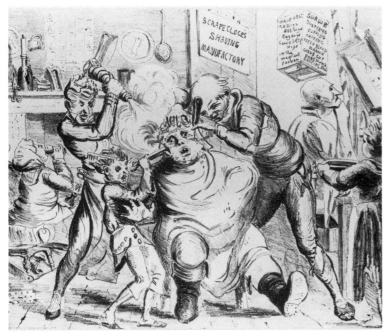

152 An English barber's shop, *c* 1820

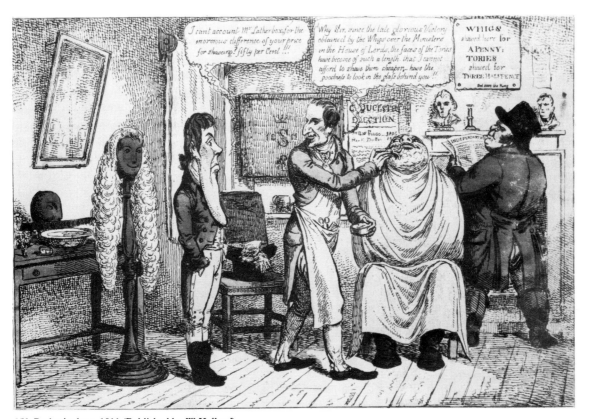

153 Barber's shop, 1811 (Published by *W Holland*)

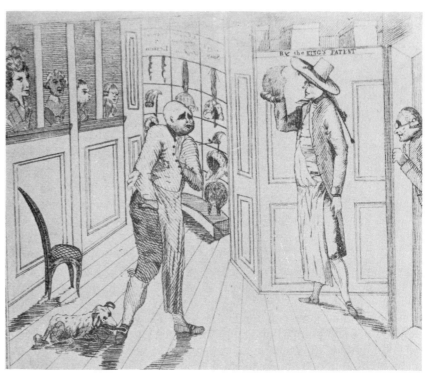

154 London Wigmaker's 1793 (After a print
published by *Fores*)

155 Barber's saloon, Richmond,
Virginia, 1861 (After *The Illustrated
London News*. Note the spitoons)

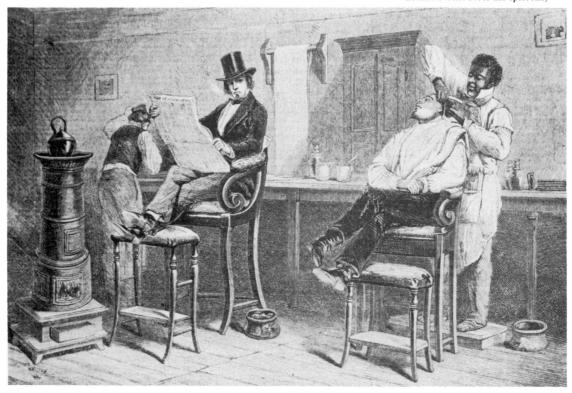

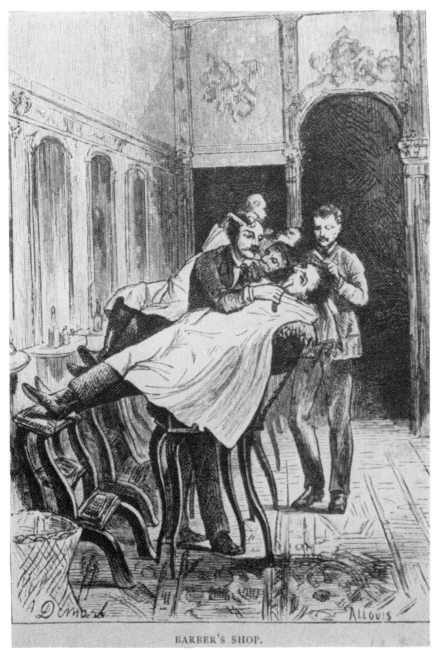

BARBER'S SHOP.

156 'At The Chair' in an American
barber's shop, *c* 1885

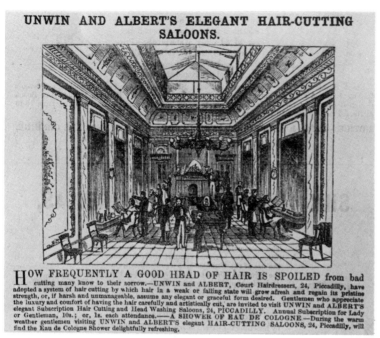

UNWIN AND ALBERT'S ELEGANT HAIR-CUTTING SALOONS.

HOW FREQUENTLY A GOOD HEAD OF HAIR IS SPOILED from bad cutting many know to their sorrow.—UNWIN and ALBERT, Court Hairdressers, 24, Piccadilly, have adopted a system of hair cutting by which hair in a weak or falling state will grow afresh and regain its pristine strength, or, if harsh and unmanageable, assume any elegant or graceful form desired. Gentlemen who appreciate the luxury and comfort of having the hair carefully and artistically cut, are invited to visit UNWIN and ALBERT'S elegant Subscription Hair Cutting and Head Washing Saloons, 24, PICCADILLY. Annual Subscription for Lady or Gentleman, 10s.; or, 1s. each attendance.——A SHOWER OF EAU DE COLOGNE—During the warm weather gentlemen visiting UNWIN and ALBERT'S elegant HAIR-CUTTING SALOONS, 24, Piccadilly, will find the Eau de Cologne Shower delightfully refreshing.

157 Hair-cutting Saloon, Piccadilly, (From an advertisement)

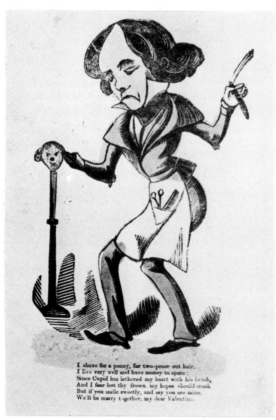

158 Valentine, c 1850. Note the Barber's apron

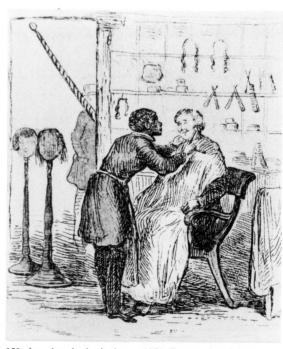

159 American barber's shop, c 1850. From a pictorial card forming part of a game called 'The Yankee Trader'

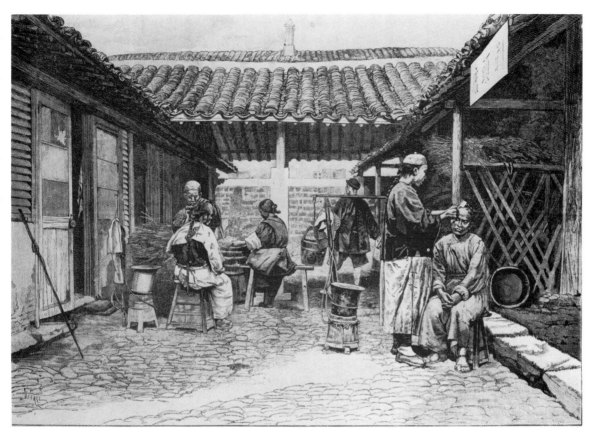

160 Chinese itinerant barber, 1876
(After *The Illustrated London News*)

161 Queue dressing. 'Pigtails and Powder'.
(From the watercolour by *Frank Dadd*, 1884)

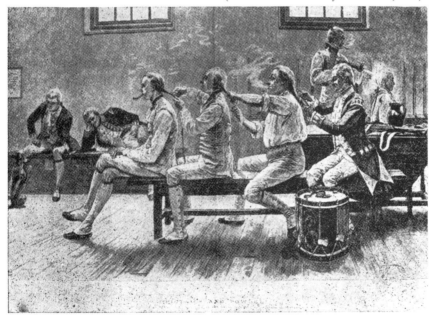

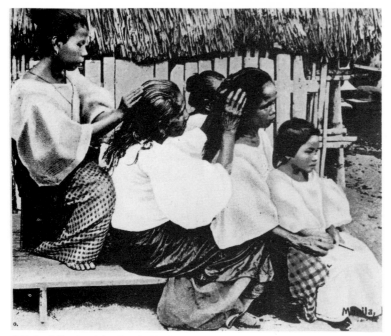

162 Squirling (or delousing) in Manilla, 1900

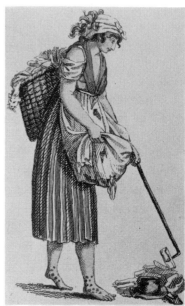

163 Chiffoniere or rag gatherer, c 1815

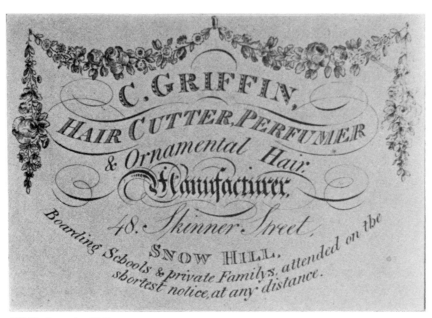

164 Trade card, c 1840

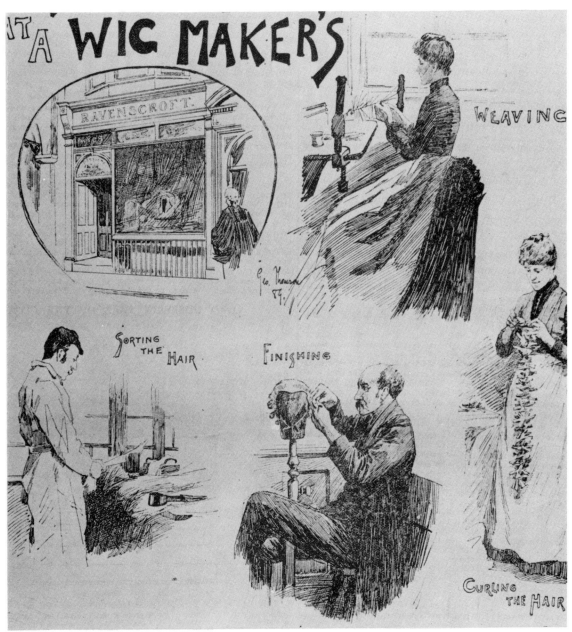

165 Ravenscroft, Wigmaker, London. Showing processes in the manufacture of a barrister's wig (From *Pall Mall Budget*, 30th May 1889)

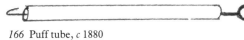

166 Puff tube, *c* 1880

167 A Pyr-pointed hairpin

PYR POINTED

Grip & Plain.

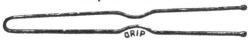

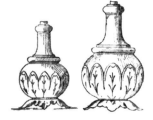

168 Decorated Nickel Shampoo Gourds, 19th cent

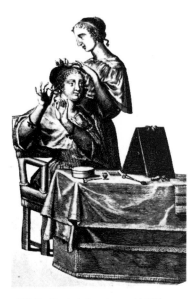

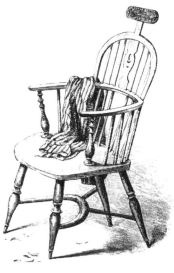

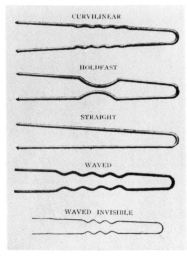

169 Ladies hairdressing, mid 17th cent

170 A barber's chair, 19th cent (After *Procter*)

171 Hairpins, *c* 1920

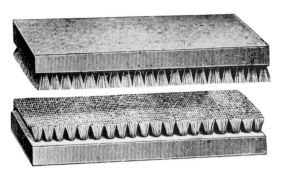

172 Drawing brushes, 19th/20th cent

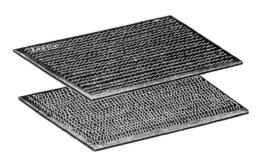

173 Wire drawing cards set in leather foundation, 19th cent

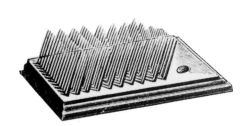

174 Card or hackle, 19th/20th cent

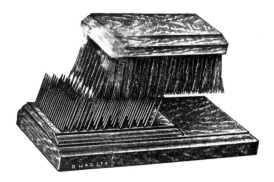

175 Card or hackle with brush guard, 19th/20th cent

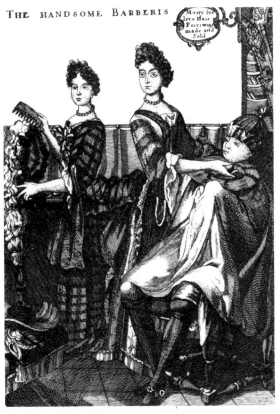

THE HANDSOME BARBERIS

Merry for live Hair Perriwigs made and Sold

176 Barberesses, 17th cent

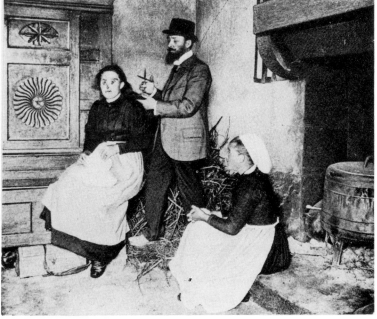

177 Barber's bowl, 17th cent.
Bristol Delft. (In the collection of the
writer)

178 Human hair collector cutting the
tresses of a peasant. Near Quintin,
Brittany, France, late 19th cent

249

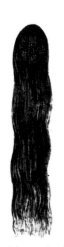

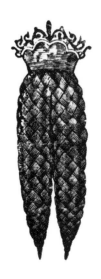

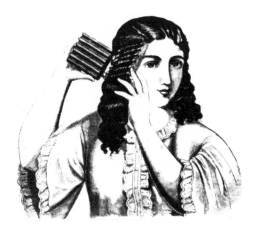

179 Postiche patch with long knotted hair

180 Seven strand double plait

181 A home hair crimper, 1862

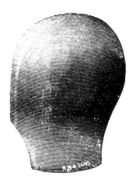

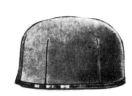

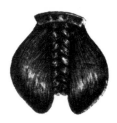

182 Wooden wig block

183 Malleable chignon block

184 Chignon of natural hair and postiche, 1863

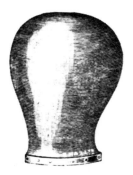

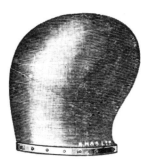

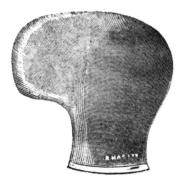

185 Malleable wig block

186 Malleable semi-transformation block

187 Malleable transformation block

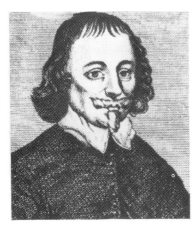

188 Roman T beard as worn by Richard Brome, poet, before 1652

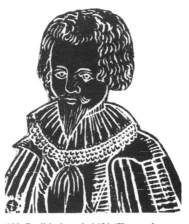

189 Bodkin beard, 1621 (From a brass rubbing by *A B Connor*)

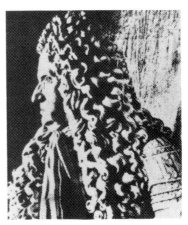

190 Allonge periwig. Baroque style, late 17th cent

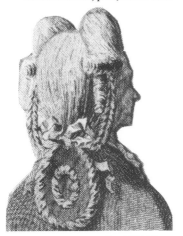

191 En Medaillon peruke, 1777 (From *The Ladies Magazine*)

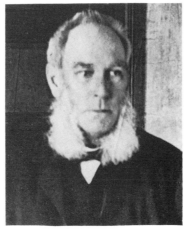

192 Mutton-chop whiskers worn by William Ludlow, farmer, Nynehead, Somerset 1875

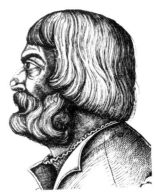

193 Bobbed natural hair, *c* 1500 (After an engraving by *Albert Dürer*)

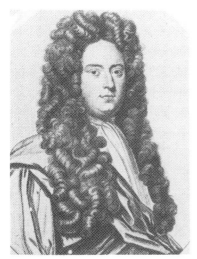

194 A full-bottom wig, *c* 1685 (After a painting by *Sir Godfrey Kneller*)

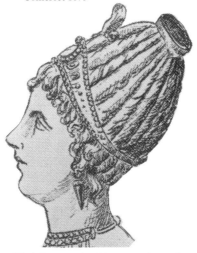

195 A Roman wig. (From a sculptured bust)

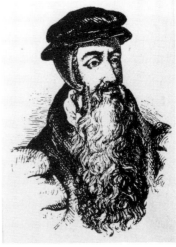

196 Full Patriarchal or Olympian beard as worn by John Knox

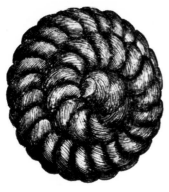 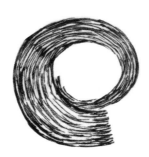 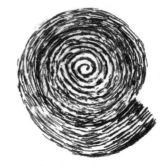

197 Coiled chignon, 36" uncoiled   *198* Barrel-spring curl   *199* Clock-spring curl

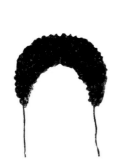 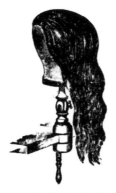 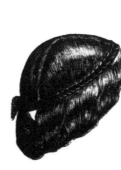 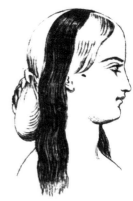

200 Frizzed diadem   *201* Malleable practice block with implanted hair, 20th cent   *202* Tour de Tête, 1863   *203* Postiche strip, 1863

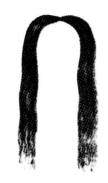 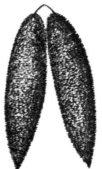 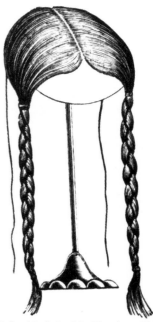

204 Twin tress, 1863   *205* Pair of side frisettes

206 Straight hair plaited bandeau, 19th cent

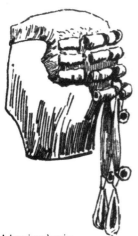

207 A barrister's wig

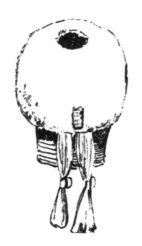

208 Back view of a Judge's wig

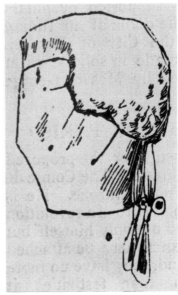

209 Judge's wig

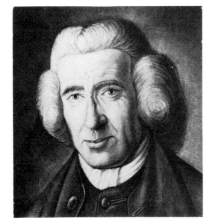

210 A long bob, as worn by James
Ferguson, FRS, 1776

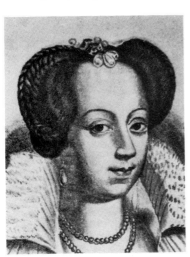

211 *Marguerite d'Angouleme coiffure,
16th cent (After Villermont)*

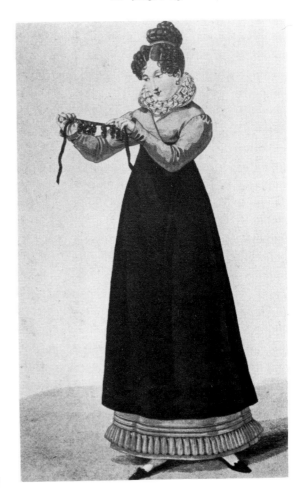

212 Tresseuse
(hair weaver)

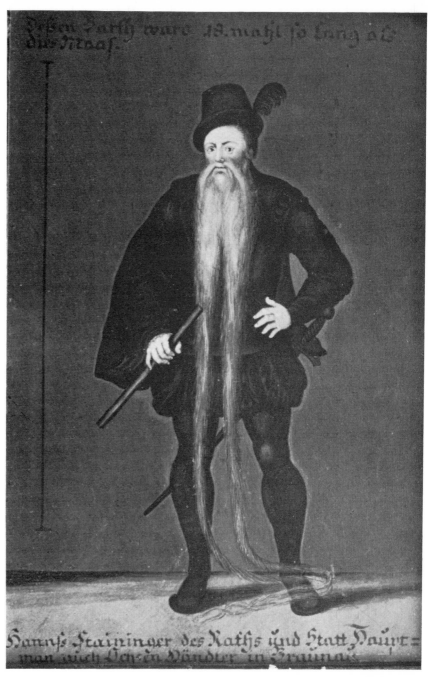

213 Hannss Staininger (d 1567),
burgomaster of Braunau. He had
one of the longest beards on record
(Original painting in the writer's
collection)

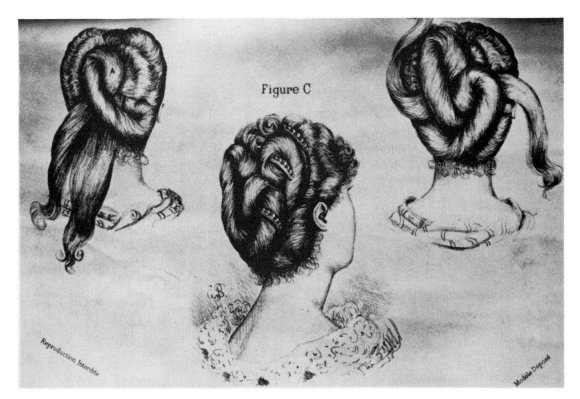

214 Method of dressing a coiffure, May
1883

215 Method of dressing a coiffure, May
1883

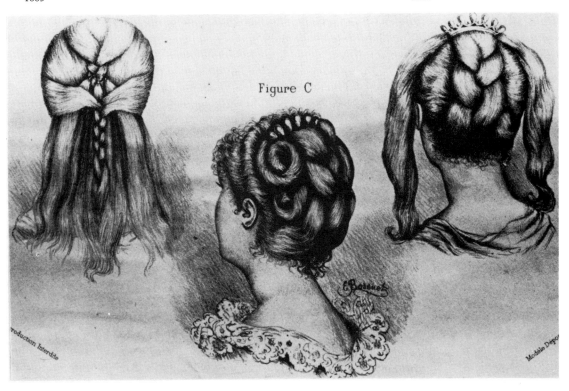

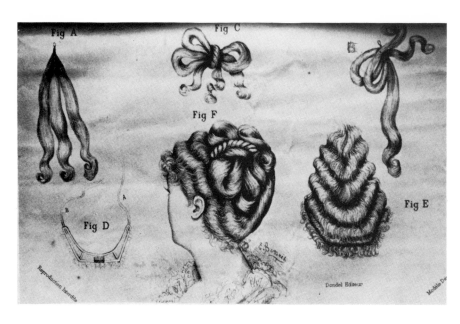

216 Coiffure of August 1883 incorporating the Countess of Pourtales knot
  A 24" three-spill switch
  B Two spills of the plait turned to form two loops
  C Completed knot with the third spill looped and the ends of the three spills gently curled
  D A postiche foundation for the neck
  E Hair arranged on the foundation shown in D
  F Finished coiffure with neck postiche shown in E and the Countess of Pourtales knot incorporated in the dressing, secured by a curved comb

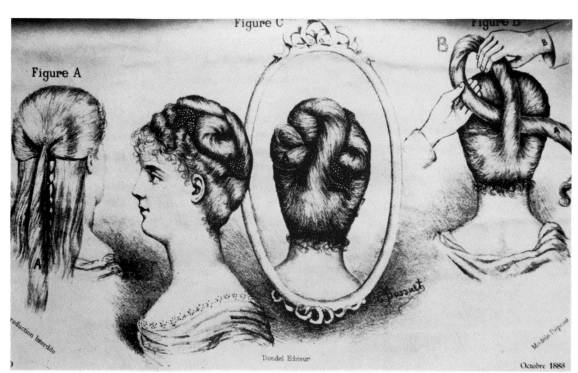

217 Method of dressing a coiffure of 1883

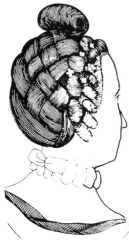

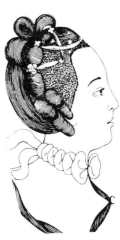

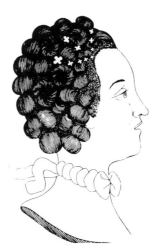

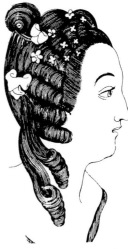

218 Style of 1768. 'Row of buckles half sloping, another in form of snails' shells, back in the manner of inlaid work' (*Legros*)

219 Style of 1768. 'Snail's shell curls and cockade'. (*Legros*)

220 Style of 1768. 'Nape frizzled or tifted in buckles, some sloping, others in the form of roses' (*Legros*)

221 Style of 1768. 'Row of buckles, dragon or serpent composed of two locks of hair with a buckle inverted' (*Legros*)

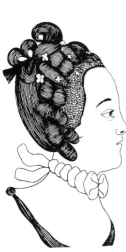

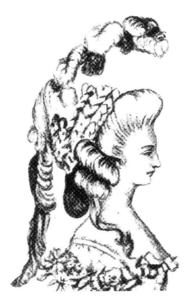

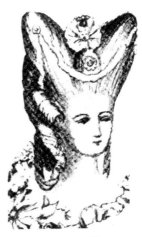

222 Style of 1768. 'Two rows of buckles in the form of shell work barred and thrown backwards, two shells and a knot tied in the form of a spindle composed of a large lock laid smooth taken from behind the head to supply the place of a plume' (*Legros*)

223 Casque à la Clorinde, 1777

224 En Soleil Levant coiffure

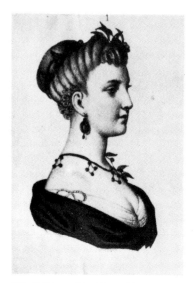

225 Coiffure with chignon Recamier, 1866

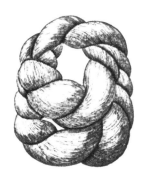

226 Spanish coil chignon

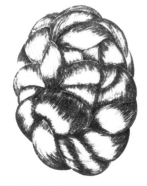

227 Beatrice chignon

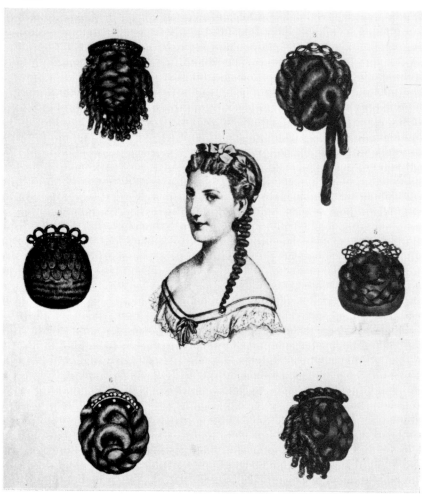

228 Coiffure of 1867
  1 Coiffure with waved bandeau over forehead
  2 Chignon of long curled hair on wire with plait in middle
  3 Chignon with curled hair forming a twist in the centre surrounded with little curls on wire and two Alexandra curls on one side
  4 Chignon Marie Antoinette covered with cap of hair on wire
  5 Chignon Marie Antoinette with a coiled plait
  6 Chignon with coil dressed in a Carman's knot on a wire foundation
  7 Chignon with coiled plait and a grape of curls on a wire foundation.

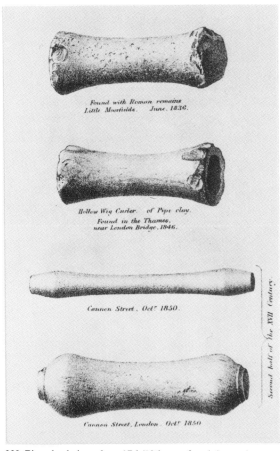

229 Pipe clay hair curlers, 17th/18th cent for piping and curling hair for postiche

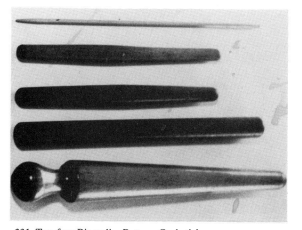

231 *Top* four Bigoudis; *Bottom* Curl stick

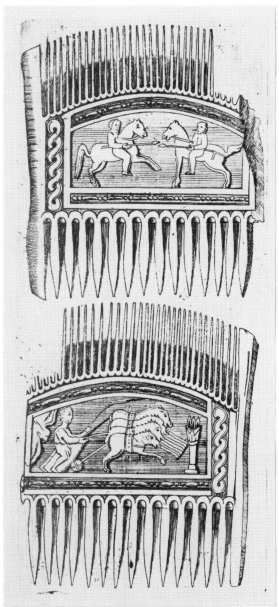

230 Roman hairdressing combs (bone), 2nd cent AD

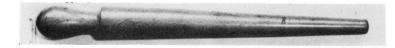

232 Large curl stick, 19th cent, for dressing long, hanging curls

233 Wigs of 1772 (From *Baratariana*, Dublin 1773)

L-R standing
1 Bob wig or bob major, also called citizen's Sunday buckle
2 Cut wig or cauliflower wig
3 Long bob
4 Knotted wig, this bouffant style also called a physical tye
5 Bob wig with the front curls dressed as in a square wig
6 A short bob or minor bob

L-R sitting
1 Physical bob wig, also called episcopal, physical bob, and parsonic (worn by bishops)
2 Short bob or minor bob
3 Physical bob

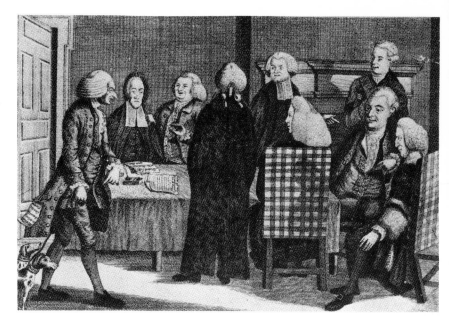

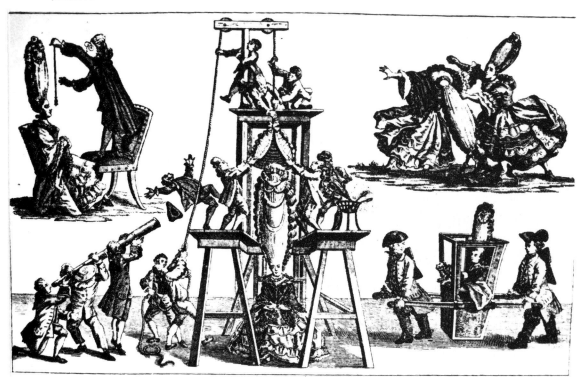

234 Caricature of hairdressing *c* 1771 (After *Villermont*)

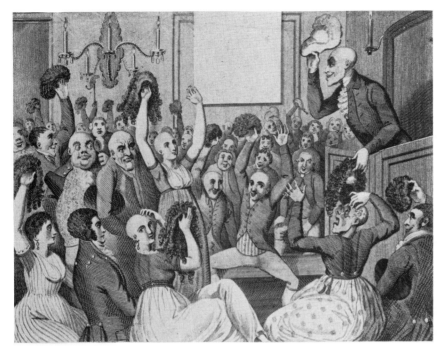

235 'Wigs are the rage, or debate on the
baldness of the times', *c* 1790 (After
R Newton)

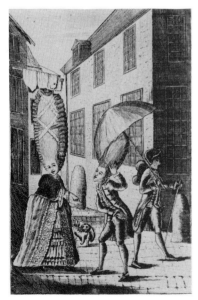

236 Paris street scene, 18th cent. The
two men are dressed à la Macaroni

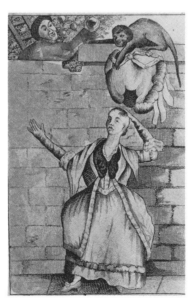

237 'Sleight of hand by a monkey or the
ladies head unloaded', 18th cent

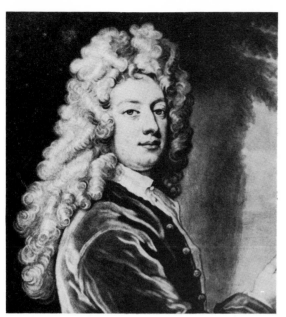

238 Full-bottom wig (After a painting by Sir Godfrey Kneller, 1710)

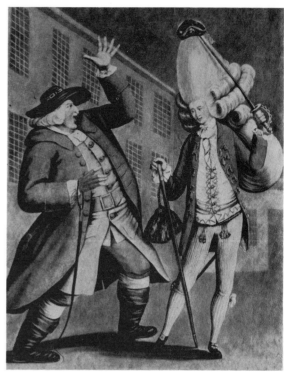

239 A Macaroni peruke, *c* 1775 (After *S Grimm*)

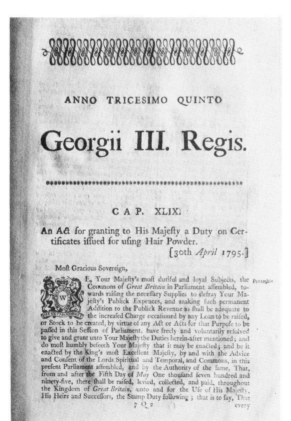

240 A Hair Powder Act, 1795

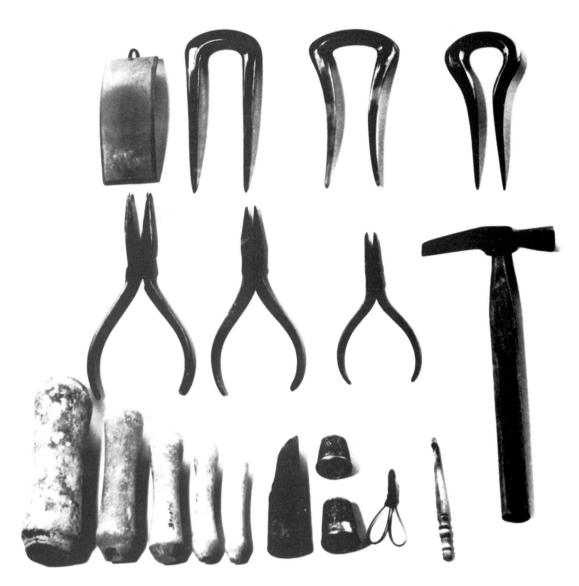

241 *Top row:* Slide and three horn pins, late 19th cent
Middle row: Block point pliers and boardwork hammer
Bottom row: 5 pipe clay hair curlers 17th/18th cent, metal finger shield, two thimbles, a jockey, bone knotting needle for knotting large pinches of hair to soft, open net

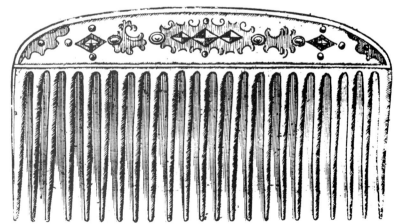

242 Roman bone hair comb, 2nd cent

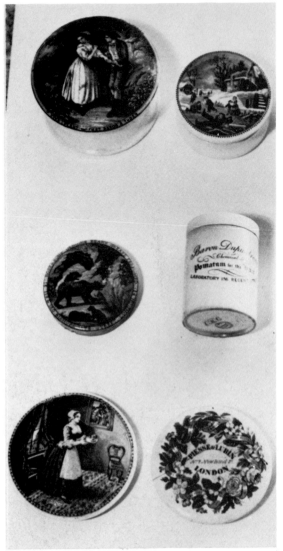

243 Bear's grease and pomatum pots

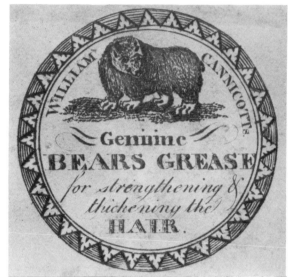

244 Bear's grease pot label

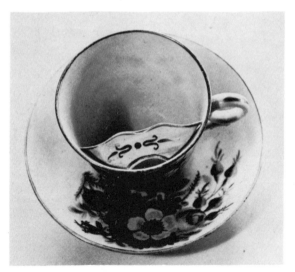

245 Moustache cup, 19th cent

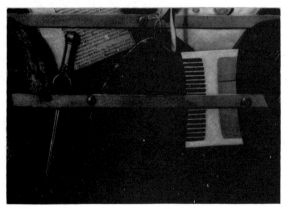

246 Hairdressing combs of 1696 (from a painting by *E Colyer*)

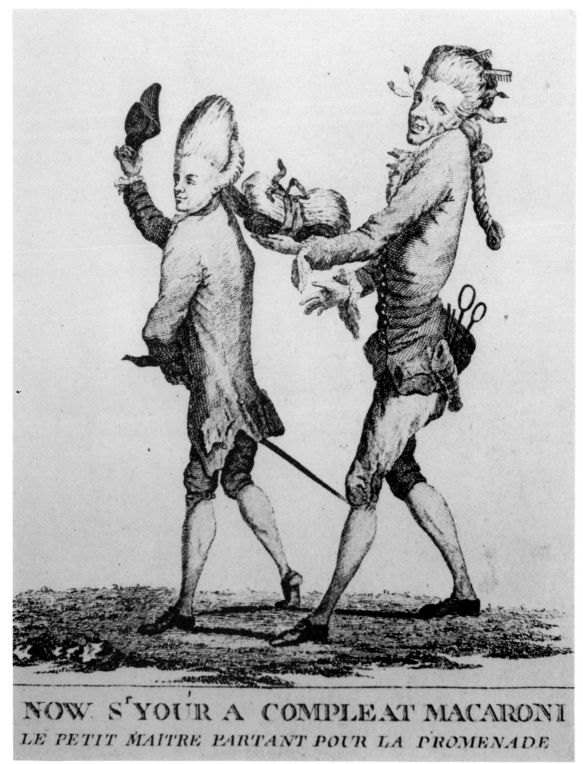

NOW S'YOUR A COMPLEAT MACARONI

LE PETIT MAITRE PARTANT POUR LA PROMENADE

247 Macaroni wig and barber with a queue wig, 18th cent. Notice the curling irons sticking out of the barber's tail pocket, also his powder puff

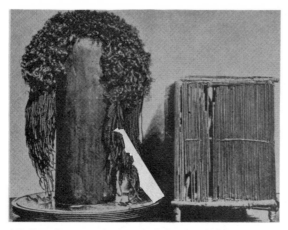

248 Egyptian woman's wig and wig box, *c* 1400 BC

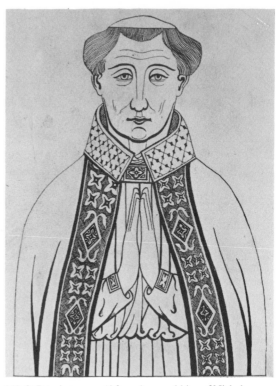

249 St Peter's tonsure (After a brass rubbing of Nicholas North, 1445, by *Arthur Connor*, FSA)

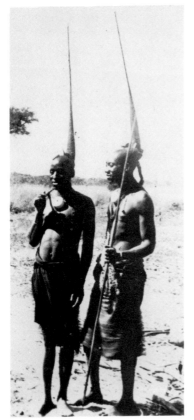

250 Cone headdresses, *qv*.

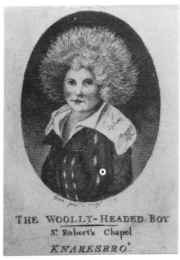

251 Woolly-headed Boy of Knaresborough, 1793

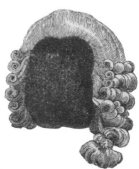

252 18th cent wig worn by Linnaeus (1707-1778), founder of modern botany

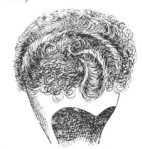

253 Semi-transformation on hollow, velvet-covered display block, late 19th cent

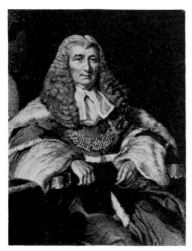

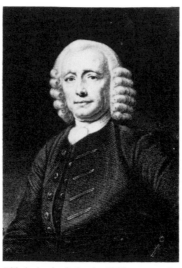

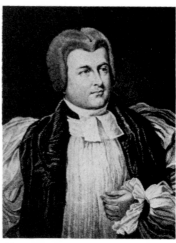

254 A Judge's full-bottom wig as worn by Baron Tenterden, *qv*

255 A six-tier bob wig, 1768, as worn by John Hamon, horologist

256 A Bishop's wig or Physical bob, also called Episcopal or Parsonic peruke

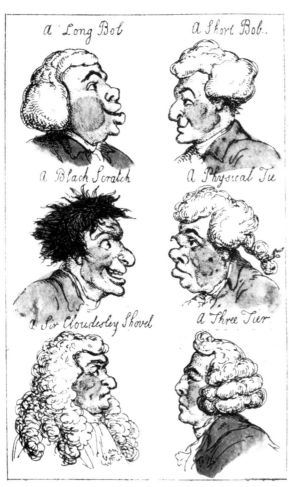

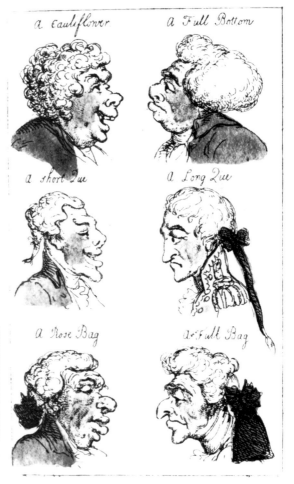

257 18th cent wigs (After *Rowlandson*)

258 18th cent wigs (After *Rowlandson*)

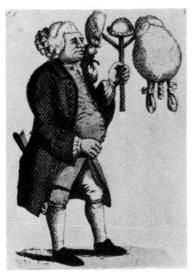

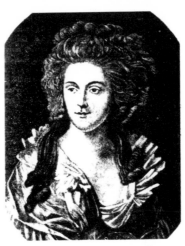

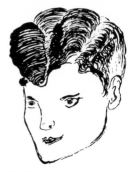

261 Cockscomb

259 18th cent perukes. Barber holding wig stand wears a Major bob; *Left:* on stand a Cadogan; *Middle:* a Minor bob; *Right:* a Physical Tye

260 La Duchesse d'Orleans coiffure, 18th cent

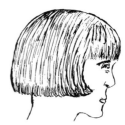

262 Egyptian bob

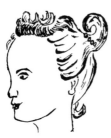

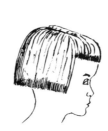

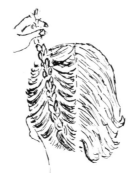

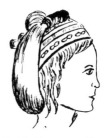

263 A la Grecque coiffure, 1742

264 Buster Brown bob

265 French braid

266 A la Grecque coiffure, 1797

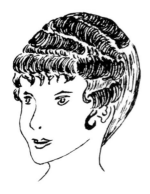

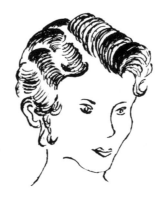

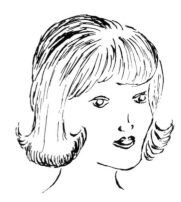

267 Gilda bob

268 Soubrette bob

269 Guiche style

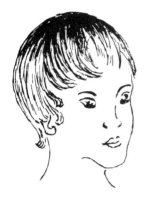

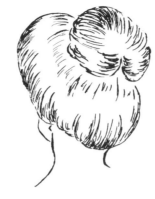

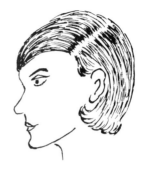

270 Faun bob

271 Brioche style

272 Marienbad style

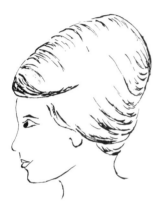

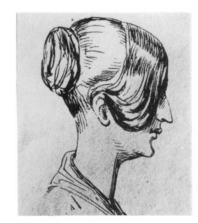

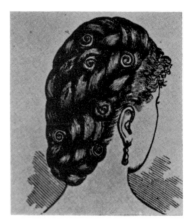

273 Beehive style, 1959-1963

274 Blinkers, 1857

275 Zephyr coiffure (After *Creer*)

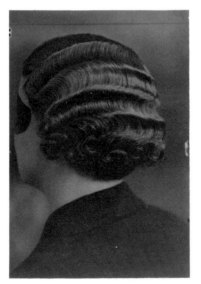

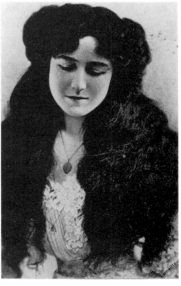

276 Permanently waved Short bob with
curled ends. Executed by the writer
using the Gallia System, 1928

277 Flowing hair. Miss Madge Crichton,
1904

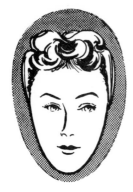

278 Oval face

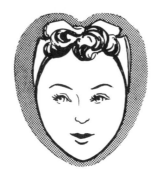

279 Heart-shaped face

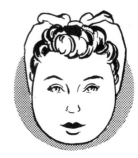

280 Round face

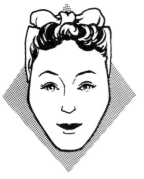

281 Diamond-shaped face

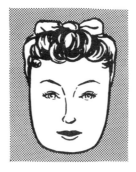

282 Square face

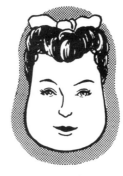

283 Pear-shaped face

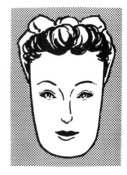

284 Oblong face

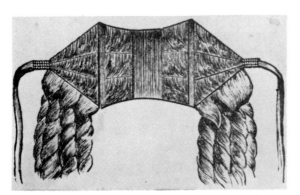

285 French ringlet front with parting, showing foundation
    (After *Creer*, 1887)

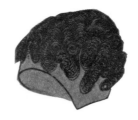

286 Eureka puff

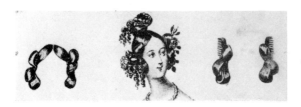

287 Postiche of 1835
    1 Band of front hair
    2 Coiffure with a cocque
    3 Hair knots worked on combs

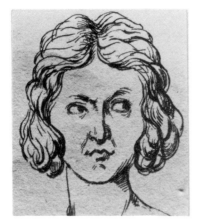

288 Square-root style, 1857

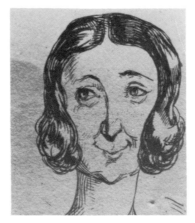

289 Door-knocker style, 1857

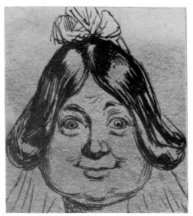

290 Pyramidal style, 1857

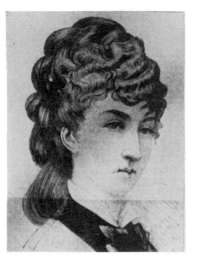

291 Style of 1876

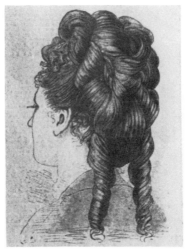

292 Hair style incorporating interlaced loops, 1876

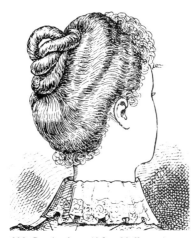

293 Grecian knot (After *Mallemont*)

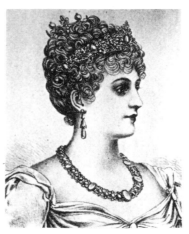

294 Coiffure of the 1st Empire (After *Vachon*)

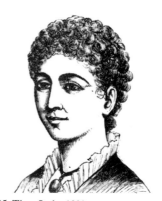

295 Titus Style, 1880s

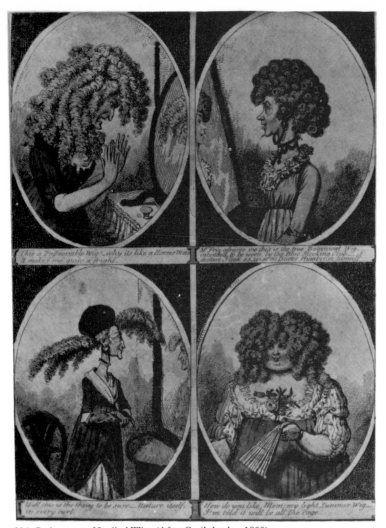

296 Caricatures of Ladies' Wigs (After *Cruikshank, c* 1800)

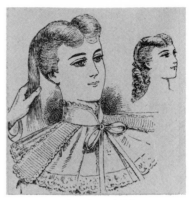

297 Empress Bandeau, 1898

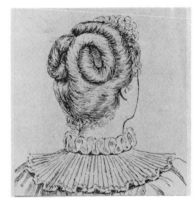

298 The Figure of Eight, 1898

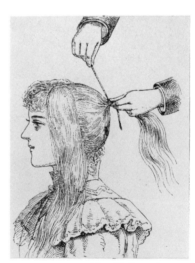

299 Hairbinder (After *Mallemont*)

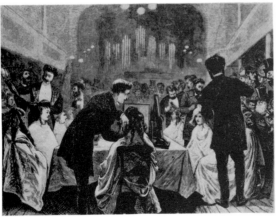

300 Hairdressing Competition and Exhibition, London 1872
(*The Graphic*)

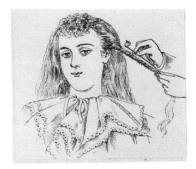

301 Method of singeing long hair with a taper, 1898 (After *Mallemont*)

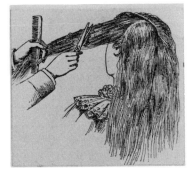

302 Cutting the points of long hair, 1898

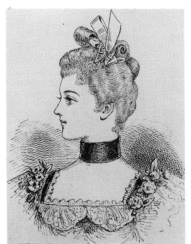

303 Puff coiffure with ribbon, *c* 1890

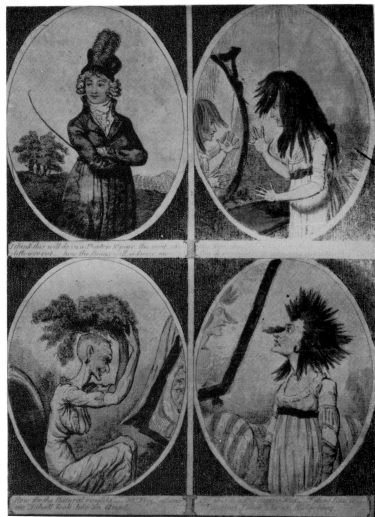

304 Caricatures of ladies' wigs (After *Cruikshank*, *c* 1800)

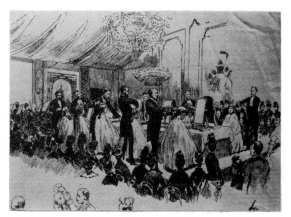

305 Hairdressing Competition and Exhibition, London 1888 (*Illustrated London News*)

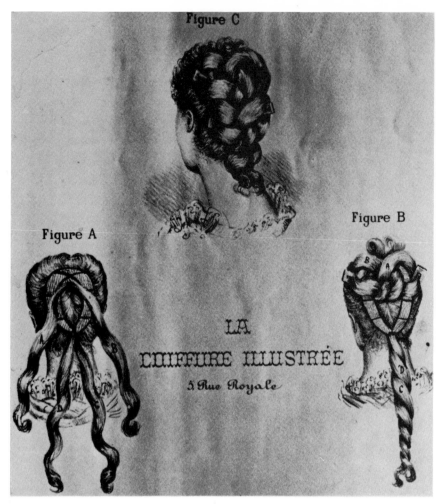

307 A Crépon with false hair
      tails
    B Method of dressing
    C Completed hairdress
      with false front and
      decorated tortoise-
      shell combs

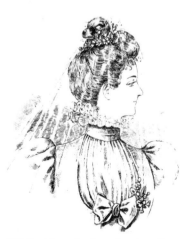

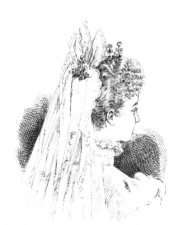

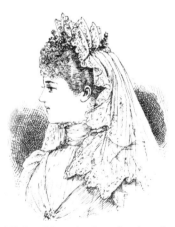

307 Jewish mode of wearing the veil,
    1898 (After *Mallemont*)

308 Renaissance mode of wearing the
    veil, 1898

309 Spanish mode of wearing the veil,
    1898

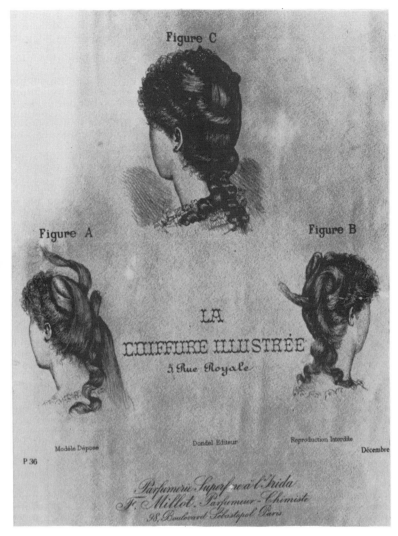

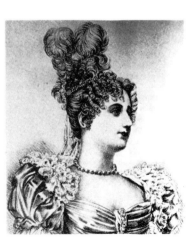

310 Method of dressing a grand evening
coiffure of 1884

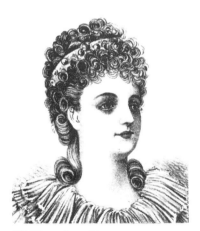

311 Directoire coiffure

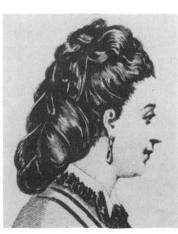

312 Hanging chignon, 1869

313 Restoration style, 1892 (After
Vachon)

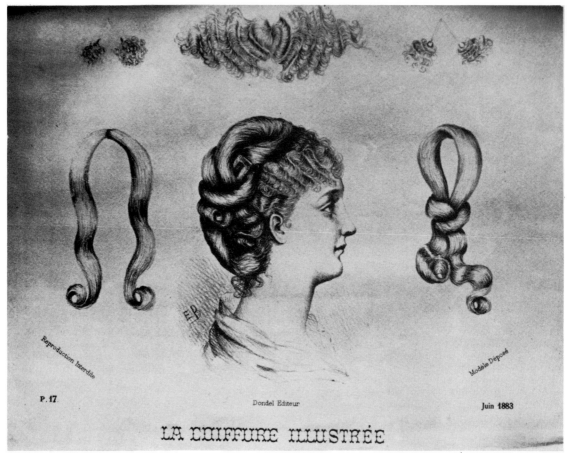

P. 17.

Dondel Editeur

Juin 1883

LA COIFFURE ILLUSTRÉE

314 A coiffure of 1883. *Top:* a Marion Bandelette with a pair of pincurls on either side; *Left side:* of the dressed head is a swathe; *Right side:* a knot of hair formed from the swathe

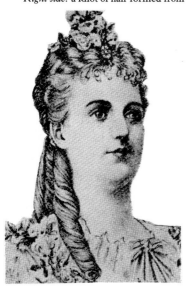

315 Style of the Second Empire (French), showing Alexandra curls

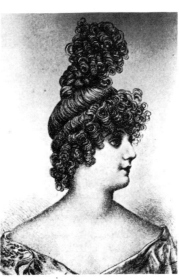

316 Coiffure Merveilleuse (After *Vachon*)

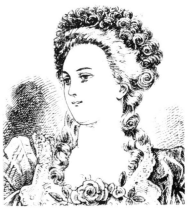

317 Powdered coiffure, time of Louis XVI

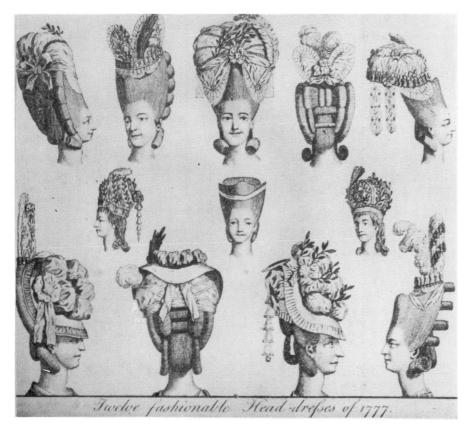

318 Hair styles of 1777

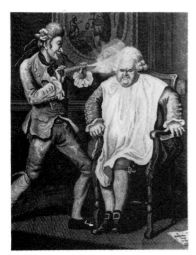

319 Powder puff in use, 1770 (after a painting by *J Collet*)

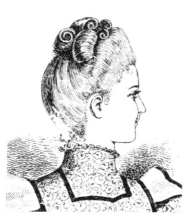

320 Upswept coiffure, Watteau style, 1898

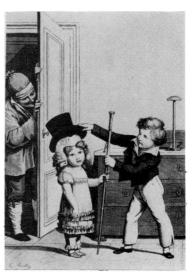

321 Grandfather's wig, 1820. Notice the mushroom upon which the wig rests when not being worn

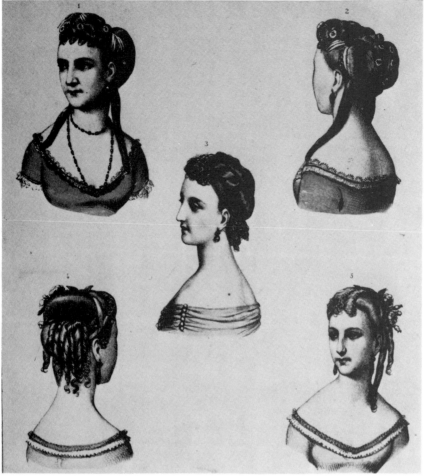

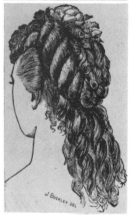

322 Hair styles of 1867:
   1 Coiffure with Alexandra curls falling over each shoulder
   2 ditto, back view
   3 note Grape of curls at the neck
   4 Coiffure with a double Marie Antoinette chignon and a grape of curls springing from between
   5 ditto, front view

323 Berthé coiffure, 1897 (After *Creer*)

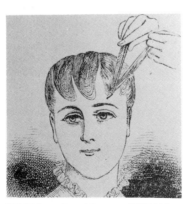

324 Hair setting with water, 1898 (After *Mallemont*)

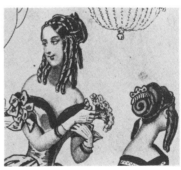

325 Style of 1843 showing front, ringlets, also called barley sugar curls, drop curls and hanging curls; back, coiled chignon

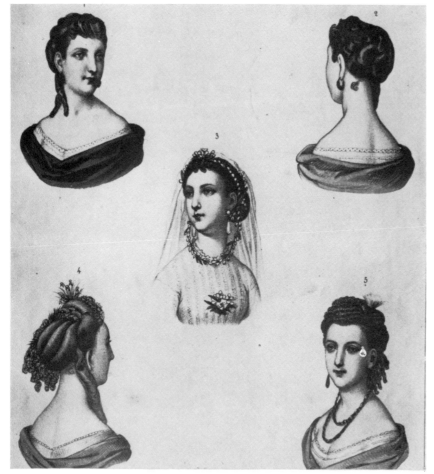

326 Hair styles of 1866:

326 Hair styles of 1866:
1 Coiffure executed by the use of water. 'This method of waving is coming into practice more every day' replacing the use of irons
2 ditto, back view
3 Wedding hairdress
4 Note the bunch of curls over the forehead and the grape of curls at the neck
5 An 1866 version of a Marie Antoinette coiffure

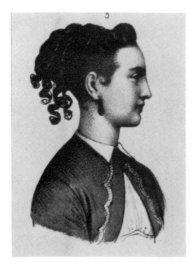

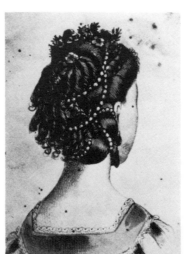

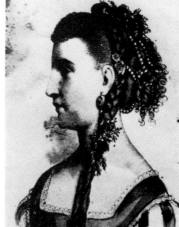

327 Coiffure in the Chinese style, 1866. Hair drawn back from the face and up from the neck

328 Coiffure of 1867

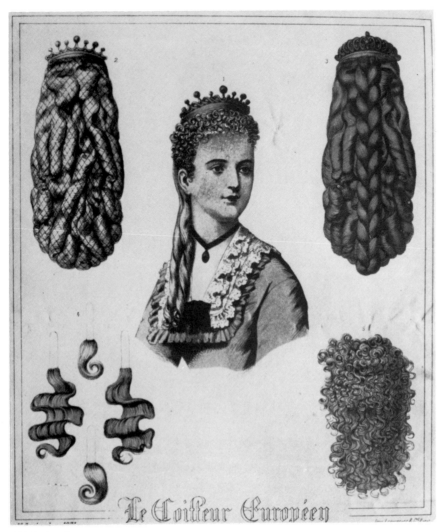

329 Styles of 1871:
Top left: Chignon of artificial curls within a demi-toilette net, with the curls free it was called a grande toilette
Top right: Chignon as previous but with added plait
Middle: Coiffure of postiche with diadem comb
Bottom left: Pincurls and pinwaves
Bottom right: Cachepeigne with artificial curls, called the Froufrou coiffure

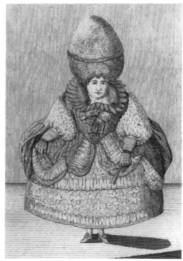

330 Hedgehog wig, 1777, also called à la Hérisson

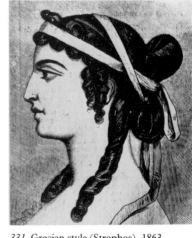

331 Grecian style (Strophos), 1863 version

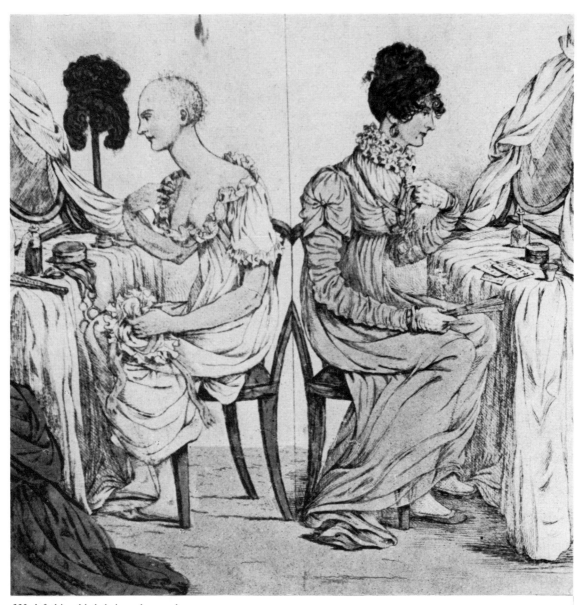

332 A fashionable lady in undress and
dress, 1807. Note wig on mushroom
wig stand

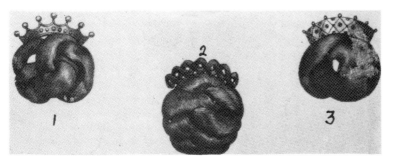

333 Chignons of 1867:
    1 Frizzed plait covered with an
      invisible net
    2 Puff curls
    3 Frizzed loose coil

334 Chignons of 1866:
Top row, L to R: Chignon Normand adorned with a figure-of-eight plait, a frizzling for wearing underneath coques, a serpentine knot constructed with four plaited locks and some frizzling in the middle.
Middle row, L to R: Chignon Normand adorned with a scarf knot and a long curl each side, coiffure of 1866, a long Cockle Shell.
Bottom row, L to R: Plaited chignon covered with curlings, chignon composed of a double figure-of-eight twist, plaited chignon with light curlings springing from the hollows of the dressing

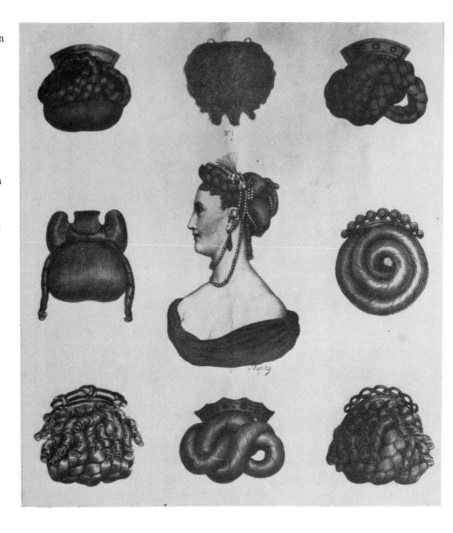

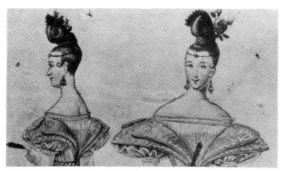

335 Coque coiffure, c 1830

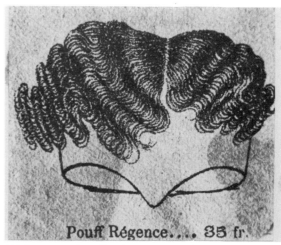

336 Regency style puff or front. Version of 1892

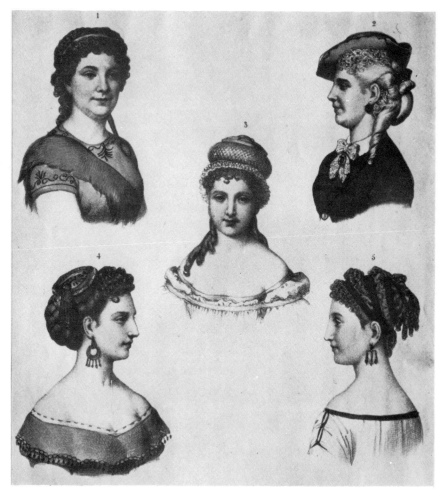

337 Styles of 1866:
1 Lightly curled
   coiffure
2 Marchioness wig.
   Louis XV style
3 Coiffure with edging
   of frizzy curls and a
   curled cachepeigne
   with long ringlets at
   the back
4 Water waved and
   curled coiffure
   dressed with a plaited
   chignon
5 Chloe hairdress. Top
   waved and curled,
   bunches of ringlets
   amongst back hair
   and bandelettes

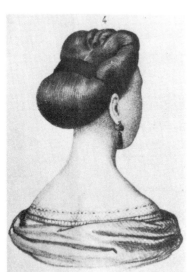

338 Coiffure with chignon Normand

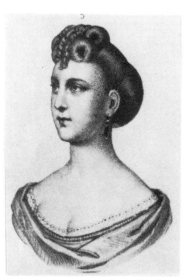

339 Front view of figure 338

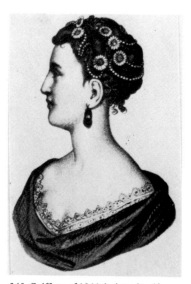

340 Coiffure of 1866 designed as 'An
    Ancient Style Coiffure'

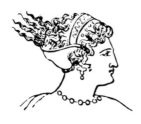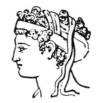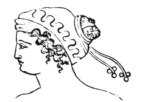

Mitra headdresses

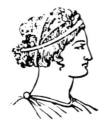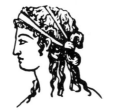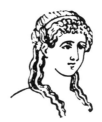

Strophos headdresses

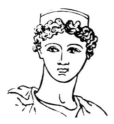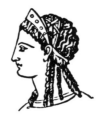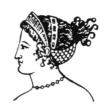

Nimbo headdresses

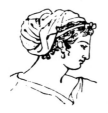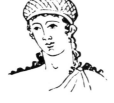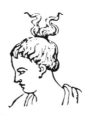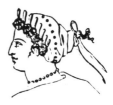

Kredemnon headdress   Sakkos headdress   Korymbos headdress   Tholia headdress

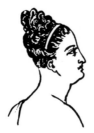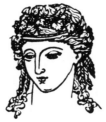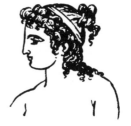

Tutulus   Nimbus   Vitta

341 Hair styles of the Greeks and Romans (After *Rimmel*)

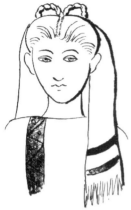

342 Hairdress of a Christian Virgin, 3rd cent

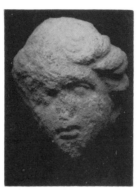
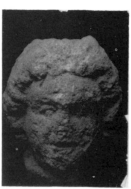

343 Romano-British hair styles of 3rd-4th cent. That on the right depicts a horned Celtic god

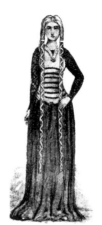

344 St Clotilde with two plaits sheathed in fouriaux, 12th cent (*Corinium Museum*)

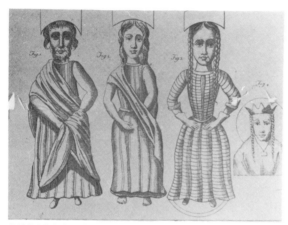

345 Irish hair styles, 9th-10th cent (*Archaeologia*, v7, 1785)

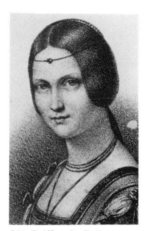

346 Coiffure La Belle Ferronnière

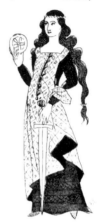

347 St Catherine with the hairdress of an unmarried girl, 12th cent

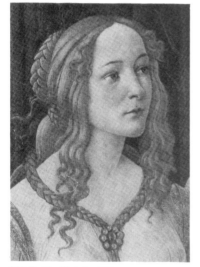

348 Botticelli style, 15th cent

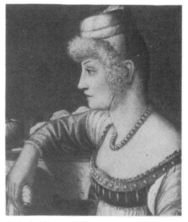

349 Coiffure of a Venetian Courtisan, 15th cent (After a painting by *Carpaccio*)

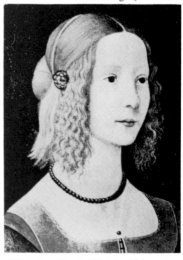

350 Italian. Botticelli style, 15th cent

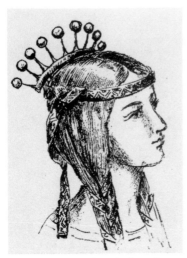

351 Freseau or backcomb of metal, 12th cent

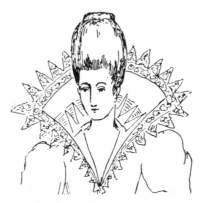

352 Coiffure of 1599

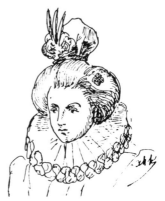

353 Coiffure of 1600

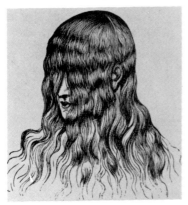

354 Natural disposition of head hair

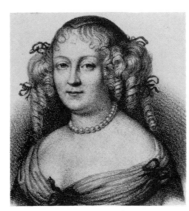

355 Sévigné coiffure, 17th cent

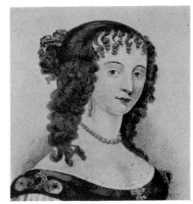

356 17th cent style with cruches

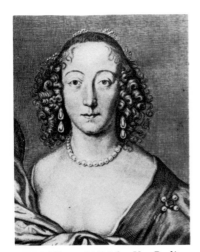

357 Coiffure, *c* 1640 (after *Van Dyck*)

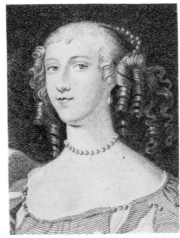

358 Coiffure of 1630 incorporating the palisade of wire sustaining hair next to the duchess or first knot

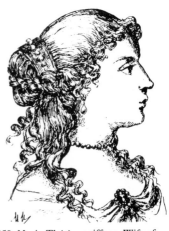

359 Marie-Thérèse coiffure, Wife of Louis XIV

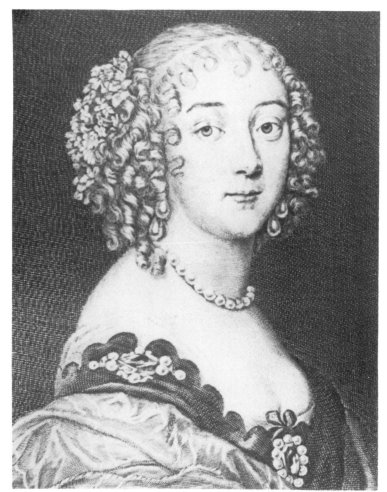

360 Coiffure, c 1650. Note the cruches, favorites, and passageres

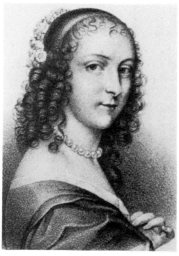

361 Ninon de l'Encos coiffure, 17th cent

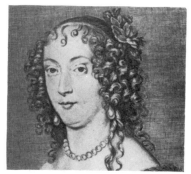

362 Style of 1646. Note love-locks hanging over the shoulder, favorites and cruches

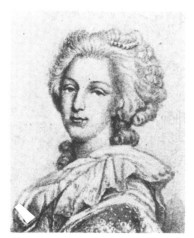

363 Marie Antoinette coiffure

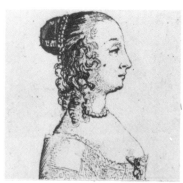

364 The Culbute or rounded chignon on the Garette coiffure. Style spread from France to England by 1640s

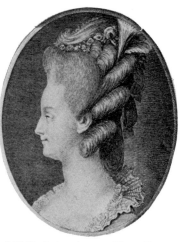

365 Marie Antoinette coiffure. 'A hundred entrancing ways did she arrange her hair . . .'

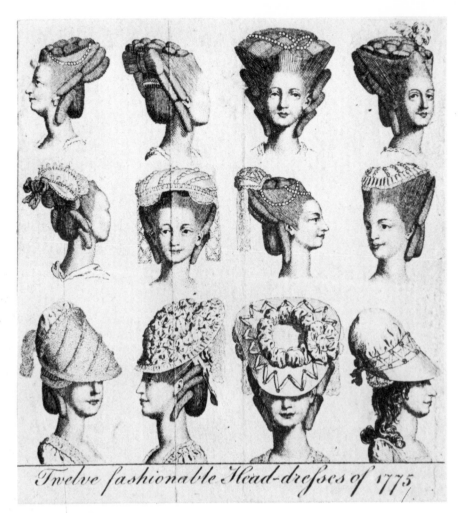

Twelve fashionable Head-dresses of 1775

366 Hair styles of 1775

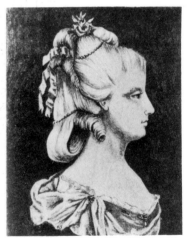

367 Coiffure Marie Christine
d'Autriche, 18th cent

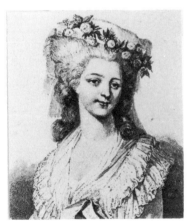

368 Coiffure La Princesse de Lamballe,
18th cent

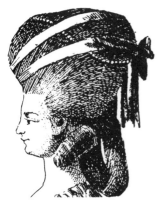

369 Coiffure Chien Couchant, 18th cent

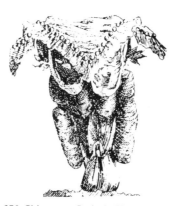

370 Chignon en Croix de Chevalier, 18th cent

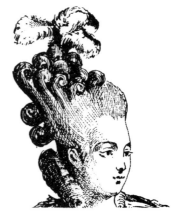

371 Coiffure en Crochets with curls and plumes, 18th cent

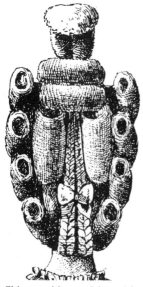

372 Chignon with two plaits and four curls à la Chancelière. 18th cent

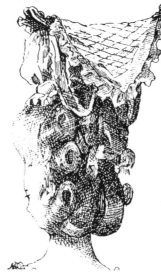

373 Chignon Noué in three parts surmounted by a bonnet of lace

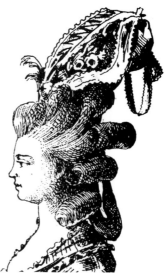

374 Coiffure en Colisée surmounted by a puff

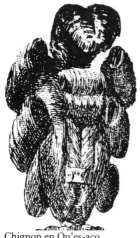

375 Chignon en Qu'es-aco

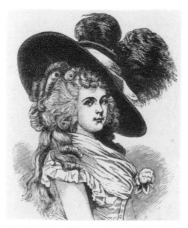

376 Duches of Devonshire coiffure, late 18th cent

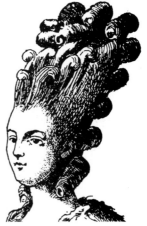

377 Coiffure en crochets with a ladder of curls

289

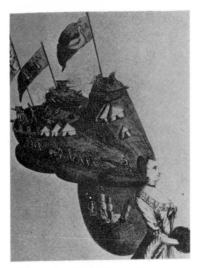

378 Bunker Hill coiffure, 18th cent

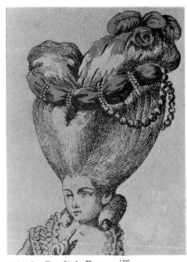

379 Le Pouf à la Puce coiffure

380 Postiches of April 1883:
Top: Fronts and semi-transformations
Bottom: Two pincurls, two chignons and a coiled double-loop marteau

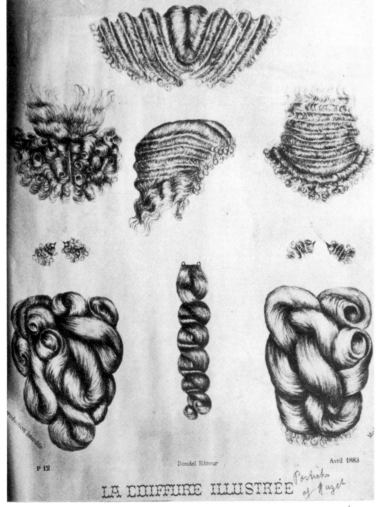

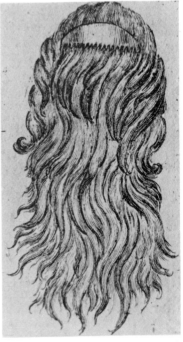

381 Natural fall of hair with a backcomb in position

The Soft Pompadour and Psyche Knot

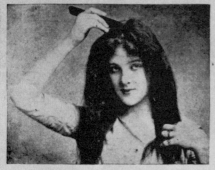

After all the tangles have been removed, a parting is made, beginning at the forehead and running backward through the centre to the top of the head, but not down the back.

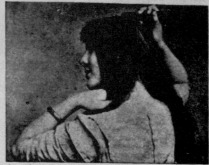

A second and third parting are now made. The second begins on the line of the first parting about two and one-half inches back from the forehead. It runs down the left side of the head and terminates an inch behind the ear. The third parting is like the second, beginning at the same point, finishing an inch behind the right ear.

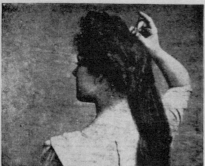

The hair is now in three divisions, the two front ones and the back portion. Before making the pompadour, all the back hair should be carefully combed and tied back so as not to be in the way. The pompadour may then be put up. First smooth the left side, brushing it forward, then up and finally back into pompadour shape. Fasten it at the top of the head with a hair-pin.

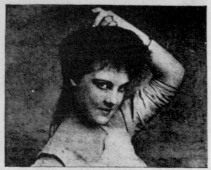

Next, the right side of the hair is smoothed out, brushed up into a pompadour and pinned securely at the top of the head, close to the place where the left side is fastened. This illustration shows the right side of the hair being pinned in place. After the pompadour is made, the hair should be carefully pulled out with the hands so as to cover all three partings.

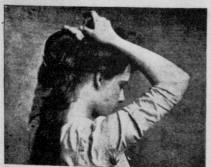

Now the hair is ready to make the psyche knot. Comb out the ends of the pompadour, untie the back hair and comb both it and the ends of the pompadour together. Brush the long hair up so that it can be tied with narrow black ribbon, close to the head, but about two inches above the nape of the neck. After the hair is tied in place, begin to twist it into coil shape.

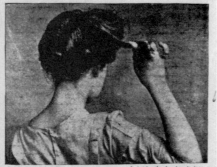

Bring the twisted coil up toward the top of the head, shaping it into a psyche effect. Fasten it securely with two or three hair-pins as shown in the fifth illustration. Then continue to twist the hair until it is all used, coiling it at the same time loosely around the first part of the psyche knot. Fasten the completed psyche knot with hair-pins.

702

382 Psyche knot and the method of
  dressing (*Girl's Own Paper*, 1911)

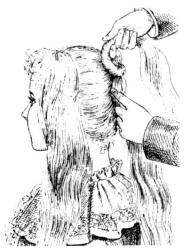

383 Dressing a twist, late 19th cent

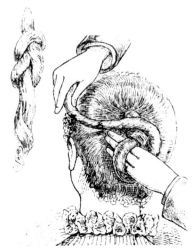

384 A Gordian knot

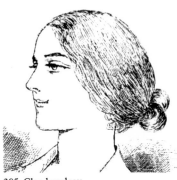

385 Cleo bandeau

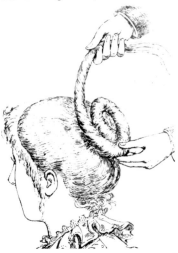

386 Dressing a coil

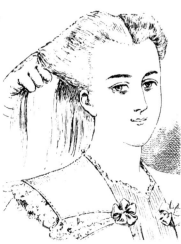

387 Forming a raised bandeau. Marie Stuart style

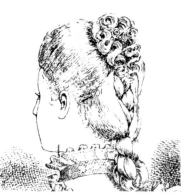

388 Interlaced Cadogan coiffure, 1898

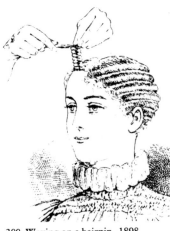

389 Waving on a hairpin, 1898

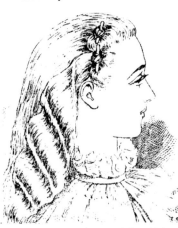

390 Waving on an ivory rod, late 19th cent

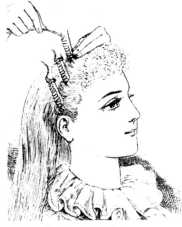

391 Waving by spiral winding on a hairpin, 1898

392 Details showing hair wound on the hairpin, 1898

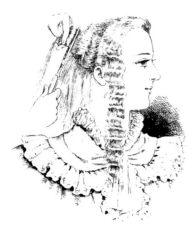

393 Marcel Waving using fingers to hold hair, 1898

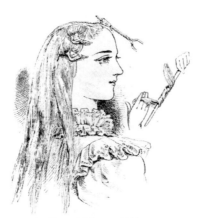

394 Curling with irons, 1898

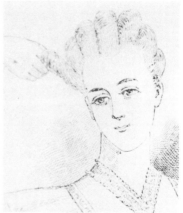

395 Raised bandeau. Louis XV style, late 19th cent version

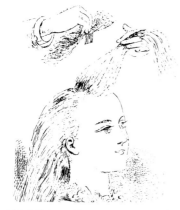

396 A Fairy puff or crêpon on a comb being added to the head hair

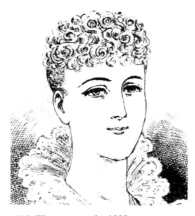

397 Water-set curls, 1898

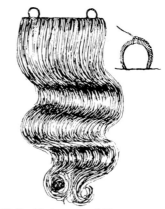

398 Double-loop waved Marteau

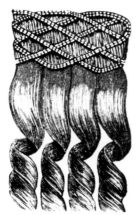

399 Ringlet bunch on diamond mesh foundation, 1887

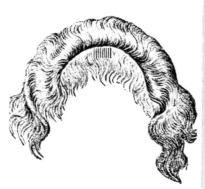

400 Weft Pompadour front on spring mount with comb attached, 19th cent

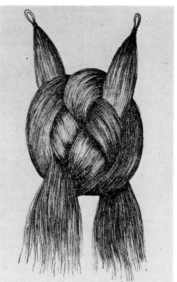

401 Interlaced single stem switches forming a knotted chignon, 1887

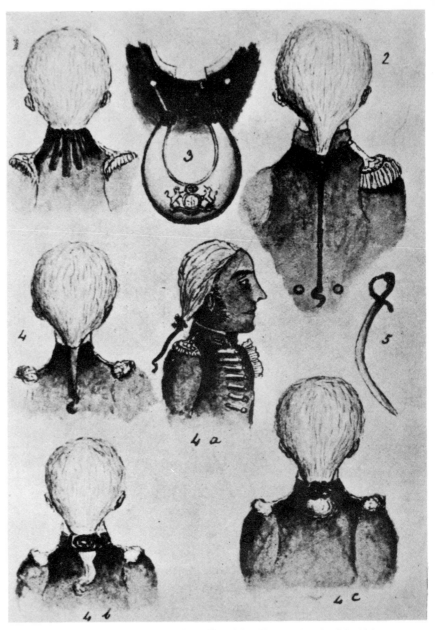

402 Types of military queues sketched from life by Lieut Thomas Austin of the 35th
Foot in 1807 (From the original sketch by kind permission of *Major R E Austin*)
1 Spread queue of 5 tails, Lieut of Household Cavalry or Footguard
2 Queue worn by Captain
3 Gorget
4, 4a, 4b, 4c Pigtail queues worn by Lieutenants of the Infantry
5 Flank Company sword of an infantry battalion. Officers wore powdered wigs,
the 'rankers' pipe-clayed their greased natural hair

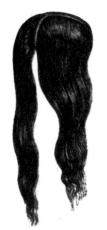

403 Bandeau with tress attached to the crown, 1863

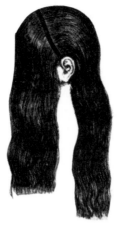

404 Postiche mounted on a velvet ribbon, 1863

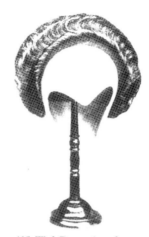

405 Weft Pompadour front on spring mount, displayed on a velvet covered, hollow wig block and stand, 19th cent

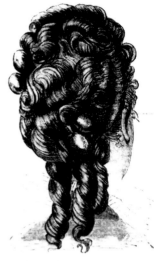

406 Style of 1876 with ringlets

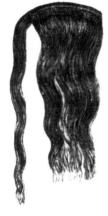

407 Bandeau with tress attached to the crown, 19th cent

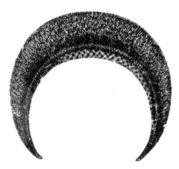

408 Waved horsehair pompadour pad, 19th cent

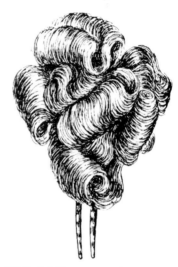

409 Curled Marteau on a pin

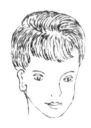

410 Coconut bob, 1920s

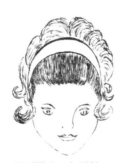

411 Wigband, 1920s

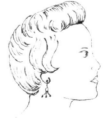

412 Cube cut, 1920s

413 Orchid bob, 1920s

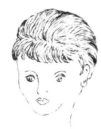

414 Moana bob, 1920s

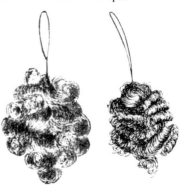

415 Pincurls, 19th cent

295

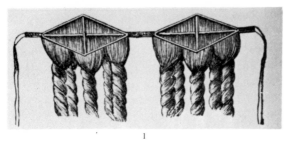

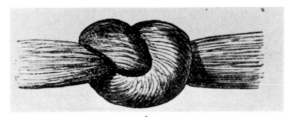

1

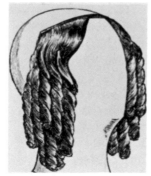

2

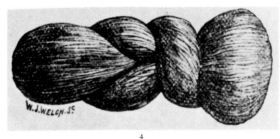

3

W.J.WELCH.SC

4

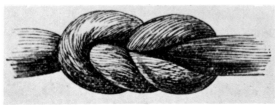

5

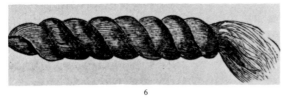

6

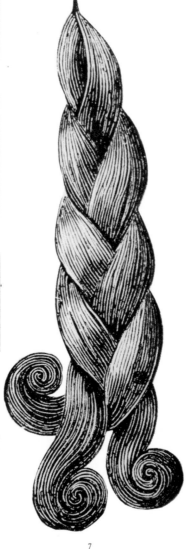

416 1 French ringlet front showing foundation
     2 French ringlet front mounted on a block
     3 Single knot
     4 Grecian knot
     5 Double Grecian knot
     6 French twist, also called torsade dondel, torsade
        gouffrée
     7 Three stem switch (After *Creer*)

7

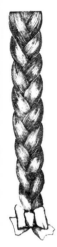

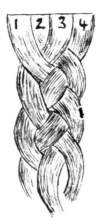

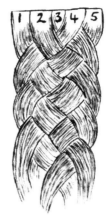

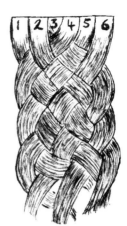

417 Marguerite plait

418 Method of forming four, five and six spill plaits

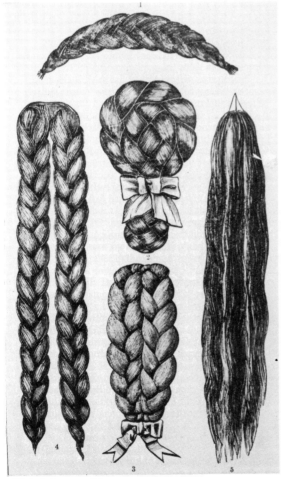

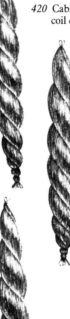

420 Cable twists for forming Spanish coil chignons, etc

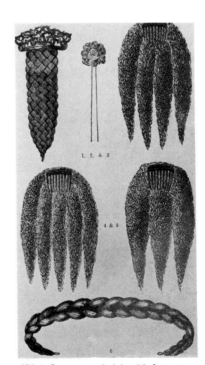

419 1 A Coronet plait
 2 Catogan chignon constructed from a four strand plait with ribbon bow
 3 Dolly Varden headdress
 4 Marguerite plaits
 5 Inserted stems for plaited coils, coronets, etc

421 1 Seven strand plait with fancy comb attached
 2 Pincurl
 3, 4 and 5 Human hair frisettes for plaited chignons
 6 Long plait for forming a coiled chignon (After *Creer*)

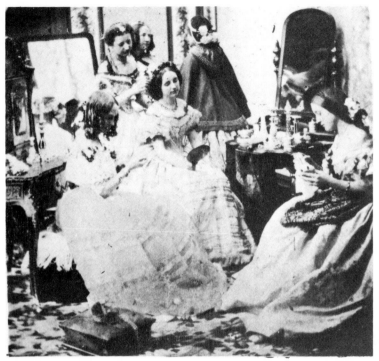

422 Home hairdressing, 1865

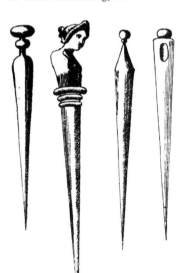

423 Romano-British bone hairpins,
2nd-3rd cent

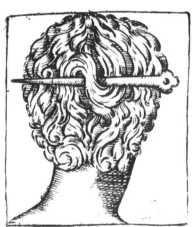

423 Romano-British bone hairpin (acus)
showing method of use

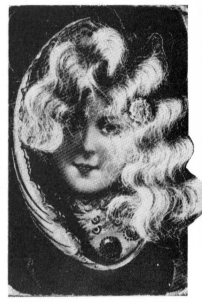

425 Postcard decorated with waved
mohair, 1904

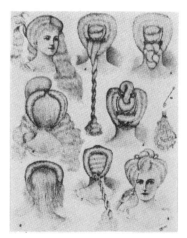

426 Method of dressing hair styles of
1903. Note the fairy puff attached to
a comb middle right of figure (*Hearth
and Home*)

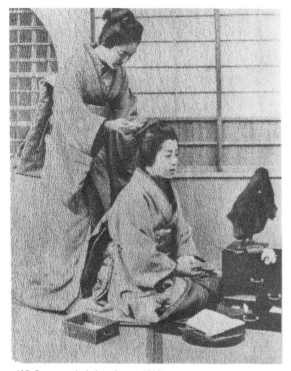

427 Japanese hairdressing, c 1908

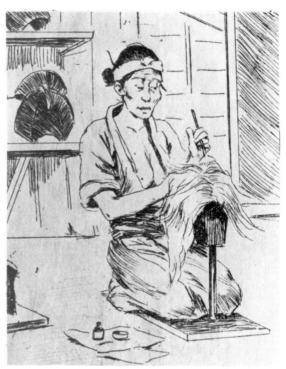

428 Japanese wigmaker, Tokyo, c 1900 (Engraving by *A Bigor*)

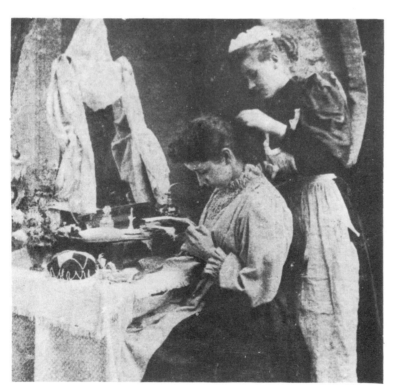

429 Lady's maid dressing her mistress's hair, c 1908

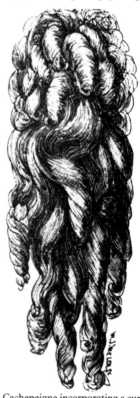

430 Cachepeigne incorporating a curled chignon

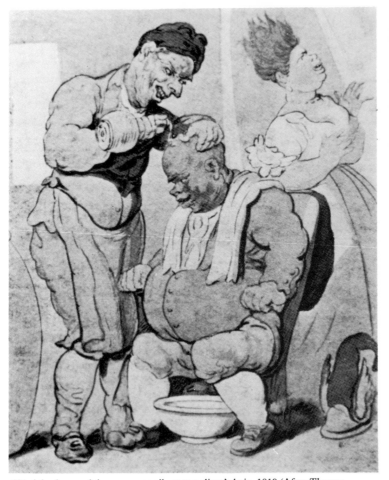

431 A barber applying macassar oil, *qv* to a client's hair, 1819 (After *Thomas Rowlandson*)

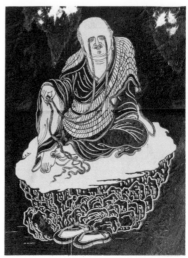

432 Trichosis of the eyebrows

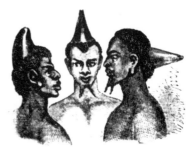

433 Bushukulompo headdress (After *Rimmel*)

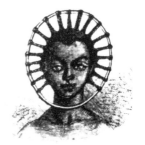

434 Astura Headdress

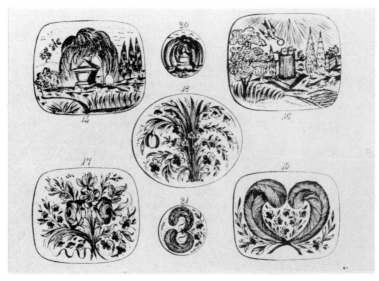

436 Hair jewellery. Victorian period

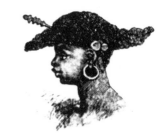

435 Londa Headdress

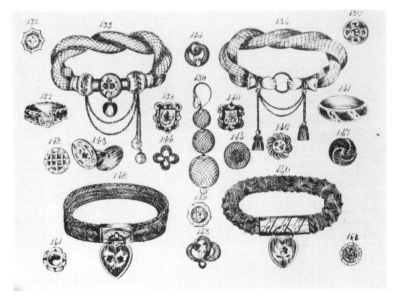

437 Hair jewellery. Victorian period

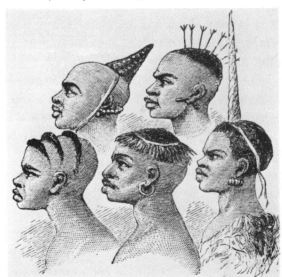

438 Headdress of the Ounyamonezi Tribe

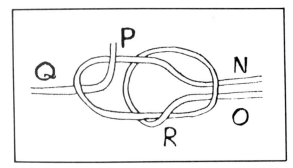

439 Hair weaver's joining knot

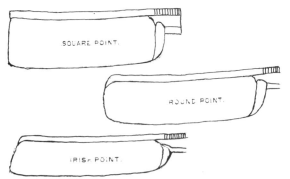

440 Types of cut-throat razor blade points

SQUARE POINT.

ROUND POINT.

IRISH POINT.

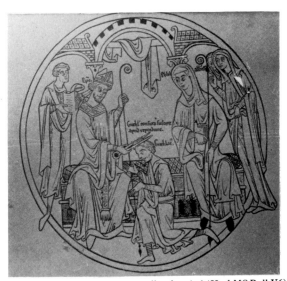

441 Conferring the tonsure, medieval period (*Harl MS* Roll Y6)

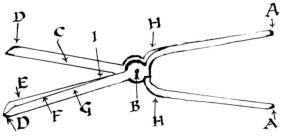

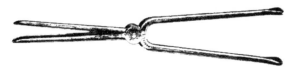

443 Marcel waving irons, 1914

442 The constituent parts of Marcel waving and curling irons.
A Handle; B Pivot or fulcrum; C Rod (shaft, prong or
tine); D point or tip; E Far-edge (of grooved shaft) ie, the
edge farther from the operator when the irons are poised
ready for use; F Near-edge (of grooved shaft) ie, the
edge nearest the operator when the irons are poised ready for
use; G Grooved or concave shaft (prong or tine); H
Shoulder; I Crutch

444 Curling irons, 1900

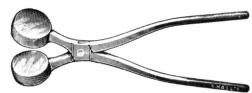

445 Pinching irons, 19th cent. In 18th cent also called curl-
paper irons

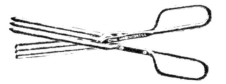

446 Pronged crimping irons, 19th cent

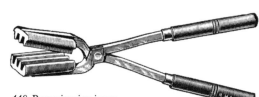

445A Pressing iron, 19th cent

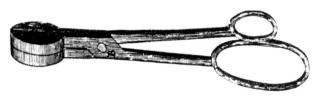

447 Pinching irons, 18th cent

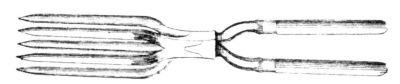

448 Box crimping irons

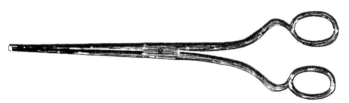

449 Pronged crimping irons with wooden handles, early 20th cent

450 Curling irons, 18th cent

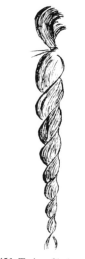

451 Twist of hair

453 Two spill switch dressed in a twist with a curl bunch at either end for wear at the nape, 1930s

BOARD-WORK;

OR

THE ART OF WIG-MAKING,

ETC.

DESIGNED FOR THE USE OF HAIRDRESSERS AND ESPECIALLY OF YOUNG MEN IN THE TRADE.

TO WHICH IS ADDED

REMARKS UPON RAZORS, RAZOR-SHARPENING, RAZOR STROPS, & MISCELLANEOUS RECIPES, SPECIALLY SELECTED.

By EDWIN CREER,

EDITOR OF "THE HAIRDRESSERS' CHRONICLE," AUTHOR OF "A POPULAR TREATISE ON THE HUMAN HAIR;" "LESSONS IN HAIRDRESSING," ETC.

WITH PORTRAIT AND NUMEROUS ILLUS-TRATIONS.

LONDON :

R. HOVENDEN & SONS,

31 & 32, BERNERS STREET, W., AND

91, 93, & 95, CITY ROAD, E.C.

1887.

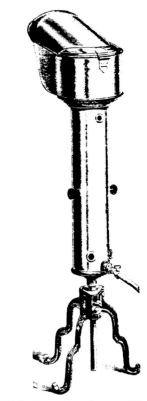

454 Gas-heated hair dryer, *c* 1895

452 Title page of the earliest comprehensive work on board-work in English, 1887

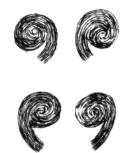

455 *Top:* Divergent curls; *Bottom: Convergent curls*

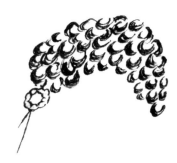

456 Pluma of hair, 17th cent

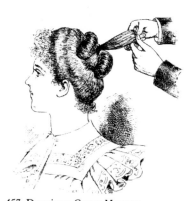

457 Dressing a Coque Marteau

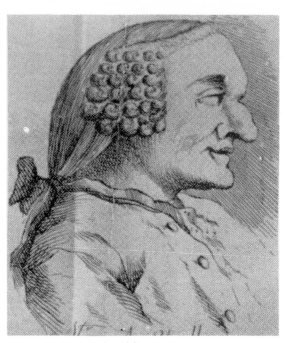

458 Au Vieillard peruke, 18th cent

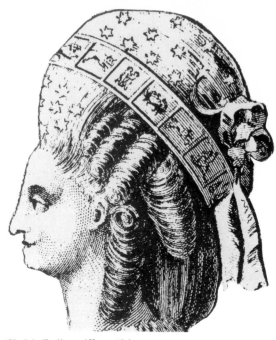

459 A la Zodiac coiffure, 18th cent

460 Trade card of a Belgian coiffure, showing a window display of the 1840s

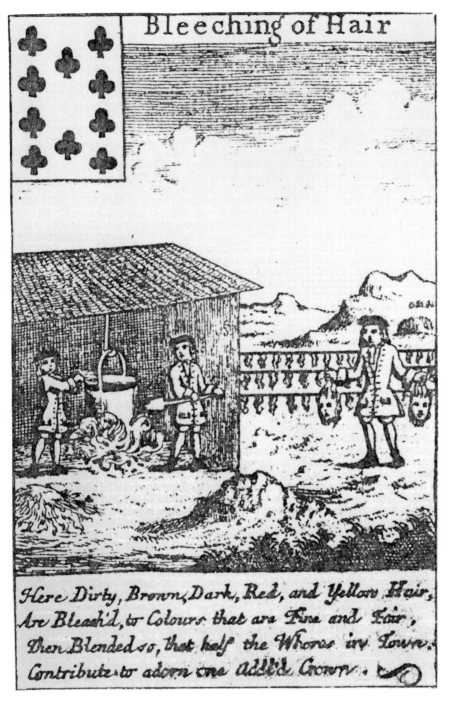

Bleeching of Hair

Here Dirty, Brown, Dark, Red, and Yellow Hair,
Are Bleach'd, to Colours that are Fine and Fair,
Then Blended so, that half the Whores in Town,
Contribute to adorn one Add'd Crown.

461 Enlarged reproduction of an English
playing card, *c* 1710, showing the
process of bleaching hair in the open
field, hence the name 'field' hair.
Note the cauldron for boiling the
hair and the heap of pearl-ash
(potassium carbonate) used in the
cauldron to degrease the hair

305

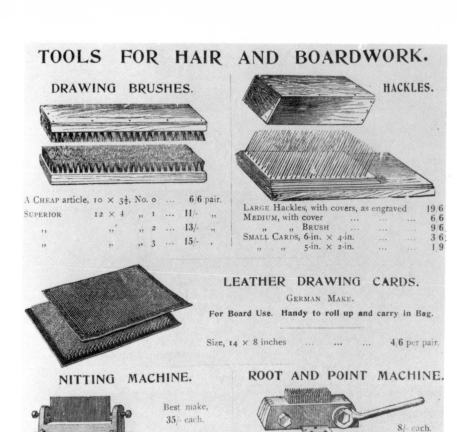

TOOLS FOR HAIR AND BOARDWORK.

DRAWING BRUSHES.

A CHEAP article, 10 × 3½, No. 0 ... 6/6 pair.
SUPERIOR   12 × 4   ,, 1 ... 11/- ,,
,,   ,,   ,, 2 ... 13/- ,,
,,   ,,   ,, 3 ... 15/- ,

HACKLES.

LARGE Hackles, with covers, as engraved   19/6
MEDIUM, with cover 6/6
  ,,   ,,   BRUSH 9/6
SMALL CARDS, 6-in. × 4-in. 3/6
  ,,   ,,   5-in. × 2-in. 1/9

LEATHER DRAWING CARDS.

GERMAN MAKE.

For Board Use. Handy to roll up and carry in Bag.

Size, 14 × 8 inches   ...   .   4/6 per pair.

NITTING MACHINE.

Best make,
35/- each.

ROOT AND POINT MACHINE.

8/- each.

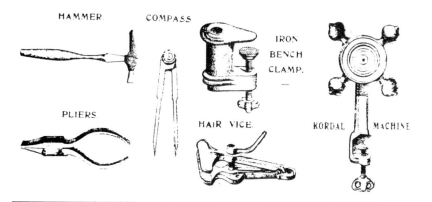

HAMMER   COMPASS

IRON
BENCH
CLAMP.

PLIERS

HAIR VICE.

KORDAL MACHINE

462 Wigmaker's tools of the 19th cent

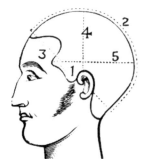

463 Measurements required by the wigmaker for a normal head:
1 The circumference of the head
2 Forehead to poll
3 Ear to ear, across the forehead
4 Ear to ear, over the top
5 Temple to temple, round the back

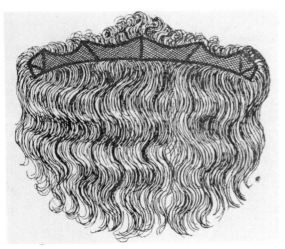

464 Foundation side of a transformation, 19th cent

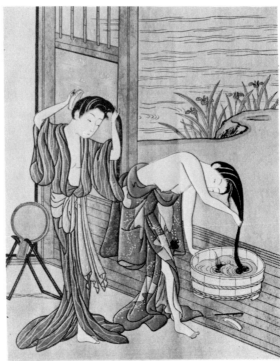

465 Japanese women shampooing their hair, 19th cent (From a print by Harunobu)

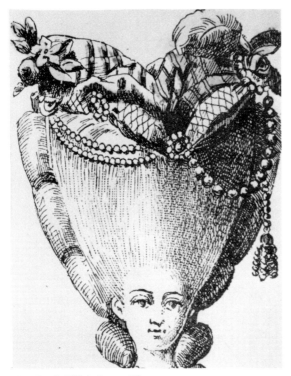

466 Pouf à L'Asiatique coiffure

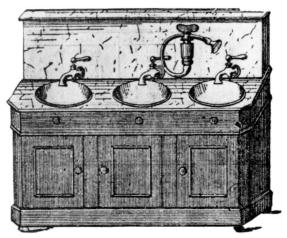

467 Shampoo basins of 1884

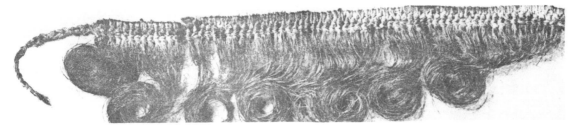

468 The oldest known extant hair weft from the tomb of Zer, Abydos, Egypt, c 3000 BC. The original weft is in the Pitt Rivers Museum, Oxford

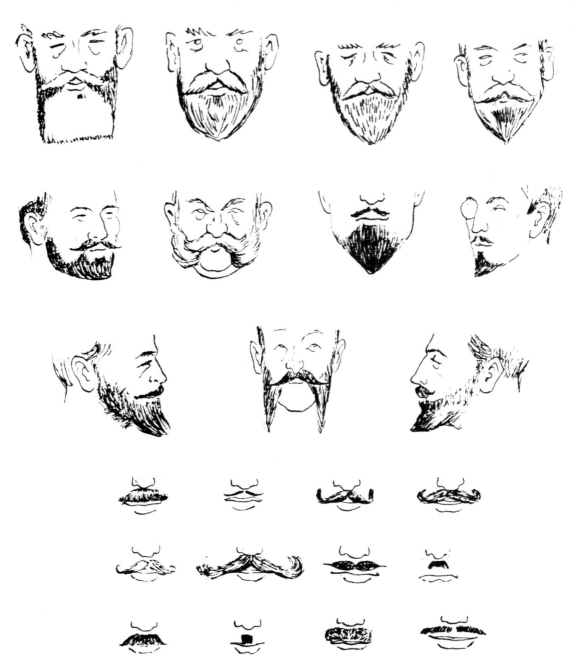

469 Beard and moustache names from *The Rules and Technical Handbook of the London Academy of Gentlemen's Hairdressing;* 1928

Beards

    Top line: The square Belgrave, The round Belgrave, The round pointed Belgrave. The pointed Belgrave

    2nd line: The Naval, The Franz Joseph, The Baker, The Count

    3rd line: The Marquis, Dundreary Whiskers, The St James

Moustaches

    4th line: The Military, The Coleman, The Kaiser, The Russian

    5th line: The Marquis, The Hindenburg, The Sergeant Major, The Grock

    6th line: The General, The Chaplin, The Brush, The Curl

470 Advertisement for the hair goods and services of Mrs F Stevens, the writer's grandmother, *c* 1900

471 Advertisement of John Stevens, the writer's grandfather, 1884

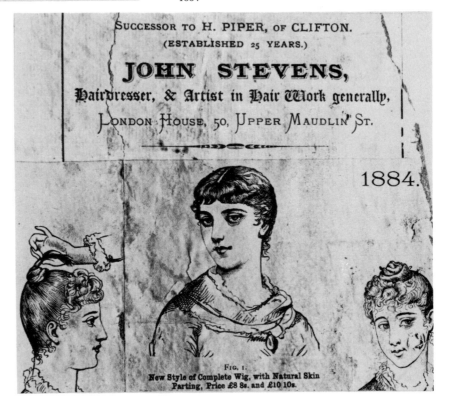

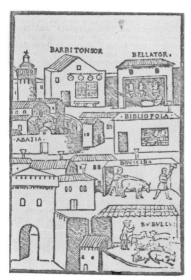

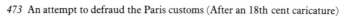
473 An attempt to defraud the Paris customs (After an 18th cent caricature)

472 Venetian print, dated 1533, depicting what is probably the earliest printed picture of a barber's shop

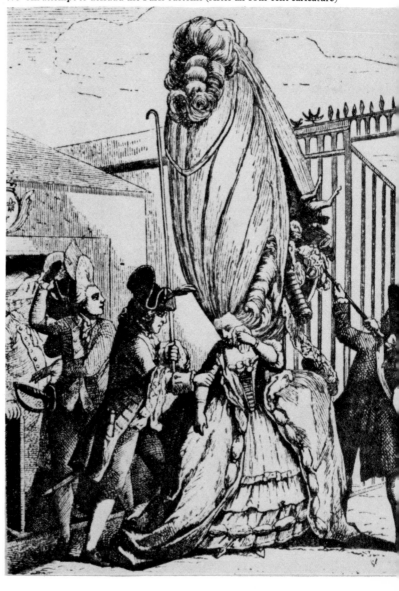

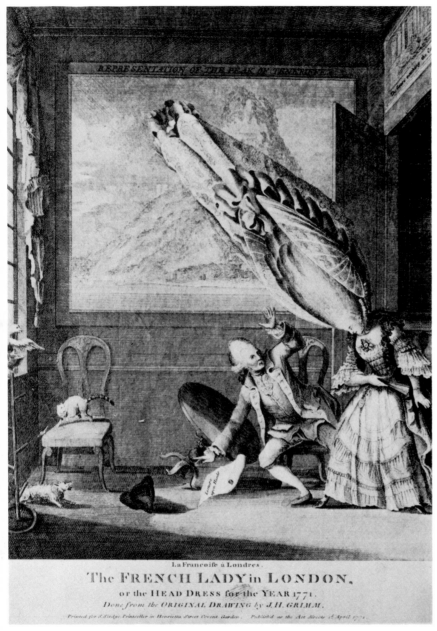

La Françoife à Londres.

The FRENCH LADY in LONDON,
or the HEAD DRESS for the YEAR 1771.
Done from the ORIGINAL DRAWING by J.H. GRIMM.

Printed for S.Sledge, Printseller in Henrietta Street Covent Garden. Publifhed, as the Act directs 15 April 1771.

474 A caricature of a high French headdress of 1771 (From a drawing by *J H Grimm*)

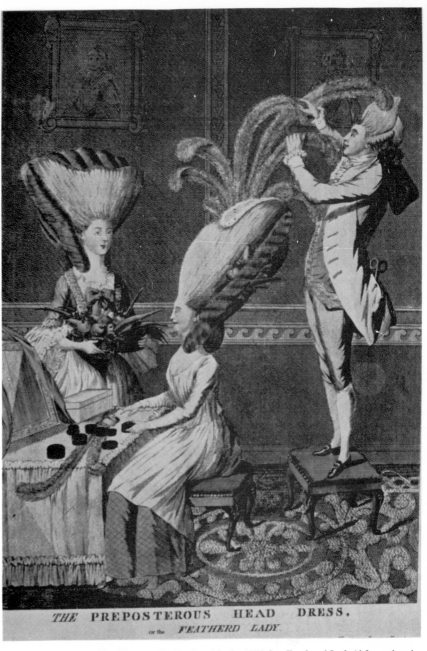

THE PREPOSTEROUS HEAD DRESS,
or the FEATHERD LADY.

475 *The Preposterous Headdress* or *The Feathered Lady*, 1778 See *Feathered Lady* (After a drawing by *Mary Darley*)